New and Evolving Infections of the 21st Century

I. W. Fong & Ken Alibek

New and Evolving Infections of the 21st Century

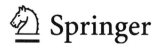 Springer

I. W. Fong
Professor of Medicine
University of Toronto
Toronto, ON MB1W8
Canada
fungi@smh.toronto.on.ca

Ken Alibeck
Executive Director, Center of Biodefense
George Mason University
Manassas, VA 20110
USA
kalibek@gmu.edu

Cover illustration: APImages

Library of Congress Control Number: 2006921352

ISBN-10: 0-387-32647-2   e-ISBN-10: 0-387-32830-0
ISBN-13: 978-0387-32647-4   e-ISBN-13: 978-0387-32830-0

Printed on acid-free paper.

9 8 7 6 5 4 3 2 1

springer.com

Contents

Section I: Evolving Infectious Diseases

1. West Nile Virus in the Americas

Lyle R. Petersen, John T. Roehrig, and James J. Sejvar

1.1. Virology	3
1.1.1. Virus Structure	3
1.1.2. Genome	3
1.1.2.1. E-protein	4
1.1.2.2. Nonstructural Proteins	6
1.1.3. Genetics and Virulence	8
1.2. Epidemiology	9
1.2.1. Ecology	9
1.2.1.1. Vectors	9
1.2.1.2. Vertebrate Hosts	11
1.2.2. Geographic Spread	12
1.2.2.1. United States and Canada	12
1.2.2.2. Latin America	12
1.2.3. Incidence of Human Infection and Illness	15
1.2.3.1. United States	15
1.2.3.2 Canada	16
1.2.4. Risk Factors for Infection, Severe Disease, and Death	17
1.2.5. Non-Mosquito Transmission Routes	18
1.2.5.1. Blood Transfusion	18
1.2.5.2. Organ Transplantation	18
1.2.5.3. Intrauterine Transmission	19
1.2.5.4. Other Transmission Modes	19
1.3. Clinical Spectrum	20
1.3.1. West Nile Fever	20
1.3.2. Neuroinvasive Disease	21
1.3.2.1. Meningitis	23
1.3.2.2. Encephalitis	23
1.3.2.3. Weakness and Paralysis	24
1.3.3. Other Clinical Manifestations	27
1.3.3.1. Ocular Manifestations	27
1.3.3.2. Miscellaneous Manifestations	28
1.3.4. Clinical Illness in Special Population Groups	28
1.3.4.1. Children	28
1.3.4.2. Immunocompromised Patients	28

1.4. Diagnosis.. 29
    1.4.1. Antibody Detection... 29
        1.4.1.1. IgM ELISA... 29
        1.4.1.2. IgG ELISA 30
        1.4.1.3. Neutralization Test 30
    1.4.2. Antigen Detection.. 31
        1.4.2.1. Antigen-Capture ELISA 31
        1.4.2.2. Immunohistochemical Staining 31
    1.4.3. Detection of Viral Genomic Sequences 31
        1.4.3.1 Nucleic Acid Amplification Test (NAAT) 31
    1.4.4. Other Laboratory, Radiologic, and Electrodiagnostic Findings 33
1.5. Management 34
1.6. Prevention 36
    1.6.1. Human Personal Protection 36
    1.6.2. Mosquito Control 37
    1.6.3. Vaccines 37
    1.6.4. Screening of Blood Donations 38
1.7. Future Directions 38
    1.7.1. Surveillance 38
    1.7.2. Diagnosis and Treatment................................... 39
    1.7.3. Prevention... 39
    References 40

2. Hantavirus Cardiopulmonary Syndrome: A New Twist to an Established Pathogen

Frederick T. Koster and Howard Levy

2.1. Virology.. 57
    2.1.1. Classification and Characteristics 57
    2.1.2. Viral Replication... 58
2.2. Pathophysiology and Animal Models 61
    2.2.1. Cell Entry.. 61
    2.2.2. Virulence 62
    2.2.3. Cellular Targets for HV 63
    2.2.4. Pathology and Pathogenesis 64
    2.2.5. Role of the T-Cell Response 65
    2.2.6. Immunity 67
    2.2.7. Animal Models 69
2.3. Epidemiology and Transmission................................... 70
    2.3.1. Epidemiology 70
    2.3.2. Transmission 70
2.4. Clinical Spectrum 73
    2.4.1. Asymptomatic or Mild Infection 73
    2.4.2. Incubation Period 74
    2.4.3. Clinical Presentation of HCPS.............................. 74
        2.4.3.1. Febrile Phase....................................... 74
        2.4.3.2. Cardiopulmonary Phase 75
        2.4.3.3. Convalescent Phase................................. 76
    2.4.4. Clinical Presentation of HFRS 76

2.5. Diagnosis of Acute Infection 77
2.6. Current Management 77
2.7. Prevention 80
2.8. Future Directions 81
References 82

3. Human Ehrlichioses and Anaplasmosis

Jere W. McBride and David H. Walker

3.1. Human Ehrlichioses (Human Monocytotropic and Ehrlichiosis Ewingii) 93
    3.1.1. Taxonomy.. 93
    3.1.2. Morphology 93
    3.1.3. Genetic, Antigenic, and Phenotypic Characteristics 96
    3.1.4. Pathogenesis and Immunity................................ 98
    3.1.5. Emergency, Epidemiology, and Transmission 102
    3.1.6. Clinical Spectrum 104
    3.1.7. Laboratory Diagnosis 105
    3.1.8. Treatment and Prevention 106
3.2. Human Anaplasmosis 107
    3.2.1. Taxonomy.. 107
    3.2.2. Morphology 107
    3.2.3. Genetic, Antigenic, and Phenotypic Characteristics 108
    3.2.4. Pathogenesis and Immunity................................ 110
    3.2.5. Emergency, Epidemiology and Transmission.................... 114
    3.2.6. Clinical Spectrum 115
    3.2.7. Laboratory Diagnosis 115
    3.2.8. Prevention and Treatment 116
3.3. Future Directions 117
References 117

4. Cross-Species Transmission of Poxviruses

Mike Bray

4.1. Introduction: The Poxvirus Family 129
    4.1.1. The Poxvirus "Survival Strategy" 134
    4.1.2. Measures and Countermeasures 135
    4.1.3. Maintenance Hosts and Cross-Species Transmission 138
    4.1.4. Barriers to Cross-Species Transmission....................... 139
4.2. Poxviruses That Cause Human Disease 140
    4.2.1. Orthopoxvirus... 141
        4.2.1.1. Variola Virus 142
        4.2.1.2. MonkeyPox Virus 143
        4.2.1.3. Vaccinia Virus 144
        4.2.1.4. CowPox Virus 145
        4.2.1.5. Ectromelia Virus 146
        4.2.1.6. CamelPox Virus 147
        4.2.1.7. Other Orthopoxviruses 147
    4.2.2. Yatapoxvirus.. 148
    4.2.3. Parapoxvirus.. 149
    4.2.4. Molluscipoxvirus 150

4.3. Genera that have not Caused Human Disease 151
        4.3.1. Leporipoxvirus 151
        4.3.2. Capripoxvirus 152
        4.3.3. Suipoxvirus 153
        4.3.4. Avipoxvirus 154
4.4. Newly Identified Poxvirus Genera 155
4.5. Conclusion 155
References 156

Section II: Newly Recognized Human Viruses

5. The Severe Acute Respiratory Syndrome

Kwok-Yung Yuen, Samson S.Y. Wong, and J.S. Malik Peiris

5.1. Introduction 163
5.2. Sequence of Events 163
5.3. Epidemiological Characteristics 164
5.4. General Virology 166
5.5. Clinical Findings 172
5.6. Laboratory Diagnostics 173
5.7. Pathology and Immunology 174
5.8. Animal Models and Koch's Postulates 175
5.9. Clinical Management 176
        5.9.1. Antivirals and Immunomodulators 177
        5.9.2. Passive and Active Immunization 178
5.10. Laboratory Safety, Community and Hospital Infection Control 182
References 183

6. Newly Identified Human Herpesviruses: HHV-6, HHV-7, and HHV-8

Laurie T. Krug, Chong-Gee Teo, Keiko Tanaka-Taya, and Naoki Inoue

6.1. HHV-6 and HHV-7 197
        6.1.1. Biology 197
                6.1.1.1. Cell Tropism and Viral Entry 197
                6.1.1.2. Gene Expression and Replication 198
                6.1.1.3. Latency and Reactivation 199
                6.1.1.4. Immune Responses and Immune Evasion 201
                6.1.1.5. Pathogenesis 202
                6.1.1.6. Animal Models 203
        6.1.2. Epidemiology 203
                6.1.2.1. Primary Infection 203
                6.1.2.2. Transmission 204
                6.1.2.3. Proposed Disease Associations 205
        6.1.3. Clinical Spectrum 205
                6.1.3.1. Exanthem Subitum (Roseola) 205
                6.1.3.2. Encephalitis 206
                6.1.3.3. Post-transplantation Disease 206

6.1.4. Management and Prevention 208
    6.1.4.1. Antivirals 208
    6.1.4.2. Transplantation Management 208
6.2. HHV-8 208
    6.2.1. Biology 208
        6.2.1.1. Cell Tropism and Viral Entry 208
        6.2.1.2. Latency and Reactivation 209
        6.2.1.3. Immune Response and Immune Evasion 210
        6.2.1.4. Pathogenesis 216
        6.2.1.5. Animal Models 222
    6.2.2. Epidemiology 226
        6.2.2.1. Seroepidemiology 226
        6.2.2.2. HHV-8 Genotypes 229
        6.2.2.3. Transmission 231
    6.2.3. Clinical Spectrum 234
        6.2.3.1. Primary Infection 234
        6.2.3.2. Kaposi's Sarcoma 235
        6.2.3.3. Primary Effusion Lymphoma (PEL) 238
        6.2.3.4. Castleman's Disease 239
        6.2.3.5. Other Lymphoproliferative Disorders 240
        6.2.3.6. Other Neoplastic Disorders 240
        6.2.3.7. Other Diseases 240
    6.2.4. Management 241
        6.2.4.1. Antivirals 241
        6.2.4.2. Anti-retroviral Protease Inhibitors 242
        6.2.4.3. Other Approaches 242
References 242

Section III: Emerging Viruses in Asia

7. Nipah and Hendra Viruses Encephalitis

Khean Jin Goh, Kum Thong Wong, and Chong Tin Tan

7.1. Introduction 279
7.2. Hendra Virus Infection 279
    7.2.1. Epidemiology 280
    7.2.2. Clinical Features 280
    7.2.3. Diagnosis 281
    7.2.4. Pathology 281
7.3. Nipah Virus Infection 281
    7.3.1. Epidemiology 282
    7.3.2. Clinical Features 284
    7.3.3. Investigations 285
    7.3.4. Treatment and Outcome 287
    7.3.5. Relapsed and Late-Onset Encephalitis 287
    7.3.6. Pathology 287
    7.3.7. Pathogenesis 289
7.4. Conclusion 290
References 290

8. Enterovirus 71 Encephalitis

Luan-Yin Chang, Shin-Ru Shih, Li-Min Huang, and Tzou-Yien Lin

8.1. Virology 295
    8.1.1. Virological Classification of Enterovirus 71 295
    8.1.2. General Characteristics of Enterovirus 296
    8.1.3. Virion Structure of Enterovirus 296
    8.1.4. Replication Cycle of Enterovirus 297
    8.1.5. Genotypes and Neurovirulence of EV71 297
8.2. Transmission and Incubation Period 298
    8.2.1. Route of Transmission 298
    8.2.2. The Rate of Household Transmission 299
    8.2.3. Incubation Period 300
8.3. Epidemiology 300
    8.3.1. Worldwide Epidemiology 300
    8.3.2. Epidemiology in Taiwan 301
8.4. Clinical Spectrum 303
    8.4.1. Asymptomatic Infection 304
    8.4.2. Stage 1: Uncomplicated EV71 Illness 304
    8.4.3. Stage 2: Complicated EV71 Illness with CNS Involvement 305
        8.4.3.1. EV71 Aseptic Meningitis 305
        8.4.3.2. EV71 Encephalitis 306
        8.4.3.3. Polio-like Syndrome 306
        8.4.3.4. Encephalomyelitis 306
        8.4.3.5. Image Studies for CNS Involvement 306
    8.4.4. Stage 3: Cardiopulmonary Failure or Pulmonary Edema 307
        8.4.4.1. Pathogenesis of EV71-related Cardiopulmonary
                Failure 308
    8.4.5. Stage 4: Convalescence and Long-term Sequelae 310
    8.4.6. Factors Associated with Complications 310
    8.4.7. EV71 Versus Coxsackievirus A16 310
8.5. Diagnosis 311
    8.5.1. Virus Isolation and Identification 311
    8.5.2. Gene Chips 311
    8.5.3. Serology Test 312
        8.5.3.1. Neutralizing Antibody 312
        8.5.3.2. EV71 IgM 312
8.6. Management 313
    8.6.1. Stage-based Management 314
    8.6.2. Antiviral Agents 314
        8.6.2.1. Inhibitors of Virion Attachment for Enteroviruses 315
        8.6.2.2. Inhibitors of Uncoating for Enteroviruses 316
        8.6.2.3. Pleconaril (VP 63843) and Novel Anti-EV71 Agents 316
8.7. Prevention 318
    8.7.1. Hand Washing and Isolation 318
    8.7.2. EV71-related Disease and Laboratory Surveillance 319
    8.7.3. Vaccination 319
8.8. Future Directions 320
References 320

9. Avian Influenza Viruses and Pandemic Influenza

Menno Douwe de Jong

9.1. Introduction 327
9.2. Virology. 328
    9.2.1. Biological Properties 328
    9.2.2. Classification 329
    9.2.3. Natural Hosts 329
    9.2.4. Determinants of Host Range 329
    9.2.5. Antigenic Variation and The Emergence of Pandemic Influenza
           Strains. 331
           9.2.5.1. Antigenic Drift 331
           9.2.5.2. Antigenic Shift 331
9.3. Pathogensis of Avian Influenza. 332
    9.3.1. Avian Influenza Virus Infections in Natural Hosts 332
    9.3.2. Viral Determinants of Pathogenicity 333
    9.3.3. Host Factors 336
9.4. Avian Influeza Viruses Infecting Humans. 337
    9.4.1. Pandemics of the 20th Century. 337
    9.4.2. H7N7 Viruses 339
    9.4.3. H7N3 Viruses 341
    9.4.4. H9N2 Viruses 342
    9.4.5. H5N1 Viruses 343
           9.4.5.1. Outbreaks of Influenza H5N1 in Poultry and
                   Humans. 343
           9.4.5.2. The Clinical Spectrum of Human H5N1 Infections 344
           9.4.5.3. The Evolution of H5N1 Viruses, 1997–2004 347
9.5. Laboratory Diagniosis of Avian Influenza. 349
    9.5.1. Virus Isolation 349
    9.5.2. Antigen Detection. 350
    9.5.3. RT-PCR. 350
    9.5.4. Serology 351
9.6. Treatment and Prevention. 352
    9.6.1. Antiviral Treatment 352
    9.6.2. Infection Control and Prophylaxis 354
    9.6.3. Vaccination 356
9.7. Pandemic Preparedness and Future Directives 356
References 359

Index 369

Contributors

Ken Alibek
Executive Director and Distinguished
 Professor of Medical Microbiology and
 Immunology
The National Centre for Biodefense
George Manson University

Mike Bray
Biodefense Clinical Research Branch, Office
 of Clinical Research
National Institute of Allergy and Infectious
 Diseases
National Institutes of Health
Bethesda, Maryland

Dr. Luan-Yin Chang
Division of Pediatric Infectious Diseases,
 Department of Pediatrics
National Taiwan University Hospital
College of Medicine
National Taiwan University
Taipei 100, Taiwan

Jeremy Farrar
FRCP DPhil
Clinical Reader University of Oxford
Director University of Oxford Research Unit
Hospital for Tropical Diseases
Ho Chi Minh Tu, Viet Nam

Ignatius Wellington (Bill) Fong
Professor of Medicine
Division of Infectious Diseases
30 Bond St.
Toronto, Ont., M5B 1W8.

Dr. Khean Jin Goh
Department of Medicine
Faculty of Medicine
University of Malaya
Pantai Valley, 50603 Kuala Lumpur,
 MALAYSIA

Li-Min Huang
Professor, Division of Pediatric Infectious
 Diseases
Dept. of Pediatrics National Taiwan University
 Hospital
College of Medicine, National Taiwan University
Taipei 100, Taiwan

Naoki Inoue, PhD
Chief, Laboratory of Herpesviruses
Department of Virology I
National Institute of Infectious Disease
Tokyo 162-8640, Japan

Dr. Menno de Jong
Oxford University Clinical Research Unit
Hospital for Tropical Diseases
Ho Chi Minh City, Viet Nam

Fred Koster
Lovelace Respiratory Research Institute
Albuquerque, NM

Dr. Laurie T. Krug
Department of Microbiology and Immunology
Yerkes National Primate Research Center
Emory University
Atlanta, GA, 30329

Howard Levy
Eli Lilly and Company
Lilly Corporate Center
Indianapolis, IN

Tzou-Yien Lin
Professor, Division of pediatric Infectious
 Disease
Dept. of Pediatrics, Chang Gung Children's
 Hospital
Chang Gung University
Taoyuan 333, Taiwan

Jere W. McBride, PhD
Department of Pathology, Center for
 Biodefense and Emerging Infectious
 Diseases
Sealy Center for Vaccine Development
 University of Texas Medical Branch
Galveston, Texas

Dr. Malik Peiris
Dept. of Microbiology, University Pathology
 bldg
Queen Mary Hospital
Hong Kong

Dr. Lyle Peterson
Division of Vector-borne Infectious Diseases
Centers for Disease Control and Prevention
Fort Collins, CO 80522

Dr. John Roehrig
Division of Vector-borne Infectious Disease
Fort Collins, CO, 80522

Dr. James Sejvar
Division of Viral and Rickettsial Diseases
Centers for Disease Control and Prevention
Atlanta, GA 30333

Shin-Ru Shih
Professor, Clinical Virology Laboratory
Chang Gung Memorial Hospital, and School of
    Medical technology
Tao-Yuan 333 Taiwan

Chong Tin Tan
Professor and Head, Division of Neurology
University of Malaya, Neurology Laboratory
Kuala Lumpur 50603

Keiko Tanaka-Taya
Infectious Disease Surveillance Centre
National Institute of Infectious Diseases
Shinjuku-ku, Tokyo, 162-8640, Japan

Chong-Gee Teo
Sexually Transmitted and Blood Borne Virus
    Laboratory
Health Protection Agency
London, UK, NW9 5HT

David H. Walker, MD
Department of Pathology
University of Texas Medical Branch-Galveston
Galveston, Texas 77555

Kum Thong Wong
Professor & Consultant, Head
Dept. of Pathology, Faculty of Medicine
University of Malaya
50603 Kuala Lumpur, Malaysia

Samson SY Wong
Department of Microbiology
The University of Hong Kong
University Pathology Building
Queen Mary Hospital, Pokfulam, Hong Kong

Kwok-Yung Yuen
Department of Microbiology
The University of Hong Kong
University Pathology Building
Queen Mary Hospital
Pokfulam, Hong Kong

Section I: Evolving Infectious Diseases

1. West Nile Virus in the Americas

LYLE R. PETERSEN, JOHN T. ROEHRIG, AND JAMES J. SEJVAR

1.1. Virology

West Nile virus (WNV) is a member of the Japanese encephalitis (JE) serocomplex, which contains four other medically important flaviviruses: JE, St. Louis encephalitis (SLE), Murray Valley encephalitis (MVE), and Kunjin (KUN) viruses (Gubler and Roehrig, 1998). Until 1999, when WNV was first identified in the United States, each of these flaviviral encephalitis viruses had relatively unique geographic distributions. Since 1999, however, WN and SLE viruses have co-circulated in North America (Lillibridge et al., 2004).

1.1.1. Virus Structure

Flaviviruses are enveloped, spherical RNA viruses, possessing an isometric core 30–35 nm in diameter, which contains capsid (C; 14 kDa) proteins complexed with single-stranded positive-sense RNA. This core is surrounded by a lipid bilayer containing an envelope (E; 50–60 kDa) protein and a membrane (M; 8 kDa) protein, giving a total virion diameter of about 45 nm (Chambers et al., 1990). The M-protein is first synthesized as a precursor protein, prM. The virion structure of WNV has recently been solved using cryoelectron microscopy (Mukhopadhyay et al., 2003). The virion envelope contains an icosahedral scaffold of 90 E-protein dimers.

1.1.2. Genome

The flavivirus genome is a single-stranded, positive-sense RNA ~11,000 nucleotides (nt) in length, which is capped at the 5′-end, but has no poly(A) tract at the 3′-end. Flavivirus RNAs have conserved noncoding sequences at the 5′- and 3′-ends. A 9 nt cyclization (5′-CYC) sequence near the 5′-end of the genome is complementary to a 3′-CYC sequence in the 3'-terminal noncoding region (NCR), and these plus 3' stem-loop and pseudoknot structures are required for initiation of RNA synthesis (Chambers et al., 1990; Khromykh et al., 2001; You et al., 2001). A model for KUNV RNA replication proposes that flavivirus RNA is synthesized asymmetrically and semiconservatively in a replicative intermediate that uses negative-sense RNA as a recycling template, and dsRNA can be detected in infected cells using anti-dsRNA antibodies (Westaway et al., 1999).

Complete nucleotide sequences have been reported for many flavivirus genomes, including all four dengue viruses (DENV) serotypes (Deubel et al., 1986; Zhao et al., 1986; Deubel et al., 1988; Hahn et al., 1988; Osatomi and Sumiyoshi, 1990; Fu et al., 1992; Kinney et al., 1997) and several isolates of WNV (Lanciotti et al., 2002). The gene order from the 5'-end of the flavivirus RNA genome is C, prM, E, NS1, NS2A, NS2B, NS3, NS4A, NS4B, NS5 (C, capsid; prM, premembrane; E, envelope; NS, nonstructural proteins). A single polyprotein is translated, then cleaved co- and post-translationally by host signalases and a viral encoded protease to produce the mature proteins. The development of infectious cDNA clone technology has been important for analyzing the genomes of DENV, yellow fever virus (YFV) and WNV (Rice et al., 1989; Kinney et al., 1997; Yamshchikov et al., 2001; Shi et al., 2002). This technology has allowed researchers to genetically manipulate RNA genomes and identify viral determinants of host range, attachment and fusion, virulence, replication, packaging, and assembly.

1.1.2.1. E-protein

The flavivirus E-protein is the most important antigen in regard to virus biology and humoral immunity. It is a class II fusion protein that interacts with cell receptors and elicits potent virus-neutralizing antibodies. The E-protein also undergoes an irreversible conformational shift when exposed to low pH, resulting in a cell-membrane fusion (CMF)-competent form. Upon viral attachment and entry via low-pH endocytic vesicles, it is assumed that this conformational shift results in fusion of the virion envelope and the endocytic vesicular membrane, releasing the nucleocapsid into the cytoplasm. During viral assembly and maturation in low-pH exocytic vesicles, it is believed that the prM protein functions as a chaperone for the E-protein, maintaining its native conformation. The prM to M-cleavage occurs late in the maturational process, presumably as the virion is released into a neutral-pH environment. Virions containing uncleaved prM protein are less infectious and not capable of efficiently initiating virus-mediated CMF.

The structure of the E-protein homodimer has been solved for tick-borne encephalitis (TBE) and DEN viruses. It is likely that the homodimeric structure of the E-protein for all other flaviviruses, including WNV, will be similar. The molecular structure of the E-protein was first defined in studies using monoclonal antibodies (MAbs) (Heinz et al., 1982; Kimura-Kuroda and Yasui, 1983; Roehrig et al., 1983; Heinz, 1986; Guirakhoo et al., 1989; Mandl et al., 1989). Heinz and co-workers identified three antigenic domains (A, B, and C) on the E-protein of TBEV. Subsequent biochemical analyses of these domains determined that the A-domain approximately included amino acids (a.a.s) 51–135 and 195–284 and was a linearly discontinuous domain divided by C-domain (approximately a.a.s 1–50 and 136–194). Domain B included a.a.s 300–395. Our understanding of the structure–function relationships of the E-protein was greatly advanced by the solving of the 2 angstrom structure of the amino-terminal 395 amino acids of the TBEV and DENV E-protein homodimer (Modis et al., 2003, 2004). The E-protein folds into three distinct domains, I, II, and III, which correlate directly with the previously defined antigenic domains C, A, and B. The locations of the E-protein disulfide bonds are conserved among all flaviviruses (Nowak and Wengler, 1987); therefore, it has been generally assumed that the E-protein structure is the same for all flaviviruses. The inability of reduced and denatured WNV E-protein to elicit antiviral neutralizing antibodies when inoculated into mice emphasizes the importance of conformation to virus neutralization (Wengler, 1989).

The regions of the E-protein involved in attachment to cell receptors were first localized through selection of viruses capable of resisting virus-neutralizing monoclonal antibodies (MAbs). These neutralization escape variants have a.a. changes that prevent the binding of the selecting neutralizing MAb. Several flaviviruses have been examined in this way (Lobigs et al., 1987; Holzmann et al., 1989; Mandl et al., 1989; Cecilia and Gould, 1991; Hasegawa et al., 1992; Jiang et al., 1993; Gao et al., 1994; Lin et al., 1994; McMinn et al., 1995; Ryman et al., 1997; Beasley and Aaskov, 2001; Lok et al., 2001; Morita et al., 2001). Most neutralization escape variants have been selected using MAbs that are either type or subtype specific, indicating a high degree of antigenic drift in the identified regions. Five neutralization regions on the E-protein have been identified: region 1, a.a.s 67–72 and 112; region 2, a.a.s 124–128; region 3, a.a.s 155, 158; region 4, a.a.s 274–279, 52, and 136; and region 5, a.a.s 307–311, 333, 384, and 385. These regions are located on the outer, upper surfaces of the E-protein primarily in domains II and III, suggesting easy access to antiviral antibody. The ability of virus neutralizing antibody to bind to the outer surfaces of the E-protein is consistent with the two mechanisms of flavivirus neutralization thus far identified: blocking virus attachment to susceptible cells (Crill and Roehrig, 2001) and blocking virus-mediated CMF (Gollins and Porterfield, 1986a; Butrapet et al., 1998; Roehrig et al., 1998).

Antibody blocking of low-pH-catalyzed virus-mediated CMF was the first well-defined mechanism of WNV neutralization (Gollins and Porterfield, 1986a, 1986b, 1986c; Kimura et al., 1986). This mechanism of neutralization has since been confirmed with other flaviviviruses (Butrapet et al., 1998; Roehrig et al., 1998). Because a.a.s 98–110 of the E-protein in all flaviviruses are strictly conserved, uncharged, or hydrophobic a.a.s, this region has been hypothesized to be the fusion peptide. Using DEN2V E-protein-derived antipeptide antibodies to probe the entire sequence of both native and low-pH-treated virions to assess the accessibility of E-protein regions at different pHs, it has been demonstrated that certain regions of the E-protein were more accessible after a low-pH-catalyzed conformational change (Roehrig, 2000). Not surprisingly, one of these newly exposed regions (a.a.s 58–121) included the putative fusion peptide and was spatially proximal to a second region (a.a.s 225–249) identified in domain II (Rey et al., 1995; Roehrig et al., 1998). These results were confirmed in a subsequent study with TBEV (Holzmann et al., 1993). Antigenic mapping of the DEN2V E-protein determined that two of the three epitopes that elicited virus fusion-blocking MAbs could be mapped to a peptide fragment composed of a.a.s 1–120 (Roehrig et al., 1998). One of these epitopes (A1) is flavivirus cross-reactive and conformation dependent (Roehrig et al., 1998). This DEN2V epitope is essentially identical to the TBEV defined epitope A1. It has subsequently been determined that the TBEV anti-A1 MAb can also block low-pH-catalyzed cell-membrane fusion mediated by TBEV recombinant subviral particles (RSPs) (Corver et al., 2000; Allison et al., 2001; Stiasny et al., 2002). TBEV or WNV RSPs with mutations at Leu-107 of the E-glycoprotein have strongly impaired or completely abrogated fusion activity and reduced reactivity of anti-A1 Mabs (Allison et al., 2001; Crill and Chang, 2004). It is unknown whether or not this a.a. is critical for DEN virus-mediated CMF.

1.1.2.2. Nonstructural Proteins

Arthropod-borne flaviviruses encode at least seven nonstructural (NS) proteins in the 3′ three-quarters of their genome RNA (Rice et al., 1985). Recent studies have attributed several essential functions in viral replication to the NS proteins. Knowledge of protein structures, functions, and interactions could pinpoint vulnerable targets for enzyme inhibition or disruption of protein–protein interactions. The RNA replication complex includes NS1, NS2A, NS3, NS4A, and NS5 proteins (Westaway et al., 1997, 1999), which are assembled on cytoplasmic membranes co- and post-translationally (Khromykh et al., 1998). Nonspecific *in vitro* RNA synthesis activity can be demonstrated for NS5 (Bartholomeusz and Wright, 1993), which has been shown to form heterodimers with NS3 (Kapoor et al., 1995). In a yeast 2-hybrid system, a.a. residues 320–368 of DEN2V NS5 and residues 303–405 in NS3 were shown to mediate protein–protein interactions (Johansson et al., 2001); however, complementation analysis with KUNV suggested that the N-terminal 316 a.a.s of NS5 and N-terminal 178 a.a.s of NS3 were required for interaction (Liu et al., 2002). The C-terminal two-thirds of the NS5 protein contains the RNA-dependent RNA polymerase (RdRP) activity (Tan et al., 1996), and an N-terminal domain is predicted to be a methyl transferase (Koonin, 1993).

The flavivirus NS1 protein elicits high-titered antibody in flavivirus-infected or -immunized animals, but its function in flavivirus replication remains an enigma (Falkler et al., 1973). It has been determined that NS1 immunization or passive transfer of anti-NS1 Mabs can protect animals from viral challenge (Schlesinger et al., 1985, 1986, 1987; Henchal et al., 1988; Iacono-Connors et al., 1996).

The NS3 protein also has multiple functions. Padmanabhan and colleagues have characterized the serine protease activity of the DEN2V NS3 protein by crystallization of the N-terminal domain (Krishna Murthy et al., 1999). Enzymatic activity was analyzed by introduction of site-specific mutations into cDNA constructs (Valle and Falgout, 1998). The 167 N-terminal a.a. residues constitute the serine protease that carries out NS2A-2B, 2B-3, 3-4A, and 4B-5 cleavages of the primary polyprotein translation product and secondary cleavages within the C, NS2A, NS3, and NS4A proteins (Krishna Murthy et al., 1999). The catalytic triad residues of DEN2V NS3 protease are His-51, Asp-75, and Ser-135, and additional a.a. residues have been implicated in specificity. Substrate cleavage sites have the positively-charged a.a.s Lys-Arg, Arg-Arg, Arg-Lys, and occasionally Gln-Arg at the P2 and P1 positions, and Gly, Ala, or Ser at the P1′ position (Krishna Murthy et al., 1999; Murthy et al., 1999). Several different flaviviral serine proteases share these structural features and cleavage sites (Krishna Murthy et al., 1999), suggesting that identification of broad-spectrum flaviviral replication inhibitors might be possible. Interaction between NS2B and NS3 is required for membrane association and efficient, specific *trans*-cleavages by this protease (Clum et al., 1997). A 40-a.a. hydrophilic region on NS2B activates the NS3 protease domain, and 3 hydrophobic regions are required for membrane insertion of the complex (Krishna Murthy et al., 1999). NS3 a.a residues 168–188, including a basic a.a-cluster (184-Arg-Lys-Arg-Lys), are required for RNA-stimulated nucleoside triphosphatase activity (Li et al., 1999). Unwinding of double-stranded RNA in replicative intermediates by the viral helicase, as well as capping during synthesis of the viral genome could require NTPase activity. The C-terminal domain of DENV NS3 contains seven motifs characteristic of DExH helicase activity (Li et al., 1999; Matusan et al., 2001). Matusan et al. mapped a.a. residues required for helicase activity and viral replication by site-specific mutagenesis of a DEN-2 infectious clone (Matusan et al., 2001).

1.1.3. Genetics and Virulence

Strains of WNV can be divided into two genetic lineages (1 and 2) by phylogenetic analysis of the complete genome sequence or of the E-protein gene sequence (Lanciotti et al., 1999, 2002). Major human outbreaks of WNV have been associated only with lineage 1 WNVs. Lineage 2 WNVs apparently maintain themselves in enzootic cycles only, primarily in Africa. Sequencing and analysis of the original North American WNV isolate (NY99) quickly implicated the Middle East as the likely source of the WNV that entered the New York City (NYC) area in 1999 (Briese et al., 1999; Jia et al., 1999; Lanciotti et al., 1999). This genotypic link was further confirmed by the similar phenotypic characteristics of the NY99 WNV and a strain of WNV isolated from storks in Israel (Lanciotti et al., 1999; Bin et al., 2001; Malkinson et al., 2001, 2002; Banet-Noach et al., 2003, 2004). Both NY99 and Israeli strains of WNV killed birds. Because birds are the primary amplifying and reservoir hosts for WNV, the high mortality in certain birds from these WNV strains was unusual. No other outbreaks of WNV have been associated with high bird mortality, including the human WNV outbreaks in Romania (1996) and Volgograd (1999) (Han et al., 1999; Platonov et al., 2001).

Mortality has been recorded in more than 280 native and captive bird species in North America (Petersen and Hayes, 2004). The NY99 strain of WNV appears to be lethal to most birds of the family Corvidae (crows, ravens, and jays) (Komar et al., 2003a; Brault et al., 2004). The substantial crow and blue jay mortality has served as the foundation for the ecological WNV surveillance based on reporting dead birds to public health officials (Brault et al., 2004; Weingartl et al., 2004; Yaremych et al., 2004). In addition to corvids, other birds such as raptors also appear to have high mortality after NY99 WNV infection. The high American crow mortality rate for the NY99 WNV strain as compared with two other lineage 1 WNV strains (KUN [a subtype of WNV circulating in Australia] and strain isolated in Kenya [KEN-3829]) has been confirmed in the laboratory (Brault et al., 2004). Four a.a. differences exist between the KEN-3829 and NY99 WNV strains. Two a.a. changes occur in the capsid (a.a.s 3 and 8), and two a.a. changes occur in the envelope protein (a.a.s 126 and 159). The changes in the E-protein occur in domain II and could affect virus-mediated CMF. Further studies using recombination of infectious cDNA clones of WNV will better elucidate the significance of these a.a. changes.

As WNV has spread westward across the United States, its genome has remained remarkably stable, with minor temporal and regional variations observed. These variations usually represent less than 0.5% of the genomic sequence and result in only a few a.a. changes in any given isolate (Beasley et al., 2003; Davis et al., 2003; Blitvich et al., 2004; Davis et al., 2004; Ebel et al., 2004; Granwehr et al., 2004).

1.2. Epidemiology

WNV is one of the most widely distributed of all arboviruses, with an extensive distribution throughout Africa, the Middle East, parts of Europe and the former Soviet Union, South Asia, and Australia (Petersen and Roehrig, 2001; Campbell et al., 2002). The virus had not been detected in North America before a human outbreak of meningitis and encephalitis and an accompanying epizootic in birds in 1999 in the New York City area (Nash et al., 2001).

1.2.1. Ecology

Birds are the primary amplifying hosts, and the virus is maintained in a bird–mosquito–bird cycle primarily involving *Culex* spp. mosquitoes (Fig. 1.1) (Hubalek and Halouzka, 1999; Hayes, 2001). Humans and other vertebrates, such as horses, do not develop a high level of viremia and, thus, are thought to be incidental hosts who play a minor role in the transmission cycle.

1.2.1.1. Vectors

The major mosquito vector in Africa and the Middle East is *Cx. univittatus*, with *Cx. picilipes*, *Cx. neavei*, *Cx. decens*, *Aedes albocephalus*, or *Mimomyia* spp. important in some areas (Hubalek and Halouzka, 1999; Solomon, 2004). In Europe, *Cx. pipiens*, *Cx. modestus*, and *Coquillettidia richiardii* are important. In Asia, *Cx. tritaeniorhynchus*, *Cx. vishnui*, and *Cx. quinquefasciatus* predominate (Hubalek and Halouzka, 1999).

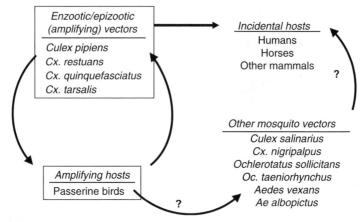

Figure 1.1. West Nile virus transmission cycle, North America.

As of December 2004, surveillance has identified 58 mosquito species infected with WNV in North America (Petersen and Hayes, 2004). WNV and SLEV appear to share the same maintenance vectors, with *Cx. pipiens* (northern house mosquito) and *Cx. restuans* the maintenance vectors in the northeastern United States and Canada, *Cx. quinquefasciatus* (southern house mosquito) the main maintenance vector in the southern United States, and *Cx. tarsalis* the main maintenance vectors in the western United States and Canada (CDC, 2002d; Solomon, 2004). *Cx. salinarius* was implicated in the epidemic on Staten Island in 2000, and, along with *Cx. nigripalpus,* may be important in Florida (Kulasekera et al., 2001; Blackmore et al., 2003).

Culex spp. mosquitoes are important for their role in overwintering the virus in temperate climates, where they hibernate as adult mosquitoes (CDC, 2000a; Nasci et al., 2001; Bugbee and Forte, 2004). The amplification cycle begins when infected overwintering mosquitoes emerge in the spring and infect birds. Amplification within the bird–mosquito–bird cycle continues until late summer and fall, when *Culex* mosquitoes begin diapause and rarely blood-feed. Vertical transmission can occur by an inefficient process in which virus enters the fully formed egg during oviposition (Baqar et al., 1993; Miller et al., 2000; Goddard et al., 2003). The importance of vertical transmission in maintaining the virus is unknown but may be an important mechanism of infection of mosquitoes entering diapause.

In temperate climates, human WNV outbreaks tend to occur during abnormally hot summers (Cornel et al., 1993). This could occur in part because environmental temperature increases the speed of infection dissemination and WNV titers in newly infected mosquitoes, which, in turn, increases the overall vector competency (Cornel et al., 1993; Dohm and Turell, 2001; Dohm et al., 2002). As with SLEV, other environmental factors that affect host and vector abundance, as well as preexisting levels of immunity in birds, likely play a major role in determining the potential for WNV outbreaks (Day, 2001).

WNV has been isolated from hard (ixodid) and soft (argasid) ticks species in regions of Europe, Africa, and Asia, but it is unclear what role they play in maintaining or disseminating the virus (Platonov, 2001). A North American argasid tick species (*Ornithodorus moubata*) was shown to harbor WNV for at least 132 days and was able to infrequently infect rodents (Lawrie et al., 2004).

1.2.1.2. Vertebrate Hosts

Wild birds develop prolonged high levels of viremia and serve as amplifying hosts (Komar et al., 2003a). Passerine birds develop high levels of viremia, are abundant, and become infected in high numbers during epizootics, suggesting that they may be the principal reservoir hosts for WNV (Komar et al., 2001; Komar, 2003; Komar et al., 2003a).

WNV transmission among caged birds suggests that direct transmission from bird to bird may occur (Langevin et al., 2001; Swayne et al., 2001; McLean et al., 2002; Komar et al., 2003a). The means of this cage mate transmission is unknown; however, the detection of WNV in oral and cloacal swabs suggests possible oral transmission (Komar et al., 2002). In experiments, birds can be infected orally via ingestion of contaminated water, dead birds and mice, and infected mosquitoes (Langevin et al., 2001; McLean et al., 2002; Komar et al., 2003a). Mathematical models suggest that bird-to-bird transmission has little impact in overall transmission dynamics in nature (Naowarat and Tang, 2004).

More than 21,000 cases of WNV disease in equines were reported from 1999 through 2004 in the United States. Incidence peaked in 2002 and subsequently decreased in 2003 and 2004 after a WNV vaccine became available. Approximately 10% of experimentally infected horses develop clinical illness (Bunning et al., 2002). Clinical series indicate a 20% to 40% mortality among clinically ill horses (Cantile et al., 2000; Porter et al., 2003; Weese et al., 2003; Salazar et al., 2004; Ward et al., 2004). Age, vaccination status, inability to rise, and female gender are associated with the risk of death (Salazar et al., 2004). Viremia in horses is low and of short duration; thus, horses are unlikely to serve as important amplifying hosts for WNV in nature (Bunning et al., 2001, 2002).

WNV has been isolated or identified serologically in many native and imported vertebrate species in North America, including bats (Pilipski et al., 2004), wolves (Lichtensteiger et al., 2003; Lanthier et al., 2004), eastern fox and gray squirrels (Kiupel et al., 2003; Heinz-Taheny et al., 2004), sheep (Tyler et al., 2003), alligators (Miller et al., 2003; Klenk et al., 2004), alpacas (Dunkel et al., 2004; Kutzler et al., 2004; Yaeger et al., 2004), black bears (Farajollahi et al., 2003), a Barbary macaque (Olberg et al., 2004), a Suffolk ewe (Yaeger et al., 2004), reindeer (Palmer et al., 2004), dogs (Lichtensteiger et al., 2003), and monkeys and baboons (Ratterree et al., 2003).

1.2.2. Geographic Spread

1.2.2.1. United States and Canada

Since its emergence in the New York City area in 1999, the virus has spread rapidly across the United States (Fig. 1.2) (Petersen and Hayes, 2004). In 2004, WNV activity was detected in every continental U.S. state except Washington State. Whereas the southern spread from the New York City area to the southeastern United States was predicted according to bird migration patterns (Lord and Calisher, 1970; Peterson et al., 2003), the means of the virus' westward spread is less certain and may be due to random bird dispersal movements (Rappole and Hubalek, 2003).

WNV was first detected in Canada in southern Ontario in 2001 and by 2002 had spread to Manitoba, Quebec, Nova Scotia, and Saskatchewan (Drebot et al., 2003). By 2003, the virus' distribution extended into New Brunswick and Alberta.

1.2.2.2. Latin America

WNV was first detected south of the United States border in 2001, when a resident of the Cayman Islands developed WNV encephalitis (CDC, 2002e). In 2002, WNV was isolated from a dead Common Raven in Tabasco State, Mexico (Estrada-Franco et al., 2003) and in 2003 was detected by genetic sequencing of cerebellar tissue from a dead horse from Nuevo Leon State, Mexico (Blitvich et al., 2004) (Table 1.1). Complete genome sequencing showed that the isolate from Tabasco State in southern Mexico included 46 nucleotide (0.42%) and 4 amino acid (0.11%) differences from the NY99 prototype strain (Beasley et al., 2004). Plaque-purified variants of the isolate with mutations at the E-protein glycosylation motif had decreased mouse virulence. Phylogenetic analysis of the genetic sequences from the horse in Nuevo Leon State showed genetic relatedness to recent isolates from Texas that do not encode mutations at the E glycosylation motif (Blitvich et al., 2004).

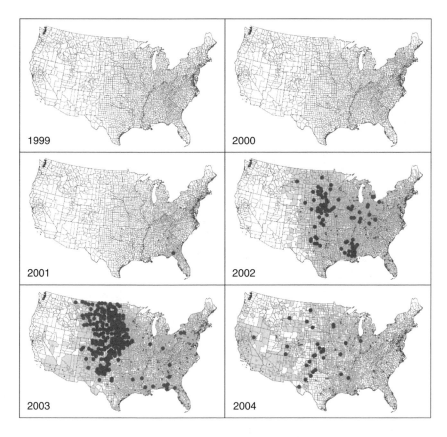

Human Neuroinvasive Disease Incidence per million
● .01-9.99   ● 10-99.99   ● >=100

Any WNV Activity (birds, mosquitoes, horses, humans)

Figure 1.2. West Nile virus in the United States, 1999–2004. The incidence of human neuroinvasive disease is indicated by county.

Serologic evidence in birds and horses suggests that WNV has circulated in the Dominican Republic (Komar et al., 2003b), Jamaica (Dupuis et al., 2003), and Guadeloupe (Quirin et al., 2004), as well as widely in Mexico (Blitvich et al., 2003b; Estrada-Franco et al., 2003; Fernandez-Salas et al., 2003; Lorono-Pino et al., 2003; Marlenee et al., 2004) (Table 1.1). In Mexico and Guadeloupe, a high proportion of tested horses had WNV antibodies. Although sampling was sometimes done in areas where equine mortality from unknown causes had been observed, substantial equine mortality from documented WNV infection has been lacking. In Guadeloupe, paired samples from horses sampled at an approximate 1-year interval indicated that 47% developed neutralizing antibodies;

Table 1.1. Published studies of West Nile virus in Latin America, 2001–2004

Location	Year	Source	Test	Comment	Reference
Cayman Islands	2001	Human	Not described	Encephalitis	CDC, (2002e)
Guadeloupe	2002/2003	Horses	IgG and IgM ELISA; PRNT80 WNV and SLEV	Forty-seven percent of 114 seroconverted (IgG) between July 2002 and January 2003. All negative by IgM. Seven of 10 tested IgG-positive horses had WNV-specific neutralizing antibody. No clinical illness.	Quirin et al. (2004)
Guadeloupe	2002/2003	Chickens	IgG and IgM ELISA; PRNT80 WNV and SLEV	Eleven of 20 IgG positive. All four IgG-positive specimens had WNV-specific neutralizing antibody. No clinical illness.	Quirin et al. (2004)
Jamaica	2002	Resident and migratory birds	Indirect ELISA; PRNT90 Ilhéus, SLEV, WNV	Twenty-seven of 348 resident birds WNV positive. One of 194 migratory birds positive.	Dupuis et al. (2003)
Mexico, Yucatan State	2002	Horses	Blocking ELISA; HI SLEV; PRNT90 Ilhéus, SLEV, WNV, Bussuquara	Three of 252 WNV positive. No clinical illness.	Lorono-Pino et al. (2003)
Mexico, Coahuila State	2002	Horses	Blocking ELISA; PRNT90 SLEV, WNV	All 5 ill horses WNV positive, 6 of 9 from same ranch as ill horses positive, 4 of 10 from other areas positive.	Blitvich et al. (2003b)
Mexico, multiple states	2002–2003	Horses	IgG ELISA, HI SLE and WNV; PRNT90 SLEV, WNV, VEE	Four hundred forty-one horses from 14 states tested. Sampling from herds with encephalitic history. Ninety-seven WNV positive from six states.	Estrada-Franco et al. (2003)
Mexico, Tamaulipas State	2003	Migratory and resident birds	Blocking ELISA; PRNT90 SLEV, WNV	Three resident and one migratory bird positive in captures March 2003. Seven hundred ninety-six birds tested from 2001 to 2003.	Fernandez-Salas et al. (2003)
Mexico, Tabasco State	2003	Bird	Virus isolation	Sample from dead common raven.	Estrada-Franco et al. (2003)
Mexico, Nuevo Leon State	2003	Horses	Blocking ELISA; PRNT90 SLEV, WNV	Twenty of 88 horses positive.	Marlenee et al. (2004)
Mexico, Nuevo Leon State	2003	Horse	Virus isolation	Brain tissue from dead horse.	Blitvich et al. (2004)

WNV, West Nile virus; SLEV, St. Louis encephalitis virus; PRNT80, plaque reduction neutralization test, 80% reduction in number of plaques; PRNT90, plaque reduction neurtralization test, 90% reduction in number of plaques.

however, clinical illness was not observed, and IgM antibodies were not detected (Quirin et al., 2004).

1.2.3. Incidence of Human Infection and Illness

1.2.3.1. United States

Despite extensive spread of WNV in nature from 1999 through 2001, human disease was infrequently reported, with only 149 cases reported in the United States during those years (Table 1.2; Fig. 1.2) (CDC, 2000b; Marfin et al., 2001; Nash et al., 2001; CDC, 2002e; Petersen and Hayes, 2004). However, in 2002, a multistate outbreak throughout the Midwest resulted in more than 4000 reported cases, of whom 2946 had reported neuroinvasive disease (Table 1.2; Fig. 1.2) (O'Leary et al., 2004). This outbreak was epidemiologically similar to a 1975 outbreak of SLEV, which involved approximately 2000 persons (Creech, 1977). In 2003, nearly 10,000 cases were reported, of whom 2866 had neuroinvasive disease. Wider availability of commercial WNV antibody detection assays resulted in increased diagnosis and reporting of patients with WN fever in 2003; however, the similar number of neuroinvasive disease cases reported in 2002 and 2003 indicated that both outbreaks were of similar magnitude (Table 1.2) (Petersen and Hayes, 2004). The incidence of WNV neuroinvasive disease was lower in 2004 compared with the two previous years (Table 1.2), with approximately one-third of the cases reported from California and Arizona (Fig. 1.2).

Serological surveys indicate that even in areas experiencing outbreaks, less than 5% of the population has been exposed to the virus (Tsai et al., 1998; CDC, 2001; Mostashari et al., 2001; Petersen and Hayes, 2004). Based on the 6849 reported cases of WNV neuroinvasive disease from 1999 through 2004 and the estimated proportions of infected persons

Table 1.2. Total number of reported cases of WNV disease and number of cases with neuroinvasive disease, United States, 1999–2004

Year	Total cases	Neuroinvasive cases	Fatalities
1999	62	54	7
2000	21	19	2
2001	66	64	9
2002	4156	2946	284
2003	9862	2866	264
2004	2539	1142	128
Total	16,706	7091	694

who develop WN fever and WNV neuroinvasive disease, approximately 1 million persons have become infected with the WNV in the United States, of whom approximately 190,000 have become ill (Petersen and Hayes, 2004). Through 2004, more than 690 deaths have been reported (Petersen and Hayes, 2004), with a fatality rate of approximately 10% among persons with neuroinvasive disease.

Human WNV infection incidence increases in early summer and peaks in August or early September (Fig. 1.3). However, an outbreak in Phoenix, Arizona, in 2004 began in May and peaked in late June and early July. In the United States, within large regional WNV epidemics, the incidence of human disease varies markedly from county to county, suggesting the importance of local ecological conditions (Fig. 1.2).

1.2.3.2. Canada

The first cases of human WNV disease in Canada occurred in 2002, with 426 reported illnesses and 20 deaths reported from Quebec and Ontario. In 2003, 1494 cases were reported, of whom 217 had neuroinvasive disease and 10 died. In 2004, there were only 26 reported cases, of whom 13 had neuroinvasive disease; none died. These incidences parallel those in the northern United States.

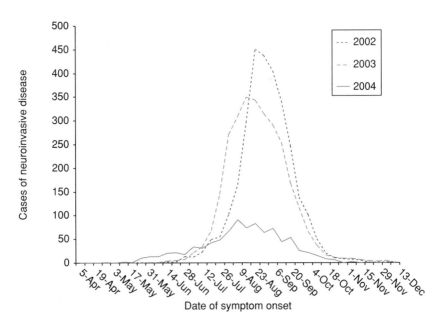

Figure 1.3. Number of reported cases of West Nile virus neuroinvasive disease by week of symptom onset, 2002–2004.

1.2.4. Risk Factors for Infection, Severe Disease, and Death

Serologic surveys in Romania (Tsai et al., 1998) and New York City (Tsai et al., 1998; Mostashari et al., 2001) indicate that WNV infection incidence is constant across all age groups during outbreaks. Surveillance data from the United States indicate that age is the most important host risk factor for development of neuroinvasive disease after infection. The incidence of neuroinvasive disease increases approximately 1.5-fold for each decade of life, resulting in a risk approximately 30 times greater for a person 80–90 years old compared with a child younger than 10 years old (O'Leary et al., 2004).

Advanced age is the most important risk factor for death. Surveillance data indicate that case fatality rates of persons with WNV neuroinvasive disease increases from 1% among persons under 40 years of age to 36% among persons 90 years and older (O'Leary et al., 2004). During outbreaks, hospitalized persons older than 70 years of age had case fatality rates of 15% in Romania (Tsai et al., 1998) and 29% in Israel (Chowers et al., 2001). Encephalitis with severe muscle weakness and change in the level of consciousness were also prominent clinical risk factors predicting fatal outcome (Chowers et al., 2001; Nash et al., 2001). Diabetes mellitus was an independent risk factor for death during the 1999 New York City outbreak (Nash et al., 2001). The incidence of neuroinvasive disease and the probability of death after acquiring neuroinvasive disease is slightly higher in men than women (O'Leary et al., 2004).

Organ transplant recipients are at extreme risk of developing neuroinvasive disease after WNV infection. The first indication that transplant recipients were at high risk of developing neuroinvasive disease was the development of WNV encephalitis in three of four recipients of organs from a WN viremic donor (Iwamoto et al., 2003). A seroprevalence study carried out in patients of Canadian outpatient transplant clinics after a WNV epidemic in 2002 indicated that the risk of neuroinvasive disease after infection was 40% (95% confidence interval 16–80%) (Kumar et al., 2004a). During that epidemic, transplant patients were approximately 40 times more likely than the population-at-large to have developed WN neuroinvasive disease (Kumar et al., 2004b).

Individual case reports or small case series have described WNV neuroinvasive disease in transplant recipients of kidney (Armali et al., 2003; Hardinger et al., 2003; Iwamoto et al., 2003; Cushing et al., 2004; DeSalvo et al., 2004; Kleinschmidt-DeMasters et al., 2004; Kumar et al., 2004b; Smith et al., 2004; Wadei et al., 2004), kidney/pancreas (Kleinschmidt-DeMasters et al., 2004; Ravindra et al., 2004), liver (Iwamoto et al., 2003; Pealer et al., 2003; Kleinschmidt-DeMasters et al., 2004; Kumar et al., 2004b), lung (Kleinschmidt-DeMasters et al., 2004), heart (Iwamoto et al., 2003; Kumar et al., 2004b), bone marrow (Hiatt et al., 2003; Pealer et al., 2003; Robertson et al., 2004), and stem cells (Hong et al., 2003; Pealer et al., 2003; Kleinschmidt-DeMasters et al., 2004; Reddy et al., 2004). Neuroinvasive disease was reported in a patient with acute myelogenous leukemia without stem cell transplantation (Pealer et al., 2003). A patient with common variable immunodeficiency developed WNV meningitis with good clinical outcome (Alonto et al., 2003). Only one person with WNV encephalitis and human immunodeficiency virus infection has been reported (Szilak and Minamoto, 2000).

The risk of death among persons with WNV infection who have underlying immunodeficiencies is unknown and cannot be ascertained from individual case reports. In a series of 11 transplant patients with WNV neuroinvasive disease, 2 died and 3 developed significant residual neurological deficits (Kleinschmidt-DeMasters et al., 2004).

1.2.5. Non-Mosquito Transmission Routes

1.2.5.1. Blood Transfusion

Nearly all human infections are due to mosquito bites. However, blood transfusion–related transmission was considered a theoretical possibility because most persons with WNV infection have a short period of viremia but remain asymptomatic. The risk of WNV transmission from blood products obtained from donors living in the epicenter of the 1999 New York City outbreak was estimated at 1.8 per 10,000 units, although no instances of transfusion transmission were documented at that time (Biggerstaff and Petersen, 2002). Transfusion-associated WNV transmission was proved during the 2002 U.S. WNV epidemic when 23 transfusion recipients became infected after receipt of platelets, red blood cells, or plasma from 16 viremic blood donors (Harrington et al., 2003; Pealer et al., 2003). The 15 recipients who developed WNV-related illness became ill 2 to 21 days (median 10) after transfusion. The implicated blood donors had low-level viremias (0.8 to 75.1 plaque-forming units per ml) and all lacked WNV IgM antibodies at the time of donation. Mathematical models indicated that the mean risk of transfusion-associated WNV transmission during the 2002 epidemic ranged from 2.1 to 4.7 per 10,000 donors in high-incidence states (Biggerstaff and Petersen, 2003).

1.2.5.2. Organ Transplantation

One instance of WNV transmission via organ transplantation has been documented (Iwamoto et al., 2003). The organ donor had become infected from a contaminated blood transfusion one day before the organs were harvested. Both recipients of the donor's kidneys and the recipient of the donor's heart developed WNV encephalitis; the recipient of the donor's liver developed WN fever. Symptoms began 7 to 17 days after transplantation.

1.2.5.3. Intrauterine Transmission

Intrauterine transmission has been documented in one case (CDC, 2002a; Alpert et al., 2003). The mother was diagnosed with WNV infection and paraparesis approximately 2 months before delivery. Cord blood and infant heel stick blood were positive for WNV-specific IgM and neutralizing antibodies. Funduscopic examination of the infant revealed chorioretinal scarring, and magnetic resonance imaging showed generalized lissencephaly, severe white matter loss in the temporal and occipital lobes, and a 2-cm cyst involving the left posterior temporal lobe.

1.2.5.4. Other Transmission Modes

Experimental studies have shown that WNV may be transmitted efficiently from lactating hamsters to suckling hamsters (Reagan et al., 1956). One possible WNV transmission via human breast milk has been reported (CDC, 2002c). The mother was infected with WNV from a contaminated blood transfusion 1 day after delivery and developed WNV meningitis 11 days later. The infant was breast-fed starting 1 day after delivery; WNV nucleic acid and WNV-specific IgM and IgG antibodies were detected in a sample of breast milk 16 days after delivery. The infant remained asymptomatic, but a serum sample obtained 25 days after delivery showed WNV-specific IgM antibodies.

Human laboratory-acquired WNV infections by the percutaneous route have been reported (CDC, 2002b). Aerosol transmission was also suspected when a laboratory worker became infected after breathing an aerosol containing infected mouse brains; subsequent experiments showed that mice, hamsters, and monkeys can be infected via the aerosol route (Nir, 1959). Mice infected by the aerosol route develop early viral replication in the lungs, followed by dissemination to the blood and other organs (Nir et al., 1965).

Dialysis-related WNV transmission has also been suspected (CDC, 2004a). Two persons developed symptomatic WNV infection 8 and 19 days after receiving dialysis on the same dialysis machine. A third person, who received dialysis between these two patients on the same machine, remained asymptomatic but had WNV IgG and neutralizing antibodies in serum 42 days after dialysis. An outbreak of WNV infection occurred among turkey farm workers; however, the means of transmission in that setting was unknown (CDC, 2003b).

1.3. Clinical Spectrum

From the virus' first isolation and identification in 1937 in the West Nile district of Uganda (Smithburn et al., 1940) until the mid-1990s, WNV outbreaks were almost always associated with mild human illness (Goldblum et al., 1954; Marberg et al., 1956; Jupp, 2001; Murgue et al., 2001; Petersen and Roehrig, 2001; Campbell et al., 2002; Murgue et al., 2002). However, 11% of the study subjects experimentally infected with WNV as a cancer therapy in the early 1950s developed encephalitis, sometimes accompanied by paralysis, involuntary twitching, and cogwheel rigidity (Southam and Moore, 1954). The first recorded instance of severe neurological disease during an outbreak occurred in Israeli nursing homes in 1957 (Spigland et al., 1958), and the virus was isolated from the brains of three children who died of encephalitis in India in 1980 and 1981 (George et al., 1984). Nevertheless, severe neurological disease during outbreaks remained uncommon until the recent outbreaks in Algeria, 1994 (Le Guenno et al., 1996); Romania, 1996 (Tsai et al., 1998); Tunisia, 1997 (Murgue et al., 2001); Russia, 1999 (Platonov et al., 2001); United States and Canada, 1999–2004 (Petersen and Hayes, 2004); Israel, 2000 (Chowers et al., 2001); and Sudan, 2002 (Depoortere et al., 2004). Investigation of these outbreaks has greatly expanded our knowledge of the clinical spectrum of illness due to WNV.

Serological surveys after contemporary outbreaks indicate that about a fifth of human WNV infections results in clinical illness without neuroinvasive disease, and 1 in 150 results in neuroinvasive disease (meningitis, encephalitis, acute flaccid paralysis) (Tsai et al., 1998; CDC, 2001; Mostashari et al., 2001).

1.3.1. West Nile Fever

The term *West Nile fever* (WN fever) was coined by Goldblum when he described the mild, febrile illnesses occurring during an Israeli outbreak in 1952 (Goldblum et al., 1954). Goldblum described the illness as one of sudden onset, characterized by malaise, general weakness, a chilly sensation with fever, drowsiness, severe frontal headache, aching of the eyes when moved, and pains mostly in the chest and lumbar regions, with a few patients having gastrointestinal disturbances, anorexia, nausea, and dryness of the throat. He noted that the acute illness lasted 3 to 6 days, but convalescence was slow, lasting 1 to 2 weeks and accompanied by general fatigue. This and subsequent investigations suggest the typical incubation period is approximately 2–14 days.

WN fever has been reported in all age groups; the median age of persons reported with WN fever during the 2002 U.S. epidemic was 49 years (O'Leary et al., 2004). Because few persons with WN fever consult a physician, are diagnosed with serologic tests, and are reported to national surveillance, age-specific incidence data and clinical descriptions of illness are subjected to considerable bias. One contemporary study has quantified the symptoms of WN fever (Watson et al., 2004). This study, based on statewide WNV virus surveillance in Illinois, was likely biased toward more severely ill patients because WNV antibody testing was not widely available at that time. Approximately one-third of the patients with WN fever were hospitalized, and those hospitalized were older than those not hospitalized (65 years vs. 46 years). As described in earlier outbreaks of WN fever, fever, headache, fatigue, myalgias, and gastrointestinal complaints were prominent symptoms (Table 1.3). The Illinois study reaffirmed early observations that complete recovery from WN fever is typical, but some symptoms, particularly fatigue, and disability may be prolonged in some patients (Watson et al., 2004).

The rash associated with WN fever is morbilliform, maculopapular, and nonpruritic and predominates over the torso and extremities, sparing the palms and soles (Anderson et al., 2004). The rash often appears several days after symptom onset and may coincide with convalescence from initial symptoms. The rash was a prominent symptom in early outbreaks of WN fever (Marberg et al., 1956) but has been less frequent in persons with neuroinvasive disease in contemporary outbreaks (Table 1.3). One explanation for this difference is that rash may be less likely to occur in more severely ill patients. The marked difference in rash between ambulatory and hospitalized patients with WN fever in the Illinois study supports this hypothesis (Table 1.3). Lymphadenopathy has been infrequently reported in contemporary outbreaks.

1.3.2. Neuroinvasive Disease

U.S. surveillance data indicate that WNV neuroinvasive disease can occur in persons of all ages; however, the incidence increases by age (O'Leary et al., 2004). WNV meningitis makes up the largest percentage of neuroinvasive disease cases in younger age groups, while the proportion of encephalitis increases in older age groups.

Table 1.3. Symptoms reported among hospitalized patients with neuroinvasive disease during outbreaks in New York (1999) (Nash et al., 2001), Romania (1996) (Tsai et al., 1998), and Israel (2000) (Chowers et al., 2001); among hospitalized patients with West Nile fever (1953) (Marberg et al., 1956); and among hospitalized and nonhospitalized patients with West Nile fever in Illinois (2002) (Watson et al., 2004)

Symptom*	New York 1999 hospitalized (n = 59), percent (%)	Romania 1996 hospitalized (n = 393), percent (%)	Israel 2000 hospitalized (n = 233), percent (%)	Israel 1953 hospitalized (n = 50), percent (%)	Illinois 2002 hospitalized (n = 30), percent (%)	Illinois 2002 outpatient (n = 68), percent (%)
Fever	90	91	98	100	93	76
Fatigue				"nearly all"	90	99
Weakness	56				70	57
Nausea	53			25		
Vomiting	51	53	31	10	43	21
Headache	47	77	58	80	50	81
Change in mental status	46	34†	40†			
Diarrhea	27		19	30	33	24
Rash	19		21	"about half"	23	72
Cough	19			8		
Stiff neck	19	57	29		43‡	60‡
Myalgia	17		15	25	50	68
Arthralgia	15				27	41
Lymphadenopathy	2		10	90		

*Some listed symptoms were not reported in all studies.
†Reported as confusion.
‡Reported as stiff neck or neck pain.

1.3.2.1. Meningitis

During the 2002 U.S. epidemic, the median age of persons reported with WNV meningitis was 46 years (O'Leary et al., 2004). WNV meningitis is clinically similar to that of other viral meningitides. Affected persons experience the abrupt onset of fever, headache, and meningeal signs, including nuchal rigidity, the presence of Kernig and/or Brudzinski signs, and photophobia or phonophobia. The associated headache may be severe, requiring hospitalization for pain control; associated gastrointestinal disturbance may result in dehydration, exacerbating head pain, and systemic symptoms (Sejvar et al., 2003a). WNV meningitis is generally associated with a favorable outcome, though, similar to WN fever, some patients experience persistent headache, fatigue, and myalgias (Sejvar et al., 2003a). During the 2002 U.S. epidemic, 2% of reported cases of meningitis from WNV were fatal (O'Leary et al., 2004).

1.3.2.2. Encephalitis

During the 2002 U.S. epidemic, the median age of persons reported with WNV encephalitis was 64 years (O'Leary et al., 2004). WNV encephalitis may range in severity from a mild, self-limited confusional state to severe encephalopathy, coma, and death. Several neurological syndromes, primarily extrapyramidal disorders, have been observed in patients with WNV encephalitis (Pepperell et al., 2003; Sejvar et al., 2003a; Burton et al., 2004; Sayao et al., 2004). Patients with WNV encephalitis frequently develop a coarse tremor, particularly in the upper extremities. The tremor tends to be postural and may have a kinetic component (Sejvar et al., 2003a; Burton et al., 2004; Emig and Apple, 2004; Sayao et al., 2004). Myoclonus, predominantly of the upper extremities and facial muscles, may occur and also may have a kinesigenic component. Features of parkinsonism, including hypomimia, bradykinesia, and postural instability, may be seen and can be associated with falls and functional difficulties (Robinson et al., 2003; Sejvar et al., 2003a). Similar to other causes of parkinsonism, a resting tremor is frequently absent. Cerebellar ataxia, with associated truncal instability and gait disturbance leading to falls, has been described (Kanagarajan et al., 2003; Burton et al., 2004; Sayao et al., 2004). Opsoclonus–myoclonis has been reported (Khosla, 2004; Sayao et al., 2004). These abnormal movements usually follow the onset of mental status changes and typically resolve over time; however, primary tremor and parkinsonism may persist in patients recovering from severe encephalitis (Pepperell et al., 2003; Sejvar et al., 2003a). Seizures are uncommon in patients with WNV encephalitis.

The development of these movement disorders is due to specific neurotropism of WNV for regions of the brain involved with control of movement. At a cellular level, it appears that WN virus has a predilection for neurons in the CNS (Doron et al., 2003) with the most consistent involvement appearing in the brain stem (particularly the medulla and pons), the deep gray nuclei, particularly the substantia nigra of the basal ganglia and the thalami, and the cerebellum (Bosanko et al., 2003; Kelley et al., 2003; Guarner et al., 2004). This clinico-pathologic correlation may be extended to the neuroimaging findings in WNV encephalitis.

Few data exist regarding the long-term neurologic and functional outcomes of WNV encephalitis. As with many other viral encephalitides, initial severe neurologic illness does not necessarily correlate with eventual outcome, and some patients with initial severe encephalopathy with associated coma may experience dramatic recovery and minimal sequelae (Sejvar et al., 2003a). However, others experience persistent neurologic dysfunction, including persistent movement disorders, headaches, fatigue, and cognitive complaints. Large hospital-based series suggest that patients with severe WNV encephalitis frequently require assistance with daily activities after acute-care discharge (Pepperell et al., 2003; Emig and Apple, 2004). Patients may frequently self-report substantial functional and cognitive difficulties up to a year after acute infection, and only 37% of patients in the 1999 New York City outbreak achieved full recovery at 1 year (Klee et al., 2004). Cognitive disturbances after WNV encephalitis have not been well characterized; however, difficulties with attention and concentration as well as neuropsychiatric problems including apathy and depression have been described (Sejvar et al., 2003a; Klee et al., 2004).

Fatality rates range from 10% to 20% among patients with severe neuroinvasive disease (Pepperell et al., 2003; O'Leary et al., 2004), and mortality is higher among the elderly and those with immunocompromising conditions. A small patient series suggested that lymphopenia may predict poor clinical outcome (Cunha et al., 2004).

1.3.2.3. Weakness and Paralysis

Acute weakness has been described as a feature of WNV infection since the 1950s (Southam and Moore, 1954) and has been variably attributed to myelitis, Guillain–Barré syndrome, or radiculopathy (Gadoth et al., 1979; Ahmed et al., 2000; Park et al., 2003). However, recent data indicate most cases of paralysis from WNV infection result from viral involvement of and damage to the lower motor neurons of the spinal cord (anterior horn cells), resulting in poliomyelitis (Glass et al., 2002; Leis et al., 2002; Jeha et al., 2003; Li et al., 2003; Sejvar et al., 2003b; Burton et al., 2004; Fratkin et al., 2004; Heresi et al., 2004), a syndrome more typically associated with poliovirus infection (Sejvar, 2004). WNV poliomyelitis frequently has clinical features that help to differentiate it from other acute, infectious causes of weakness (Table 1.4). WNV poliomyelitis generally develops soon after illness onset, usually within the first 24 to 48 hours. Limb paralysis generally develops rapidly and may be abrupt, occasionally raising clinical concern for stroke (Berner et al., 2002; Kulstad and Wichter, 2003). The weakness is usually asymmetric and often results in monoplegia. Patients with severe and extensive spinal cord involvement will develop a more symmetric dense quadriplegia. Central facial weakness, frequently bilateral, can also be seen (Jeha et al., 2003). While sensory loss or numbness is generally absent, patients will often experience intense pain in the affected limbs just before or during the onset of weakness.

Diffuse involvement by WNV of the lower brain stem, including the motor nuclei of the vagus and glossopharyngeal nerves, and high cervical spinal cord may result in diaphragmatic and intercostal muscle paralysis and subsequent neuromuscular respiratory failure requiring emergent endotracheal intubation (Doron et al., 2003; Betensley et al., 2004). Respiratory involvement in WNV poliomyelitis is associated with high morbidity and mortality, and among survivors, prolonged ventilatory support may be required (Betensley et al., 2004; Fan et al., 2004; Marciniak et al., 2004). Inability to wean off ventilatory support, and withdrawal of this support, may be a frequent cause of death among persons with respiratory involvement. Patients developing early dysarthria and dysphagia are at greater risk for subsequent respiratory failure, and patients with early bulbar findings in the setting of suspected WNV infection should be monitored closely.

WNV infection may cause other forms of acute weakness, including brachial plexopathy (Almhanna et al., 2003) as well as radiculopathy and a predominantly demyelinating peripheral neuropathy similar to Guillain–Barré syndrome (Ahmed et al., 2000; Park et al., 2003), but these are infrequent and may be recognized by their clinical and electrophysiologic features (Table 1.4). The weakness associated with the Guillain–Barré-like syndrome is usually symmetric and ascending in nature and is associated with sensory and autonomic dysfunction. Additionally, cerebrospinal fluid examination will generally show cytoalbuminologic dissociation (elevated protein in the absence of pleocytosis), and electodiagnostics will be consistent with a predominantly demyelinating polyneuropathy.

The long-term functional outcome in patients with WNV poliomyelitis has not yet been characterized; however, preliminary data indicate generally incomplete recovery of limb strength resulting in profound residual deficits

Table 1.4. Comparison of clinical characteristics in patients with various forms of acute weakness; West Nile poliomyelitis, Guillain–Barré syndrome, West Nile virus–associated fatigue, acute stroke, and myopathy

Characteristic	West Nile poliomyelitis	Guillain–Barré syndrome	West Nile virus–associated fatigue	Stroke	Acute myopathy
Timing of onset	Acute phase of infection; sudden onset	One to 4 weeks after acute infection; gradual progression	Acute phase of infection	Abrupt, sudden onset	Generally subacute and progressive
Fever and leukocytosis	Present	Generally absent	Present	Absent	Generally absent
Weakness distribution	Asymmetric; occasional monoplegia	Generally symmetric; ascending distally to proximally	Generalized; subjective, but neurologic examination normal	Asymmetric or focal; may result in hemiplegia; other concurrent neurologic signs	Proximal weakness greater than distal, generally symmetric
Sensory symptoms	Absence of numbness, paresthesias, or sensory loss; pain often present in affected limbs	Painful distal paresthesias and sensory loss	Generally absent	Present or absent, depending on localization	Generally absent
Bowel/bladder involvement	Often present	May be present	Absent	Absent	Absent
Concurrent encephalopathy	Often present	Generally absent	May be seen with fever, meningitis, or encephalitis	Generally absent	Absent
CSF profile	Pleocytosis and elevated protein	Absence of pleocytosis; elevated protein (albuminocytologic dissociation)	Pleocytosis and elevated protein in the setting of meningitis/encephalitis	Generally normal (increased red blood cells in hemorrhagic stroke)	Generally normal
Electrodiagnostics	Reduction of compound muscle action potentials; preservation of sensory action potentials	Conduction block, prolonged F-wave latencies; decreased motor unit recruitment	Normal studies	Normal studies	Reduced amplitude and duration of motor unit potentials; early recruitment

(Burton et al., 2004; Marciniak et al., 2004). However, some persons experience total or near-total recovery of strength, particularly among those with milder initial weakness. Electrodiagnostic determinants of prognosis and outcome are currently unknown. Quadriplegia and respiratory failure are associated with high morbidity and mortality, and recovery is slow and almost invariably incomplete (Betensley et al., 2004).

1.3.3. Other Clinical Manifestations

Although the severe manifestations of WNV infection generally result from central nervous system involvement, other non-neurological manifestations have been increasingly recognized. However, these manifestations have been mostly described in case reports or small case series, and a definitive causal relationship with WNV infection is less substantiated.

1.3.3.1. Ocular Manifestations

Ocular manifestations, including chorioretinitis and vitritis, are commonly reported (Adelman et al., 2003; Bains et al., 2003; Hershberger et al., 2003; Kuchtey et al., 2003; Vandenbelt et al., 2003; Shaikh and Trese, 2004). The chorioretinal lesions have been described as multifocal and with a "target-like" appearance (Adelman et al., 2003); retinal hemorrhages have also been noted. Lesions tend to be clustered primarily in the temporal and nasal regions of the periphery of the fundus. An inflammatory vitritis has occurred concomitantly with the chorioretinitis and may be significant enough to obscure the optic disk. Symptomatic persons describe gradual visual blurring and loss, floaters, and flashes. Although experience with management is limited, improvement both in symptoms and in underlying chorioretinal lesions has been observed after treatment with intraocular corticosteroids (Adelman et al., 2003). Retinal occlusive vasculitis without chorioretinal findings (Kaiser et al., 2003), anterior uveitis (Kuchtey et al., 2003), and optic neuritis (Vaispapir et al., 2002; Anninger et al., 2003; Gilad et al., 2003; Anninger and Lubow, 2004) have been noted.

A prospective study of ocular changes among consecutively enrolled patients presenting to a hospital with WNV infection during an outbreak in Tunisia indicated that 80% had multifocal chorioretinitis with mild vitreous inflammatory reaction on presentation or during follow-up (Khairallah et al., 2004). Other common findings included intraretinal hemorrhages in 72%, white-centered retinal hemorrhages in 24%, focal retinal vascular sheathing in 10%, and retinal vascular leakage in 17%. Most patients were asymptomatic, and symptoms were self-limited.

1.3.3.2. Miscellaneous Manifestations

Rhabdomyolysis, suggesting a viral myositis, has been reported during WNV infection (Jeha et al., 2003; Kulstad and Wichter, 2003). Presence of WNV in skeletal muscle has been noted (Southam and Moore, 1954). Hepatitis and pancreatitis have been reported (Perelman and Stern, 1974; Doron et al., 2003; Yim et al., 2004), and WNV has been identified in hepatic and pancreatic specimens at pathology, suggesting that viscerotropic WNV disease may occur (Southam and Moore, 1954). Myocarditis has been seen pathologically in WNV infection (Sampson et al., 2000), but clinical correlation with cardiac dysfunction in humans remains to be demonstrated. One case of stiff-person syndrome, a rare autoimmune disorder associated with antibodies against glutamic acid decarboxylase, has been reported after WNV infection (Hassin-Baer et al., 2004). One person with central diabetes insipidus compli-cating WNV encephalitis has been reported (Sherman-Weber and Axelrod, 2004).

1.3.4. Clinical Illness in Special Population Groups

1.3.4.1. Children

The incidence of symptomatic WNV infection is lower in children than in adults. Of more than 9000 cases of WNV infection reported nationally during the 2003 epidemic, less than 6% were in persons aged 19 years (Hayes and O'Leary, 2004). Most cases of pediatric WNV illness are WN fever, and neuroinvasive disease, when it occurs, is predomi-nantly meningitis (Hayes and O'Leary, 2004). It is unknown whether the neurological features and clinical outcome of neuroinvasive disease in children is similar to that of adults. Poliomyelitis (Vidwan et al., 2003; Heresi et al., 2004), fatal encephalitis (Carey et al., 1968), rhomboen-cephalitis (Nichter et al., 2000), and hepatitis (Yim et al., 2004) have been described in children with WNV infection. Similar to adults, children with immunocompromised status may be more susceptible to more severe illness (Ravindra et al., 2004).

1.3.4.2. Immunocompromised Patients

The incubation period may be prolonged in immunocompromised patients. The incubation period ranged from 7 to 17 days among four recipients of WNV-infected organs (Iwamoto et al., 2003). Organ transplant recipients who later received WNV infected blood transfusions had a median 13.5-day incubation period, compared with a median 8-day incubation period among recipients of WNV-infected blood transfusions who did not have obvious immunocompromising conditions (Pealer et al., 2003).

Information about the clinical spectrum of WNV infection in immunocompromised patients is derived from case reports or small case series and, thus, is potentially biased toward more severe illness. Nevertheless, the largest case series to date (11 transplant patients) indicated that the clinical findings were similar to those of non-immunocompromised patients but at the severe end of the spectrum of severity (Kleinschmidt-DeMasters et al., 2004).

1.4. Diagnosis

WNV disease diagnosis is based on identification either of antiviral IgM or IgG antibodies in serum or cerebrospinal fluid or of infectious virus or viral RNA from tissue specimens. The standard assays used to detect antiviral antibody are the IgM-capture enzyme-linked immunosorbent assay (MAC-ELISA), the indirect IgG ELISA, and the plaque-reduction neutralization test (PRNT) (Johnson et al., 2000; Martin et al., 2000, 2002). Viruses isolated in a variety of mammalian or invertebrate cells can be identified with virus-specific or cross-reactive monoclonal antibodies (Mabs), Mab-based antigen capture assays, or with a variety of nucleic acid detection polymerase chain reaction (PCR) assays (Tsai et al., 1987; Tsai et al., 1988; Lanciotti et al., 2000; Lanciotti and Kerst, 2001; Hunt et al., 2002). Whereas the PCR assays are amenable to automation and detection of multiple viruses, the serological assays have yet to be multiplexed and automated. In addition, ELISA has the requirement of species-specific capture or detector antibodies. The introduction of WNV into North America has reemphasized the need for assays capable of rapidly detecting antibodies to many viruses in many species (Gubler et al., 2000; Petersen and Roehrig, 2001; Gubler, 2002; Roehrig et al., 2002). To circumvent the need for many species-specific capture antibodies for detecting anti-WNV antibodies in animal species, a blocking ELISA has been designed and employed (Blitvich et al., 2003a; Blitvich et al., 2003c).

1.4.1. Antibody Detection

1.4.1.1. IgM ELISA

Assays that detect virus-elicited immunoglobulin M (IgM) are useful because they detect antibodies produced within days of a primary viral infection. IgM antibody capture enzyme-linked immunosorbent assay (MAC-ELISA) is the preferred approach to IgM detection because it is simple, sensitive, and applicable to serum and cerebrospinal fluid (CSF) samples. Whereas most ELISAs are based on a 96-well microplate format, assays are being developed and adapted to microsphere-based systems (Wong et al., 2003, 2004).

Approximately 75% of patients with WNV encephalitis have detectable IgM in serum or CSF in the first 4 days of illness, and nearly 100% are reactive by 7 days. The timing of development of IgM antibody in patients presenting with WN fever has not been well documented. Patients with immunocompromising conditions may have delayed or absent development of IgM antibody (Fan et al., 2004; Guarner et al., 2004). Although levels of IgM antibodies generally decline after 2 to 4 weeks and are absent after 90 to 120 days, IgM persists in serum for a year or more after infection in some patients with neuroinvasive disease (Roehrig et al., 2003). Detectable IgM antibody has also been shown to persist in CSF for at least 199 days in some patients (Hassin-Baer et al., 2004; Kapoor et al., 2004).

Whereas cross-reactivity of WNV and SLEV antibodies is a potential problem for interpretation of serological test results, studies have shown that the WNV MAC-ELISA has high predictive value for diagnosis of primary WNV infection in humans (Martin et al., 2002, 2004).

1.4.1.2. IgG ELISA

IgG ELISA has replaced the hemagglutination-inhibition (HI) test for the diagnosis of WNV infections. The sensitivities of IgG ELISAs generally are similar to or greater than those of HI tests, and their specificities correspondingly are equal or lower. The IgG ELISA has limited utility in diagnosis of acute human infections.

1.4.1.3. Neutralization Test

The serum neutralization test is the most virus-specific test for serologic diagnosis and is used confirm other serologic testing results. The serum dilution-plaque reduction neutralization test (PRNT) performed in cell culture is the standard method. Neutralizing-antibody levels generally rise within days of the onset of illness, peak in the second week, and decline slowly to moderate or low levels, where they persist for years and often a lifetime. The sensitivity of the test is high, but most importantly, no other approach is as virus-specific.

1.4.2. Antigen Detection

1.4.2.1. Antigen-Capture ELISA

Antigen-capture ELISA has been used to directly detect antigens of WNV in environmental specimens (Hunt et al., 2002). Generally, an overnight incubation of antigen maximizes sensitivity, which approaches 10^3 plaque-forming units (PFU)/0.1 ml. Antigen-capture ELISA also has proved useful in epidemiologic surveillance of arbovirus infection rates in vector mosquitoes. A single infected mosquito in a pool can be detected rapidly and cheaply by the direct detection of antigen, allowing greater flexibility and time to implement emergency vector control measures. For WNV, the antigen-capture technique has been successfully converted to a dipstick format (Nasci et al., 2003; Ryan et al., 2003).

1.4.2.2. Immunohistochemical Staining

Certain arbovirus infections can be rapidly diagnosed by directly detecting virus-infected cells by immunofluorescence (IF) or other histochemical techniques. Immunohistochemical staining was useful in the diagnosis of the first human cases of WNV in New York City in 1999 as well as in other unusual circumstances when tissue samples were available (Shieh et al., 2000; Iwamoto et al., 2003; Cushing et al., 2004).

1.4.3. Detection of Viral Genomic Sequences

1.4.3.1. Nucleic Acid Amplification Test (NAAT)

Several nucleic acid amplification platforms have been successfully utilized for the detection of arboviruses, including standard reverse transcriptase (RT)-PCR (with agarose gel analysis), real-time RT-PCR using fluorescent probes, nucleic acid sequence–based amplification (NASBA), and transcription-mediated amplification (TMA) (Giachetti et al., 2002). These techniques have recently been reviewed (Lanciotti, 2003). In general, the NAAT assays have a sensitivity in identifying arboviruses equal to or greater than the most sensitive viral isolation procedures while providing equal specificity in identifying specific viruses. The dynamics of *in vivo* viral replication and tissue tropisms must be carefully considered so that the utility of a NAAT assay to a particular arbovirus can be properly applied and interpreted.

WNV produces a short viremia that is low or absent at the time of clinical presentation of CNS symptoms. For clinical diagnosis, detection of virus in serum by NAAT or other methods has low sensitivity, and a negative result is not informative. Detection of virus nucleic acid in CSF of patients with encephalitis or meningitis often has higher sensitivity than detection in serum. In one study of patients with WNV encephalitis, virus was detected by a real-time RT-PCR in 14% of acute serum specimens and 57% of CSF specimens (Lanciotti et al., 2000).

The use of NAAT assays for the detection of arboviruses in environmental surveillance protocols is highly successful, particularly testing of field-collected mosquitoes. In this application, NAAT has often demonstrated superior sensitivity when compared with virus isolation or antigen detection assays. With the addition of automation, these NAAT approaches have been used to test hundreds of mosquito specimens in a single day (Shi et al., 2001). NAAT assays have also been successfully utilized in environmental surveillance by detecting arboviruses from tissues obtained from field-collected vertebrate hosts.

1.4.3.1.1. Reverse Transcriptase–Polymerase Chain Reaction (RT-PCR). Standard RT-PCR–based assays (as compared with real-time assays described below) to detect arbovirus genomic sequences have been developed for a number of agents (Kuno, 1998). These assays use either virus-specific primers or consensus primers that are designed to amplify genetically related viruses that detect RT-PCR product by agarose gel electrophoresis and staining with ethidium bromide. It is important to note that nonspecific amplification occasionally can generate DNA products with similar or identical mobility, which would lead to a false-positive interpretation of results. Greater specificity can be achieved by using sequence-specific approaches for detecting and confirming the identity of the amplified DNA. When consensus primers are utilized, a sequence-specific detection method such as one of those described above must be employed to specifically identify the resulting DNA, because by the design of the assay all related viruses would all be amplified. A consensus RT-PCR assay has been described for flaviviruses (Scaramozzino et al., 2001).

1.4.3.1.2. Real-time 5′ Exonuclease Fluorogenic Assays (TaqMan). TaqMan RT-PCR assays combine RT-PCR amplification with fluorescent-labeled virus-specific probes able to detect amplified DNA during the amplification reaction. These assays offer numerous advantages over standard RT-PCR; namely, increased sensitivity and specificity, quantitation of initial target RNA, high throughput, and rapid turnaround of results. The increased specificity of the TaqMan assay compared with standard RT-PCR is due to the use of the virus-specific internal probe during the amplification. A variety of TaqMan assays for the detection of WNV have been developed (Briese et al., 2000; Lanciotti et al., 2000).

1.4.3.1.3. Nucleic Acid Sequence–based Amplification (NASBA). Another
amplification technology that has successfully been used for the detection and identification of WNV is NASBA (Lanciotti and Kerst, 2001).
This approach shares some similarities with RT-PCR at the initial
stages; however, the final amplification product is single-stranded
RNA. Amplified RNA can be detected in a sequence-specific manner
either by utilizing an electrochemiluminescence (ECL) probe detection format or in real time using a fluorescent-labeled molecular beacon probe.

1.4.4. Other Laboratory, Radiologic, and Electrodiagnositic Findings

Total leukocyte counts in peripheral blood are usually normal or elevated (Asnis et al., 2001; Chowers et al., 2001; Sejvar et al., 2003a).
Lymphopenia can be observed in patients with WNV neuroinvasive disease (Chowers et al., 2001), and one small case series suggested that the
degree of lymphopenia may have prognostic importance (Cunha et al.,
2004). Anemia and thrombocytopenia have also been noted in some
patients (Chowers et al., 2001). In persons with WNV neuroinvasive disease, CSF examination is generally characterized by elevated protein and
a modest pleocytosis (Chowers et al., 2001; Pepperell et al., 2003; Burton
et al., 2004; Sayao et al., 2004). Although this pleocytosis is generally
lymphocytic, CSF obtained soon after symptom onset may show a neutrophilic predominance (Pepperell et al., 2003; Crichlow et al., 2004; Fan
et al., 2004; Sayao et al., 2004). The presence of plasma cells in CSF may
suggest WNV infection (Carson et al., 2003). Mollaret-like cells have also
been observed in the CSF of patients with WNV encephalitis (Procop
et al., 2004).

Computed tomography (CT) of the brain in WNV encephalitis is
generally normal and not helpful in diagnosis, except to exclude other
etiologies of encephalopathy (Chowers et al., 2001; Nash et al., 2001;
Weiss et al., 2001; Pepperell et al., 2003). Magnetic resonance imaging
(MRI) may frequently be normal, even in severe encephalitis (Brilla
et al., 2004). In approximately one-third of patients, magnetic resonance
(MR) imaging shows enhancement of the leptomeninges, the periventricular areas, or both. Hyperintensity on T2-weighed MR images may
be seen in regions such as the basal ganglia, thalami, caudate nuclei,
brain stem, and spinal cord (Fig. 1.4) (Rosas and Wippold, 2003; Al-
Shekhlee and Katirji, 2004; Gea-Banacloche et al., 2004). Cerebellar
lesions are sometimes also seen (Agid et al., 2003; Rosas and Wippold,
2003; Sejvar et al., 2003a; Brilla et al., 2004). An initially normal MR

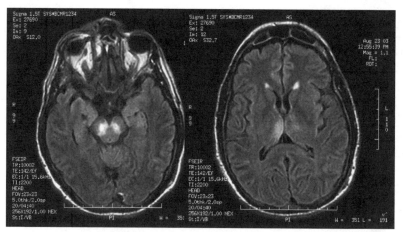

Figure 1.4. Fluid-attenuated inversion recovery magnetic resonance imaging sequence of the brain in a patient with West Nile virus encephalitis with associated parkinsonism and tremor, displaying signal abnormality in the substantia nigra, the mesial temporal lobe, and the right posterior thalamus.

can evolve to show evidence of deep gray matter involvement (Gea-Banacloche et al., 2004).

Electroencephalography in patients with meningitis or encephalitis generally shows generalized, continuous slowing, which is more prominent in the frontal or temporal regions (Gandelman-Marton et al., 2003). One report suggests that an anterior predominance of slow waves may be characteristic of WNV (Brilla et al., 2004).

Patients with acute flaccid paralysis due to WNV poliomyelitis have electromyography/nerve conduction velocity studies (EMG/NCS) that display findings consistent with a motor axonopathy, with diminished compound muscle action potentials with little or no demyelinating changes and preservation of sensory nerve potentials (Leis et al., 2002; Pepperell et al., 2003; Al-Shekhlee and Katirji, 2004; Marciniak et al., 2004). Spinal magnetic resonance imaging may show signal abnormalities in the anterior spinal cord (Heresi et al., 2004), consistent with anterior horn cell damage; ventral nerve root enhancement may be seen as well.

1.5. Management

Patients with otherwise uncomplicated WN fever generally do not require specific intervention. Patients with severe WNV meningitis may require pain control for severe headache, and rehydration may be required if associated nausea and vomiting are severe. Patients with WNV encephalitis require assessment of level of consciousness, and airway protection is important if severe obtundation develops. Controlled clinical trials have not assessed the benefits of antiepileptic medications, hyperosmotics, or steroids in cases where seizures and increased intracranial pressure are present.

In persons developing acute asymmetric paralysis, CSF evaluation and electrodiagnostic studies should be conducted. Patients with WNV virus infection who develop early dysarthria and dysphagia are at higher risk for subsequent acute respiratory failure; for this reason, hospitalization and monitoring is advised. Experience with the management of WNV poliomyelitis is limited; however, initiation of aggressive physical activity during the acute febrile period of illness due to poliovirus infection has historically been associated with more profound and persistent weakness (Guyton, 1949), and without additional data, aggressive physical activity during the acute febrile illness or during the initial 48–72 hours of weakness in WNV poliomyelitis is not advised.

There are no specific, proven treatments for WNV infection. The fact that WN viremia in humans is short-lived and is usually cleared by the time of clinical presentation presents a substantial theoretical obstacle for specific antiviral therapies. However, studies in monkeys and humans indicate that WNV may persist in the CNS or other organs for prolonged periods (Southam and Moore, 1954; Pogodina et al., 1983). The variability in clinical outcome of WNV infection complicates interpretation of nonrandomized clinical trials.

The antiviral agent ribavirin has had demonstrated *in vitro* activity against WNV infection (Jordan et al., 2000; Anderson and Rahal, 2002), but therapeutic efficacy has not yet been demonstrated in animal models. Ribavirin was used in an uncontrolled, nonblinded fashion in patients with WNV neuroinvasive disease in Israel in 2000, where it was found to be ineffective and potentially detrimental (Chowers et al., 2001). Ribavirin increased mortality in Syrian golden hamsters when administered 2 days after WNV inoculation (Morrey et al., 2004).

Interferon reduced viremia and slightly impoved mortality in Syrian golden hamsters when administered 2 days after WNV inoculation and before development of symptoms (Morrey et al., 2004). No synergistic effect was noted with coadministration of ribavirin. Placebo-controlled trials of interferon-α-2a in the treatment of the closely related flavivirus, JEV, failed to demonstrate a beneficial effect (Solomon et al., 2003). Case reports of patients with WNV encephalitis have suggested a possible clinical benefit of interferon α-2b (Sayao et al., 2004; Kalil et al., 2005). Nevertheless, two patients receiving interferon α-2b and ribavirin for hepatitis C infection developed WN fever after mosquito exposure (Hrnicek and Mailliard, 2004).

Animal models have suggested the efficacy of high-titer WNV-specific intravenous immune globulin (IVIG), particularly when administered before or shortly after WNV challenge (Camenga et al., 1974; Shimoni et al., 2001; Tesh et al., 2002; Agrawal and Petersen, 2003; Ben-Nathan et al., 2003; Diamond et al., 2003). Several patients with underlying immunodeficiencies who have been treated with IVIG have been reported with variable outcome (Shimoni et al., 2001; Hamdan et al., 2002; Haley et al., 2003).

Controlled trials of third-generation anti-sense compounds are underway. The use of angiotensin-receptor blockers in the United States as definitive therapy for WNV infection has not been assessed in a controlled fashion. Improvement in clinical condition after administration of high-dose steroids was noted in one patient with encephalitis and acute flaccid paraysis (Pyrgos and Younus, 2004).

1.6. Prevention

1.6.1. Human Personal Protection

Avoidance of mosquito exposure by using repellants is a mainstay of prevention. However, evaluation of the effectiveness of repellents in community settings has been complicated by difficulties in quantifying mosquito exposure in relation to repellant use. Repellents using DEET (*N,N*-diethyl-meta-toluamide or *N,N*-diethyl-3-methylbenzamide) have been used by the general public in the United States since 1957. DEET is available in many products, and its duration of mosquito repellent action relates to its concentration, with concentrations above 50% providing no added benefit (Buescher et al., 1983). DEET has an outstanding safety profile, and most data relating to its toxic effects relate to inappropriate use, such as ingestion of the chemical (Fradin, 1998). DEET has proved to be safe in children (Bell et al., 2002) and pregnant women (McGready et al., 2001).

Other repellents available in the United States, such as picaridin (1-methyl-propyl 2-[2-hydroxyethyl]-1-piperidinecarboxylate), oil of lemon eucalyptus (*p*-menthane-3,8-diol [PMD]), and a mixture of soybean oil and vanillin and other ingredients have efficacies similar to DEET (Frances et al., 2002; Barnard and Xue, 2004; Costantini et al., 2004; Frances et al., 2004). Many other products for use on skin are marketed but have shorter duration of action or lower efficacy (Fradin, 1998; Barnard and Xue, 2004). Permethrin is an effective repellent approved for use on clothing or fabrics but not on skin.

Other personal measures advocated to reduce mosquito bite exposure include avoidance of outdoor activities at dawn and dusk when mosquito activity is high and wearing protective clothing, including long sleeves and pants, during periods of likely mosquito exposure.

1.6.2. Mosquito Control

Reduction of vector populations by public mosquito control programs is another mainstay of WNV prevention in North America. These programs emphasize an integrated pest management approach, which combines surveillance, source reduction, larvicide (*Bacillus thuringiensis* var. *israelensis* [Bti], *Bacillus sphaericus* [Bs], methoprene), adulticide (organophosphates, pyrethroids), and other biological control, as well as public relations and education (Rose, 2001). Evaluation of these programs on reducing the incidence of human WNV infection is complicated by the focal and sporadic nature of epidemics.

Ultralow-volume application of adulticides is used during epidemics or when surveillance indicators suggest an impending epidemic; however, concern over environmental effects or adverse impact on public health makes their use controversial in many communities. Acute illness after application of adulticides is rare (CDC, 2003a; Karpati et al., 2004). Studies have shown that adulticide applications must cover a large geographic area and must involve multiple treatments, otherwise vector mosquito populations will quickly rebound (Mitchell et al., 1970; Reisen et al., 1984; Andis et al., 1987).

1.6.3. Vaccines

Two equine WNV vaccines have been licensed in the United States. A formalin-inactivated, whole-virus WNV vaccine licensed in the United States became available in 2001 and was fully licensed in 2003 (Hall and Khromykh, 2004). More recently, a recombinant canarypox virus vaccine expressing the prM/E proteins of a 1999 WNV isolate has been licensed (Minke et al., 2004; Siger et al., 2004). A DNA vaccine containing the preM/E genes of WNV has been shown to protect against mosquito-borne challenge of WNV in mice and horses (Davis et al., 2001).

The candidate human WNV vaccine furthest in development is a chimeric virus containing the nonstructural genes of the live attenuated YFV 17D vaccine virus backbone and the PrM/E genes of WNV (Arroyo et al., 2001; Monath, 2001; Arroyo et al., 2004). A candidate chimeric vaccine using an attenuated DENV-4 backbone has also been developed (Pletnev et al., 2002; Pletnev et al., 2003). Other vaccine strategies are under development but are likely years away from clinical practice.

Controversy exists whether vaccination with a related flavivirus can protect against WNV (Monath, 2002).

1.6.4. Screening of Blood Donations

Since 2003, all blood donations in the United States and Canada have been screened using WNV nucleic acid–amplification tests. These tests are conducted on minipools of samples from 6 or 16 blood donations, depending on the test format (CDC, 2004c). Screening identified more than 1000 viremic blood donors in the United States in 2003 and 2004 (Petersen and Hayes, 2004). However, at least seven IgM-negative blood donors with very low level viremias (0.06–0.5 PFU/ml) were not detected by minipool screening, which resulted in transfusion-associated WNV infection in recipients (CDC, 2004b, 2004c). For that reason, in 2004, blood centers implemented algorithms to switch to single-unit screening in areas experiencing outbreaks. The estimated effectiveness in eliminating the residual risk of transfusion transmission using various criteria to switch from minipool screening to single-unit testing ranged from 57% to 100% (Custer et al., 2004).

1.7. Future Directions

1.7.1. Surveillance

Dead bird surveillance currently forms the cornerstone of ecological surveillance because it has been shown to be a very sensitive indicator of WNV activity in an area. However, questions remain regarding the long-term sustainability and utility of dead bird surveillance. Dead bird reporting relies on public participation, which could wane in coming seasons as WNV becomes a routine summertime event. The system could also become less sensitive if susceptible bird populations dwindle. Dead bird reporting was invaluable for detecting the incursion of WNV into new areas; however, its continuing value in triggering public health response remains uncertain. Whereas the density of bird deaths may highlight areas of high human risk (Mostashari et al., 2003), monitoring the density of bird deaths may not prove practical or useful in many locations over a sustained time period. The long-term utility of other surveillance indicators, such as mosquito infection rates, sentinel chicken seroconversions, and viremic blood donors, for public health decision-making also requires evaluation. Equine surveillance will remain important for monitoring WNV vaccination efforts.

The apparent widespread distribution of WNV in Mexico, Central America, and the Caribbean as determined by serological studies in birds and horses contrasts with the paucity of widespread human or animal disease. Whether this discrepancy is due to cross-reactivity of other flaviviruses, lack of intensive surveillance, or some other biological reason is an important public health question. Intensive surveillance of dead birds, sick equines, and humans with WNV-compatible neuroinvasive disease in sentinel locations in Latin America will provide direct evidence for the virus' presence and will help to monitor its impact on health.

1.7.2. Diagnosis and Treatment

The presence of multiple flaviviruses such as dengue, yellow fever, and rocio will invariably complicate serological diagnosis in Latin America. Development of flavivirus-specific antigens that can be used in serologic tests is urgently needed.

Controlled clinical trials to evaluate new therapies and vaccines are needed. However, the fact that WNV has highly variable incidence, is geographically dispersed and sporadic, and often affects rural or suburban areas makes the traditional paradigm of conducting clinical trials in established urban academic clinical centers ineffective and expensive. New procedures, where clinical trials could be rapidly implemented in rural or suburban hospitals in epidemic areas, would greatly enhance our ability to conduct clinical trials for WNV and other emerging infections.

1.7.3. Prevention

A significant challenge will be to maintain public support for sustainable mosquito-control programs given the highly sporadic and focal nature of WNV epidemics. Because controlled community trials of mosquito-control interventions are extremely difficult to conduct, a concerted long-term effort is required to evaluate the efficacy of various mosquito-control efforts, as has been done for SLEV in the United States.

Development and evaluation of behavioral intervention programs to increasing use of personal protective measures, such as the use of insect repellents, to reduce WNV risk is imperative. These programs must go beyond education, as surveys indicate that knowledge of WNV may not translate into behavioral change, particularly in areas where mosquitoes are not thought to be a problem (McCarthy et al., 2001).

It is likely that an effective WNV vaccine for humans can be developed. However, the eventual commercial viability of such a vaccine remains unclear as the eventual public health need, and cost–benefit, of such a vaccine cannot yet be determined. Although the future incidence of WNV infection cannot be determined, studies of the estimated cost-effectiveness of a vaccine may help determine if such a substantial investment in developing a vaccine is likely to be returned.

References

Adelman, R. A., Membreno, J. H., Afshari, N. A. and Stoessel, K. M. (2003). West Nile virus chorioretinitis. *Retina* 23(1): 100–1.

Agid, R., Ducreux, D., Halliday, W. C., Kucharczyk, W., terBrugge, K. G. and Mikulis, D. J. (2003). MR diffusion-weighted imaging in a case of West Nile virus encephalitis. *Neurology* 61(12): 1821–3.

Agrawal, A. G. and Petersen, L. R. (2003). Human immunoglobulin as a treatment for West Nile virus infection. [comment] *J Infect Dis* 188(1): 1–4.

Ahmed, S., Libman, R., Wesson, K., Ahmed, F. and Einberg, K. (2000). Guillain-Barre syndrome: An unusual presentation of West Nile virus infection. *Neurology* 55(1): 144–6.

Allison, S. L., Schalich, J., Stiasny, K., Mandl, C. W. and Heinz, F. X. (2001). Mutational evidence for an internal fusion peptide in flavivirus envelope protein E. *J Virol* 75(9): 4268–75.

Almhanna, K., Palanichamy, N., Sharma, M., Hobbs, R. and Sil, A. (2003). Unilateral brachial plexopathy associated with West Nile virus meningoencephalitis. *Clin Infect Dis* 36(12): 1629–30.

Alonto, A. M., Aronoff, D. M. and Malani, P. N. (2003). West Nile virus meningitis in patient with common variable immunodeficiency. *Emerg Infect Dis* 9(10): 1353–4.

Alpert, S. G., Fergerson, J. and Noel, L. P. (2003). Intrauterine West Nile virus: Ocular and systemic findings. *Am J Ophthalmol* 136(4): 733–5.

Al-Shekhlee, A. and Katirji, B. (2004). Electrodiagnostic features of acute paralytic poliomyelitis associated with West Nile virus infection. *Muscle Nerve* 29(3): 376–80.

Anderson, J. F. and Rahal, J. J. (2002). Efficacy of interferon alpha-2b and ribavirin against West Nile virus in vitro. *Emerg Infect Dis* 8(1): 107–8.

Anderson, R. C., Horn, K. B., Hoang, M. P., Gottlieb, E. and Bennin, B. (2004). Punctate exanthem of West Nile Virus infection: Report of 3 cases. *J Am Acad Dermatol* 51(5): 820–3.

Andis, M. D., Sackett, S. R., Carroll, M. K. and Bordes, E. S. (1987). Strategies for the emergency control of arboviral epidemics in New Orleans. *J Am Mosq Control Assoc* 3(2): 125–30.

Anninger, W. and Lubow, M. (2004). Visual loss with West Nile virus infection: A wider spectrum of a "new" disease. *Clin Infect Dis* 38(7): e55–6.

Anninger, W. V., Lomeo, M. D., Dingle, J., Epstein, A. D. and Lubow, M. (2003). West Nile virus–associated optic neuritis and chorioretinitis. *Am J Ophthalmol* 136(6): 1183–5.

Armali, Z., Ramadan, R., Chlebowski, A. and Azzam, Z. S. (2003). West Nile meningo–encephalitis infection in a kidney transplant recipient. *Transplant Proc* 35(8): 2935–6.

Arroyo, J., Miller, C., Catalan, J., Myers, G. A., Ratterree, M. S., Trent, D. W. and Monath, T. P. (2004). ChimeriVax-West Nile virus live-attenuated vaccine: Preclinical evaluation of safety, immunogenicity, and efficacy. *J Virol* 78(22): 12497–507.

Arroyo, J., Miller, C. A., Catalan, J. and Monath, T. P. (2001). Yellow fever vector live-virus vaccines: West Nile virus vaccine development. *Trends Mol Med* 7(8): 350–4.

Asnis, D. S., Conetta, R., Waldman, G. and Teixeira, A. A. (2001). The West Nile virus encephalitis outbreak in the United States (1999–2000): From Flushing, New York, to beyond its borders. *Ann N Y Acad Sci* 951: 161–71.

Bains, H. S., Jampol, L. M., Caughron, M. C. and Parnell, J. R. (2003). Vitritis and chorioretinitis in a patient with West Nile virus infection. *Arch Ophthalmol* 121(2): 205–7.

Banet–Noach, C., Gantz, A. Y., Lublin, A. and Malkinson, M. (2004). A twelve-month study of West Nile virus antibodies in a resident and a migrant species of kestrels in Israel. *Vector Borne Zoonotic Dis* 4(1): 15–22.

Banet-Noach, C., Malkinson, M., Brill, A., Samina, I., Yadin, H., Weisman, Y., Pokamunski, S., King, R., Deubel, V. and Stram, Y. (2003). Phylogenetic relationships of West Nile viruses isolated from birds and horses in Israel from 1997 to 2001. *Virus Genes* 26(2): 135–41.

Baqar, S., Hayes, C. G., Murphy, J. R. and Watts, D. M. (1993). Vertical transmission of West Nile virus by Culex and Aedes species mosquitoes. *Am J Trop Med Hyg* 48(6): 757–62.

Barnard, D. R. and Xue, R. (2004). Laboratory evaluation of mosquito repellents against *Aedes albopictus, Culex nigripalpus,* and *Ochelerotatus triseriatus* (Diptera: Culicidae). *J Med Entomol* 41(4): 726–30.

Bartholomeusz, A. I. and Wright, J. C. (1993). Synthesis of dengue virus RNA in vitro: Initiation and the involvement of proteins NS3 and NS5. *Arch Virol* 279(1–2): 111–21.

Beasley, D. W. and Aaskov, J. G. (2001). Epitopes on the dengue 1 virus envelope protein recognized by neutralizing IgM monoclonal antibodies. *Virology* 279(2): 447–58.

Beasley, D. W., Davis, C. T., Estrada-Franco, J., Navarro-Lopez, R., Campomanes-Cortes, A., Tesh, R. B., Weaver, S. C. and Barrett, A. D. (2004). Genome sequence and attenuating mutations in West Nile virus isolate from Mexico. *Emerg Infect Dis* 10(12): 2221–4.

Beasley, D. W., Davis, C. T., Guzman, H., Vanlandingham, D. L., Travassos da Rosa, A. P., Parsons, R. E., Higgs, S., Tesh, R. B. and Barrett, A. D. (2003). Limited evolution of West Nile virus has occurred during its southwesterly spread in the United States. *Virology* 309(2): 190–5.

Bell, J. W., Veltri, J. C. and Page, B. C. (2002). Human Exposures to N,N-diethyl-m-toluamide insect repellents reported to the American Association of Poison Control Centers 1993–1997. *Int J Toxicol* 21(5): 341–52.

Ben-Nathan, D., Lustig, S., Tam, G., Robinzon, S., Segal, S. and Rager-Zisman, B. (2003). Prophylactic and therapeutic efficacy of human intravenous immunoglobulin in treating West Nile virus infection in mice. [see comment] *J Infect Dis* 188(1): 5–12.

Berner, Y. N., Lang, R. and Chowers, M. Y. (2002). Outcome of West Nile fever in older adults. *J Am Geriatr Soc* 50(11): 1844–6.

Betensley, A. D., Jaffery, S. H., Collins, H., Sripathi, N. and Alabi, F. (2004). Bilateral diaphragmatic paralysis and related respiratory complications in a patient with West Nile virus infection. *Thorax* 59(3): 268–9.

Biggerstaff, B. J. and Petersen, L. R. (2002). Estimated risk of West Nile virus transmission through blood transfusion during an epidemic in Queens, New York City. *Transfusion* 42(8): 1019–26.

Biggerstaff, B. J. and Petersen, L. R. (2003). Estimated risk of transmission of the West Nile virus through blood transfusion in the US, 2002. *Transfusion* 43(8): 1007–17.

Bin, H., Grossman, Z., Pokamunski, S., Malkinson, M., Weiss, L., Duvdevani, P., Banet, C., Weisman, Y., Annis, E., Gandaku, D., Yahalom, V., Hindyieh, M., Shulman, L. and Mendelson, E. (2001). West Nile fever in Israel 1999-2000: From geese to humans. *Ann N Y Acad Sci* 951: 127–42.

Blackmore, C. G., Stark, L. M., Jeter, W. C., Oliveri, R. L., Brooks, R. G., Conti, L. A. and Wiersma, S. T. (2003). Surveillance results from the first West Nile virus transmission season in Florida, 2001. *Am J Trop Med Hyg* 69(2): 141–50.

Blitvich, B. J., Bowen, R. A., Marlenee, N. L., Hall, R. A., Bunning, M. L. and Beaty, B. J. (2003a). Epitope-blocking enzyme-linked immunosorbent assays for detection of west nile virus antibodies in domestic mammals. *J Clin Microbiol* 41(6): 2676–9.

Blitvich, B. J., Fernandez-Salas, I., Contreras-Cordero, J. F., Lorono-Pino, M. A., Marlenee, N. L., Diaz, F. J., Gonzalez-Rojas, J. I., Obregon-Martinez, N., Chiu-Garcia, J. A., Black, W. C. t. and Beaty, B. J. (2004). Phylogenetic analysis of West Nile virus, Nuevo Leon State, Mexico. *Emerg Infect Dis* 10(7): 1314–7.

Blitvich, B. J., Fernandez-Salas, I., Contreras-Cordero, J. F., Marlenee, N. L., Gonzalez-Rojas, J. I., Komar, N., Gubler, D. J., Calisher, C. H. and Beaty, B. J. (2003b). Serologic evidence of West Nile virus infection in horses, Coahuila State, Mexico. *Emerg Infect Dis* 9(7): 853–6.

Blitvich, B. J., Marlenee, N. L., Hall, R. A., Calisher, C. H., Bowen, R. A., Roehrig, J. T., Komar, N., Langevin, S. A. and Beaty, B. J. (2003c). Epitope-blocking enzyme-linked immunosorbent assays for the detection of serum antibodies to west nile virus in multiple avian species. *J Clin Microbiol* 41(3): 1041–7.

Bosanko, C. M., Gilroy, J., Wang, A. M., Sanders, W., Dulai, M., Wilson, J. and Blum, K. (2003). West nile virus encephalitis involving the substantia nigra: Neuroimaging and pathologic findings with literature review. *Arch Neurol* 60(10): 1448–52.

Brault, A. C., Langevin, S. A., Bowen, R. A., Panella, N. A., Biggerstaff, B. J., Miller, B. R. and Komar, N. (2004). Differential virulence of West Nile strains for American crows. *Emerg Infect Dis* 10(12): 2161–8.

Briese, T., Glass, W. G. and Lipkin, W. I. (2000). Detection of West Nile virus sequences in cerebrospinal fluid. [see comment] *Lancet* 355(9215): 1614–5.

Briese, T., Jia, X. Y., Huang, C., Grady, L. J. and Lipkin, W. I. (1999). Identification of a Kunjin/West Nile-like flavivirus in brains of patients with New York encephalitis. *Lancet* 354(9186): 1261–2.

Brilla, R., Block, M., Geremia, G. and Wichter, M. (2004). Clinical and neuroradiologic features of 39 consecutive cases of West Nile Virus meningoencephalitis. *J Neurol Sci* 220(1–2): 37–40.

Buescher, M. D., Rutledge, L. C., Wirtz, R. A. and Nelson, J. H. (1983). The dose-persistence relationship of DEET against *Aedes aegypti*. *Mosq News* 43: 364–6.

Bugbee, L. M. and Forte, L. R. (2004). The discovery of West Nile virus in overwintering Culex pipiens (Diptera: Culicidae) mosquitoes in Lehigh County, Pennsylvania. *J Am Mosq Control Assoc* 20(3): 326–7.

Bunning, M. L., Bowen, R. A., Cropp, B., Sullivan, K., Davis, B., Komar, N., Godsey, M., Baker, D., Hettler, D., Holmes, D. and Mitchell, C. J. (2001). Experimental infection of horses with West Nile virus and their potential to infect mosquitoes and serve as amplifying hosts. *Ann N Y Acad Sci* 951: 338–9.

Bunning, M. L., Bowen, R. A., Cropp, C. B., Sullivan, K. G., Davis, B. S., Komar, N., Godsey, M. S., Baker, D., Hettler, D. L., Holmes, D. A., Biggerstaff, B. J. and Mitchell, C. J. (2002). Experimental infection of horses with West Nile virus. *Emerg Infect Dis* 8(4): 380–6.

Burton, J. M., Kern, R. Z., Halliday, W., Mikulis, D., Brunton, J., Fearon, M., Pepperell, C. and Jaigobin, C. (2004). Neurological manifestations of West Nile virus infection. *Can J Neurol Sci* 31(2): 185–93.

Butrapet, S., Kimura-Kuroda, J., Zhou, D. S. and Yasui, K. (1998). Neutralizing mechanism of a monoclonal antibody against Japanese encephalitis virus glycoprotein E. *Am J Trop Med Hyg* 58(4): 389–98.

Camenga, D. L., Nathanson, N. and Cole, G. A. (1974). Cyclophosphamide-potentiated West Nile viral encephalitis: Relative influence of cellular and humoral factors. *J Infect Dis* 130(6): 634–41.

Campbell, G. L., Marfin, A. A., Lanciotti, R. S. and Gubler, D. J. (2002). West Nile virus. *Lancet Infect Dis* 2(9): 519–29.

Cantile, C., Di Guardo, G., Eleni, C. and Arispici, M. (2000). Clinical and neuropathological features of West Nile virus equine encephalomyelitis in Italy. *Equine Vet J* 32(1): 31–5.

Carey, D. E., Rodrigues, F. M., Myers, R. M. and Webb, J. K. (1968). Arthropod-borne viral infections in children in Vellore, South India, with particular reference to dengue and West Nile viruses. *Indian Pediatrics* 5(7): 285–96.

Carson, P. J., Steidler, T., Patron, R., Tate, J. M., Tight, R. and Smego, R. A., Jr. (2003). Plasma cell pleocytosis in cerebrospinal fluid in patients with West Nile virus encephalitis. *Clin Infect Dis* 37(1): e12–5.

CDC (2000a). Update: Surveillance for West Nile virus in overwintering mosquitoes—New York, 2000. *MMWR Morb Mortal Wkly Rep* 49(9): 178–9.

CDC (2000b). Update: West Nile Virus activity—Eastern United States, 2000. *MMWR Morb Mortal Wkly Rep* 49(46): 1044–7.

CDC (2001). Serosurveys for West Nile virus infection—New York and Connecticut counties, 2000. *MMWR Morb Mortal Wkly Rep* 50(3): 37–9.

CDC (2002a). Intrauterine West Nile virus infection—New York, 2002. *MMWR Morb Mortal Wkly Rep* 51(50): 1135–6.

CDC (2002b). Laboratory-acquired West Nile virus infections—United States, 2002. *MMWR Morb Mortal Wkly Rep* 51(50): 1133–5.

CDC (2002c). Possible West Nile virus transmission to an infant through breast-feeding—Michigan, 2002. *MMWR Morb Mortal Wkly Rep* 51(39): 877–8.

CDC (2002d). Provisional surveillance summary of the West Nile virus epidemic—United States, January–November 2002. *MMWR Morb Mortal Wkly Rep* 51(50): 1129–33.

CDC (2002e). West Nile Virus activity—United States, 2001. *MMWR Morb Mortal Wkly Rep* 51(23): 497–501.

CDC (2003a). Surveillance for acute insecticide-related illness associated with mosquito-control efforts—nine states, 1999–2002. *MMWR Morb Mortal Wkly Rep* 52(27): 629–34.

CDC (2003b). West Nile virus infection among turkey breeder farm workers—Wisconsin, 2002. *MMWR Morb Mortal Wkly Rep* 52(42): 1017–9.

CDC (2004a). Possible dialysis-related west nile virus transmission—Georgia, 2003. *MMWR Morb Mortal Wkly Rep* 53(32): 738–9.

CDC (2004b). Transfusion-associated transmission of West Nile virus—Arizona, 2004. *MMWR Morbid Mortal Wkly Rep* 53(36): 842–4.

CDC (2004c). Update: West Nile virus screening of blood donations and transfusion-associated transmission—United States, 2003. *MMWR Morb Mortal Wkly Rep* 53(13): 281–4.

Cecilia, D. and Gould, E. A. (1991). Nucleotide changes responsible for loss of neuroinvasiveness in Japanese encephalitis virus neutralization-resistant mutants. *Virology* 181(1): 70–7.

Chambers, T. J., Hahn, C. S., Galler, R. and Rice, C. M. (1990). Flavivirus genome organization, expression, and replication. *Annu Rev Microbiol* 44: 649–88.

Chowers, M. Y., Lang, R., Nassar, F., Ben-David, D., Giladi, M., Rubinshtein, E., Itzhaki, A., Mishal, J., Siegman-Igra, Y., Kitzes, R., Pick, N., Landau, Z., Wolf, D., Bin, H., Mendelson, E., Pitlik, S. D. and Weinberger, M. (2001). Clinical characteristics of the West Nile fever outbreak, Israel, 2000. *Emerg Infect Dis* 7(4): 675–8.

Clum, S., Ebner, K. E. and Padmanabhan, R. (1997). Cotranslational membrane insertion of the serine proteinase precursor NS2B-NS3(Pro) of dengue virus type 2 is required for efficient in vitro processing and is mediated through the hydrophobic regions of NS2B. *J Biol Chem* 272(49): 30715–23.

Cornel, A. J., Jupp, P. G. and Blackburn, N. K. (1993). Environmental temperature on the vector competence of Culex univittatus (Diptera: Culicidae) for West Nile virus. *J Med Entomol* 30(2): 449–56.

Corver, J., Ortiz, A., Allison, S. L., Schalich, J., Heinz, F. X. and Wilschut, J. (2000). Membrane fusion activity of tick-borne encephalitis virus and recombinant subviral particles in a liposomal model system. *Virology* 269(1): 37–46.

Costantini, C., Badolo, A. and Ilboudo-Sanogo, E. (2004). Field evaluation of the efficacy and persistence of insect repellents DEET, IR3535, and KBR 3023 against Anopheles gambiae complex and other Afrotropical vector mosquitoes. *Trans R Soc Trop Med Hyg* 98: 644–52.

Creech, W. B. (1977). St. Louis encephalitis in the United States, 1975. *J Infect Dis* 135(6): 1014–6.

Crichlow, R., Bailey, J. and Gardner, C. (2004). Cerobrospinal fluid neutrophilic pleocytosis in hospitalized West Nile virus patients. *J Am Board Fam Pract* 17: 470–2.

Crill, W. D. and Chang, G. J. (2004). Localization and characterization of flavivirus envelope glycoprotein cross–reactive epitopes. *J Virol* 78(24): 13975–86.

Crill, W. D. and Roehrig, J. T. (2001). Monoclonal antibodies that bind to domain III of dengue virus E glycoprotein are the most efficient blockers of virus adsorption to Vero cells. *J Virol* 75(16): 7769–73.

Cunha, B. A., McDermott, B. P. and Mohan, S. S. (2004). Prognostic importance of lymphopenia in West Nile encephalitis. *Am J Med* 117(9): 710–1.

Cushing, M. M., Brat, D. J., Mosunjac, M. I., Hennigar, R. A., Jernigan, D. B., Lanciotti, R., Petersen, L. R., Goldsmith, C., Rollin, P. E., Shieh, W. J., Guarner, J. and Zaki, S. R. (2004). Fatal West Nile virus encephalitis in a renal transplant recipient. *Am J Clin Pathol* 121(1): 26–31.

Custer, B., Tomasulo, P. A., Murphy, E. L., Caglioti, S., Harpool, D., McEvoy, P. and Busch, M. P. (2004). Triggers for switching from minipool testing by nucleic acid technology to individual-donation nucleic acid testing for West Nile virus: Analysis of 2003 data to inform 2004 decision making. *Transfusion* 44(11): 1547–54.

Davis, B. S., Chang, G. J., Cropp, B., Roehrig, J. T., Martin, D. A., Mitchell, C. J., Bowen, R. and Bunning, M. L. (2001). West Nile virus recombinant DNA vaccine protects mouse and horse from virus challenge and expresses in vitro a noninfectious recombinant antigen that can be used in enzyme-linked immunosorbent assays. *J Virol* 75(9). 4040–7.

Davis, C. T., Beasley, D. W., Guzman, H., Raj, R., D'Anton, M., Novak, R. J., Unnasch, T. R., Tesh, R. B. and Barrett, A. D. (2003). Genetic variation among temporally and geographically distinct West Nile virus isolates, United States, 2001, 2002. *Emerg Infect Dis* 9(11): 1423–9.

Davis, C. T., Beasley, D. W., Guzman, H., Siirin, M., Parsons, R., Tesh, R. and Barrett, A. D. (2004). Emergence of attenuated West Nile virus variants in Texas. *Virology* 330(1): 342–50.

Day, J. F. (2001). Predicting St. Louis encephalitis virus epidemics: Lessons from recent, and not so recent, outbreaks. *Annu Rev Entomol* 46: 111–38.

Depoortere, E., Kavle, J., Keus, K., Zeller, H., Murri, S. and Legros, D. (2004). Outbreak of West Nile virus causing severe neurological involvement in children, Nuba Mountains, Sudan, 2002. *Trop Med Int Health* 9(6): 730–6.

DeSalvo, D., Roy-Chaudhury, P., Peddi, R., Merchen, T., Konijetti, K., Gupta, M., Boardman, R., Rogers, C., Buell, J., Hanaway, M., Broderick, J., Smith, R. and Woodle, E. S. (2004). West Nile virus encephalitis in organ transplant recipients: Another high-risk group for meningoencephalitis and death. [see comment] *Transplantation* 77(3): 466–9.

Deubel, V., Kinney, R. M. and Trent, D. W. (1986). Nucleotide sequence and deduced amino acid sequence of the structural proteins of dengue type 2 virus, Jamaica genotype. *Virology* 155(2): 365–77.

Deubel, V., Kinney, R. M. and Trent, D. W. (1988). Nucleotide sequence and deduced amino acid sequence of the nonstructural proteins of dengue type 2 virus, Jamaica genotype: Comparative analysis of the full-length genome. *Virology* 165(1): 234–44.

Diamond, M. S., Sitati, E. M., Friend, L. D., Higgs, S., Shrestha, B. and Engle, M. (2003). A critical role for induced IgM in the protection against West Nile virus infection. *J Exp Med* 198(12): 1853–62.

Dohm, D. J., O'Guinn, M. L. and Turell, M. J. (2002). Effect of environmental temperature on the ability of Culex pipiens (Diptera: Culicidae) to transmit West Nile virus. *J Med Entomol* 39(1): 221–5.

Dohm, D. J. and Turell, M. J. (2001). Effect of incubation at overwintering temperatures on the replication of West Nile Virus in New York Culex pipiens (Diptera: Culicidae). *J Med Entomol* 38(3): 462–4.

Doron, S. I., Dashe, J. F., Adelman, L. S., Brown, W. F., Werner, B. G. and Hadley, S. (2003). Histopathologically proven poliomyelitis with quadriplegia and loss of brainstem function due to West Nile virus infection. *Clin Infect Dis* 37(5): e74–7.

Drebot, M. A., Lindsay, R., Barker, I. K., Buck, P. A., Fearon, M., Hunter, F., Sockett, P. and Artsob, H. (2003). West Nile virus surveillance and diagnostics: A Canadian perspective. *Can J Infect Dis* 14(2): 105–14.

Dunkel, B., F., D. P., Wotman, K. L., Johns, I. C., Beech, J. and Wilkins, P. A. (2004). Encephalomyelitis from West Nile flavivirus in 3 alpacas. *J Vet Intern Med* 18: 365–7.

Dupuis, A. P., 2nd, Marra, P. P. and Kramer, L. D. (2003). Serologic evidence of West Nile virus transmission, Jamaica, West Indies. *Emerg Infect Dis* 9(7): 860–3.

Ebel, G. D., Carricaburu, J., Young, D., Bernard, K. A. and Kramer, L. D. (2004). Genetic and phenotypic variation of West Nile virus in New York, 2000-2003. *Am J Trop Med Hyg* 71(4): 493–500.

Emig, M. and Apple, D. J. (2004). Severe West Nile virus disease in healthy adults. *Clin Infect Dis* 38(2): 289–92.

Estrada-Franco, J. G., Navarro-Lopez, R., Beasley, D. W., Coffey, L., Carrara, A. S., Travassos da Rosa, A., Clements, T., Wang, E., Ludwig, G. V., Cortes, A. C., Ramirez, P. P., Tesh, R. B., Barrett, A. D. and Weaver, S. C. (2003). West Nile virus in Mexico: Evidence of widespread circulation since July 2002. *Emerg Infect Dis* 9(12): 1604–7.

Falkler, W. A., Jr., Diwan, A. R. and Halstead, S. B. (1973). Human antibody to dengue soluble complement-fixing (SCF) antigens. *J Immunol* 111(6): 1804–9.

Fan, E., Needham, D. M., Brunton, J., Kern, R. Z. and Stewart, T. E. (2004). West Nile virus infection in the intensive care unit: A case series and literature review. *Can Respir J* 11(5): 354–8.

Farajollahi, A., Panella, N. A., Carr, P., Crans, W., Burguess, K. and Komar, N. (2003). Serologic evidence of West Nile virus infection in black bears (Ursus americanus) from New Jersey. *J Wildlife Dis* 39(4): 894–6.

Fernandez-Salas, I., Contreras-Cordero, J. F., Blitvich, B. J., Gonzalez-Rojas, J. I., Cavazos-Alvarez, A., Marlenee, N. L., Elizondo-Quiroga, A., Lorono-Pino, M. A., Gubler, D. J., Cropp, B. C.,

Calisher, C. H. and Beaty, B. J. (2003). Serologic evidence of West Nile Virus infection in birds, Tamaulipas State, Mexico. *Vector Borne Zoonotic Dis* 3(4): 209–13.

Fradin, M. S. (1998). Mosquitoes and mosquito repellents: A clinician's guide. *Ann Intern Med* 128(11): 931–40.

Frances, S. P., Van Dung, N., Beebe, N. W. and Debboun, M. (2002). Field evaluation of repellent formulations against daytime and nighttime biting mosquitoes in a tropical rainforest in northern Australia. *J Med Entomol* 39(3): 541–4.

Frances, S. P., Waterson, D. G., Beebe, N. W. and Cooper, R. D. (2004). Field evaluation of repellent formulations containing deet and picaridin against mosquitoes in Northern Territory, Australia. *J Med Entomol* 41(3): 414–7.

Fratkin, J. D., Leis, A. A., Stokic, D. S., Slavinski, S. A. and Geiss, R. W. (2004). Spinal cord neuropathology in human West Nile virus infection. *Arch Pathol Lab Med* 128(5): 533–7.

Fu, J., Tan, B. H., Yap, E. H., Chan, Y. C. and Tan, Y. H. (1992). Full-length cDNA sequence of dengue type 1 virus (Singapore strain S275/90). *Virology* 188(2): 953–8.

Gadoth, N., Weitzman, S. and Lehmann, E. E. (1979). Acute anterior myelitis complicating West Nile fever. *Arch Neurol* 36(3): 172–3.

Gandelman-Marton, R., Kimiagar, I., Itzhaki, A., Klein, C., Theitler, J. and Rabey, J. M. (2003). Electroencephalography findings in adult patients with West Nile virus-associated meningitis and meningoencephalitis. *Clin Infect Dis* 37(11): 1573–8.

Gao, G. F., Hussain, M. H., Reid, H. W. and Gould, E. A. (1994). Identification of naturally occurring monoclonal antibody escape variants of louping ill virus. *J Gen Virol* 75 (Pt 3): 609–14.

Gea-Banacloche, J., Johnson, R. T., Bagic, A., Butman, J. A., Murray, P. R. and Agrawal, A. G. (2004). West Nile virus: pathogenesis and therapeutic options. *Ann Intern Med* 140(7): 545–53.

George, S., Gourie-Devi, M., Rao, J. A., Prasad, S. R. and Pavri, K. M. (1984). Isolation of West Nile virus from the brains of children who had died of encephalitis. *Bull World Health Organ* 62(6): 879–82.

Giachetti, C., Linnen, J. M., Kolk, D. P., Dockter, J., Gillotte-Taylor, K., Park, M., Ho-Sing-Loy, M., McCormick, M. K., Mimms, L. T. and McDonough, S. H. (2002). Highly sensitive multiplex assay for detection of human immunodeficiency virus type 1 and hepatitis C virus RNA. *J Clin Microbiol* 40(7): 2408–19.

Gilad, R., Lampl, Y., Sadeh, M., Paul, M. and Dan, M. (2003). Optic neuritis complicating west nile virus meningitis in a young adult. *Infection* 31(1): 55–6.

Glass, J. D., Samuels, O. and Rich, M. M. (2002). Poliomyelitis due to West Nile virus. *N Engl J Med* 347(16): 1280–1.

Goddard, L. B., Roth, A. E., Reisen, W. K. and Scott, T. W. (2003). Vertical transmission of West Nile Virus by three California Culex (Diptera: Culicidae) species. *J Med Entomol* 40(6): 743–6.

Goldblum, N., Sterk, V. V. and Paderski, B. (1954). West Nile fever: The clinical features of the disease and the isolation of West Nile virus from the blood of nine human cases. *Am J Hyg* 59: 89–103.

Gollins, S. W. and Porterfield, J. S. (1986a). A new mechanism for the neutralization of enveloped viruses by antiviral antibody. *Nature* 321(6067): 244–6.

Gollins, S. W. and Porterfield, J. S. (1986b). pH-dependent fusion between the flavivirus West Nile and liposomal model membranes. *J Gen Virol* 67 (Pt 1): 157–66.

Gollins, S. W. and Porterfield, J. S. (1986c). The uncoating and infectivity of the flavivirus West Nile on interaction with cells: Effects of pH and ammonium chloride. *J Gen Virol* 67 (Pt 9): 1941–50.

Granwehr, B. P., Li, L., Davis, C. T., Beasley, D. W. and Barrett, A. D. (2004). Characterization of a West Nile virus isolate from a human on the Gulf Coast of Texas. *J Clin Microbiol* 42(11): 5375–7.

Guarner, J., Shieh, W. J., Hunter, S., Paddock, C. D., Morken, T., Campbell, G. L., Marfin, A. A. and Zaki, S. R. (2004). Clinicopathologic study and laboratory diagnosis of 23 cases with West Nile virus encephalomyelitis. *Hum Pathol* 35(8): 983–90.

Gubler, D. J. (2002). The global emergence/resurgence of arboviral diseases as public health problems. *Arch Med Res* 33(4): 330–42.

Gubler, D. J., Campbell, G. L., Nasci, R., Komar, N., Petersen, L. and Roehrig, J. T. (2000). West Nile virus in the United States: guidelines for detection, prevention, and control. *Viral Immunol* 13(4): 469–75.

Gubler, D. J. and Roehrig, J. T. (1998). Togaviridae and Flaviviridae. *Topley and Wilson's Microbiology and Microbial Infections*. A. B. L. Collier and M. Sussman. London, Arnold Publishing. 1: 579–600.

Guirakhoo, F., Heinz, F. X. and Kunz, C. (1989). Epitope model of tick-borne encephalitis virus envelope glycoprotein E: analysis of structural properties, role of carbohydrate side chain, and conformational changes occurring at acidic pH. *Virology* 169(1): 90–9.

Guyton, A. (1949). Reaction of the body to poliomyelitis and the recovery process. *Arch Int Med* 83: 27.

Hahn, Y. S., Galler, R., Hunkapiller, T., Dalrymple, J. M., Strauss, J. H. and Strauss, E. G. (1988). Nucleotide sequence of dengue 2 RNA and comparison of the encoded proteins with those of other flaviviruses. *Virology* 162(1): 167–80.

Haley, M., Retter, A. S., Fowler, D., Gea-Banacloche, J. and O'Grady, N. P. (2003). The role for intravenous immunoglobulin in the treatment of West Nile virus encephalitis. *Clin Infect Dis* 37(6): e88–90.

Hall, R. A. and Khromykh, A. A. (2004). West Nile virus vaccines. *Expert Opin Biol Ther* 4(8): 1295–305.

Hamdan, A., Green, P., Mendelson, E., Kramer, M. R., Pitlik, S. and Weinberger, M. (2002). Possible benefit of intravenous immunoglobulin therapy in a lung transplant recipient with West Nile virus encephalitis. *Transplant Infect Dis* 4(3): 160–2.

Han, L. L., Popovici, F., Alexander, J. P., Jr., Laurentia, V., Tengelsen, L. A., Cernescu, C., Gary, H. E., Jr., Ion-Nedelcu, N., Campbell, G. L. and Tsai, T. F. (1999). Risk factors for West Nile virus infection and meningoencephalitis, Romania, 1996. *J Infect Dis* 179(1): 230–3.

Hardinger, K. L., Miller, B., Storch, G. A., Desai, N. M. and Brennan, D. C. (2003). West Nile virus–associated meningoencephalitis in two chronically immunosuppressed renal transplant recipients. *Am J Transplant* 3(10): 1312–5.

Harrington, T., Kuehnert, M. J., Kamel, H., Lanciotti, R. S., Hand, S., Currier, M., Chamberland, M. E., Petersen, L. R. and Marfin, A. A. (2003). West Nile virus infection transmitted by blood transfusion. *Transfusion* 43(8): 1018–22.

Hasegawa, H., Yoshida, M., Shiosaka, T., Fujita, S. and Kobayashi, Y. (1992). Mutations in the envelope protein of Japanese encephalitis virus affect entry into cultured cells and virulence in mice. *Virology* 191(1): 158–65.

Hassin-Baer, S., Kirson, E. D., Shulman, L., Buchman, A. S., Bin, H., Hindiyeh, M., Markevich, L. and Mendelson, E. (2004). Stiff-person syndrome following West Nile fever. *Arch Neurol* 61(6): 938–41.

Hayes, C. G. (2001). West Nile virus: Uganda, 1937, to New York City, 1999. *Ann N Y Acad Sci* 951: 25–37.

Hayes, E. B. and O'Leary, D. R. (2004). West Nile virus infection: A pediatric perspective. *Pediatrics* 113(5): 1375–81.

Heinz, F. X. (1986). Epitope mapping of flavivirus glycoproteins. *Adv Virus Res* 31: 103–68.

Heinz, F. X., Berger, R., Majdic, O., Knapp, W. and Kunz, C. (1982). Monoclonal antibodies to the structural glycoprotein of tick-borne encephalitis virus. *Infect Immun* 37(3): 869–74.

Heinz-Taheny, K. M., Andrews, J. J., Kinsel, M. J., Pessier, A. P., Pinkerton, M. E., Lemberger, K. Y., Novak, R. J., Dizikes, G. J., Edwards, E. and Komar, N. (2004). West Nile virus infection in free-ranging squirrels in Illinois. *J Vet Diagn Invest* 16(3): 186–90.

Henchal, E. A., Henchal, L. S. and Schlesinger, J. J. (1988). Synergistic interactions of anti-NS1 monoclonal antibodies protect passively immunized mice from lethal challenge with dengue 2 virus. *J Gen Virol* 69 (Pt 8): 2101–7.

Heresi, G. P., Mancias, P., Mazur, L. J., Butler, I. J., Murphy, J. R. and Cleary, T. G. (2004). Poliomyelitis-like syndrome in a child with West Nile virus infection. *Pediatr Infect Dis J* 23(8): 788–9.

Hershberger, V. S., Augsburger, J. J., Hutchins, R. K., Miller, S. A., Horwitz, J. A. and Bergmann, M. (2003). Chorioretinal lesions in nonfatal cases of West Nile virus infection. *Ophthalmology* 110(9): 1732–6.

Hiatt, B., DesJardin, L., Carter, T., Gingrich, R., Thompson, C. and de Magalhaes-Silverman, M. (2003). A fatal case of West Nile virus infection in a bone marrow transplant recipient. *Clin Infect Dis* 37(9): e129–31.

Holzmann, H., Mandl, C. W., Guirakhoo, F., Heinz, F. X. and Kunz, C. (1989). Characterization of antigenic variants of tick-borne encephalitis virus selected with neutralizing monoclonal antibodies. *J Gen Virol* 70 (Pt 1): 219–22.

Holzmann, H., Utter, G., Norrby, E., Mandl, C. W., Kunz, C. and Heinz, F. X. (1993). Assessment of the antigenic structure of tick-borne encephalitis virus by the use of synthetic peptides. *J Gen Virol* 74 (Pt 9): 2031–5.

Hong, D. S., Jacobson, K. L., Raad, II, de Lima, M., Anderlini, P., Fuller, G. N., Ippoliti, C., Cool, R. M., Leeds, N. E., Narvios, A., Han, X. Y., Padula, A., Champlin, R. E. and Hosing, C. (2003). West Nile encephalitis in 2 hematopoietic stem cell transplant recipients: case series and literature review. *Clin Infect Dis* 37(8): 1044–9.

Hrnicek, M. J. and Mailliard, M. E. (2004). Acute west nile virus in two patients receiving interferon and ribavirin for chronic hepatitis C. *Am J Gastroenterol* 99(5): 957.

Hubalek, Z. and Halouzka, J. (1999). West Nile fever–a reemerging mosquito-borne viral disease in Europe. *Emerg Infect Dis* 5(5): 643–50.

Hunt, A. R., Hall, R. A., Kerst, A. J., Nasci, R. S., Savage, H. M., Panella, N. A., Gottfried, K. L., Burkhalter, K. L. and Roehrig, J. T. (2002). Detection of West Nile virus antigen in mosquitoes and avian tissues by a monoclonal antibody-based capture enzyme immunoassay. *J Clin Microbiol* 40(6): 2023–30.

Iacono-Connors, L. C., Smith, J. F., Ksiazek, T. G., Kelley, C. L. and Schmaljohn, C. S. (1996). Characterization of Langat virus antigenic determinants defined by monoclonal antibodies to E, NS1 and preM and identification of a protective, non-neutralizing preM-specific monoclonal antibody. *Virus Res* 43(2): 125–36.

Iwamoto, M., Jernigan, D. B., Guasch, A., Trepka, M. J., Blackmore, C. G., Hellinger, W. C., Pham, S. M., Zaki, S., Lanciotti, R. S., Lance-Parker, S. E., DiazGranados, C. A., Winquist, A. G., Perlino, C. A., Wiersma, S., Hillyer, K. L., Goodman, J. L., Marfin, A. A., Chamberland, M. E. and Petersen, L. R. (2003). Transmission of West Nile virus from an organ donor to four transplant recipients. *N Engl J Med* 348(22): 2196–203.

Jeha, L. E., Sila, C. A., Lederman, R. J., Prayson, R. A., Isada, C. M. and Gordon, S. M. (2003). West Nile virus infection: A new acute paralytic illness. *Neurology* 61(1): 55–9.

Jia, X. Y., Briese, T., Jordan, I., Rambaut, A., Chi, H. C., Mackenzie, J. S., Hall, R. A., Scherret, J. and Lipkin, W. I. (1999). Genetic analysis of West Nile New York 1999 encephalitis virus. *Lancet* 354(9194): 1971–2.

Jiang, W. R., Lowe, A., Higgs, S., Reid, H. and Gould, E. A. (1993). Single amino acid codon changes detected in louping ill virus antibody-resistant mutants with reduced neurovirulence. *J Gen Virol* 74 (Pt 5): 931–5.

Johansson, M., Brooks, A. J., Jans, D. A. and Vasudevan, S. G. (2001). A small region of the dengue virus-encoded RNA-dependent RNA polymerase, NS5, confers interaction with both the nuclear transport receptor importin-beta and the viral helicase, NS3. *J Gen Virol* 82 (Pt 4): 735–45.

Johnson, A. J., Martin, D. A., Karabatsos, N. and Roehrig, J. T. (2000). Detection of anti-arboviral immunoglobulin G by using a monoclonal antibody-based capture enzyme-linked immunosorbent assay. *J Clin Microbiol* 38(5): 1827–31.

Jordan, I., Briese, T., Fischer, N., Lau, J. Y. and Lipkin, W. I. (2000). Ribavirin inhibits West Nile virus replication and cytopathic effect in neural cells. *J Infect Dis* 182(4): 1214–7.

Jupp, P. G. (2001). The ecology of West Nile virus in South Africa and the occurrence of outbreaks in humans. *Ann N Y Acad Sci* 951: 143–52.

Kaiser, P. K., Lee, M. S. and Martin, D. A. (2003). Occlusive vasculitis in a patient with concomitant West Nile virus infection. *Am J Ophthalmol* 136(5): 928–30.

Kalil, A. C., Devetten, M. P., Singh, S., Lesiak, B., Poage, D. P., Bargenquast, K., Fayad, P. and Freifeld, A. G. (2005). Use of interferon-alpha in patients with West Nile encephalitis: Report of 2 cases. *Clin Infect Dis* 40(5): 764–6.

Kanagarajan, K., Ganesh, S., Alakhras, M., Go, E. S., Recco, R. A. and Zaman, M. M. (2003). West Nile virus infection presenting as cerebellar ataxia and fever: Case report. *South Med J* 96(6): 600–1.

Kapoor, H., Signs, K., Somsel, P., Downes, F. P., Clark, P. A. and Massey, J. P. (2004). Persistence of West Nile Virus (WNV) IgM antibodies in cerebrospinal fluid from patients with CNS disease. *J Clin Virol* 31(4): 289–91.

Kapoor, M., Zhang, L., Ramachandra, M., Kusukawa, J., Ebner, K. E. and Padmanabhan, R. (1995). Association between NS3 and NS5 proteins of dengue virus type 2 in the putative RNA replicase is linked to differential phosphorylation of NS5. *J Biol Chem* 270(32): 19100–6.

Karpati, A. M., Perrin, M. C., Matte, T., Leighton, J., Schwartz, J. and Barr, R. G. (2004). Pesticide spraying for West Nile virus control and emergency department asthma visits in New York City, 2000. *Environ Health Perspect* 112(11): 1183–7.

Kelley, T. W., Prayson, R. A., Ruiz, A. I., Isada, C. M. and Gordon, S. M. (2003). The neuropathology of West Nile virus meningoencephalitis. A report of two cases and review of the literature. *Am J Clin Pathol* 119(5): 749–53.

Khairallah, M., Ben Yahia, S., Ladjimi, A., Zeghidi, H., Ben Romdhane, F., Besbes, L., Zaouali, S. and Messaoud, R. (2004). Chorioretinal involvement in patients with West Nile virus infection. *Ophthalmology* 111(11): 2065–70.

Khosla, J. (2004). West Nile encephalitis presenting as opsoclonus-myoclonus-cerebellar ataxia. *Ann Neurol* 56(Suppl. 8): S70.

Khromykh, A. A., Kenney, M. T. and Westaway, E. G. (1998). trans-Complementation of flavivirus RNA polymerase gene NS5 by using Kunjin virus replicon-expressing BHK cells. *J Virol* 72(9): 7270–9.

Khromykh, A. A., Meka, H., Guyatt, K. J. and Westaway, E. G. (2001). Essential role of cyclization sequences in flavivirus RNA replication. *J Virol* 75(14): 6719–28.

Kimura, T., Gollins, S. W. and Porterfield, J. S. (1986). The effect of pH on the early interaction of West Nile virus with P388D1 cells. *J Gen Virol* 67 (Pt 11): 2423–33.

Kimura-Kuroda, J. and Yasui, K. (1983). Topographical analysis of antigenic determinants on envelope glycoprotein V3 (E) of Japanese encephalitis virus, using monoclonal antibodies. *J Virol* 45(1): 124–32.

Kinney, R. M., Butrapet, S., Chang, G. J., Tsuchiya, K. R., Roehrig, J. T., Bhamarapravati, N. and Gubler, D. J. (1997). Construction of infectious cDNA clones for dengue 2 virus: strain 16681 and its attenuated vaccine derivative, strain PDK–53. *Virology* 230(2): 300–8.

Kiupel, M., Simmons, H. A., Fitzgerald, S. D., Wise, A., Sikarskie, J. G., Cooley, T. M., Hollamby, S. R. and Maes, R. (2003). West Nile virus infection in Eastern fox squirrels (Sciurus niger). *Vet Pathol* 40(6): 703–7.

Klee, A. L., Maidin, B., Edwin, B., Poshni, I., Mostashari, F., Fine, A., Layton, M. and Nash, D. (2004). Long–term prognosis for clinical West Nile virus infection. *Emerg Infect Dis* 10(8): 1405–11.

Kleinschmidt-DeMasters, B. K., Marder, B. A., Levi, M. E., Laird, S. P., McNutt, J. T., Escott, E. J., Everson, G. T. and Tyler, K. L. (2004). Naturally acquired West Nile virus encephalomyelitis in transplant recipients: Clinical, laboratory, diagnostic, and neuropathological features. *Arch Neurol* 61(8): 1210–20.

Klenk, K., Snow, J., Morgan, K., Bowen, R., Stephens, M., Foster, F., Gordy, P., Beckett, S., Komar, N., Gubler, D. and Bunning, M. (2004). Alligators as West Nile virus amplifiers. *Emerg Infect Dis* 10(12): 2150–5.

Komar, N. (2003). West Nile virus: Epidemiology and ecology in North America. *Adv Virus Res* 61: 185–234.

Komar, N., Lanciotti, R., Bowen, R., Langevin, S. and Bunning, M. (2002). Detection of West Nile virus in oral and cloacal swabs collected from bird carcasses. *Emerg Infect Dis* 8(7): 741–2.

Komar, N., Langevin, S., Hinten, S., Nemeth, N., Edwards, E., Hettler, D., Davis, B., Bowen, R. and Bunning, M. (2003a). Experimental infection of North American birds with the New York 1999 strain of West Nile virus. *Emerg Infect Dis* 9(3): 311–22.

Komar, N., Panella, N. A., Burns, J. E., Dusza, S. W., Mascarenhas, T. M. and Talbot, T. O. (2001). Serologic evidence for West Nile virus infection in birds in the New York City vicinity during an outbreak in 1999. *Emerg Infect Dis* 7(4): 621–5.

Komar, O., Robbins, M. B., Klenk, K., Blitvich, B. J., Marlenee, N. L., Burkhalter, K. L., Gubler, D. J., Gonzalvez, G., Pena, C. J., Peterson, A. T. and Komar, N. (2003b). West Nile virus transmission in resident birds, Dominican Republic. *Emerg Infect Dis* 9(10): 1299–302.

Koonin, E. V. (1993). Computer-assisted identification of a putative methyltransferase domain in NS5 protein of flaviviruses and lambda 2 protein of reovirus. *J Gen Virol* 74 (Pt 4): 733–40.

Krishna Murthy, H. M., Judge, K., DeLucas, L., Clum, S. and Padmanabhan, R. (1999). Crystallization, characterization and measurement of MAD data on crystals of dengue virus NS3 serine protease complexed with mung-bean Bowman-Birk inhibitor. *Acta Crystallogr D Biol Crystallogr* 55 (Pt 7): 1370–2.

Kuchtey, R. W., Kosmorsky, G. S., Martin, D. and Lee, M. S. (2003). Uveitis associated with West Nile virus infection. *Arch Ophthalmol* 121(11): 1648–9.

Kulasekera, V. L., Kramer, L., Nasci, R. S., Mostashari, F., Cherry, B., Trock, S. C., Glaser, C. and Miller, J. R. (2001). West Nile virus infection in mosquitoes, birds, horses, and humans, Staten Island, New York, 2000. *Emerg Infect Dis* 7(4): 722–5.

Kulstad, E. B. and Wichter, M. D. (2003). West Nile encephalitis presenting as a stroke. *Ann Emerg Med* 41(2): 283.

Kumar, D., Drebot, M. A., Wong, S. J., Lim, G., Artsob, H., Buck, P. and Humar, A. (2004a). A seroprevalence study of west nile virus infection in solid organ transplant recipients. *Am J Transplant* 4(11): 1883–8.

Kumar, D., Prasad, G. V., Zaltzman, J., Levy, G. A. and Humar, A. (2004b). Community-acquired West Nile virus infection in solid-organ transplant recipients. *Transplantation* 77(3): 399–402.

Kuno, G. (1998). Universal diagnostic RT-PCR protocol for arboviruses. *J Virol Methods* 72(1): 27–41.

Kutzler, M. A., R.J., B., Garder-Graff, K., Baker, R. J., Delay, J. P. and Mattson, D. E. (2004). West Nile virus infection in two alpacas. *J Am Veterinary Med Assoc* 225(6): 921–4.

Lanciotti, R. S. (2003). Molecular amplification assays for the detection of flaviviruses. *Adv Virus Res* 61: 67–99.

Lanciotti, R. S., Ebel, G. D., Deubel, V., Kerst, A. J., Murri, S., Meyer, R., Bowen, M., McKinney, N., Morrill, W. E., Crabtree, M. B., Kramer, L. D. and Roehrig, J. T. (2002). Complete genome sequences and phylogenetic analysis of West Nile virus strains isolated from the United States, Europe, and the Middle East. *Virology* 298(1): 96–105.

Lanciotti, R. S. and Kerst, A. J. (2001). Nucleic acid sequence-based amplification assays for rapid detection of West Nile and St. Louis encephalitis viruses. *J Clin Microbiol* 39(12): 4506–13.

Lanciotti, R. S., Kerst, A. J., Nasci, R. S., Godsey, M. S., Mitchell, C. J., Savage, H. M., Komar, N., Panella, N. A., Allen, B. C., Volpe, K. E., Davis, B. S. and Roehrig, J. T. (2000). Rapid detection of west nile virus from human clinical specimens, field-collected mosquitoes, and avian samples by a TaqMan reverse transcriptase-PCR assay. *J Clin Microbiol* 38(11): 4066–71.

Lanciotti, R. S., Roehrig, J. T., Deubel, V., Smith, J., Parker, M., Steele, K., Crise, B., Volpe, K. E., Crabtree, M. B., Scherret, J. H., Hall, R. A., MacKenzie, J. S., Cropp, C. B., Panigrahy, B., Ostlund, E., Schmitt, B., Malkinson, M., Banet, C., Weissman, J., Komar, N., Savage, H. M., Stone, W., McNamara, T. and Gubler, D. J. (1999). Origin of the West Nile virus responsible for an outbreak of encephalitis in the northeastern United States. *Science* 286(5448): 2333–7.

Langevin, S. A., Bunning, M., Davis, B. and Komar, N. (2001). Experimental infection of chickens as candidate sentinels for West Nile virus. *Emerg Infect Dis* 7(4): 726–9.

Lanthier, I., Hebert, M., Tremblay, D., Harel, J., Dallaire, A. D. and Girard, C. (2004). Natural West Nile virus infection in a captive juvenile Arctic wolf (Canis lupus). *J Vet Diagn Invest* 16(4): 326–9.

Lawrie, C. H., Uzcategui, N. Y., Gould, E. A. and Nuttall, P. A. (2004). Ixodid and argasid tick species and west nile virus. *Emerg Infect Dis* 10(4): 653–7.

Le Guenno, B., Bougermouh, A., Azzam, T. and Bouakaz, R. (1996). West Nile: A deadly virus? *Lancet* 348(9037): 1315.

Leis, A. A., Stokic, D. S., Polk, J. L., Dostrow, V. and Winkelmann, M. (2002). A poliomyelitis-like syndrome from West Nile virus infection. *N Engl J Med* 347(16): 1279–80.

Li, H., Clum, S., You, S., Ebner, K. E. and Padmanabhan, R. (1999). The serine protease and RNA-stimulated nucleoside triphosphatase and RNA helicase functional domains of dengue virus type 2 NS3 converge within a region of 20 amino acids. *J Virol* 73(4): 3108–16.

Li, J., Loeb, J. A., Shy, M. E., Shah, A. K., Tselis, A. C., Kupski, W. J. and Lewis, R. A. (2003). Asymmetric flaccid paralysis: A neuromuscular presentation of West Nile virus infection. [see comment] *Ann Neurol* 53(6): 703–10.

Lichtensteiger, C. A., Heinz-Taheny, K., Osborne, T. S., Novak, R. J., Lewis, B. A. and Firth, M. L. (2003). West Nile virus encephalitis and myocarditis in wolf and dog. *Emerg Infect Dis* 9(10): 1303–6.

Lillibridge, K. M., Parsons, R., Randle, Y., Travassos da Rosa, A. P., Guzman, H., Siirin, M., Wuithiranyagool, T., Hailey, C., Higgs, S., Bala, A. A., Pascua, R., Meyer, T., Vanlandingham, D. L. and Tesh, R. B. (2004). The 2002 introduction of West Nile virus into Harris County, Texas, an area historically endemic for St. Louis encephalitis. *Am J Trop Med Hyg* 70(6): 676–81.

Lin, B., Parrish, C. R., Murray, J. M. and Wright, P. J. (1994). Localization of a neutralizing epitope on the envelope protein of dengue virus type 2. *Virology* 202(2): 885–90.

Liu, W. J., Sedlak, P. L., Kondratieva, N. and Khromykh, A. A. (2002). Complementation analysis of the flavivirus Kunjin NS3 and NS5 proteins defines the minimal regions essential for formation of a replication complex and shows a requirement of NS3 in cis for virus assembly. *J Virol* 76(21): 10766–75.

Lobigs, M., Dalgarno, L., Schlesinger, J. J. and Weir, R. C. (1987). Location of a neutralization determinant in the E protein of yellow fever virus (17D vaccine strain). *Virology* 161(2): 474–8.

Lok, S. M., Ng, M. L. and Aaskov, J. (2001). Amino acid and phenotypic changes in dengue 2 virus associated with escape from neutralisation by IgM antibody. *J Med Virol* 65(2): 315–23.

Lord, R. D. and Calisher, C. H. (1970). Further evidence of southward transport of arboviruses by migratory birds. *Am J Epidemiol* 92(1): 73–8.

Lorono-Pino, M. A., Blitvich, B. J., Farfan-Ale, J. A., Puerto, F. I., Blanco, J. M., Marlenee, N. L., Rosado-Paredes, E. P., Garcia-Rejon, J. E., Gubler, D. J., Calisher, C. H. and Beaty, B. J. (2003). Serologic evidence of West Nile virus infection in horses, Yucatan State, Mexico. *Emerg Infect Dis* 9(7): 857–9.

Malkinson, M., Banet, C., Weisman, Y., Pokamunski, S., King, R., Drouet, M. T. and Deubel, V. (2002). Introduction of West Nile virus in the Middle East by migrating white storks. *Emerg Infect Dis* 8(4): 392–7.

Malkinson, M., Weisman, Y., Pokamonski, S., King, R. and Deubel, V. (2001). Intercontinental transmission of West Nile virus by migrating white storks. *Emerg Infect Dis* 7(3 Suppl): 540.

Mandl, C. W., Guirakhoo, F., Holzmann, H., Heinz, F. X. and Kunz, C. (1989). Antigenic structure of the flavivirus envelope protein E at the molecular level, using tick-borne encephalitis virus as a model. *J Virol* 63(2): 564–71.

Marberg, K., Goldblum, N., Sterk, V. V., Jasinska-Klingberg, W. and Klingberg, M. A. (1956). The natural history of West Nile Fever. I. Clinical observations during an epidemic in Israel. *Am J Hyg* 64(3): 259–69.

Marciniak, C., Sorosky, S. and Hynes, C. (2004). Acute flaccid paralysis associated with West Nile virus: motor and functional improvement in 4 patients. *Arch Phys Med Rehabil* 85(12): 1933–8.

Marfin, A. A., Petersen, L. R., Eidson, M., Miller, J., Hadler, J., Farello, C., Werner, B., Campbell, G. L., Layton, M., Smith, P., Bresnitz, E., Cartter, M., Scaletta, J., Obiri, G., Bunning, M., Craven, R. C., Roehrig, J. T., Julian, K. G., Hinten, S. R., Gubler, D. J. and Arbo, N. E. T. C. S. G. (2001). Widespread West Nile virus activity, eastern United States, 2000. *Emerg Infect Dis* 7(4): 730–5.

Marlenee, N. L., Lorono-Pino, M. A., Beaty, B. J. and Blitvich, B. J. (2004). Detection of antibodies to West Nile and Saint Louis encephalitis viruses in horses. *Salud Publica Mexico* 46(5): 373–5.

Martin, D. A., Biggerstaff, B. J., Allen, B., Johnson, A. J., Lanciotti, R. S. and Roehrig, J. T. (2002). Use of immunoglobulin m cross-reactions in differential diagnosis of human flaviviral encephalitis infections in the United States. *Clin Diagn Lab Immunol* 9(3): 544–9.

Martin, D. A., Muth, D. A., Brown, T., Johnson, A. J., Karabatsos, N. and Roehrig, J. T. (2000). Standardization of immunoglobulin M capture enzyme-linked immunosorbent assays for routine diagnosis of arboviral infections. *J Clin Microbiol* 38(5): 1823–6.

Martin, D. A., Noga, A., Kosoy, O., Johnson, A. J., Petersen, L. R. and Lanciotti, R. S. (2004). Evaluation of a diagnostic algorithm using immunoglobulin M enzyme-linked immunosorbent assay to differentiate human West Nile virus and St. Louis encephalititis virus infections during the 2002 West Nile virus epidemic in the United States. *Clin Diagn Lab Immunol* 11(6): 1130–3.

Matusan, A. E., Pryor, M. J., Davidson, A. D. and Wright, P. J. (2001). Mutagenesis of the Dengue virus type 2 NS3 protein within and outside helicase motifs: Effects on enzyme activity and virus replication. *J Virol* 75(20): 9633–43.

McCarthy, T. A., Hadler, J. L., Julian, K., Walsh, S. J., Biggerstaff, B. J., Hinten, S. R., Baisley, C., Iton, A., Brennan, T., Nelson, R. S., Achambault, G., Marfin, A. A. and Petersen, L. R. (2001). West Nile virus serosurvey and assessment of personal prevention efforts in an area with intense epizootic activity: Connecticut, 2000. *Ann N Y Acad Sci* 951: 307–16.

McGready, R., Hamilton, K. A., Simpson, J. A., Cho, T., Luxemburger, C., Edwards, R., Looareesuwan, S., White, N. J., Nosten, F. and Lindsay, S. W. (2001). Safety of the insect repellent N,N-diethyl-M-toluamide (DEET) in pregnancy. *Am J Trop Med Hyg* 65(4): 285–9.

McLean, R. G., Ubico, S. R., Bourne, D. and Komar, N. (2002). West Nile virus in livestock and wildlife. *Curr Topics Microbiol Immunol* 267: 271–308.

McMinn, P. C., Lee, E., Hartley, S., Roehrig, J. T., Dalgarno, L. and Weir, R. C. (1995). Murray valley encephalitis virus envelope protein antigenic variants with altered hemagglutination properties and reduced neuroinvasiveness in mice. *Virology* 211(1): 10–20.

Miller, B. R., Nasci, R. S., Godsey, M. S., Savage, H. M., Lutwama, J. J., Lanciotti, R. S. and Peters, C. J. (2000). First field evidence for natural vertical transmission of West Nile virus in Culex univittatus complex mosquitoes from Rift Valley province, Kenya. *Am J Trop Med Hyg* 62(2): 240–6.

Miller, D. L., Mauel, M. J., Baldwin, C., Burtle, G., Ingram, D., Hines, M. E., 2nd and Frazier, K. S. (2003). West Nile virus in farmed alligators. *Emerg Infect Dis* 9(7): 794–9.

Minke, J. M., Siger, L., Karaca, K., Austgen, L., Gordy, P., Bowen, R., Renshaw, R. W., Loosmore, S., Audonnet, J. C. and Nordgren, B. (2004). Recombinant canarypoxvirus vaccine carrying the prM/E genes of West Nile virus protects horses against a West Nile virus-mosquito challenge. *Arch Virol Suppl* (18): 221–30.

Mitchell, C. J., Kilpatrick, J. W., Hayes, R. O. and Curry, H. W. (1970). Effects of ultra-low volume applications of malathion in Hale County, Texas. II. Mosquito populations in treated and untreated areas. *J Med Entomol* 7(1): 85–91.

Modis, Y., Ogata, S., Clements, D. and Harrison, S. C. (2003). A ligand-binding pocket in the dengue virus envelope glycoprotein. *Proc Natl Acad Sci U S A* 100(12): 6986–91.

Modis, Y., Ogata, S., Clements, D. and Harrison, S. C. (2004). Structure of the dengue virus envelope protein after membrane fusion. *Nature* 427(6972): 313–9.

Monath, T. P. (2001). Prospects for development of a vaccine against the West Nile virus. *Ann N Y Acad Sci* 951: 1–12.

Monath, T. P. (2002). Editorial: Jennerian vaccination against West Nile virus. [comment] *Am J Trop Med Hyg* 66(2): 113–4.

Morita, K., Tadano, M., Nakaji, S., Kosai, K., Mathenge, E. G., Pandey, B. D., Hasebe, F., Inoue, S. and Igarashi, A. (2001). Locus of a virus neutralization epitope on the Japanese encephalitis virus envelope protein determined by use of long PCR-based region-specific random mutagenesis. *Virology* 287(2): 417–26.

Morrey, J. D., Day, C. W., Julander, J. G., Blatt, L. M., Smee, D. F. and Sidwell, R. W. (2004). Effect of interferon–alpha and interferon-inducers on West Nile virus in mouse and hamster animal models. *Antivir Chem Chemother* 15(2): 101–9.

Mostashari, F., Bunning, M. L., Kitsutani, P. T., Singer, D. A., Nash, D., Cooper, M. J., Katz, N., Liljebjelke, K. A., Biggerstaff, B. J., Fine, A. D., Layton, M. C., Mullin, S. M., Johnson, A. J., Martin, D. A., Hayes, E. B. and Campbell, G. L. (2001). Epidemic West Nile encephalitis, New York, 1999: Results of a household-based seroepidemiological survey. *Lancet* 358(9278): 261–4.

Mostashari, F., Kulldorff, M., Hartman, J. J., Miller, J. R. and Kulasekera, V. (2003). Dead bird clusters as an early warning system for West Nile virus activity. *Emerg Infect Dis* 9(6): 641–6.

Mukhopadhyay, S., Kim, B. S., Chipman, P. R., Rossmann, M. G. and Kuhn, R. J. (2003). Structure of West Nile virus. *Science* 302(5643): 248.

Murgue, B., Murri, S., Triki, H., Deubel, V. and Zeller, H. G. (2001). West Nile in the Mediterranean basin: 1950–2000. *Ann N Y Acad Sci* 951: 117–26.

Murgue, B., Zeller, H. and Deubel, V. (2002). The ecology and epidemiology of West Nile virus in Africa, Europe and Asia. *Curr Topics Microbiol Immunol* 267: 195–221.

Murthy, H. M., Clum, S. and Padmanabhan, R. (1999). Dengue virus NS3 serine protease. Crystal structure and insights into interaction of the active site with substrates by molecular modeling and structural analysis of mutational effects. *J Biol Chem* 274(9): 5573–80.

Naowarat, S. and Tang, I. M. (2004). Effect of bird-to-bird transmission of the West Nile virus on the dynamics of the transmission of this disease. *Southeast Asian J Trop Med Public Health* 35(1): 162–6.

Nasci, R. S., Gottfried, K. L., Burkhalter, K. L., Ryan, J. R., Emmerich, E. and Dave, K. (2003). Sensitivity of the VecTest antigen assay for eastern equine encephalitis and western equine encephalitis viruses. *J Am Mosq Control Assoc* 19(4): 440–4.

Nasci, R. S., Savage, H. M., White, D. J., Miller, J. R., Cropp, B. C., Godsey, M. S., Kerst, A. J., Bennett, P., Gottfried, K. and Lanciotti, R. S. (2001). West Nile virus in overwintering Culex mosquitoes, New York City, 2000. *Emerg Infect Dis* 7(4): 742–4.

Nash, D., Mostashari, F., Fine, A., Miller, J., O'Leary, D., Murray, K., Huang, A., Rosenberg, A., Greenberg, A., Sherman, M., Wong, S. and Layton, M. (2001). The outbreak of West Nile virus infection in the New York City area in 1999. *N Engl J Med* 344(24): 1807–14.

Nichter, C. A., Pavlakis, S. G., Shaikh, U., Cherian, K. A., Dobrosyzcki, J., Porricolo, M. E. and Chatturvedi, I. (2000). Rhombencephalitis caused by West Nile fever virus. *Neurology* 55(1): 153.

Nir, Y., Beemer, A. and Goldwasser, R. A. (1965). West Nile virus infection in mice following exposure to a viral aerosol. *Br J Exp Pathol* 46(4): 443–9.

Nir, Y. D. (1959). Airborne West Nile virus infection. *Am J Trop Med Hyg* 8: 537–9.

Nowak, T. and Wengler, G. (1987). Analysis of disulfides present in the membrane proteins of the West Nile flavivirus. *Virology* 156(1): 127–37.

Olberg, R. A., Barker, I. K., Crawshaw, G. J., Bertelsen, M. F., Drebot, M. A. and Andonova, M. (2004). West Nile virus encephalitis in a Barbary macaque (Macaca sylvanus). *Emerg Infect Dis* 10(4): 712–4.

O'Leary, D. R., Marfin, A. A., Montgomery, S. P., Kipp, A. M., Lehman, J. A., Biggerstaff, B. J., Elko, V. L., Collins, P. D., Jones, J. E. and Campbell, G. L. (2004). The epidemic of West Nile virus in the United States, 2002. *Vector Borne Zoonotic Dis* 4(1): 61–70.

Osatomi, K. and Sumiyoshi, H. (1990). Complete nucleotide sequence of dengue type 3 virus genome RNA. *Virology* 176(2): 643–7.

Palmer, M. V., Stoffregen, W. C., Rogers, D. G., Hamir, A. N., Richt, J. A., Pedersen, D. D. and Waters, W. R. (2004). West Nile virus infection in reindeer (Rangifer tarandus). *J Vet Diagn Invest* 16(3): 219–22.

Park, M., Hui, J. S. and Bartt, R. E. (2003). Acute anterior radiculitis associated with West Nile virus infection. *J Neurol Neurosurg Psychiatry* 74(6): 823–5.

Pealer, L. N., Marfin, A. A., Petersen, L. R., Lanciotti, R. S., Page, P. L., Stramer, S. L., Stobierski, M. G., Signs, K., Newman, B., Kapoor, H., Goodman, J. L. and Chamberland, M. E. (2003). Transmission of West Nile virus through blood transfusion in the United States in 2002. *N Engl J Med* 349(13): 1236–45.

Pepperell, C., Rau, N., Krajden, S., Kern, R., Humar, A., Mederski, B., Simor, A., Low, D. E., McGeer, A., Mazzulli, T., Burton, J., Jaigobin, C., Fearon, M., Artsob, H., Drebot, M. A., Halliday, W. and Brunton, J. (2003). West Nile virus infection in 2002: Morbidity and mortality among patients admitted to hospital in southcentral Ontario. *CMAJ* 168(11): 1399–405.

Perelman, A. and Stern, J. (1974). Acute pancreatitis in West Nile Fever. *Am J Trop Med Hyg* 23(6): 1150–2.

Petersen, L. R. and Hayes, E. B. (2004). Westward ho?—The spread of West Nile virus. *N Engl J Med* 351(22): 2257–9.

Petersen, L. R. and Roehrig, J. T. (2001). West Nile virus: A reemerging global pathogen. *Emerg Infect Dis* 7(4): 611–4.

Peterson, A. T., Vieglais, D. A. and Andreasen, J. K. (2003). Migratory birds modeled as critical transport agents for West Nile Virus in North America. *Vector Borne Zoonotic Dis* 3(1): 27–37.

Pilipski, J., Pilipski, L. and Risley, L. (2004). West Nile virus antibodies in bats from New Jersey and New York. *J Wildlife Dis* 40(2): 335–7.

Platonov, A. E. (2001). West Nile encephalitis in Russia 1999-2001: Were we ready? Are we ready? *Ann N Y Acad Sci* 951: 102–16.

Platonov, A. E., Shipulin, G. A., Shipulina, O. Y., Tyutyunnik, E. N., Frolochkina, T. I., Lanciotti, R. S., Yazyshina, S., Platonova, O. V., Obukhov, I. L., Zhukov, A. N., Vengerov, Y. Y. and Pokrovskii,

V. I. (2001). Outbreak of West Nile virus infection, Volgograd Region, Russia, 1999. *Emerg Infect Dis* 7(1): 128–32.

Pletnev, A. G., Claire, M. S., Elkins, R., Speicher, J., Murphy, B. R. and Chanock, R. M. (2003). Molecularly engineered live-attenuated chimeric West Nile/dengue virus vaccines protect rhesus monkeys from West Nile virus. *Virology* 314(1): 190–5.

Pletnev, A. G., Putnak, R., Speicher, J., Wagar, E. J. and Vaughn, D. W. (2002). West Nile virus/dengue type 4 virus chimeras that are reduced in neurovirulence and peripheral virulence without loss of immunogenicity or protective efficacy. [Erratum appears in *Proc Natl Acad Sci U S A* 2002;99(10):7184] *Proc Natl Acad Sci U S A* 99(5): 3036–41.

Pogodina, V. V., Frolova, M. P., Malenko, G. V., Fokina, G. I., Koreshkova, G. V., Kiseleva, L. L., Bochkova, N. G. and Ralph, N. M. (1983). Study on West Nile virus persistence in monkeys. *Arch Virol* 75(1–2): 71–86.

Porter, M. B., Long, M. T., Getman, L. M., Giguere, S., MacKay, R. J., Lester, G. D., Alleman, A. R., Wamsley, H. L., Franklin, R. P., Jacks, S., Buergelt, C. D. and Detrisac, C. J. (2003). West Nile virus encephalomyelitis in horses: 46 cases (2001). *J Am Vet Med Assoc* 222(9): 1241–7.

Procop, G. W., Yen-Lieberman, B., Prayson, R. A. and Gordon, S. M. (2004). Mollaret-like cells in patients with West Nile virus infection. *Emerg Infect Dis* 10(4): 753–4.

Pyrgos, V. and Younus, F. (2004). High-dose steroids in the management of acute flaccid paralysis due to West Nile virus infection. *Scand J Infect Dis* 36(6–7): 509–12.

Quirin, R., Salas, M., Zientara, S., Zeller, H., Labie, J., Murri, S., Lefrancois, T., Petitclerc, M. and Martinez, D. (2004). West Nile virus, Guadeloupe. *Emerg Infect Dis* 10(4): 706–8.

Rappole, J. H. and Hubalek, Z. (2003). Migratory birds and West Nile virus. *J Appl Microbiol* 94 (Suppl): 47S–58S.

Ratterree, M. S., da Rosa, A. P., Bohm, R. P., Jr., Cogswell, F. B., Phillippi, K. M., Caillouet, K., Schwanberger, S., Shope, R. E. and Tesh, R. B. (2003). West Nile virus infection in nonhuman primate breeding colony, concurrent with human epidemic, southern Louisiana. *Emerg Infect Dis* 9(11): 1388–94.

Ravindra, K. V., Freifeld, A. G., Kalil, A. C., Mercer, D. F., Grant, W. J., Botha, J. F., Wrenshall, L. E. and Stevens, R. B. (2004). West Nile virus-associated encephalitis in recipients of renal and pancreas transplants: Case series and literature review. *Clin Infect Dis* 38(9): 1257–60.

Reagan, R. L., Yancey, F. S., Chang, S. C. and Brueckner, A. L. (1956). Transmission of West Nile virus (B956 strain) and Semliki Forest virus (MBB26146-M-404744-958 strain) to suckling hamsters during lactation. *J Immunol* 76(3): 243–245.

Reddy, P., Davenport, R., Ratanatharathorn, V., Reynolds, C., Silver, S., Ayash, L., Ferrara, J. L. and Uberti, J. P. (2004). West Nile virus encephalitis causing fatal CNS toxicity after hematopoietic stem cell transplantation. *Bone Marrow Transplant* 33(1): 109–12.

Reisen, W. K., Yoshimura, G., Reeves, W. C., Milby, M. M. and Meyer, R. P. (1984). The impact of aerial applications of ultra-low volume adulticides on Culex tarsalis populations (Diptera: Culicidae) in Kern County, California, USA, 1982. *J Med Entomol* 21(5): 573–85.

Rey, F. A., Heinz, F. X., Mandl, C., Kunz, C. and Harrison, S. C. (1995). The envelope glycoprotein from tick-borne encephalitis virus at 2 A resolution. *Nature* 375(6529): 291–8.

Rice, C. M., Grakoui, A., Galler, R. and Chambers, T. J. (1989). Transcription of infectious yellow fever RNA from full-length cDNA templates produced by in vitro ligation. *New Biol* 1(3): 285–96.

Rice, C. M., Lenches, E. M., Eddy, S. R., Shin, S. J., Sheets, R. L. and Strauss, J. H. (1985). Nucleotide sequence of yellow fever virus: Implications for flavivirus gene expression and evolution. *Science* 229(4715): 726–33.

Robertson, K. B., Barron, M. A. and Nieto, Y. (2004). West Nile virus infection in bone marrow transplant patients. *Bone Marrow Transplant* 34(9): 823–4.

Robinson, R. L., Shahida, S., Madan, N., Rao, S. and Khardori, N. (2003). Transient parkinsonism in West Nile virus encephalitis. *Am J Med* 115(3): 252–3.

Roehrig, J. T. (2000). Arboviruses. *Clinical Virology Manual*. S. Specter, R. L. Hodinka and S. A. Young. Washington, DC, ASM: 356–73.

Roehrig, J. T., Bolin, R. A. and Kelly, R. G. (1998). Monoclonal antibody mapping of the envelope glycoprotein of the dengue 2 virus, Jamaica. *Virology* 246(2): 317–28.

Roehrig, J. T., Layton, M., Smith, P., Campbell, G. L., Nasci, R. and Lanciotti, R. S. (2002). The emergence of West Nile virus in North America: Ecology, epidemiology, and surveillance. *Curr Topics Microbiol Immunol* 267: 223–40.

Roehrig, J. T., Mathews, J. H. and Trent, D. W. (1983). Identification of epitopes on the E glycoprotein of Saint Louis encephalitis virus using monoclonal antibodies. *Virology* 128(1): 118–26.

Roehrig, J. T., Nash, D., Maldin, B., Labowitz, A., Martin, D. A., Lanciotti, R. S. and Campbell, G. L. (2003). Persistence of virus-reactive serum immunoglobulin m antibody in confirmed west nile virus encephalitis cases. *Emerg Infect Dis* 9(3): 376–9.

Rosas, H. and Wippold, F. J., 2nd (2003). West Nile virus: Case report with MR imaging findings. *AJNR Am J Neuroradiol* 24(7): 1376–8.

Rose, R. I. (2001). Pesticides and public health: integrated methods of mosquito management. *Emerg Infect Dis* 7(1): 17–23.

Ryan, J., Dave, K., Emmerich, E., Fernandez, B., Turell, M., Johnson, J., Gottfried, K., Burkhalter, K., Kerst, A., Hunt, A., Wirtz, R. and Nasci, R. (2003). Wicking assays for the rapid detection of West Nile and St. Louis encephalitis viral antigens in mosquitoes (Diptera: Culicidae). *J Med Entomol* 40(1): 95–9.

Ryman, K. D., Ledger, T. N., Weir, R. C., Schlesinger, J. J. and Barrett, A. D. (1997). Yellow fever virus envelope protein has two discrete type-specific neutralizing epitopes. *J Gen Virol* 78 (Pt 6): 1353–6.

Salazar, P., Traub-Dargatz, J. L., Morley, P. S., Wilmot, D. D., Steffen, D. J., Cunningham, W. E. and Salman, M. D. (2004). Outcome of equids with clinical signs of West Nile virus infection and factors associated with death. *J Am Vet Med Assoc* 225(2): 267–74.

Sampson, B. A., Ambrosi, C., Charlot, A., Reiber, K., Veress, J. F. and Armbrustmacher, V. (2000). The pathology of human West Nile Virus infection. *Hum Pathol* 31(5): 527–31.

Sayao, A. L., Suchowersky, O., Al-Khathaami, A., Klassen, B., Katz, N. R., Sevick, R., Tilley, P., Fox, J. and Patry, D. (2004). Calgary experience with West Nile virus neurological syndrome during the late summer of 2003. *Can J Neurol Sci* 31(2): 194–203.

Scaramozzino, N., Crance, J. M., Jouan, A., DeBriel, D. A., Stoll, F. and Garin, D. (2001). Comparison of flavivirus universal primer pairs and development of a rapid, highly sensitive heminested reverse transcription-PCR assay for detection of flaviviruses targeted to a conserved region of the NS5 gene sequences. *J Clin Microbiol* 39(5): 1922–7.

Schlesinger, J. J., Brandriss, M. W., Cropp, C. B. and Monath, T. P. (1986). Protection against yellow fever in monkeys by immunization with yellow fever virus nonstructural protein NS1. *J Virol* 60(3): 1153–5.

Schlesinger, J. J., Brandriss, M. W. and Walsh, E. E. (1985). Protection against 17D yellow fever encephalitis in mice by passive transfer of monoclonal antibodies to the nonstructural glycoprotein gp48 and by active immunization with gp48. *J Immunol* 135(4): 2805–9.

Schlesinger, J. J., Brandriss, M. W. and Walsh, E. E. (1987). Protection of mice against dengue 2 virus encephalitis by immunization with the dengue 2 virus non-structural glycoprotein NS1. *J Gen Virol* 68 (Pt 3): 853–7.

Sejvar, J. J. (2004). West Nile virus and "poliomyelitis." *Neurology* 63(2): 206–7.

Sejvar, J. J., Haddad, M. B., Tierney, B. C., Campbell, G. L., Marfin, A. A., Van Gerpen, J. A., Fleischauer, A., Leis, A. A., Stokic, D. S. and Petersen, L. R. (2003a). Neurologic manifestations and outcome of West Nile virus infection. *JAMA* 290(4): 511–5.

Sejvar, J. J., Leis, A. A., Stokic, D. S., Van Gerpen, J. A., Marfin, A. A., Webb, R., Haddad, M. B., Tierney, B. C., Slavinski, S. A., Polk, J. L., Dostrow, V., Winkelmann, M. and Petersen, L. R. (2003b). Acute flaccid paralysis and West Nile virus infection. *Emerg Infect Dis* 9(7): 788–93.

Shaikh, S. and Trese, M. T. (2004). West Nile virus chorioretinitis. *Br J Ophthalmol* 88(12): 1599–60.

Sherman-Weber, S. and Axelrod, P. (2004). Central diabetes insipidus complicating West Nile encephalitis. *Clin Infect Dis* 38(7): 1042–3.

Shi, P. Y., Kauffman, E. B., Ren, P., Felton, A., Tai, J. H., Dupuis, A. P., 2nd, Jones, S. A., Ngo, K. A., Nicholas, D. C., Maffei, J., Ebel, G. D., Bernard, K. A. and Kramer, L. D. (2001). High-throughput detection of West Nile virus RNA. *J Clin Microbiol* 39(4): 1264–71.

Shi, P. Y., Tilgner, M., Lo, M. K., Kent, K. A. and Bernard, K. A. (2002). Infectious cDNA clone of the epidemic West Nile virus from New York City. *J Virol* 76(12): 5847–56.

Shieh, W. J., Guarner, J., Layton, M., Fine, A., Miller, J., Nash, D., Campbell, G. L., Roehrig, J. T., Gubler, D. J. and Zaki, S. R. (2000). The role of pathology in an investigation of an outbreak of West Nile encephalitis in New York, 1999. *Emerg Infect Dis* 6(4): 370–2.

Shimoni, Z., Niven, M. J., Pitlick, S. and Bulvik, S. (2001). Treatment of West Nile virus encephalitis with intravenous immunoglobulin. *Emerg Infect Dis* 7(4): 759.

Siger, L., Bowen, R. A., Karaca, K., Murray, M. J., Gordy, P. W., Loosmore, S. M., Audonnet, J. C., Nordgren, R. M. and Minke, J. M. (2004). Assessment of the efficacy of a single dose of a recombinant vaccine against West Nile virus in response to natural challenge with West Nile virus-infected mosquitoes in horses. *Am J Vet Res* 65(11): 1459–62.

Smith, R. D., Konoplev, S., DeCourten-Myers, G. and Brown, T. (2004). West Nile virus encephalitis with myositis and orchitis. *Hum Pathol* 35(2): 254–8.

Smithburn, K. C., Hughes, T. P., Burke, A. W. and Paul, J. H. (1940). A neurotropic virus isolated from the blood of a native of Uganda. *Am J Trop Med Hyg* 20: 470–92.

Solomon, T. (2004). Flavivirus encephalitis. *N Engl J Med* 351(4): 370–8.

Solomon, T., Dung, N. M., Wills, B., Kneen, R., Gainsborough, M., Diet, T. V., Thuy, T. T., Loan, H. T., Khanh, V. C., Vaughn, D. W., White, N. J. and Farrar, J. J. (2003). Interferon alfa-2a in Japanese encephalitis: A randomised double-blind placebo-controlled trial. *Lancet* 361(9360): 821–6.

Southam, C. M. and Moore, A. E. (1954). Induced virus infections in man by the Egypt isolates of West Nile virus. *Am J Trop Med Hyg* 3(1): 19–50.

Spigland, I., Jasinska-Klingberg, W., Hofshi, E. and Goldblum, N. (1958). Clinical and laboratory observations in an outbreak of West Nile fever in Israel in 1957. *Harefuah* 54(11): 275–81.

Stiasny, K., Allison, S. L., Schalich, J. and Heinz, F. X. (2002). Membrane interactions of the tick–borne encephalitis virus fusion protein E at low pH. *J Virol* 76(8): 3784–90.

Swayne, D. E., Beck, J. R., Smith, C. S., Shieh, W. J. and Zaki, S. R. (2001). Fatal encephalitis and myocarditis in young domestic geese (Anser anser domesticus) caused by West Nile virus. *Emerg Infect Dis* 7(4): 751–3.

Szilak, I. and Minamoto, G. Y. (2000). West Nile viral encephalitis in an HIV-positive woman in New York. *N Engl J Med* 342(1): 59–60.

Tan, B. H., Fu, J., Sugrue, R. J., Yap, E. H., Chan, Y. C. and Tan, Y. H. (1996). Recombinant dengue type 1 virus NS5 protein expressed in Escherichia coli exhibits RNA-dependent RNA polymerase activity. *Virology* 216(2): 317–25.

Tesh, R. B., Arroyo, J., Travassos Da Rosa, A. P., Guzman, H., Xiao, S. Y. and Monath, T. P. (2002). Efficacy of killed virus vaccine, live attenuated chimeric virus vaccine, and passive immunization for prevention of West Nile virus encephalitis in hamster model. *Emerg Infect Dis* 8(12): 1392–7.

Tsai, T. F., Bolin, R. A., Montoya, M., Bailey, R. E., Francy, D. B., Jozan, M. and Roehrig, J. T. (1987). Detection of St. Louis encephalitis virus antigen in mosquitoes by capture enzyme immunoassay. *J Clin Microbiol* 25(2): 370–6.

Tsai, T. F., Happ, C. M., Bolin, R. A., Montoya, M., Campos, E., Francy, D. B., Hawkes, R. A. and Roehrig, J. T. (1988). Stability of St. Louis encephalitis viral antigen detected by enzyme immunoassay in infected mosquitoes. *J Clin Microbiol* 26(12): 2620–5.

Tsai, T. F., Popovici, F., Cernescu, C., Campbell, G. L. and Nedelcu, N. I. (1998). West Nile encephalitis epidemic in southeastern Romania. *Lancet* 352(9130): 767–71.

Tyler, J. W., Turnquist, S. E., David, A. T., Kleiboeker, S. B. and Middleton, J. R. (2003). West Nile virus encephalomyelitis in a sheep. *J Vet Int Med* 17(2): 242–4.

Vaispapir, V., Blum, A., Soboh, S. and Ashkenazi, H. (2002). West Nile virus meningoencephalitis with optic neuritis. *Arch Int Med* 162(5): 606–7.

Valle, R. P. and Falgout, B. (1998). Mutagenesis of the NS3 protease of dengue virus type 2. *J Virol* 72(1): 624–32.

Vandenbelt, S., Shaikh, S., Capone, A., Jr. and Williams, G. A. (2003). Multifocal choroiditis associated with West Nile virus encephalitis. *Retina* 23(1): 97–9.

Vidwan, G., Bryant, K. K., Puri, V., Stover, B. H. and Rabalais, G. P. (2003). West Nile virus encephalitis in a child with left-side weakness. *Clin Infect Dis* 37(6): e91–4.

Wadei, H., Alangaden, G. H., Sillix, D. H., El-Amm, J. M., Gruber, S. A., West, M. S., Granger, D. K., Garnick, J., Chandrasekar, P., Migdal, S. D. and Haririan, A. (2004). West Nile virus encephalitis: An emerging disease in renal transplant recipients. *Clin Transplant* 18: 753–8.

Ward, M. P., Levy, M., Thacker, H. L., Ash, M., Norman, S. K., Moore, G. E. and Webb, P. W. (2004). Investigation of an outbreak of encephalomyelitis caused by West Nile virus in 136 horses. *J Am Vet Med Assoc* 225(1): 84–9.

Watson, J. T., Pertel, P. E., Jones, R. C., Siston, A. M., Paul, W. S., Austin, C. C. and Gerber, S. I. (2004). Clinical characteristics and functional outcomes of West Nile fever. *Ann Intern Med* 141(5): 360–5.

Weese, J. S., Baird, J. D., DeLay, J., Kenney, D. G., Staempfli, H. R., Viel, L., Parent, J., Smith–Maxie, L. and Poma, R. (2003). West Nile virus encephalomyelitis in horses in Ontario: 28 cases. *Can Vet J* 44(6): 469–73.

Weingartl, H. M., Neufeld, J. L., Copps, J. and Marszal, P. (2004). Experimental West Nile virus infection in blue jays (Cyanocitta cristata) and crows (Corvus brachyrhynchos). *Vet Pathol* 41(4): 362–70.

Weiss, D., Carr, D., Kellachan, J., Tan, C., Phillips, M., Bresnitz, E., Layton, M. and West Nile Virus Outbreak Response Working, G. (2001). Clinical findings of West Nile virus infection in hospitalized patients, New York and New Jersey, 2000. *Emerg Infect Dis* 7(4): 654–8.

Wengler, G. (1989). An analysis of the antibody response against West Nile virus E protein purified by SDS-PAGE indicates that this protein does not contain sequential epitopes for efficient induction of neutralizing antibodies. *J Gen Virol* 70 (Pt 4): 987–92.

Westaway, E. G., Khromykh, A. A. and Mackenzie, J. M. (1999). Nascent flavivirus RNA colocalized in situ with double-stranded RNA in stable replication complexes. *Virology* 258(1): 108–17.

Westaway, E. G., Mackenzie, J. M., Kenney, M. T., Jones, M. K. and Khromykh, A. A. (1997). Ultrastructure of Kunjin virus-infected cells: Colocalization of NS1 and NS3 with double-stranded RNA, and of NS2B with NS3, in virus-induced membrane structures. *J Virol* 71(9): 6650–61.

Wong, S. J., Boyle, R. H., Demarest, V. L., Woodmansee, A. N., Kramer, L. D., Li, H., Drebot, M., Koski, R. A., Fikrig, E., Martin, D. A. and Shi, P. Y. (2003). Immunoassay targeting nonstructural protein 5 to differentiate West Nile virus infection from dengue and St. Louis encephalitis virus infections and from flavivirus vaccination. *J Clin Microbiol* 41(9): 4217–23.

Wong, S. J., Demarest, V. L., Boyle, R. H., Wang, T., Ledizet, M., Kar, K., Kramer, L. D., Fikrig, E. and Koski, R. A. (2004). Detection of human anti-flavivirus antibodies with a West Nile virus recombinant antigen microsphere immunoassay. *J Clin Microbiol* 42(1): 65–72.

Yaeger, M., Yoon, K. J., Schwartz, K. and Berkland, L. (2004). West Nile virus meningoencephalitis in a Suri alpaca and Suffolk ewe. *J Vet Diagn Invest* 16(1): 64–6.

Yamshchikov, V. F., Wengler, G., Perelygin, A. A., Brinton, M. A. and Compans, R. W. (2001). An infectious clone of the West Nile flavivirus. *Virology* 281(2): 294–304.

Yaremych, S. A., Warner, R. E., Mankin, P. C., Brawn, J. D., Raim, A. and Novak, R. (2004). West Nile virus and high death rate in American crows. *Emerg Infect Dis* 10(4): 709–11.

Yim, R., Posfay-Barbe, K. M., Nolt, D., Fatula, G. and Wald, E. R. (2004). Spectrum of clinical manifestations of West Nile virus infection in children. *Pediatrics* 114(6): 1673–5.

You, S., Falgout, B., Markoff, L. and Padmanabhan, R. (2001). In vitro RNA synthesis from exogenous dengue viral RNA templates requires long range interactions between 5'- and 3'-terminal regions that influence RNA structure. *J Biol Chem* 276(19): 15581–91.

Zhao, B., Mackow, E., Buckler-White, A., Markoff, L., Chanock, R. M., Lai, C. J. and Makino, Y. (1986). Cloning full-length dengue type 4 viral DNA sequences: Analysis of genes coding for structural proteins. *Virology* 155(1): 77–88.

2. Hantavirus Cardiopulmonary Syndrome: A New Twist to an Established Pathogen

FREDERICK T. KOSTER AND HOWARD LEVY

Human disease due to hantaviruses (HV) worldwide are virus strain–dependent variations on the theme of vascular leak syndrome. In the Americas, hantaviruses cause a syndrome called hantavirus pulmonary syndrome (HPS), or hantavirus cardiopulmonary syndrome (HCPS), the latter to recognize the central role of cardiac involvement in fatal disease. In Asia and Europe, hantaviruses cause the hemorrhagic fever renal syndrome (HFRS) and the milder variant nephropathia epidemica (NE). HFRS was described during the Korean conflict and the virus first isolated in 1978, but in retrospect the disease was described in China centuries earlier (Johnson, 2001). The field was reinvigorated by the discovery of HPS and Sin Nombre (SN) virus in 1993 in the American Southwest (Nichol et al., 1993; Duchin et al., 1994), but in retrospect aspects of the disease were probably described in Navajo legend centuries earlier. Two comprehensive reviews cover broad aspects of hantaviruses (Nichol, 2001; Schmaljohn and Hooper, 2001), and other excellent reviews focus on particular aspects of the pathogen and disease (Johnson, 2001; Plyusnin and Morzunov, 2001; Bausch and Ksiazek, 2002; Hjelle, 2002; Khaiboullina and St. Jeor, 2002; Vapalahti et al., 2003; Maes et al., 2004; Pini, 2004). This review synthesizes recent information on the pathophysiology and treatment of hantaviral infections focusing primarily on HCPS and highlighting the parallels and contrasts with HFRS.

2.1. Virology

2.1.1. Classification and Characteristics

Hantavirus is a genus of enveloped, tripartite, negative-sense RNA viruses in the Bunyaviridae family (Table 2.1) and is the only group in this family that is not a naturally arthropod-borne virus. Since the isolation in 1978 of its prototype Hantaan virus (HTN) (Lee et al., 1978), the genus has grown to include more than 20 different viruses, as distinguished by amino acid sequence differences or the more classic plaque reduction neutralization test (PRNT) (Chu et al., 1995). Viruses commonly associated with human infection and disease in Asia and Europe include Hantaan (HTN), Seoul (SEO), Dobrava (DOB), and Puumala (PUU) and in the Americas include sin nombre (SN), New York (NY), Choclo (CHO), Andes (AND), Laguna Negra (LN), the Oran clade in Argentina, Juquitiba (JUQ), Araraquara (ARA), and others in Brazil (Table 2.1). Other hantaviruses have been isolated from natural hosts but have not been associated with human infection, including Topografov (TOP), Isla Vista (ISLA), El Moro Canyon (ELMC), Rio Segundo (RIOS), Muleshoe (MUL), Rio Mamore (RIOM), Bloodland Lake (BLL), Delgadito (DEL), Maporal (MAP), and Calabazo (CAL) viruses (Zeier et al., 2005). Each virus has a specific primary natural rodent host (Table 2.1), although spillover into related species is frequently documented. Why some hantaviruses cause human infection and others do not is not understood.

The hantaviruses are relatively stable in nature (Schmaljohn, 1996). M genomic sequences of Sweetwater canyon virus isolated from deer mice in 1983 in California compared with two strains of SN virus causing HCPS in 1993 in New Mexico showed nucleotide sequence variation of less than 14%, and the deduced amino acid sequences varied less than 2% despite a 10-year span and 500-mile separation (Hjelle et al., 1994a; Jay et al., 1997). Evidence of high amino acid conservation (about 95%) in M segments also has been shown in NY virus and the recently described Oligoryzomys-borne genotypes in Argentina, despite variation of nucleotide sequences of 10–20% in strains isolated from different geographic locations (Levis et al., 1998; Morzunov et al., 1998). Phylogenetic relatedness of the hantaviruses generally mirrors that of their natural host, supporting the hypothesis of hantavirus–host coevolution or cospeciation (Yates et al., 2002).

2.1.2. Viral Replication

Hantavirus is lipid solvent sensitive and acid labile (pH <5) but can remain infectious for several days after excretion by rodents into the environment (Schmaljohn, 1996). Hantavirus virions appear spherical to slightly oval in shape with a diameter ranging from 71 to 200 nm, averaging 100 nm (Goldsmith et al., 1995). The virions have a dense, bilayered lipid membrane encasing the granulofilamentous nucleocapsid,

Table 2.1. The hantaviruses associated with human infection

Hantavirus strain (abbr.)	Host rodent (species)	Geographic range	Syndrome	Case:infection ratio	Annual incidence (n)/mortality rate (%)
Eurasian					
Hantaan (HTN)	Striped field mouse (*Apodemus agrarius*)	Eastern, central Asia	HFRS	1:1.5	100,000/1–5%
Seoul (SEO)	Common rat (*Rattus norvegicus*)	Urban worldwide	HFRS	Unknown	Unknown/1–2%
Puumala (PUU)	Bank vole (*Clethrionomys glareolus*)	Northern, central Europe	NE	1:20	30,000/0.1–1.0%
Dobrava (DOB)	Yellow-necked field mouse (*Apodemus falvicollis*)	Balkans	HFRS	Unknown	100/15%
Tula (TUL)	European common voles (*Microtus arvalis, M. agrestis*)	Central, northern Europe	NE	Unknown	Unknown/0%
Saaremaa (SAA)	Striped field mouse (*Apodemus agyarius*)	Northern Europe	NE	Unknown	Unknown/0%
American					
Sin nombre (SN)	Deer mouse (*Peromyscus maniculatus*)	Western North America	HCPS	2:1	20–80/35–40%
New York (NY)	White-footed mouse (*Peromyscus leucopus*)	Eastern North America	HCPS	Unknown	3 cases/1 fatal
Black Creek Canal (BCC)	Cotton rat (*Sigmodon hispidus*)	Florida	HCPS	Unknown	1 case/0
Bayou (BAY)	Rice rat (*Oryzomys palustris*)	Louisiana, eastern Texas	HCPS	Unknown	5 cases/1 fatal
Andes (AND)	Long-tailed rice rat (*Oligoryzomys longicaudatus*)	Argentina, Chile	HCPS	1:2	50–200/35–40%
Laguna Negra (LN)	Small vesper mouse, large vesper mouse (*Calomys laucha, C. callosus*)	Western Paraguay, northwestern Argentina, southern Bolivia	HCPS	1:10	2–30/9%
Choclo (CHO)	Costa Rican rice rat (*O. fulvesens*)	Western Panama	HCPS	1:20	2–30/10%
Bermejo (BMJ)	Yellow pigmy rice rat (*O. flavescens* or *O. chacoensis*)	Northern Argentina, southern Bolivia	HCPS	Unknown	Unknown/20%
Oran (ORN)	Long-tailed rice rat (*O. longicaudatus*)	Northwestern Argentina, southern Bolivia	HCPS	Unknown	Unknown/35%
Lechiguanes (LEC)	Yellow pigmy rice rat (*O. flavescens*)	Central Argentina	HCPS	Unknown	Unknown/30%
Juquitibé (JUQ)	Black-footed pygmy rice rat (*O. nigripos*)	Southern Brazil	HCPS	Unknown	Unknown/25%
Araraquara (ARA)	Hairy-tailed bolo mouse (*Bolomys lasiurus*)	Central Brazil	HCPS	Unknown	20–50/25%
Castelo dos Sonkos (CAS)	Unknown	Central Brazil	HCPS	Unknown	Unknown/25%

HFRS, hemorrhage fever renal syndrome; NE, nephropathia epidemica; HCPS, hantavirus cardiopulmonary syndrome.

often appearing as parallel filaments or coils, and like all members of the Bunyaviridae family, but unlike other negative-sense RNA virus families, lack an internal matrix protein.

The hantavirus genome consists of three segments of single-stranded, negative-sense RNA, denoted long (L), medium (M), and short (S) segments, respectively. Complete genome sequences have been determined for seven hantaviruses: HTN, SEO, PUU, Prospect Hill (PH), SN, AND, and Tula (TUL). The 5' and 3' termini of all three RNA segments have highly conserved regions that are complementary to each other and are thought to serve as a panhandle structure (Chizhikov et al., 1995; Plyusnin et al., 1996).

S segments range in size from 1.7 to 2.1 kb and contain regions of conserved and variable sequences. S-cRNA has an open reading frame (ORF) that encodes a nucleocapsid (N) protein of about 430 amino acids (aa) with molecular weight approximately 48 kDa. The 3' non-coding region (NCR) in S-cRNA is long (331–730 bp). The function (s) of NCRs is unknown but may have some roles in the regulation of viral transcription and replication. A potential ORF has been found in some viral sequences, either sharing the same ORF for N protein or overlapping with the N-ORF, but no protein has been found. The 3.6–3.7 kb M-segment contains a single ORF that encodes a glycoprotein precursor polypeptide (GPC) of about 1135 aa. GPC is processed by co-translational cleavage to produce two surface glycoproteins G1 and G2, coded in the order of 5' G1–G2 3' and consisting of approximately 652 and 488 aa, calculated to be 64 and 54 kDa, respectively. Common structural features are found in the G1 and G2 proteins, including a specific five-amino-acid sequence WAASA preceding the co-translational cleavage site, three potential N-glycosylation sites in all G1 proteins at amino acids 142, 358, and 410 and in all G2 proteins at aa 939, and 57 conserved cysteine residues (Spiropoulou et al., 1994). The 6.5–6.6 kb L segment contains a large single ORF in the cRNA that encodes the RNA-dependent RNA polymerase of approximately 2150 amino acids, with a molecular weight of about 250 kDa. The 3' and 5' termini are short (about 40 bp).

Complementary mRNAs and genomic RNAs are synthesized from the negative-sense viral RNA genomes. Hantavirus mRNAs are not polyadenylated, and the exact length of these mRNAs has not been determined. Similar to other bunyaviruses, HTN mRNAs contain heterogeneous 5' terminal extensions adopted from the host. A "prime-and-realign" mechanism of initiation has been proposed for both mRNA and genomic RNA synthesis, and a comprehensive description of the mechanism is described in Schmaljohn and Hooper (2001).

2.2. Pathophysiology and Animal Models

2.2.1. Cell Entry

Cell entry of pathogenic hantaviruses is dependent on β3 integrin. Cells expressing recombinant αvβ3 or αIIbβ3 on surfaces facilitated SNV and NY-1 virus infection, but not for the nonpathogenic Prospect Hill virus (PH) (Gavrilovskaya et al., 1998). Cell entry of SNV and NY-1 viruses can be inhibited by antibodies to β3 integrins and by the β3-integrin ligand vitronectin in an arginine–glycine–aspartic acid directed ligand (RGD)-independent fashion, and infection by PH virus is reduced by β1-integrin antibodies and fibronectin. Mackow and colleagues have elegantly demonstrated HV-specific, RGD-independent binding to an apical domain (the plexin–semaphorin–integrin domain) of the bent, inactive conformation of $\alpha_V\beta_3$ integrin (Raymond et al., 2005). HV-β3 interaction is likely to lock the integrin in a bent conformation and inhibit endothelial cell movement (Gavrilovskaya et al., 2002). The thrombocytopenia and vascular permeability defects seen in multiple bleeding disorders that involve β3-integrin dysfunction are similar to those defects in HCPS. Innovative strategies are needed to test the role of β3-integrin dysfunction in HV pathogenesis discussed below.

Studies in other bunyaviruses showed that N proteins can be detected within 2 h after infection and the surface glycoproteins shortly thereafter, indicating that viral mRNAs are transcribed and translated very rapidly (Bishop, 1996). Cytoplasmic inclusion bodies consisting of N protein are usually found closely associated with rough endoplasmic reticulum and Golgi complex (Goldsmith et al., 1995). The carboxyterminal domains of HTN N-proteins form multimers in mammalian cells (Yoshimatsu et al., 2003). Trimers of SN N-protein bind with high affinity the panhandle structure of the three hantaviral RNAs, are able to distinguish viral from nonviral RNA, and are required for encapsidation of the three viral RNAs (Mir and Panganiban, 2004, 2005) . The N proteins of Black Creek Canal (BCC) localize to actin microfilaments, suggesting that actin microfilaments may be involved in hantavirus assembly and release (Ravkov et al., 1998). In polarized kidney epithelial (Vero) cells, both SN and BCC are more efficiently taken up and released from the apical surface, unlike other members of Bunyaviridae (Goldsmith et al., 1995; Ravkov et al., 1997).

Envelope G1 and G2 proteins are N-linked glycosylated transmembrane proteins existing as a heterodimer first dimerizing in the endoplasmic reticulum, then targeting to the Golgi complex (Ruusala et al., 1992). SN buds at the plasma membrane of infected cells (Goldsmith et al., 1995). G1 and G2 proteins contain neutralizing epitopes. The G1 protein contains immunoreceptor typrosine-based activation motifs (ITAMs) that bind

T cell, B cell, and endothelial cell signaling kinases (Geimonen et al., 2003). The conservation of these motifs among pathogenic American HV and their role in signaling regulation in vascular endothelia suggest a role in HV pathogenesis, as discussed below.

2.2.2. Virulence

Reverse genetics technology has begun to provide the opportunity to study the molecular pathogenesis of virulence of bunyaviruses (Flick and Pettersson, 2001; Flick et al., 2002) and hantaviruses (Flick et al., 2003). Clues for virulence characteristics derives from reassortant variants, loss-of-function mutations, and interactions with the interferon-induced proteins in eukaryotic cells. As in many negative-sense RNA viruses (Chare et al., 2003), reassortment of segments occurs in nature in Sin Nombre virus (Henderson et al., 1995; Li et al., 1995), Puumala virus (Sironen et al., 2001), and Tula virus (Sibold et al., 1999). An S-segment recombinant Tula virus was not competitive with the wild-type virus over multiple cell passages, but the observed survival time would theoretically permit transmission of recombinant hantaviruses in nature (Plyusnina and Plyusnin, 2005). *In vitro* double infection resulting in segment shuffling between Andes and SN virus infections suggests that the M segment is not the primary site of virulence expression for Andes virus (McElroy et al., 2004).

As seen in RNA viruses (Domingo and Holland, 1997), alternation-of-phenotype mutations have been located in the L, M, and S segments. Loss of a potential N-glycosylation site in the G2 protein at position 900 was found in a PUU strain associated with a more severe form of nephropathia epidemica in Germany (Pilaski et al., 1994). Replacement of serine with glycine at position 1124 of the G2 protein was associated with a reduction of viral virulence, perhaps as a result of altered palmitoylation reducing fusion activity (Isegawa et al., 1994). A single amino acid change in the G1 glycoprotein of an HTN strain virulent in neonatal mice resulted in decreased virulence and reduced invasion of the central nervous system (Ebihara et al., 2000). Adaptation of rodent-derived hantavirus strains to serial passage in primate cell cultures has resulted in multiple mutations primarily in coding and non-coding regions of the L and S segments (Chizhikov et al., 1995; Lundkvist et al., 1997; Nemirov et al., 2003), but no unifying principles have yet emerged. Relating genetic determinants to pathogenesis is difficult when there are many nucleotide differences between strains of different virulence, and the field awaits the application of reverse genetics technology.

2.2.3. Cellular Targets for HV

HV infect primarily endothelial cells (ECs) *in vivo* but also infect alveolar macrophages and follicular dendritic cells, and some HV infect renal tubular epithelial cells. Evidence for infection of circulating T cells is not yet conclusive. Histopathological studies find viral antigen in capillary endothelial cells systemically, but it is not known how much this represents replicating virus. Highest levels of antigen are found in the lung with lesser amounts in heart, kidney, liver, and spleen (Nolte et al., 1995; Zaki et al., 1995; Green et al., 1998). No cytopathic effects are seen *in vitro* or *in vivo*. HV infects dendritic cells (DCs) expressing β3 integrins in the mature or immature phenotype, without inducing cytopathic effect or apoptosis (Raftery et al., 2002). Moreover, infection does not inhibit the differentiation to a mature phenotype nor inhibit the ability to sensitize T lymphocytes, suggesting that DCs are at least permissive for HV replication.

The absence of interferon-α/β induced Mx proteins appears to render Vero cells permissive for HV growth, and Mx gene products inhibit HV replication (Frese et al., 1996; Kanerva et al., 1996; Jin et al., 2001). In human respiratory type II epithelial cell line A549, HTN was inhibited by Mx1 and 2′,5′-oligoadenylated synthetase genes, but not by RNA-dependent protein kinase R (PKR) (Nam et al., 2003). The pathogenic NY-1 and HTN viruses appeared to suppress many early cellular interferon responses in endothelial cells, responses not suppressed by the non-pathogenic PH virus (Geimonen et al., 2002). In human umbilical vein endothelial cells (HUVECs), HTN replicated efficiently for 48 h prior to delayed induction of MxA protein, whereas the less pathogenic TUL virus replicated inefficiently in HUVECs accompanied by early MxA protein expression (Kraus et al., 2004). These results link virulence to interferon-stimulated gene suppression, as documented for many RNA viruses, and awaits the application of RNAi and reverse genetics technologies to elucidate the details.

Infection of endothelial cell monolayers by HV, without added factors, does not induce monolayer permeability (Sundstrom et al., 2001). Tumor necrosis factor-α (TNF-α) alone may initiate endothelial cell monolayer permeability (Goldblum et al., 1993), and low levels of TNF added to endothelial cells infected with SN virus (Khaiboullina et al., 2000) or Hantaan virus (Niikura et al., 2004) will induce modest increases in monolayer permeability. This increase in permeability is not associated with apoptosis, intercellular gap formation, nitric oxide production, or prostaglandin production (Niikura et al., 2004). In general, infection of HUVECs induces variable arrays of gene transcription, with upregulation of chemokine genes but not cytokine genes, and pathogenic hantaviruses induce different patterns from nonpathogenic strains (Geimonen et al., 2002; Khaiboullina et al., 2004). Although HV may induce apoptosis in Vero cells (Kang et al., 1999), there is currently no immunohistochemical evidence that apoptosis of endothelial cells in the human pulmonary vasculature accounts for the vascular leak.

2.2.4. Pathology and Pathogenesis

The evidence for altered vascular permeability has been recognized for years in HFRS with widespread capillary engorgement, focal hemor-rhage, and interstitial edema in many organs (Lukes, 1954). Retroperi-toneal edema is massive in some cases, with histologic evidence for renal medullary congestion, pituitary necrosis, and adrenal hemorrhage and necrosis in many fatal cases. In HCPS, the most striking finding at autopsy is edematous lungs with pleural effusions as large as 8 L (Nolte et al., 1995; Zaki et al., 1995). Pulmonary edema fluid has an identical protein electrophoresis pattern to that of serum, documenting the severity of loss of reflection coefficient of the alveolar-capillary membrane (Levy and Simpson, 1994; Bustamente et al., 1997). Also striking is the low cell count in bronchoalveolar lavage samples, the near absence of red cell con-tamination, and the large volume generated, often exceeding 1.0 L of straw-colored fluid aspirated each hour from the endotracheal tube. The heart, kidneys, brain, and adrenals are grossly and histologically normal. The liver may be slightly enlarged and has microscopic evidence of tria-ditis. In fatal cases, histologically the pulmonary alveoli are filled with acellular proteinaceous fluid with hyaline-like membranes. The modestly thickened septa contain primarily large mononuclear cells, including immunoblasts, monocytes, and plasma cells but few polymorphonuclear leukocytes, and the alveolar epithelial cells are intact. This picture is in marked contrast with acute respiratory distress syndrome, characterized by thickened septa, hyaline membranes, and neutrophilic inflammatory infiltrate in the septa and alveoli, and to typical viral pneumonitis, characterized by mixed cellular infiltrate in interstitium and alveoli and disrupted alveolar epithelial cell layer.

In HFRS, circulating immune complexes are detected (Luo et al., 1985), and the classical complement pathway is activated (Yan et al., 1981). Moreover, the kidney in the acute phase of nephropathia epi-demica contains deposits of immunoglobulin and complement beneath the basement membrane, suggesting that immune complexes may have a role in the immunopathogenesis of the renal lesion in HFRS (Jokinen et al., 1978). In contrast, in HCPS, circulating immune complexes have not been detected by several assay, and serum levels of activated complement components are normal or slightly depressed, and electron microscopy of lung and kidney have not revealed typical immune complex deposits. The coagulopathy of HFRS is represented as an imbalance of coagulation over fibrinolysis combined with platelet dysfunction (Cosgriff, 1991). In addition to thrombocytopenia, coagulation defects in HCPS due to SN virus are more subtle than HFRS but include reduced activated partial thromboplastin time, marked decrease in plasminogen activator inhibitor-1 (PAI-1), and inverse correlation between PAI-1 and activated protein C (H. Levy, unpublished data). High PAI-1 preventing a switch from procoagulant state to profibrinolytic state is also observed in lethal dengue hemorrhagic fever (Van Gorp et al., 2002).

The role of the virus in directly mediating tissue injury has been questioned in light of the absence of cytopathic effect. There are, however, two lines of evidence implicating the virus in SN disease. First, a semiquantitative assay for plasma viral RNA found a positive correlation between high viral load and hemoconcentration and thrombocytopenia, with a trend toward fatal disease (Terajima et al., 1999). Second, a clear relationship exists between survival and higher neutralizing antibody titers in HCPS (Bharadwaj et al., 2000), and this relationship has been confirmed for Andes virus infection in Chile (H. Galeno, unpublished data). Finally, the binding of pathogenic HVs to $\beta3$ integrins and the similarities of HCPS to a group of bleeding disorders characterized by dysregulated $\beta3$ integrins suggests key events at the virus–endothelial cell membrane interaction (Raymond et al., 2005).

2.2.5. Role of the T-Cell Response

A number of lines of evidence have implicated cellular immune responses, particularly CD8+ T cells, in the pathogenesis of both HFRS and HCPS. In HFRS, the presence of activated T cells, soluble interleukin-2 receptors, and interferon-γ-producing cells in peripheral blood is evidence of highly activated T cells (Huang et al., 1994). The immunoblasts populating the lung, pleural effusion, liver, spleen, lymph nodes, and bloodstream are a striking feature of HCPS (Nolte et al., 1995). Immunoperoxidase studies document monocytes and T cells in lung parenchyma (Zaki et al., 1995). Flow cytometry studies identified the large blast-like cells in blood and pleural fluid as predominantly activated CD8+ T cells, but also included CD4+ T cells and B cells. Elevated plasma levels of interleukin-2, interleukin-2 receptors, interferon-γ, interleukin-6, interleukin-10, TNF-α, and soluble receptors for TNF-α suggest marked cytokine activation (F. Koster, unpublished data). Most striking in

SN infection was the relationship between high TNF levels and severity, and high IL-8 levels found only in severe HCPS. A similar array of elevated serum cytokines are found in PUU infection (Linderholm et al., 1996). In fatal cases of SN infection, abundant mononuclear cells in lung and spleen tissue secreted TNF-α, IL-1, IL-6, and IL-2 (Mori et al., 1999). Activated immunoblastic cells are few or absent infiltrating the kidney, heart, and most other tissues, in spite of the presence of viral antigen in endothelial cells in these organs, supporting the speculation that the cellular infiltrate, not the virus, is responsible for tissue injury in the lung in HCPS (Zaki et al., 1995; Mori et al., 1999).

Compelling evidence is pointing to a critical role for virus-specific T cells, particularly CD8+ T cells, in pathogenesis using HLA allelic-specific disease associations and enumeration of HV-specific T cells. Shock and renal failure in PUU infection is associated with the major histocompatibility complex (MHC) extended haplotype HLA-B8-DR3, and mild disease is associated with the class I allele HLA-B27 (Mustonen et al., 1996, 2004). The C4A null allele and the TNF2 hyperproducer phenotype allele are in linkage disequilibrium with the B8 allele and may passively contribute to the severe disease phenotype (Makela et al., 2002). In HCPS, preliminary data from 75 patients indicate that severe disease with cardiogenic shock and requirement for mechanical ventilation is associated with the MHC class I allele HLA-B*3501, and mild disease is associated with the B*27 allele (R. Olson et al., unpublished data). Allele associations cannot indicate which linked gene or genes are responsible for disease phenotype, but these associations do implicate MHC class I restricted antigen-specific responses mediated by CD8+ T cells.

Epitopes of SN, HTN, and PUU virus, described with in vitro– expanded, cloned CD4+ and CD8+ T cells, and interferon-γ secretion screening, have illustrated strain-specific epitopes in general (Ennis et al., 1997; Van Epps et al., 1999; Terajima et al., 2002; Van Epps et al., 2002; Kilpatrick et al., 2004; Terajima et al., 2004). Circulating numbers of epitope-specific T cells years after infection compare with other viral infections such as influenza. During the acute phase of SN infection as severely ill patients are entering the cardiopulmonary phase, the numbers of circulating epitope-specific, HLA-B*3501-restricted CD8+ T cells are high (Kilpatrick et al., 2004). Moreover, although numbers of moderately ill patients was small, there was a significant relationship between disease severity and higher numbers of SN-specific T cells for all three epitopes studied. Thus multiple lines of evidence implicates the contribution of specific CD8+ T cells in the evolution of disease severity. Whether the more vigorous CD8+ T-cell responses are linked to the deficits or delays in generating an effective neutralizing antibody response through the complexities of immunoregulation should be the subject of intensive investigation for this and other viral diseases.

We can construct an hypothesis of events leading to massive capillary leak in the lung in HCPS (Fig. 2.1). An early viremia prior to symptom onset seeds the lung endothelial cells with virus, resulting in secretion of chemokines but not cytopathology. The endothelial cells become targets for attack by virus-specific cytolytic T cells when this arm of the immune response matures several days later than the virus-specific IgM and IgG antibodies. Local production of interferon-α/β and T-cell secretion of interferon-γ and TNF-α may control viral replication, but the TNF-α contribution may injure the infected and bystander endothelial cells, creating temporary paracellular gaps for escaping plasma fluid but not cells. The complex relationships between TNF-α, tissue factor (TF), extrinsic clotting factors (Friedl et al., 2002), endothelial cell membrane expression of αVβ3 integrins, and alterations of these by hantaviruses (Raymond et al., 2005) may mediate synergistic effects between multiple factors resultling in massive capillary leak. High levels of IL-8 may impair the local interferon-α/β response (Khabar et al., 1997) and nitric oxide synthetase induction (McCall et al., 1992) while attracting large numbers of neutrophils into the circulation and lungs. In the absence of studies in animal models, these hypothesized events remain speculative, along with the existence of other mediators inducing paracellular gaps and the coagulopathy.

The mechanisms of acute reversible myocardial dysfunction (not shown in Fig. 2.1) also remain speculative, but a role for excessive nitric oxide (Davis et al., 2002) may result in nitrosylated ryanodine receptors and excitation–contraction uncoupling in the myocardium (Finkel et al., 1992; Iqbal et al., 2002). Elevated circulating TNF-α has also been implicated in myocardial dysfunction (Bozkurt et al., 1998). Hantavirus nucleocapsid antigen may exert a direct hypotensive effect on cardiac function (D. Goade and M. Campen, unpublished data).

2.2.6. Immunity

There is no evidence that an individual has been infected twice with a hantavirus, suggesting lifelong immunity, with the caveat in the Americas that rare infections rarely strike twice and critical observations may be in the future. Antibodies to G1 appear early in infection shortly after the appearance of antibodies to N protein, do not cross-react among hantavirus species, recognize conformational, amino-terminal epitopes (aa 59–89 in SN virus), and functionally neutralize the viral infections *in vitro* (Schmaljohn et al., 1990; Lundkvist and Niklasson, 1992; Jenison

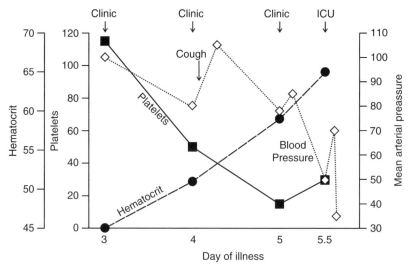

Figure 2.1. Disease course after presentation to health care after 3 days of prodromal symptoms, showing the typical rapid fall in platelet count, increasing hemoconcentration, increasing granulocyte count to 56,000/mm³, and appearance of circulating immunoblasts on day 5 (data not shown). Hypotension documented on day 4 at the second clinic visit was completely corrected by 2 L intravenous crystalloid fluids; however, the hypotension documented on day 5 did not respond to intravenous fluids, shock in the ICU responded only temporarily to maximum vasopressor doses, and the patient expired in irreversible shock.

et al., 1994; Heiskanen et al., 2004). Neutralizing antibodies demonstrated by focus reduction neutralization test (FRNT) correlate with the ability to block experimental infection but require the Fc portion of the antibody to clear the virus *in vivo* (Liang et al., 1996). Both G1 and G2 are required for higher antibody titers and efficient immunity, as protection afforded by immunity to both envelope proteins was greater than that provided by the response to either alone (Schmaljohn et al., 1990).

N proteins are highly immunogenic, and IgM antibodies are present in serum as early as the first day of systemic symptoms, peak in early convalescence, and persist at lower titers for decades. The dominant antigenic domains are localized to the N-terminus, and extensive cross-reaction occurs among the members of the American clades and EuroAsian clades (Jenison et al., 1994; Elgh et al., 1995; Yamada et al., 1995; Elgh et al., 1997). Although there is no evidence for antibody-mediated enhancement of cell infection analogous to dengue, this possibility cannot be ruled out (Morens, 1994).

Long-term circulation of memory T cells have been demonstrated after HTN (Van Epps et al., 1999, 2002) and PUU infection (Terajima et al., 2004), but their role in mediating immunity is unknown.

2.2.7. Animal Models

Suckling mice and immunodeficient mice have been used for years for assessing antibody responses and therapeutic responses to HTN virus, as the only fatal end-point assay, but such mice do not express disease similar to humans (Kim and McKee, 1985; Huggins et al., 1986). Adult immunocompetent mice of certain strains infected intraperitoneally with 5 log PFU of HTN virus do develop fatal infection with acute encephalitis, systemic endothelial cell infection, and prolonged incubation period similar to human disease (Wichmann et al., 2002). Alpha/beta interferon knockout mice were even more susceptible, confirming the central role of interferon antiviral defense.

Inoculation of adult Syrian golden hamsters (*Mesocricetus* auratus) with HTN, SEO, and SN viruses induces infection without disease, whereas inoculation of AND and MAP viruses induce disease with many features of human disease (Hooper et al., 2001b; Milazzo et al., 2002). The explanation for these striking differences in host-specific virulence is unknown. After intramuscular injection of AND, hamster died 11 to 24 days later, with onset of apparent illness with rapidly progressive respiratory distress coming 5–18 h before death (Hooper et al., 2001b). The calculated LD_{50} was 8 PFU and the ID_{50} was 3 PFU. Many histopathologic features mimicked human disease, including large pleural effusions and congested lungs, an interstitial pneumonitis with predominantly mononuclear cell infiltrate, a subacute hepatitis, and expanded splenic red pulp containing large round mononuclear cells similar to those described in HCPS (Koster et al., 2001). Viral antigen was localized to capillary endothelial cells, alveolar macrophages, mid-zonal hepatocytes, and splenic red pulp and follicular marginal zones populated by dendritic cells (Hooper et al., 2001b). Viremia peaked between days 8 and 12, and neutralizing antibody first appeared on days 12 to 14. Infection of the hamster with MAP virus induced similar histopathologic features, incubation period, viremia, and neutralizing antibody response (Milazzo et al., 2002). This virus, found in *Oligoryzomys fulvescens* in central Venezuela (Fulhorst et al., 2004), is not yet associated with human infection and was associated with a higher LD_{50} above 3 log_{10} PFU of intramuscular virus. As with the AND model, the MAP infection displayed abundant viral antigen, but no inflammation, in the myocardium. Preliminary studies have demonstrated in MAP-infected hamsters a correlation between severity of pulmonary inflammation, reduced systolic ejection fraction, and fall in mean arterial blood pressure measured in telemetered ambulatory animals (Koster, Campen, Fulhorst, and Milazzo, unpublished data). Thus the hamster may be a useful model for studies of pathogenesis and therapeutic intervention.

Rhesus macaques are suitable models for testing immunogenicity of candidate vaccines but do not develop disease (Custer et al., 2003; Hooper et al., 2003). However, intratracheal inoculation of cynomolgus macaques with PUU virus resulted in a subacute infection with histopathology confined to the medullary tubular cells of the kidneys (Groen et al., 1995).

2.3. Epidemiology and Transmission

2.3.1. Epidemiology

Hantavirus illness tends to be sporadic, accentuated by periodic outbreaks associated with burgeoning numbers of the host rodent and increased human contact (Yates et al., 2002). Mild winters allowing *P. maniculatus* survival have been associated with SNV HCPS outbreaks in the Southwest United States. In contrast, the majority of cases in Scandinavia occur during the fall and winter months, attributed to the movement of *C. glareolus* into homes, barns, and outbuildings (Niklasson and LeDuc, 1987). Cases of NE are correlated with the abundance of *C. glareolus* occurring in 3- to 4-year cycles of abundance, the prevalence of hantavirus infection in these hosts, and reports of small mammals indoors. In Korea, cases of Hantaan HFRS peak in the late spring and in the fall and winter, times that coincide with the dry season, increased number of gravid female rodents, and peak frequency of virus prevalence in *A. agrarius*. During a 12-year period in China, the annual incidence of HFRS closely correlated with the decreasing field density of *A. agrarius* in the fall, the increasing indoor density in November, and the peak incidence of human disease in November and December (Dai et al., 1981).

HCPS cases due to SNV demonstrate a year-round sporadic incidence with clusters around the spring and early summer (Hjelle and Glass, 2000). Unusually heavy rains attributed to the El Niño Southern Oscillation (ENSO) phenomenon fell several months before two outbreaks of HCPS in the Americas, the 1993 outbreak in the Four Corners area (Yates et al., 2002) and the 1995 outbreak in Paraguay (Williams et al., 1997).

2.3.2. Transmission

Inhalation of aerosolized virus particles present in the urine, feces, or saliva of rodents is the natural route of human infection. The most compelling evidence for aerosol transmission is found in laboratory outbreaks. For example, during one outbreak in a research facility in Russia housing recently acquired field-caught rodents, 18 out of 24 visitors within 5 min to 4 h of exposure became infected without direct contact with the rodents (Tsai, 1987). Percutaneous infection has been documented after direct exposure of open skin lesions to the blood of acutely ill HFRS patients (Xu et al., 1985) and after rodent bites.

Direct exposure to rodent excreta accounts for the vast majority of human infections and is related to variations in rodent density, rodent behavior invading peridomestic environments, and human behavior invading rodent environments. Increased numbers of rodents in or around households is a risk factor identified for SNV infection (Childs et al., 1995). Activities likely to attract rodents to human living areas, such as storing grain in the house or straw sacks outside the house, are associated with a higher incidence of Korean hemorrhagic fever (KHF) (Ruo et al., 1994) and HCPS in Panama (Armien et al., 2004). The numbers and density of rodents in the natural environment are dramatically influenced by fluctuations in rainfall and in anthropogenic changes in the environment. The trophic cascade hypothesis posits that increased rainfall increases rodent food resulting in a rodent population surge, followed by a delayed increase in human infection (Yates et al., 2002). The rodent population surge is accompanied by increased incidence of rodent infection through home-range competition among males with aggression (Klein et al., 2004) and wounding (Hinson et al., 2004). Actual risk to humans is localized and dependent on a complex interplay of variables including landscape and microclimate heterogeneity, local rodent food abundance, competition and predation, and adjacent human-dominated ecosystems. Refinements in predicting human infection risk is likely by intensive study of local and longitudinal rodent population dynamics (Kuenzi et al., 1999; Mills et al., 1999; Abramson and Kenkre, 2002; Ruedas et al., 2004), mathematical modeling of rodent movement and population structure (Abramson and Kenkre, 2002; Abramson et al., 2003), and remote sensing of environmental changes (Glass et al., 2002).

Human behaviors such as animal husbandry close to home (Armien et al., 2004) and living in outdoor camps or makeshift structures by shepherds, woodcutters, and farmers are also risk factors (LeDuc, 1987). Forestry workers in The Netherlands have a 2–3% annual seroconversion rate (Moll van Charante et al., 1998). Entering and cleaning unused outbuildings is the activity most frequently associated with SNV infection (Zeitz et al., 1995; Jay et al., 1996). In western Panama, exposure to Choclo virus is linked primarily to animal husbandry in peridomestic outbuildings (Armien et al., 2004). Comparison of viral nucleotide sequences in hypervariable M segments derived from human cases and epidemiologically linked rodents has provided compelling support for peridomestic exposures in most cases of SN infection studied (Hjelle et al., 1996). Unfortunately interventions to decrease rodent exposure around the home may not have a favorable impact (Douglass et al., 2003). More studies using molecular epidemiology techniques and rodent behavior modifications are needed both to improve our public health message and to engineer the environment discouraging rodent invasion.

Person-to-person transmission of hantavirus infection has been suggested only for Andes virus, and this observation has important implications for prevention. Tens of thousands of cases of HFRS occur in Eurasia every year, and yet no evidence for nosocomial or person-to-person transmission has been reported (Lee, 1989; Ruo et al., 1994). In the United States, analyses of family clusters and serologic study of exposed health care workers found no evidence for nosocomial or intrafamilial transmission of SN virus (Vitek et al., 1996; Wells et al., 1998).

In contrast, during the outbreak in southwestern Argentina in 1993 (Wells et al., 1997a), 16 of the 20 cases were linked to each other epidemiologically in three- to four-person transmission chains. Five physicians developed HCPS, one of whom had never left Buenos Aires. In another case without reported rodent exposure, the sole exposure occurred during the 20-h car ride to Buenos Aires with a symptomatic patient.

Molecular analysis of viral RNA found identical sequences for the 16 epidemiologically linked cases but nonidentical sequences among the four contemporaneous but nonepidemiologically related cases (Padula et al., 1998). Subsequent HCPS cases in Argentina, however, have not demonstrated any evidence of person-to-person transmission (Yadon, 1998).

In Chile, though serologic studies have failed to find evidence for nosocomial transmission (Castillo et al., 2004), household intrafamilial transmission, particularly among sexual partners, is suggested by serologic studies, 2-week intervals between index and secondary family case, and infection of a woman whose sole exposure was caring for her infected husband (Toro et al., 1998).

The mechanism of person-to-person transmission by aerosolization of virus from patient lungs is suggested by the presence of viral antigen in pulmonary macrophages in fatal cases (Toro et al., 1998) and viral genome detected by RT-PCR in the tracheal aspirates from patients with Andes virus HCPS. Regardless of the mechanisms, preventing intrafamilial transmission is a current focus of research in Chile (M Ferrer, P Vial, G Mertz, personal communication).

2.4. Clinical Spectrum

2.4.1. Asymptomatic or Mild Infection

Different viruses appear to be responsible for differing ratios of hospitalized disease to mild disease or asymptomatic disease. Although there have been more than 300 cases of HCPS reported to the CDC in the United States during the past 11 years, few cases of acute febrile hantavirus infection have been identified (Zavasky et al., 1999). Reporting bias may be significant, and few diagnostic assays are performed in the absence of pulmonary involvement. In North America, overall seroprevalence rates are less than 0.1% in the endemic Western states. In an HCPS case-control study in 1993 in the southwestern United States, seroprevalence among neighborhood control families was 1.3% (Zeitz et al., 1995). The extrapolated hospitalized:mild ratio in this region is calculated to be greater than 20:1. The mortality rate of reported SN virus infections is 35% (Khan et al., 1996). The seroprevalence of 0.3% in inner cities of the eastern United States is due to infection with Seoul virus from rat exposure (Glass et al., 1993; Wasser et al., 1997). In South America, there appears to be a wider range of ratios. In Argentina where at least four different hantaviruses are endemic, seroprevalence rates vary from 0.1% to 1.5% (Wells et al., 1997a). In an endemic region in southern Chile, the seroprevalence rate was found to be 2.3% (Castillo et al., 2002), where the mortality rate of hospitalized Andes infections is 38%. Seroprevalence rates in southern Brazil have been documented as high as 15% (Figueiredo et al., 2003). In western Paraguay, seroprevalence rates range from 45% among indigenous peoples to 35% among European descendants (Ferrer et al., 1998). The observation that almost all cases of HCPS occur among nonindigenous people, and rarely among indigenous people, suggests that host genetics may influence infection outcome. In western Panama, in a region dominated by Choclo virus infection with a mortality rate of 10%, seroprevalence rates vary from 3% to 45% (Armien et al., 2004). In the endemic province of Los Santos with overall seroprevalence rates of approximately 20%, in a region with 30 reported cases in a 5-year interval, the extrapolated ratio of hospitalized to mild/asymptomatic cases is calculated to be less than 1:20, in striking contrast with the estimated ratio for SN virus above.

In Europe, the overall seroprevalence rate is 2.1% (Lee, 1989) and is 8.9% in the endemic region of Sweden with annual incidence ranging from <0.8 to 30 per 100,000 population (Niklasson and LeDuc, 1987). In China, seroprevalence ranges from 1.2% to 12% depending on location, and 40,000 to 100,000 cases are reported per year, with an annual incidence of 150 per 100,000 in one rural county (Ruo et al., 1994). The reported mortality rate in China of 2% varies by location, year, and season according to the ratio of Hantaan virus infection and the milder Seoul virus infection (Chen et al., 1986).

2.4.2. Incubation Period

In small numbers of cases where the exposure has been identified by molecular epidemiologic identification of the rodent source, the incubation period for SN infection was a mean of 12 days with a range of 7 to 25 days (Wells et al., 1997b) and for Andes infection in Chile was a mean of 10 days and a range of 7 to 22 days (Ferres and Vial , 2004). Two boys bitten by an infected rodent both developed clinical disease 21 days later (Smith and St. Jeor, 2004).

2.4.3. Clinical Presentation of HCPS

All human hantavirus disease involves four primary organs: lung, kidney, heart and hematological organs. Because hantaviruses infect capillary endothelial cells, all organs are potentially infected and in fatal cases many organs are, with variations according to the viral strain involved. The disease is divided into four phases based on clinical manifestations and pathophysiology—febrile, pulmonary, diuretic, and convalescent phases—with variations between the primary location of the capillary leak syndrome in HCPS and HFRS, respectively (Koster and Hjelle, 2004).

2.4.3.1. Febrile Phase

The 2- to 7-day-long febrile phase is characterized by the typically sudden onset of fever, chills, dizziness, malaise, headaches, backache, and myalgias (Duchin et al., 1994), symptoms common to many other febrile illnesses (Moolenaar et al., 1995). The fever is usually over 39°C, the headaches and occasional photophobia may be severe suggesting meningitis, and the myalgias primarily involve the large muscles including the back, thighs, and shoulders. Ocular pain and conjunctival suffusion are uncommon, conjunctival hemorrhage is rare, and conjunctivitis does not occur. Nausea and vomiting and abdominal pain occur in more than 50% of cases, and the most common clinical diagnosis during the febrile phase is gastroenteritis. Diarrhea occurs in less than 10%, is rarely bloody, and gastric hemorrhage was found at autopsy in few cases

(Nolte et al., 1995). Anorexia is common but thirst is uncommon. Sore throat is prominent in 10–20%, but rash, petechiae, and lymphadenopathy are rare. In some episodes, the febrile phase is a crescendo illness with fever beginning insidiously during the first day and all symptoms worsening until the rapid transition into the cardiopulmonary phase.

2.4.3.2. Cardiopulmonary Phase

Dry cough followed by dyspnea and tachypnea heralds the onset of the cardiopulmonary (cardiogenic shock–pulmonary edema) phase, preceding the onset of radiographically detected pulmonary edema by as much as 12 h. Radiographically, infiltrates are almost always bilateral and may be interstitial, alveolar, or a mixed pattern (Ketai et al., 1994, 1998). Pleural effusions are common in SNV infection but less common in ANDV infection (Riquelme et al., 2003). Hypoxemia rapidly reaches a nadir rapidly over 6–12 h after onset of cough (Fig. 2.1). In 10% of patients, supplemental oxygen is not required (mild disease); 30–40% require oxygen by nasal cannula or face-mask or continuous positive airway pressure (CPAP)-mask (moderate disease); and 50–60% require mechanical ventilation (severe). Among those requiring mechanical ventilation, 70% is initiated at admission and the other 30% within 24 h of admission. The pulmonary edema is noncardiogenic in origin and may be manifest in the most severe cases by greater than 1.0 L of frothy yellow fluid, with a protein content equal to serum, aspirated from the intratracheal tube every hour for several days.

A rapid pulse rate greater than 130 beats/min is an ominous first sign of hemodynamic instability. Approximately 75–93% of patients requiring mechanical ventilation also develop hemodynamic instability with hypotension due to cardiogenic shock and, finally, electromechanical dissociation and/or terminal ventricular fibrillation (Levy and Simpson, 1994; Hallin et al., 1996; Simpson, 1998). Five percent of patients with shock do not present with or develop severe pulmonary edema. Hypotension is due to cardiogenic shock compounded by intravascular volume depletion due to vomiting and capillary leak syndrome, and to hypovolemic shock, often occurring sequentially in many patients (Fig. 2.2). Initial hypotension may be postural hypotension, accompanying a history of vomiting, and responds to volume repletion with crystalloids. Subsequent hypotension does not respond to volume repletion alone and requires vasopressor therapy. Approximately 20% of patients experience unremitting vasopressor-unresponsive hypotension and survive only with extracorporeal membrane oxygenation (ECMO) intervention (Crowley et al., 1998).

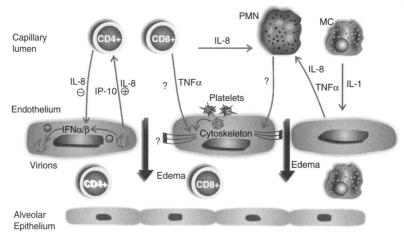

Figure 2.2. Hypothesis for cellular participants in the pathogenesis of capillary leak syndrome in HCPS. All cells and protein mediators included here are speculative based on immunohistology, because no animal model data with deletion of cells or proteins exists to clearly implicate their participation. Cell types in the interstitium (T cells and monocytes but rarely neutrophils) are also found in pleural fluid.

2.4.3.3. Convalescent Phase

Most patients experience exertional dyspnea and fatigue for 2–4 weeks after recovery from infection with SNV (Goade, D. unpublished data), AND (Castillo, H. unpublished data), and CHO viruses (Koster, F. unpublished data). Pulmonary function testing reveals persistent defects in carbon monoxide diffusing capacity for up to 1 year and in small airways expiratory flow rates for up to 3 years or more for each of these three viruses, but resolution of symptoms may occur during persistence of the measured deficits. Appearance of proteinuria alone more than 3 years after recovery from SNV infection has been repeatedly documented (Goade, D. unpublished data), contrasting with persistence of urine concentrating capacity, but not proteinuria, for years after HTN and PUU infection (Rubini et al., 1960; Niklasson et al., 1994).

2.4.4. Clinical Presentation of HFRS

The features of fever chills, headache, myalgias, backache, nausea, vomiting, and abdominal pain are common features among all prodromal illness in hantavirus infection. KHF is distinctive in the increased incidence of photophobia and ocular pain, conjunctival injection and hemorrhage, excessive thirst, facial flush, enanthem, skin-fold petechiae, and nontender lymphadenopathy, features that are rare or unreported among American hemisphere cases. Hypotension develops by the fifth to seventh day of illness, persists for up to 3 days, progresses to shock in 30–50% of episodes, and refractory shock accounts for a 30% of the mortality all due to refractory shock (Giles et al., 1954). Systemic symptoms are reported by some authors to abate prior to the onset of hypotension and to worsen in other reports with shock heralded by tachycardia. During hypotension, the cardiac index is normal or low, and with progression to shock the cardiac index decreases markedly with concomitant rise in peripheral vascular resistance (PVR) (Cugell, 1954; Entwisle and Hale, 1957). Plasma expansion with albumin results in an increase in cardiac index and decrease in PVR. Echocardiography of patients in shock from PUU infection has not indicated myocardial dysfunction (Linderholm et al., 1997), leaving the impression that shock in HFRS is due primarily to severe vascular fluid shifts into extravascular compartments.

2.5. Diagnosis of Acute Infection

Laboratory diagnosis is almost always by serologic assay (Koster and Hjelle, 2004), because antibodies are usually found in serum on the first day of symptoms. Two assays are in common use: the EIA provided by the CDC and State Laboratories (Rossi and Ksiazek, 1999) and the strip immunoblot provided by TriCore Laboratories/University of New Mexico (Hjelle et al., 1997). Viral antigen detection with immunohistochemistry in fixed tissue samples is sensitive and specific (Zaki et al., 1995, 1996; Green et al., 1998). Reverse transcriptase–polymerase chain reaction (RT-PCR) can detect viral RNA from serum or plasma or tissues (Hjelle et al., 1994b; Hjelle, 1999). Viral isolation has rarely been accomplished by tissue culture from human specimens and has no role in diagnosis.

Requests for serologic diagnosis and appropriate therapy require a high index of suspicion. Patients in the prodromal phase will complain of a flu-like illness often with gastrointestinal symptoms. Although almost all patients live in rural areas, only half offer a history of rodent or rodent dropping exposure. The key laboratory abnormality during the prodromal phase, even after 1 day of symptoms, is thrombocytopenia almost always less than 130,000 mm^{-3} (Koster et al., 2001). As the patient transitions into the cardiopulmonary phase with dyspnea and hypotension, a triad of peripheral smear findings permits a presumptive diagnosis to be made, with thrombocytopenia, circulating immunoblasts, and a left shift in the myeloid series.

2.6. Current Management

Management of patients with HCPS is greatly facilitated by early diagnosis, as the mortality rate of the patient arriving to hospital in cardiogenic shock exceeds 70%. Often, the decision for transport to a regional intensive care unit must be based solely on symptoms and early laboratory features, particularly thrombocytopenia, consistent with HCPS, because patients frequently progress precipitously into respiratory failure and shock. Platelet counts should be measured at 12-h intervals, at a minimum, as disease severity partially parallels platelet counts, and counts that remain above 100,000/mm^3 predict mild disease or an alternative diagnosis. Patient stabilization and preparation for transport includes obtaining baseline chest radiography, arterial blood gases, plasma lactate, serum electrolytes, and electrocardiogram. Although there is no evidence for person-to-person transmission of SNV infection, in contrast with Andes virus infection, we maintain universal precautions and respiratory isolation because plague should be in the differential diagnosis.

Initial fluid resuscitation should attempt to minimize crystalloid volume used as this may reduce any pulmonary edema that would occur. Current guidelines for severe sepsis patient resuscitation can be administered as long as oxygenation can be easily maintained. When advanced pulmonary edema is present, even colloids may leak into the alveoli as the pulmonary capillary–endothelial barrier is so abnormal that all plasma proteins leak. We maintain as low a wedge pressure as is compatible with satisfactory cardiac indices because of the extreme capillary leak. Even if the patient is hemodynamically stable, dobutamine should be prepared and available for use in transport if the patient deteriorates. All drugs used in advanced cardiac life support should be available. High-flow oxygen masks should be used when desaturation occurs and the trachea intubated if simple measures fail to provide adequate oxygen saturation. Although ribavirin inhibits hantavirus replication *in vitro* and was efficacious in a large trial of HFRS in China (Huggins et al., 1991), intravenous ribavirin is not likely to offer significant benefit (Mertz et al., 2004), as there is usually insufficient time for antiviral drugs alone to alter the fulminant course of HCPS. Cardiogenic rather than vasodilatory hemodynamic profile of patients in shock differs from the typical profile of septic shock (Parrillo, 1993), yet we routinely administer broad-spectrum antibiotics until the diagnosis is clear.

Dobutamine is the best inotrope to support cardiac output and mean blood pressure as it allows afterload reduction, typically elevated in the cardiogenic shock phase. A flow-directed pulmonary artery catheter should be placed even in milder presentations of the disease, as the decrease in cardiac function is frequently underestimated. Transthoracic echocardiography may allow early detection of severely decreased myocardial contractility. In the absence of any specific therapy, we have managed HCPS patients in a similar manner to those with sepsis, except as detailed. Recombinant human activated Protein C [drotrecogin alfa (activated); Xigris) is approved for the treatment of severe sepsis at high risk of death. This medication has documented benefits of more rapid normalization of blood pressure, reduced need for vasopressors, and fewer deaths due to septic shock than placebo (Ely et al., 2003). In a small case series, there appears to be less need for extracorporeal membrane oxygenation (ECMO) and fewer deaths due to HCPS than expected (H. Levy, unpublished data). We recommend initiation of therapy with drotrecogin alfa (activated) as soon as hemodynamic compromise is documented. A continuous cardiac output measuring pulmonary artery catheter is preferable to intermittent manual estimates. When dobutamine alone is insufficient to support cardiovascular function, dopamine and norepinephrine in high dose should be used. When terminal shock supervenes, we have used epinephrine boluses of 0.5 to 1 mg every 3 to 5 min while instituting ECMO therapy. ECMO is used when cardiac output falls in the face of rapidly increased vasopressor therapy, cardiogenic shock (cardiac index <2.2 L min^{-1} m^{-2}), ventricular arrhythmias, particularly ventricular tachycardia or fibrillation, or electromechanical dissociation (Crowley et al., 1998). Venoarterial ECMO allows the provision of up to 6 L/min cardiac output and has been successfully applied, increasing hospital survival of patients in shock to more than 50%. Cardiac arrhythmias, particularly episodes of electromechanical dissociation, portend a poor outcome and are aggressively treated. Thrombocytopenia has not required support with platelet transfusion in SNV infection, and a rising platelet count is an early sign of recovery. Red blood cells are given to maintain oxygen delivery if hemoglobin concentration falls. Plasma lactate levels are monitored every 4 to 8 h, and a level exceeding 4 mmol/L is an indicator for ECMO.

Close monitoring of oxygenation is extremely important so that timely intubation and mechanical ventilation can be provided when intractable hypoxemia occurs. We use high inspired oxygen concentrations and positive end expiratory pressure (PEEP) at levels above 12 cm H_2O to minimize pulmonary edema production. Pressure controlled ventilation with paralysis is preferred, usually without inverse ratio ventilation. Although gas exchange abnormalities frequently become quite severe, usually patients can be adequately oxygenated throughout the course of their illness. Inhaled nitric oxide therapy has been used in one surviving case (Rosenberg et al., 1998) but cannot be recommended until further use substantiates its efficacy and safety.

Recovery in survivors is as rapid as the initial decline, and there have been few deaths in patients who have survived for 48 h after hospital admission. After the cardiopulmonary phase, the spontaneous diuresis may be brisk, and loop diuretics need not be used to initiate diuresis.

The use of B-type natriuretic peptide has not yet been studied for efficacy and safety in this syndrome. The typical severe sepsis manifestations of multiple organ failure, renal failure, or hepatic failure are rare and imply coincident nosocomial infection. Whereas pulmonary hemorrhage or hemothorax is not uncommon in Andes virus infection, it is rare in SNV infection with only two such cases known to the authors.

2.7. Prevention

The Centers for Disease Control and Prevention has issued guidelines for reducing the risk for transmission of hantavirus infections (CDC, 2002). These guidelines, available from state and local health departments, emphasize practical recommendations for preventing rodent infestations, for cleaning up rodent-infested sites, and for trapping and disposing of rodents. Removal of deer mice from non-rodent-proofed buildings may paradoxically increase the number of resident mice (Douglass et al., 2003), emphasizing the need for rodent-proofing first.

Vaccines for hantavirus infections have been recently reviewed (Hooper and Li, 2001; Hjelle, 2002). Passive transfer of neutralizing antibody confers protection. Immunization with HTNV glycoproteins (G1 and G2) induces neutralizing antibody responses and protection (Schmaljohn et al., 1990), results that have focused attention on neutralizing antibodies as the standard surrogate marker of potential protection. Recombinant protein vaccines have been developed for HTN, and rodent brain vaccines have been used in Korea and China (Cho and Howard, 1999). HTNV amplified in rodent brain will result in 99% human seroconversion if given as three closely spaced doses, but only one-third of recipients elicited neutralizing antibody (Sohn et al., 2001). Vaccinia virus-recombinant HTNV vaccine stimulated neutralizing antibody in 72% of vaccinia-naïve individuals but uncommonly in vaccinia-immune individuals (McClain et al., 2000). It is conceivable that recombinant SNV glycoprotein vaccines could be useful when the risk for SNV transmission is high. Gene fragments of the SNV glycoproteins that elicit strong immune responses in rodent models have recently been shown to be capable of preventing infection in the deer mouse model (Bharadwaj et al., 1999). DNA vaccination with HTN M genes elicited neutralizing antibodies and protected hamsters against HTN, SEO, and DOB infection and elicited high-titered neutralizing antibodies in rhesus macaques (Hooper et al., 2001a). DNA vaccination of macaques with AND M genes also elicited high-titered neutralization antibodies that passively protected hamsters from lethal disease, even when given 5 days after challenge (Custer et al., 2003). The role of immune T cells in protection is not yet clear but has been suggested in rodent protection studies with recombinant N proteins (de Carvalho Nicacio et al., 2002). Although most vaccine development has appropriately focused on the more common HFRS viruses, it is conceivable that SNV and AND vaccines could be useful when the occupational risk for transmission is high.

2.8. Future Directions

What does the clinician need to know to improve the survival chances of the HV-infected patient? Given the rarity of disease in the Americas, and consequent difficulty in testing candidate therapies in a randomized, blinded clinical trial format, greater burden is placed on the hamster and non-human primate models to sift through candidate therapies and find the few worth the effort of a long-term clinical trial.

Postexposure immunoprophylaxis with hyperimmune sera has the greatest immediate promise and will be tested in animals and humans within the next few years. The hamster model can provide insights into several critical points during the evolution of disease, including the early events after inhalation of virus and interaction with lung dendritic cells, the anatomic correlates to a long incubation period, the relationship between viremia, pneumonitis, and immune system activation, and the etiology of shock partitioned between vascular leak and myocardial dysfunction. There are a multitude of potential mediators of vascular leak that should be explored. Several lines of evidence have implicated TNF-α, suggesting that potential interventions to be tested in the hamster model include anti-TNF monoclonal antibodies and TNF receptor–mediated blockade. As the network of regulators controlling tight-junction integrity is elucidated, this knowledge needs to be applied to the massive leak associated with HV infection in endothelial cells *in vitro* and *in vivo*. If T cells do play a major role in immunopathogenesis, selective temporary blockade of T-cell function might be explored. If HV survival is dependent on interferon-stimulated gene suppression paralleling other RNA viruses, strategies for subverting the suppression of host defenses should be explored. Nitric oxide may have a role as antiviral therapy (Reiss and Komatsu, 1998), and HV replication is suppressed *in vitro* by NO donors (F. Koster, unpublished data), but NO may also mediate tissue damage, particularly myocardial depression (Finkel et al., 1992), so the Janus faces of NO demand exploration. Finally, novel antiviral agents should be sought for targets other than viral proteases, and RNA interference offers promise.

What does the public health official need to know about HV transmission to initiate more effective prevention campaigns at the community level? Markers of increased peridomestic rodent invasion need to be identified for each environment and education strategies tested to convince the public to heed warnings of increased risk. We need to identify the man-manipulated environments, home constructions, agricultural practices, animal husbandry, deforestation, and loss of biodiversity that favor rodent population explosion and rodent invasions. Details of rodent behaviors and transmission routes may help engineer the human environment to discourage rodent contact.

References

Abramson, G., and Kenkre, V. M. (2002). Spatio-temporal patterns in the hantavirus infection. *Physical review. E. Statistical, nonlinear and soft matter physics. 66* (1PT.I): 011912. E pub. 2002, July 24.

Abramson, G., Kenkre, V. M., Yates, T. L., and Parmenter, R. R. (2003). Traveling waves of infection in the hantavirus epidemics. *Bull Math Biol 65*, 519–534.

Armien, B., Pascale, J. M., Bayard, V., Munoz, C., Mosca, I., Guerrero, G., Armien, A., Quiroz, E., Castillo, Z., Zaldivar, Y., Gracia, F., Hjelle, B., and Koster, F. (2004). High seroprevalence of hantavirus infection on the Azuero peninsula of Panama. *Am J Trop Med Hyg 70*, 682–687.

Bausch, D. G., and Ksiazek, T. G. (2002). Viral hemorrhagic fevers including hantavirus pulmonary syndrome in the Americas. *Clin Lab Med 22*, 981–1020.

Bharadwaj, M., Lyons, C. R., Wortman, I. A., and Hjelle, B. (1999). Intramuscular inoculation of Sin Nombre hantavirus cDNAs induces cellular and humoral immune responses in BALB/c mice. *Vaccine 17*, 2836–2843.

Bharadwaj, M., Nofchissey, R., Goade, D., Koster, F., and Hjelle, B. (2000). Humoral immune responses in the hantavirus cardiopulmonary syndrome. *J Infect Dis 182*, 43–48.

Bishop, D. H. (1996). Biology and molecular biology of Bunyaviruses. In: The Bunyaviridae, R. M. Elliott, ed. (New York and London, Plenum Press), pp. 19–53.

Bozkurt, B., Kribbs, S. B., Clubb, K. F. J., Michael, L. H., Didenko, V. V., Harnsby, P. J., Seta, Y., Oral, H., Spinale, F. G., and Mann, D. L. (1998). Pathophysiologically relevant concentrations of tumor necrosis factor–α promote progressive left ventricular dysfunction and remodelling in rats. *Circulation 97*, 1382–1391.

Bustamente, E. A., Levy, H., and Simpson, S. Q. (1997). Pleural fluid characteristics in hantavirus pulmonary syndrome. *Chest 112*, 1133–1136.

Castillo H, C., Sanhueza H, L., Tager F, M., Munoz N, S., Ossa A, G., and Vial C, P. (2002). Seroprevalence of antibodies against hantavirus in 10 communities of the IX region of Chile where hantavirus cardiopulmonary syndrome cases were reported. *Rev med Chil 130*, 1–10.

Castillo H, C., Villagra, E., Sanhueza H, L., Ferres, M. G., Mardones, J., and Mertz, G. (2004). Prevalence of antibodies to hantavirus among family and health care worker contacts of persons with hantavirus cardiopulmonary syndrome: lack of evidence from nosocomial transmission of Andes virus to health care workers in Chile. *Am J Trop Med Hyg 70*, 302–304.

CDC (2002). Hantavirus Pulmonay Syndrome – United States: updated recommendations for risk reduction. *Morb Mortal Wkly Rep 51*, 1–13.

Chare, E. R., Gould, E. A., and Holmes, E. C. (2003). Phylogenetic analysis reveals a low rate of homologous recombination in negative-sense RNA viruses. *J Gen Virol 84*, 2691–2703.

Chen, H. X., Qui, F. X., Dong, B. J., Ji, S. Z., Li, Y. T., Wang, Y., Wang, H. M., Zuo, G. F., Tao, X. X., and Gao, S. Y. (1986). Epidemiologic studies on hemorrhagic fever with renal syndrome in China. *J Infect Dis 154*, 394–398.

Childs, J. E., Krebs, J. W., Ksiazek, T. G., Maupin, G. O., Gage, K. L., Rollin, P. E., Zeitz, P. S., Sarisky, J., Enscore, R. E., Butler, J. C., Cheek, J. E., Glass, G. E., and Peters, C. J. (1995). A household-based, case-control study of environmental factors associated with hantavirus pulmonary syndrome in the southwestern United States. *Am J Trop Med Hyg 52*, 393–397.

Chizhikov, V., Spiropoulou, C. F., Morzunov, S., Monroe, M., Peters, C. J., and Nichol, S. T. (1995). Complete genetic characterization and analysis of isolation of Sin Nombre virus. *J Virol* *69*, 8132–8136.

Cho, H. W., and Howard, C. R. (1999). Antibody responses in humans to an inactivated hantavirus vaccine (Hantavax). *Vaccine 17*, 2569–2575.

Chu, Y. K., Jennings, G., Schmaljohn, A. L., Elgh, F., Hjelle, B., Lee, H. W., Jenison, S., Ksiazek, T. G., Peters, C. J., Rollin, P. E., and Schmaljohn, C. S. (1995). Cross-neutralization of hantaviruses with immune sera from experimentally infected animals and from hemorrhagic fever with renal syndrome and hantavirus pulmonary syndrome patients. *J Infect Dis 172*, 1581–1584.

Cosgriff, T. M. (1991). Mechanisms of disease in Hantavirus infection: pathophysiology of hemorrhagic fever with renal syndrome. *Rev Infect Dis 13*, 97–107.

Crowley, M. R., Katz, R. W., Kessler, R., Simpson, S. Q., Levy, H., Hallin, G. W., Cappon, J., Krahling, J. B., and Wernly, J. (1998). Successful treatment of adults with severe hantavirus pulmonary syndrome with extracorporeal membrane oxygenation. *Crit Care Med 26*, 409–414.

Cugell, D. W. (1954). Cardiac output in epidemic hemorrhagic fever. *Am J Med 16*, 668–670.

Custer, D. M., Thompson, E., Schmaljohn, C. S., Ksiazek, T. G., and Hooper, J. W. (2003). Active and passive vaccination against hantavirus pulmonary syndrome with Andes virus M genome segment-based DNA vaccine. *J Virol 77*, 9894–9905.

Dai, Z. Y., Xu, Z. Y., Wang, J. R., and Yang, P. Z. (1981). Epidemiologic and clinical studies of epidemic hemorrhagic fever. *Clin Med J (Engl) 94*, 143–148.

Davis, I. C., Zajac, A. J., Nolte, K. B., Botten, J., Hjelle, B., and Matalon, S. (2002). Elevated generation of reactive oxygen/nitrogen species in hantavirus cardiopulmonary syndrome. *J Virol 76*, 8347–8359.

de Carvalho Nicacio, C., Gonzalez Della Valle, M., Padula, P., Bjorling, E., Plyusnin, A., and Lundkvist, A. (2002). Cross-protection against challenge with Puumala virus after immunization with nucleocapsid proteins from different hantaviruses. *J Virol 76*, 6669–6677.

Domingo, E., and Holland, J. J. (1997). RNA virus mutations and fitness for survival. *Annu Rev Microbiol 51*, 151–178.

Douglass, R. J., Kuenzi, A. J., Williams, C. Y., Douglass, S. J., and Mills, J. N. (2003). Removing deer mice from buildings and the risk for human exposure to sin nombre virus. *Emerg Infect Dis 9*, 390–392.

Duchin, J. S., Koster, F. T., Peters, C. J., Simpson, G. L., Tempest, B., Zaki, S. R., Ksiazek, T. G., Rollin, P. E., Nichol, S., Umland, E. T., Moolenaar, R. L., Reef, S. E., Nolte, K. B., Gallaher, M. M., Bulter, J. C., and Breiman, R. F, for The Hantavirus Study Group. (1994). Hantavirus pulmonary syndrome: a clinical description of 17 patients with a newly recognized disease. *N Engl J Med 330*, 949–955.

Ebihara, H., Yoshimatsu, K., Ogino, M., Araki, K., Ami, Y., Kariwa, H., Takashima, I., Li, D., and Arikawa, J. (2000). Pathogenicity of Hantaan virus in newborn mice: genetic reassortant study demonstrating that a single amino acid change in glycoprotein G1 is related to virulence. *J Virol 74*, 9245–9255.

Elgh, F., Lundkvist, A., Alexeyev, O. A., Stenlund, H., Avsic-Zupanc, T., Hjelle, B., Lee, H. W., Smith, K. J., Vainionpaa, R., Wiger, D., Waddell, G., and Juto, P. (1997). Serological diagnosis of hantavirus infections by an enzyme-linked immunosorbent assay based on detection of immunoglobulin G and M responses to recombinant nucleocapsid proteins of five viral serotypes. *J Clin Microbiol 35*, 1122–1130.

Elgh, F., Wadell, G., and Juto, P. (1995). Comparison of the kinetics of Puumala virus specific IgM and IgG antibody responses in nephropathia epidemica as measured by a recombinant antigen-based enzyme-linked immunosorbent assay and an immunofluorescence test. *J Med Virol 45*, 146–150.

Ely, W. E., Laterre, P.-F., Angus, d. C., Helterbrand, J. D., Levy, H., Dhainaut, J.-F., Vincent, J.-L., Macias, W. L., and Bernard, G. R. (2003). Drotrecogin alfa (activated) administration across clinically important subgroups of patients with severe sepsis. *Crit Care Med 31*, 12–19.

Ennis, F. A., Cruz, J., Spiropoulou, C. F., Waite, D., Peters, C. J., Nichol, S. T., Kariwa, H., and Koster, F. T. (1997). Hantavirus pulmonary syndrome: CD8+ and CD4+ cytotoxic T lymphocytes to epitopes on Sin Nombre virus nucleocapsid protein isolated during acute illness. *Virology 238*, 380–390.

Entwisle, G., and Hale, E. (1957). Hemodynamic alteration in hemorrhagic fever. *Circulation 15*, 414–425.

Ferrer, J. F., Jonsson, C. B., Esteban, E., Galligan, D., Basombrio, M. A., Peralta-Ramos, M., Bharadwaj, M., Torrez-Martinez, N., Callahan, J., Segovia, A., and Hjelle, B. (1998). High prevalence of hantavirus infection in Indian communities of the Paraguayan and Argentinean Gran Chaco. *Am J Trop Med Hyg 59*, 438–444.

Ferres, M. G., and Vial C. P. (2004). Hantavirus in children. *Curr Opin Pediatr 16*, 70–75.

Figueiredo, L. T. M., Moreli, M. L., Campos, G. M., and Sousa, R. L. M. (2003). Hantaviruses in Sao Paulo State, Brazil. *Emerg Infect Dis 9*, 891–892.

Finkel, M. S., Oddis, C. V., Jacob, T. D., Watkins, S. C., Hattler, B. G., and Simmons, R. L. (1992). Negative inotropic effects of cytokines on the heart mediated by nitric oxide. *Science 257*, 387–389.

Flick, K., Hooper, J. W., Schmaljohn, C. S., Pettersson, R. F., Feldmann, H., and Flick, R. (2003). Rescue of Hantaan virus minigenomes. *Virology 306*, 219–224.

Flick, R., Elgh, F., Hobom, G., and Pettersson, R. F. (2002). Mutational analysis of the Uukuniemi virus (Bunyaviridae family) promoter reveals two elements of functional importance. *J Virol 76*, 10849–10860.

Flick, R., and Pettersson, R. F. (2001). Reverse genetics system for Uukuniemi virus (*Bunyaviridae*): RNA polymerase I-catalyzed expression of chimeric viral RNAs. *J Virol 75*, 1643–1655.

Frese, M., Kochs, G., Feldmann, H., Hertkorn, C., and Haller, O. (1996). Inhibition of Bunyaviruses, Phleboviruses, and Hantaviruses by human MxA protein. *J Virol 70*, 915–923.

Friedl, J., Puhlmann, M., Bartlett, D. L., Libutti, S. K., Turner, E. N., Gnant, M. F., and Alexander, H. R. (2002). Induction of permeability across endothelial cell monolayers by tumor necrosis factor (TNF) occurs via a tissue factor-dependent mechanism: relationship between the procoagulant and permeability effects of TNF. *Blood 100*, 1334–1339.

Fulhorst, C. F., Cajimat, M. N. B., Utrera, A., Milazzo, M. L., and Duno, G. M. (2004). Maporal virus, a hantavirus associated with the fulvous pygmy rice rat (Oligoryzomys fulvescens) in western Venezuela. *Virus Res 104*, 139–144.

Gavrilovskaya, I. N., Peresleni, T., Geimonen, E., and Mackow, E. R. (2002). Pathogenic hantaviruses selectively inhibit beta3 integrin directed endothelial cell migration. *Arch Virol 147*, 1913–1931.

Gavrilovskaya, I. N., Shepley, M., Shaw, R., Ginsberg, M. H., and Mackow, E. R. (1998). Beta3 integrins mediate the cellular entry of hantaviruses that cause respiratory failure. *Proc Natl Acad Sci U S A 95*, 7074–7079.

Geimonen, E., LaMonica, R., Springer, K., Farooqui, Y., Gavrilovskaya, I., and Mackow, E. R. (2003). Hantavirus pulmonary syndrome-associated hantaviruses contain conserved and functional ITAM signaling elements. *J Virol 77*, 1638–1643.

Geimonen, E., Neff, S., Raymond, T., Kocer, S. S., Gavrilovskaya, I. N., and Mackow, E. R. (2002). Pathogenic and nonpathogenic hantaviruses differentially regulate endothelial cell responses. *Proc Natl Acad Sci U S A 99*, 13837–13842.

Giles, R. B., Sheedy, J. A., Ekman, C. N., Froeb, H. F., Conley, C. C., Stockard, J. L., Cugell, D. W., Vester, J. W., Kiyasu, R. K., Entwisle, G., and Yoe, R. H. (1954). The sequelae of epidemic hemorrhagic fever: with a note on causes of death. *Am J Med 16*, 629–638.

Glass, G. G., Watson, A. J., LeDuc, J. W., Kelen, G. D., Quinn, T. C., and Childs, J. E. (1993). Infection with a ratborne hantavirus in US residents is consistently associated with hypertensive renal disease. *J Infect Dis 167*, 614–620.

Glass, G. G., Yates, T. L., Fine, J. B., Shields, T. M., Kendall, J. B., Hope, A. G., Parmenter, C. A., Peters, C. J., Ksiazek, T. G., Li, C. S., Patz, J. A., Mills, J. N. (2002). Satellite imagery characterizes local animal reservoir populations of Sin Nombre virus in Southwestern United States. *Proc Natl Acad Sci U S A 99*, 16817–16822.

Goldblum, S. E., Ding, X., and Campbell-Washington, J. (1993). Tumor necrosis factorα induces endothelial cell F-actin depolymerization, new actin synthesis, and barrier dysfunction. *Am J Physiol (Cell Physiol: 33) 264*, C894–C905.

Goldsmith, C. S., Elliott, L. H., Peters, C. J., and Zaki, S. R. (1995). Ultrastructural characteristics of Sin Nombre virus, causative agent of hantavirus pulmonary syndrome. *Arch Virol 140*, 2107–2122.

Green, W., Feddersen, R., Yousef, O., Behr, M., Smith, K., Nestler, J., Jenison, S., Yamada, T., and Hjelle, B. (1998). Tissue distribution of hantavirus antigen in naturally infected humans and deer mice. *J Infect Dis 177*, 1696–1700.

Groen, J., Gerding, M. N., Koeman, J. P., Roholl, P. J., van Amerongen, G., Jordans, H. G., Niesters, H. G., and Osterhaus, A. D. (1995). A macaque model for hantavirus infection. *J Infect Dis 172*, 38–44.

Hallin, G. W., Simpson, S. Q., Crowell, R. E., James, D. S., Koster, F. T., Mertz, G. J., and Levy, H. (1996). Cardiopulmonary manifestations of hantavirus pulmonary syndrome. *Crit Care Med 24*, 252–258.

Heiskanen, T., Li, X. D., Hepojoki, J., Gustafsson, E., Lundkvist, A., Vaheri, A., and Lankinen, H. (2004). Improvement of binding of Puumala virus neutralization site resembling peptide with a second-generation phage library. *Protein Eng 16*, 443–450.

Henderson, W. W., Monroe, M. C., St. Jeor, S. C., Thayer, W. P., Rowe, J. E., Peters, C. J., and Nichol, S. T. (1995). Naturally occurring Sin Nombre virus genetic reassortants. *Virology 214*, 602–610.

Hinson, E. R., Shone, S. M., Zink, M. C., Glass, G. G., and Klein, S. L. (2004). Wounding: the primary mode of Seoul virus transmission among male Norway rats. *Am J Trop Med Hyg 70*, 310–317.

Hjelle, B. (1999). Virus detection and identification with genetic tests. In: Manual of hemorrhagic fever with renal syndrome and hantavirus pulmonary syndrome, H. W. Lee, C. H. Calisher, and C. S. Schmaljohn, eds. (Seoul, WHO Collaborating Center for Virus Reference and Research (Hantaviruses)), pp. 132–137.

Hjelle, B. (2002). Review: Vaccines against hantaviruses. *Expert Rev Vaccines 1*, 373–384.

Hjelle, B., Chavez-Giles, F., Torrez-Martinez, N., Yates, T. L., Sarisky, J., Webb, J., and Ascher, M. (1994a). Genetic identification of a novel hantavirus of the harvest mouse Reithrodontomys megalotis. *J Virol 68*, 6751–6754.

Hjelle, B., and Glass, G. G. (2000). Outbreak of hantavirus infection in the Four Corners region of the US in the wake of the 1997–98 El Nino-Southern Oscillation. *J Infect Dis 181*, 1569–1573.

Hjelle, B., Jenison, S., Torrez-Martinez, N., Herring, B., Quan, S., Polito, A., Pichuantes, S., Yamada, T., Morris, C., Elgh, F., Lee, H. W., Artsob, H., and Dinello, R. (1997). Rapid and specific detection of Sin Nombre virus antibodies in patients with hantavirus pulmonary syndrome by a strip immunoblot assay suitable for field diagnosis. *J Clin Microbiol 35*, 600–608.

Hjelle, B., Spiropoulou, C. F., Torrez-Martinez, N., Morzunov, S., Peters, C. J., and Nichol, S. T. (1994b). Detection of Muerto Canyon virus RNA in peripheral blood mononuclear cells from patients with hantavirus pulmonary syndrome. *J Infect Dis 170*, 1013–1017.

Hjelle, B., Torrez-Martinez, N., Koster, F. T., Jay, M., Ascher, M. S., Brown, T., Reynolds, P., Ettestad, P., Voorhees, R. E., Sarisky, J., Enscore R. E., Sands L., Mosley, D. G., Kioski, C., Bryan R. T., and Sewell, C. M. (1996). Epidemiologic linkage of rodent and human hantavirus genomic sequences in case investigations of hantavirus pulmonary syndrome. *J Infect Dis 173*, 781–786.

Hooper, J. W., Custer, D. M., and Thompson, E. (2003). Four-gene combination DNA vaccine protects mice against a lethal vaccinia virus challenge and elicits appropriate antibody responses in non-human primates. *Virology 306*, 181–195.

Hooper, J. W., Custer, D. M., Thompson, E., and Schmaljohn, C. S. (2001a). DNA vaccination with the Hantaan virus M gene protects hamsters against three of four HFRS hantaviruses and elicits a high-titer neutralizing antibody response in rhesus monkeys. *J Virol 75*, 8469–8477.

Hooper, J. W., Larsen, T., Custer, D. M., and Schmaljohn, C. S. (2001b). A lethal disease model for hantavirus pulmonary syndrome. *Virology 289*, 6–14.

Hooper, J. W., and Li, D. (2001). Vaccines against hantaviruses. *Curr Top Microbiol Immunol 256*, 171–191.

Huang, C., Jin, B., Wang, M., Li, E., and Sun, C. (1994). Hemorrhagic fever with renal syndrome: relationship between pathogenesis and cellular immunity. *J Infect Dis 169*, 868–870.

Huggins, J. W., Hsiang, C. M., Cosgriff, T. M., Guang, M. Y., Smith, J. I., Wu, Z. O., LeDuc, J. W., Zheng, Z. M., Meegan, J. M., Wang, Q. N., Oland, D. D., Gui, X. E., Gibbs, P. H., Yuan, G. H., and Zhang, T. M. (1991). Prospective, double-blind, concurrent, placebo-controlled clinical trial of intravenous ribavirin therapy of hemorrhagic fever with renal syndrome. *J Infect Dis 164*, 1119–1127.

Huggins, J. W., Kim, G. R., Brand, O. M., and McKee, K. T., Jr (1986). Ribavirin therapy for Hantaan virus infection in suckling mice. *J Infect Dis 153*, 489–497.

Iqbal, M., Cohen, R. I., Marzouk, K., and Liu, S. F. (2002). Time course of nitric oxide, peroxynitrite, and antioxidants in the endotoxemic heart. *Crit Care Med 30*, 1291–1296.

Isegawa, Y., Tanishita, O., Ueda, S., and Yamanishi, K. (1994). Association of serine in position 1124 of Hantaan virus glycoprotein with virulence in mice. *J Gen Virol 75*, 3273–3278.

Jay, M., Ascher, M. S., Chomel, B. B., Madon, M., Sesline, D., Enge, B. A., Hjelle, B., Ksiazek, T. G., Rollin, P. E., Kass, P. H., and Reilly, K. (1997). Seroepidemiologic studies of hantavirus infection among wild rodents in California. *Emerg Infect Dis 3*, 183–190.

Jay, M., Hjelle, B., Davis, R., Ascher, M., Baylies, H. N., Reilly, K., and Vugia, D. (1996). Occupational exposure leading to hantavirus pulmonary syndrome in a utility company employee. *Clin Infect Dis 22*, 841–844.

Jenison, S., Yamada, T., Morris, C., Anderson, B., Torrez-Martinez, N., Keller, N., and Hjelle, B. (1994). Characterization of human antibody responses to four corners hantavirus infections among patients with hantavirus pulmonary syndrome. *J Virol 68*, 3000–3006.

Jin, H. K., Yoshimatsu, K., Takeda, A., Ogino, M., Asano, A., Arikawa, J., and Watanabe, T. (2001). Mouse Mx2 protein inhibits hantavirus but not influenza virus replication. *Arch Virol 146*, 41–49.

Johnson, K. M. (2001). Hantaviruses: history and overview. *Curr Top Microbiol Immunol 256*, 1–14.

Jokinen, E. J., Lahdevirta, J., and Collan, Y. (1978). Nephropathia epidemica: immunohistochemical study of pathogenesis. *Clin Nephrol 9*, 1–5.

Kanerva, M., Melen, K., Vaheri, A., and Julkunen, I. (1996). Inhibition of puumala and tula hantaviruses in Vero cells by MxA protein. *Virology 224*, 55–62.

Kang, J.-I., Park, S.-H., Lee, P.-W., and Ahn, B.-Y. (1999). Apoptosis is induced by hantaviruses in cultured cells. *Virology 264*, 99–105.

Ketai, L. H., Kelsey, C. A., Jordan, K., Levin, D. L., Sullivan, L. M., Williamson, M. R., Wiest, P. W., and Sell, J. J. (1998). Distinguishing hantavirus pulmonary syndrome from acute respiratory distress syndrome by chest radiography: are there different radiographic manifestations of increased alveolar permeability? *J Thorac Imaging 13*, 172–177.

Ketai, L. H., Williamson, M. R., Telepak, R. J., Levy, H., Koster, F. T., Nolte, K. B., and Allen, S. E. (1994). Hantavirus pulmonary syndrome: radiographic findings in 16 patients. *Radiology 191*, 665–668.

Khabar, K. S. A., Al-Zoghaibi, F., Al-Ahdal, M. N., Murayama, T., Dhalla, M., Mukaida, M., Taha, M., Al-Sedairy, S. T., Siddiqui, Y., Kessie, G., and Matsushima, K. (1997). The α chemokine, interleukin 8, inhibits the antiviral action of interferon α. *J Exp Med 186*, 1077–1085.

Khaiboullina, S. F., Netski, D. M., Krumpe, P., and St. Jeor, S. C. (2000). Effects of tumor necrosis factor alpha on Sin Nombre virus infection in vitro. *J Virol 74*, 11966–11971.

Khaiboullina, S. F., Rizvanov, A. A., Otteson, E., Miyazato, A., Maciejewski, J., and St. Jeor, S. C. (2004). Regulation of cellular gene expression in endothelial cells by sin nombre and prospect hill viruses. *Viral Immunol 17*, 234–251.

Khaiboullina, S. F., and St. Jeor, S. C. (2002). Hantavirus Immunology. *Viral Immunol 15*, 609–625.

Khan, A. S., Khabbaz, R. F., Armstrong, L. R., Holman, R. C., Bauer, S. P., Graber, J., Strine, T., Miller, G., Reef, S., Tappero, J., Rollin P. E., Nichol, S. T., Zaki, S. R., Bryan, R. T., Chapman, L. E., Peters, C. J., and Ksiazek, T. G. (1996). Hantavirus pulmonary syndrome: the first 100 cases. *J Infect Dis 173*, 1297–1303.

Kilpatrick, E. D., Terajima, M., Koster, F., Catalina, M. D., and Ennis, F. A. (2004). Role of specific CD8 + T cells in the severity of a fulminant zoonotic viral hemorrhagic fever, hantavirus pulmonary syndrome. *J Immunol 172*, 3297–3304.

Kim, G. R., and McKee, K. T., Jr (1985). Pathogenesis of Hantaan virus infection in suckling mice: clinical, virologic, and serologic observations. *Am J Trop Med Hyg 34*, 388–395.

Klein, S. L., Zink, M. C., and Glass, G. G. (2004). Seoul virus increases aggressive behaviour in male Norway rats. *Anim Behav 67*, 421–429.

Koster, F., Foucar, K., Hjelle, B., Scott, A., Chong, Y.-Y., Larson, R. A., and McCabe, M. (2001). Rapid presumptive diagnosis of hantavirus cardiopulmonary syndrome by peripheral blood smear review. *Am J Clin Pathol 116*, 665–672.

Koster, F. T., and Hjelle, B. (2004). Hantaviruses. In: Infectious Diseases, S. L. Gorbach, J. G. Bartlett, and N. R. Blacklow, eds. (Philadelphia, Lippincott Williams & Wilkins), pp. 2023–2031.

Kraus, A. A., Raftery, M. J., Giese, T., Ulrich, R., Zawatzky, R., Hippenstiel, S., Suttorp, N., Kruger, D. H., and Schonrich, G. (2004). Differential antiviral response of endothelial cells after infection with pathogenic and nonpathogenic hantaviruses. *J Virol 78*, 6143–6150.

Kuenzi, A. J., Morrison, M. L., Swann, D. E., Hardy, P. C., and Downard, G. T. (1999). A longitudinal study of Sin Nombre Virus prevalence in rodents, Southeastern Arizona. *Emerg Infect Dis 5*, 113–117.

LeDuc, J. W. (1987). Epidemiology of Hantaan and related viruses. *Lab Anim Sci 37*, 413–418.

Lee, H. W. (1989). Hemorrhagic fever with renal syndrome in Korea. *Rev Infect Dis 11*, S864–S876.

Lee, H. W., Lee, P. W., and Johnson, K. M. (1978). Isolation of the etiologic agent of Korean hemorrhagic fever. *J Infect Dis 137*, 298–308.

Levis, S., Morzunov, S. P., Rowe, J. E., Enria, D. A., Pini, N., Calderon, G., Sabattini, M., and St. Jeor, S. C. (1998). Genetic diversity and epidemiology of hantaviruses in Argentina. *J Infect Dis 177*, 529–538.

Levy, H., and Simpson, S. Q. (1994). Hantavirus Pulmonary Syndrome. *Am J Respir Crit Care Med 149*, 1710–1713.

Li, D., Schmaljohn, A. L., Anderson, K. K., and Schmaljohn, C. S. (1995). Complete nucleotide sequences of the M and S segments of two hantavirus isolates from California: evidence for reassortment in nature among viruses related to hantavirus pulmonary syndrome. *Virology 206*, 973–983.

Liang, M., Chu, Y. K., and Schmaljohn, C. S. (1996). Bacterial expression of neutralizing mouse monoclonal antibody Fab fragments to Hantaan virus. *Virology 217*, 262–271.

Linderholm, M., Ahlm, C., Settergren, B., Waage, A., and Tarnvik, A. (1996). Elevated plasma levels of tumor necrosis factor (TNF)-α, soluble TNF receptors, interleukin (IL)-6, and IL-10 in patients with hemorrhagic fever with renal syndrome. *J Infect Dis 173*, 38–43.

Linderholm, M., Sandstrom, T., Rinnstrom, O., Groth, S., Blomberg, A., and Tarnvik, A. (1997). Impaired pulmonary function in patients with hemorrhagic fever with renal syndrome. *Clin Infect Dis 25*, 1084–1089.

Lukes, R. J. (1954). The pathology of thirty-nine fatal cases of epidemic hemorrhagic fever. *Am J Med 16*, 639–650.

Lundkvist, A., cheng, Y., Sjolander, K. B., Niklasson, B., Vaheri, A., and Plyusnin, A. (1997). Cell culture adaptation of Puumala hantavirus changes the infectivity for its natural reservoir, Clethrionomys glareolus, and leads to accumulation of mutants with altered genomic RNA S segment. *J Virol 71*, 9515–9523.

Lundkvist, A., and Niklasson, B. (1992). Bank vole monoclonal antibodies against Puumala virus envelope glycoproteins: identification of epitopes involved in neutralization. *Arch Virol 126*, 93–105.

Luo, D. D., Wang, X. H., Jin, W. E., and Fan, J. Z. (1985). Detection and analysis of specific circulating immune complexes in epidemic hemorrhagic fever. *Clin J Infect Dis 3*, 86–90.

Maes, P., Clement, J., Gavrilovskaya, I., and Van Ranst, M. (2004). Hantaviruses: immunology, treatment, and prevention. *Viral Immunol 17*, 481–497.

Makela, S., Mustonen, J., Ala-Houhala, I., Hurme, M., Partanen, J., Vapalahti, O., Vaheri, A., and Pasternack, A. (2002). Human leukocyte antigen-B8-DR3 is a more important risk factor for severe Puumala hantavirus infection than the tumor necrosis factor-alpha(-308) G/A polymorphism. *J Infect Dis 186*, 843–846.

McCall, T. B., Palmer, R. M. J., and Moncada, S. (1992). Interleukin-8 inhibits the induction of nitric oxide synthase in rat peritoneal neutrophils. *Biochem Biophys Res Commun 186*, 680–685.

McClain, D. J., Summers, P. L., Harrison, S. A., Schmaljohn, A. L., and Schmaljohn, C. S. (2000). Clinical evaluation of a vaccinia-vectored Hantaan virus vaccine. *J Med Virol 60*, 77–85.

McElroy, A. K., Smith, J. M., Hooper, J. W., and Schmaljohn, C. S. (2004). Andes virus M genome segment is not sufficient to confer the virulence associated with Andes virus in Syrian hamsters. *Virology 326*, 130–139.

Mertz, G. J., Miedzinski, L., Goade, D., Pavia, A. T., Hjelle, B., Hansbarger, C. O., Levy, H., Koster, F. T., Baum, K., Lindemulder, A., Wang, W., Riser, L., Fernandez, H., Whitley, R. J., for the Collaborative Antiviral Study Group. (2004). Placebo-controlled, double blind trial of intravenous ribavirin for hantavirus cardiopulmonary syndrome in North America. *Clin Infect Dis 39*, 1307–1313.

Milazzo, M. L., Eyzaguirre, E. J., Molina, C. P., and Fulhorst, C. F. (2002). Maporal viral infection in the Syrian Golden Hamster: A model of hantavirus pulmonary syndrome. *J Infect Dis 186*, 1390–1395.

Mills, J. N., Yates, T. L., Ksiazek, T. G., Peters, C. J., and Childs, J. E. (1999). Long-term studies of hantavirus reservoir populations in the Southwestern United States: rationale, potential and methods. *Emerg Infect Dis 5*, 95–101.

Mir, M. A., and Panganiban, A. T. (2004). Trimeric hantavirus nucleocapsid protein binds specifically to the viral RNA panhandle. *J Virol 78*, 8281–8288.

Mir, M. A., and Panganiban, A. T. (2005). The Hantavirus Nucleocapsid Protein Recognizes Specific Features of the Viral RNA Panhandle and Is Altered in Conformation upon RNA Binding. *J Virol 79*, 1824–1835.

Moll van Charante, A. W., Groen, J., Mulder, P. G., Rijpkema, S. G., and Osterhaus, A. D. (1998). Occupational risks of zoonotic infections in Dutch forestry workers and muskrat catchers. *Eur J Epidemiol 14*, 109–116.

Moolenaar, R. L., Dalton, C., Lipman, H. B., Umland, E. T., Gallaher, M., Duchin, J. S., Chapman, L. E., Zaki, S. R., Ksiazek, T. G., Rollin, P. E., Nichol, S., Cheek, J. E., Butler, J. C., Peters, C. J., Brieman, R. F. (1995). Clinical features that differentiate hantavirus pulmonary syndrome from three other acute respiratory illnesses. *Clin Infect Dis 21*, 643–649.

Morens, D. M. (1994). Antibody-dependent enhancement of infection and the pathogenesis of viral disease. *Clin Infect Dis 19*, 500–512.

Mori, M., Rothman, A. L., Kurane, I., Montoya, J. M., Nolte, K. B., Norman, J. E., Waite, D. C., Koster, F. T., and Ennis, F. A. (1999). High levels of cytokine-producing cells in the lung tissues of patients with fatal hantavirus pulmonary syndrome. *J Infect Dis 179*, 295–302.

Morzunov, S., Rowe, J. E., Ksiazek, T. G., Peters, C. J., St. Jeor, S. C., and Nichol, S. T. (1998). Genetic analysis of the diversity and origin of hantaviruses in Peromyscus leucopus mice in North *America. J Virol 72*, 57–64.

Mustonen, J., Huttunen, N. P., Partanen, J., Baer, M., Paakkala, A., Vapalahti, O., and Uhari, M. (2004). Human leukocyte antigens B8-DRB1*03 in pediatric patients with nephropathia epidemica caused by Puumala hantavirus. *Pediatr Infect Dis J 23*, 959–961.

Mustonen, J., Partanen, J., Kanerva, M., Pietila, K., Vapalahti, O., Pasternack, A., and Vaheri, A. (1996). Genetic susceptibility to severe course of nephropathia epidemica caused by Puumala hantavirus. *Kidney Int 49*, 217–221.

Nam, J.-H., Hwang, K.-A., Yu, C.-H., Kang, T.-H., Shin, J.-Y., Choi, W.-Y., Kim, I.-B., Joo, Y.-R., Cho, H.-W., and Park, K.-Y. (2003). Expression of interferon inducible genes following Hantaan virus infection as a mechanism of resistance in A549 cells. *Virus Genes 26*, 31–38.

Nemirov, K., Lundkvist, A., Vaheri, A., and Plyusnin, A. (2003). Adaptation of Puumala hantavirus to cell culture is associated with point mutations in the coding region of the L segment and in the noncoding regions of the S segment. *J Virol 77*, 8793–8800.

Nichol, S. T. (2001). Bunyaviruses. In: Fields Virology, D. M. Knipe, and P. M. Howley, eds. (Philadelphia, Lippincott Williams & Wilkins), pp. 1603–1633.

Nichol, S. T., Spiropoulou, C. F., Morzunov, S., Rollin, P. E., Ksiazek, T. G., Feldmann, H., Sanchez, J. L., Childs, J. E., Zaki, S. R., and Peters, C. J. (1993). Genetic identification of a novel hantavirus associated with an outbreak of acute respiratory illness in the Southwestern United States. *Science 262*, 914–917.

Niikura, M., Maeda, A., Ikegami, T., Saijo, M., Kurane, I., and Morikawa, S. (2004). Modifications of endothelial cell functions by Hantaan virus infection: prolonged hyper-permeability induced by TNF-alpha of hantaan virus-infected endothelial cell monolayers. *Arch Virol 149*, 1279–1292.

Niklasson, B., Hellsten, G., and LeDuc, J. W. (1994). Hemorrhagic fever with renal syndrome: a study of sequelae following nephropathia epidemica. *Arch Virol 137*, 241–247.

Niklasson, B., and LeDuc, J. W. (1987). Epidemiology of nephropathia epidemica in Sweden. *J Infect Dis 155*, 269–276.

Nolte, K. B., Feddersen, R. M., Foucar, K., Zaki, S. R., Koster, F. T., Madar, D., Merlin, T. L., McFeeley, P. J., Umland, E. T., and Zumwalt, R. E. (1995). Hantavirus pulmonary syndrome in the United States: a pathological description of a disease caused by a new agent. *Hum Pathol 26*, 110–120.

Padula, P., Edelstein, A., Miguel, S. D., Lopez, N. M., Rossi, C. M., and Rabinovich, R. D. (1998). Hantavirus pulmonary syndrome outbreak in Argentina: molecular evidence of person-to-person transmission of Andes virus. *Virology 241*, 323–330.

Parrillo, J. E. (1993). Pathogenetic mechanisms of septic shock. *New Engl J Med 328*, 1471–1477.

Pilaski, J., Feldmann, H., Morzunov, S., Rollin, P. E., Ruo, S. L., Lauer, B., Peters, C. J., and Nichol, S. T. (1994). Genetic identification of a new Puumala virus strain causing severe hemorrhagic fever with renal syndrome in Germany. *J Infect Dis 170*, 1456–1462.

Pini, N. (2004). Hantavirus pulmonary syndrome in Latin America. *Curr Opin Infect Dis 17*, 427–431.

Plyusnin, A., and Morzunov, S. (2001). Virus evolution and genetic diversity of hantaviruses and their rodent hosts. *Curr Top Microbiol Immunol 256*, 47–75.

Plyusnin, A., Vapalahti, O., and Vaheri, A. (1996). Hantaviruses: genome structure, expression, and evolution. *J Gen Virol 77*, 2677–2687.

Plyusnina, A., and Plyusnin, A. (2005). Recombinant Tula hantavirus showed reduced fitness but is able to survive in the presence of a parental virus: analysis of consecutive passages in a cell culture. *Virol J 2*, 1–5.

Raftery, M. J., Kraus, A. A., Ulrich, R., Kruger, D. H., and Schonrich, G. (2002). Hantavirus infection in dendritic cells. *J Virol 76*, 10724–10733.

Ravkov, E. V., Nichol, S. T., and Compans, R. W. (1997). Polarized enry and release in epithelial cells of Black Creek Canal virus, a New World hantavirus. *J Virol 71*, 1147–1154.

Ravkov, E. V., Nichol, S. T., Peters, C. J., and Compans, R. W. (1998). Role of actin microfilaments in Black Creek Canal virus morphogenesis. *J Virol 72*, 2865–2870.

Raymond, T., Gorbunova, E., Gavrilovskaya, I. N., and Mackow, E. R. (2005). Pathogenic hantaviruses bind plexin-semaphorin-integrin domains present at the apex of inactive, bent αVβ3 integrin conformers. *Proc Natl Acad Sci U S A 102*, 1163–1168.

Reiss, C. S., and Komatsu, T. (1998). Does Nitric Oxide Play a Critical Role in Viral Infections? *J Virol 72*, 4547–4551.

Riquelme, R., Riquelme, M., Torres, A., Rioseco, M. L., Vergara, J. A., Scholz, L., and Carriel, A. (2003). Hantavirus Pulmonary Syndrome, Southern Chile. *Emerg Infect Dis 9*, 1438–1443.

Rosenberg, R. B., Waagner, D. C., Romano, M. J., Kanase, H. N., and Young, R. B. (1998). Hantavirus pulmonary syndrome treated with inhaled nitric oxide. *Pediatr Infect Dis* J *17*, 749–752.

Rossi, C. A., and Ksiazek, T. G. (1999). Virus detection and identification with serologic tests. 2. Enzyme-linked immunosorbent assay (ELISA). In: Manual of hemorrhagic fever with renal syndrome and hantavirus pulmonary syndrome, H. W. Lee, C. H. Calisher, and C. Schmaljohn, eds. (Seoul, WHO Collaborating Center for Virus Reference and Research (Hantaviruses), Asian Institute for Life Sciences), pp. 87–91.

Rubini, M. E., Jablon, S., and McDowell, M. E. (1960). Renal residuals of acute epidemic hemorrhagic fever. *Arch Intern Med 106*, 378–387.

Ruedas, L. A., Salazar-Bravo, J., Tinnin, D. S., Armién, B., Caceres, L., Garcia, A., Avila Diaz, M., Gracia, F., Suzán, G., Peters, C. J., Yates, T. L., and Mills, J. N. (2004). Community ecology of small mammal populations in Panama following an outbreak of hantavirus pulmonary syndrome. *J Vector Ecol 29*, 177–188.

Ruo, S. L., Li, Y. L., Tong, Z., Ma, Q. R., Liu, Z. L., Tang, Y. W., Ye, K. L., McCormick, J. B., Fisher-Hoch, S., and Xu, Z. Y. (1994). Retrospective and prospective studies of hemorrhagic fever with renal syndrome in rural China. *J Infect Dis 170*, 527–534.

Ruusala, A., Persson, R., Schmaljohn, C. S., and Pettersson, R. F. (1992). Coexpression of the membrane glycoproteins G1 and G2 of Hantaan virus is required for targeting to the Golgi complex. *Virology 186*, 53–64.

Schmaljohn, C. S. (1996). Molecular biology of Hantaviruses. In: The Bunyaviridae, R. M. Elliott, ed. (New York, Plenum Press), pp. 63–86.

Schmaljohn, C. S., Chu, Y. K., Schmaljohn, A. L., and Dalrymple, J. M. (1990). Antigenic subunits of Hantaan virus expressed by baculovirus and vaccinia virus recombinants. *J Virol 64*, 3162–3170.

Schmaljohn, C. S., and Hooper, J. W. (2001). Bunyaviridae: The Viruses and Their Replication. In: Fields Virology, D. M. Knipe, and P. M. Howley, eds. (Philadelphia, Lippincott Williams & Wilkins), pp. 1581–1602.

Sibold, C., Meisel, H., Kruger, D. H., Labuda, M., Lysy, J., Kozuch, O., Pejcoch, M., Vaheri, A., and Plyusnin, A. (1999). Recombination in Tula hantavirus evolution: analysis of genetic lineages from Slovakia. *J Virol 73*, 667–675.

Simpson, S. Q. (1998). Hantavirus pulmonary syndrome. *Heart Lung 27*, 51–57.

Sironen, T., Vaheri, A., and Plyusnin, A. (2001). Molecular evolution of Puumala hantaviruses. *J Virol 75*, 11803–11810.

Smith, J. J., and St. Jeor, S. C. (2004). Three-week incubation period for hantavirus infection. *Pediatr Infect Dis J 23*, 974–975.

Sohn, Y. M., Rho, H. O., Park, M. S., Kim, J. S., and Summers, P. L. (2001). Primary humoral immune responses to formalin inactivated hemorrhagic fever with renal syndrome vaccine (Hantavax): consideration of active immunization in South Korea. *Yonsei Med J 42*, 278–284.

Spiropoulou, C. F., Morzunov, S., Feldmann, H., Sanchez, A., Peters, C. J., and Nichol, S. T. (1994). Genome structure and variability of a virus causing hantavirus pulmonary syndrome. *Virology 200*, 715–723.

Sundstrom, J. B., McMullan, L. K., Spiropoulou, C. F., Hooper, W. C., Ansari, A. A., Peters, C. J., and Rollin, P. E. (2001). Hantavirus infection induces the expression of RANTES and IP-10 without causing increased permeability in human lung microvascular endothelial cells. *J Virol 75*, 6070–6085.

Terajima, M., Hendershot, J. D., Kariwa, H., Koster, F. T., Hjelle, B., Goade, D., DeFronzo, M. C., and Ennis, F. A. (1999). High levels of viremia in patients with the Hantavirus pulmonary syndrome. *J Infect Dis 180*, 2030–2034.

Terajima, M., Van Epps, H. L., Li, D., Leporati, A. M., Juhlin, S. E., Mustonen, J., Vaheri, A., and Ennis, F. A. (2002). Generation of recombinant vaccinia viruses expressing Puumala virus proteins and use in isolating cytotoxic T cells specific for Puumala virus. *Virus Res 84*, 67–77.

Terajima, M., Vapalahti, O., Van Epps, H. L., Vaheri, A., and Ennis, F. A. (2004). Immune responses to Puumala virus infection and the pathogenesis of nephropathic epidemica. *Microbes Infect 6*, 238–245.

Toro, J., Vega, J. D., Khan, A. S., Mills, J. N., Padula, P., Terry, W., Yadon, Z., Valderrama, R., Ellis, B. A., Pavletic, C., Cerda, R., Zaki, S., Wun-Ju, S., Meyer, R., Tapia, M., Mansilla, C., Baro, M., Vergara, J. A., Concha, M., Calderon, G., Enria, D., Peters, C. J., and Ksiazek, T. G. (1998). An outbreak of hantavirus pulmonary syndrome, Chile, 1997. *Emerg Infect Dis 4*, 687–694.

Tsai, T. F. (1987). Hemorrhagic fever with renal syndrome: mode of transmission to humans. *Lab Anim Sci 37*, 428–430.

Van Epps, H. L., Schmaljohn, C. S., and Ennis, F. A. (1999). Human memory cytotoxic T-lymphocyte (CTL) responses to Hantaan virus infection: identification of virus-specific and cross-reactive CD8+ CTL epitopes on nucleocapsid protein. *J Virol 73*, 5301–5308.

Van Epps, H. L., Terajima, M., Mustonen, J., Arstila, T. P., Corey, E. A., Vaheri, A., and Ennis, F. A. (2002). Long-lived Memory T Lymphocyte Responses After Hantavirus Infection. *J Exp Med 196*, 579–588.

Van Gorp, E. C., Setiati, T. E., Mairuhu, A. T., Suharti, C., Cate, H. H., Dolmans, W. M., Van der Meer, J. W., Hack, C. E., and Brandjes, D. P. (2002). Impaired fibrinolysis in the pathogenesis of dengue hemorrhagic fever. *J Med Virol 67*, 549–554.

Vapalahti, O., Mustonen, J., Lundkvist, A., Henttonen, H., Plyusnin, A., and Vaheri, A. (2003). Hantavirus infections in Europe. *Lancet Infect Dis 3*, 752–754.

Vitek, C. R., Breiman, R. F., Ksiazek, T. G., Rollin, P. E., McLaughlin, J. C., Umland, E. T., Nolte, K. B., Loera, A., Sewell, C. M., and Peters, C. J. (1996). Evidence against person-to-person transmission of hantavirus to health care workers. *Clin Infect Dis 22*, 824–826.

Wasser, W. G., Rossi, C. A., and Glass, G. G. (1997). Hantavirus antibodies in New York [letter]. *Ann Intern Med 127*, 166–167.

Wells, R. M., Estani, S. S., Yadon, Z. E., Enria, D. A., Padula, P., Pini, N., Della Valle, M. G., Mills, J. N., and Peters, C. J. (1998). Seroprevalence of antibodies to hantavirus in health care workers and other residents of southern Argentina. *Clin Infect Dis 27*, 895–896.

Wells, R. M., Sosa Estani, S., Yadon, Z. E., Enria, D. A., Padula, P., Pini, N., Mills, J. N., Peters, C. J., and Segura, E. L. (1997a). An unusual hantavirus outbreak in southern Argentina: person-to-person transmission? Hantavirus Pulmonary Study Group for Patagonia. *Emerg Infect Dis 3*, 171–174.

Wells, R. M., Young, J. C., Williams, R. J., Armstrong, L. R., Busico, K., Khan, A. S., Ksiazek, T. G., Rollin, P. E., Zaki, S. R., Nichol, S. T., and Peters, C. J. (1997b). Hantavirus transmission in the United States. *Emerg Infect Dis 3*, 361–365.

Wichmann, D., Grone, H.-J., Frese, M., Pavlovic, J., Anheier, B., Haller, O., Klenk, H.-D., and Feldmann, H. (2002). Hantaan virus infection causes an acute neurological disease that is fatal in adult laboratory mice. *J Virol 76*, 8890–8899.

Williams, R. J., Bryan, R. T., Mills, J. N., Palma, R. E., Vera, I., De Velasquez, F., Baez, E., Schmidt, W. E., Figueroa, R. E., Peters, C. J., Zaki, S. R., Khan, A. S., and Ksiazek, T. G. (1997). An outbreak of hantavirus pulmonary syndrome in western Paraguay. *Am J Trop Med Hyg 57*, 274–282.

Xu, Z. Y., Guo, C. S., Wu, Y. L., Zhang, X. W., and Liu, K. (1985). Epidemiological studies of hemorrhagic fever with renal syndrome: analysis of risk factors and mode of transmission. *J Infect Dis 152*, 137–144.

Yadon, Z. (1998). Epidemiology of hantavirus pulmonary syndrome in Argentina (1991–1997). *Medicina (Buenos Aires) 58*, 25–26.

Yamada, T., Hjelle, B., Lanzi, R., Morris, C., Anderson, B., and Jenison, S. (1995). Antibody responses to Four Corners hantavirus infections in the deer mouse (*Peromyscus maniculatus*): identification of an immunodominant region of the viral nucleocapsid protein. *J Virol 69*, 1939–1943.

Yan, D. Y., Gu, X. S., Wang, D. Q., and Yang, S. H. (1981). Studies on immunopathognesis in epidemic hemorrhagic fever: sequential observations on activation of the first complement component in sera from patients with epidemic hemorrhagic fever. *J Immunol 127*, 1064–1067.

Yates, T., Mills, J. N., Parmenter, C. A., Ksiazek, T. G., Parmenter, R. R., Vande Castle, J. R., Calisher, C. H., Nichol, S. T., Abbott, K. D., Young, J. C., Morrison, M. L., Beaty, B. J., Dunnum, J. L., Baker, R. J., Salazar-Bravo, J., and Peters, C. L. (2002). The ecology and evolutionary history of an emergent disease: hantavirus pulmonary syndrome. *Bioscience 52*, 989–998.

Yoshimatsu, K., Lee, B.-H., Ariki, K., Morimatsu, M., Ogino, M., Ebihara, H., and Arikawa, J. (2003). The multimerization of hantavirus nucleocapsid protein depends on type-specific epitopes. *J Virol 77*, 943–952.

Zaki, S. R., Greer, P. W., Coffield, L. M., Goldsmith, C. S., Nolte, K. B., Foucar, K., Feddersen, R., Zumwalt, R. E., Miller, G. L., and Khan, A. S. (1995). Hantavirus pulmonary syndrome. Pathogenesis of an emerging infectious disease. *Am J Pathol 146*, 552–579.

Zaki, S. R., Khan, A. S., Goodman, R. A., Armstrong, L. R., Greer, P. W., Coffield, L. M., Ksiazek, T. G., Rollin, P. E., Peters, C. J., and Khabbaz, R. F. (1996). Retrospective diagnosis of hantavirus pulmonary syndrome, 1978–1993: implications for emerging infectious diseases. *Arch Pathol Lab Med 120*, 134–139.

Zavasky, D. M., Hjelle, B., Peterson, M. C., Denton, R. W., and Reimer, L. (1999). Acute infection with Sin Nombre hantavirus without pulmonary edema. *Clin Infect Dis 29*, 664–666.

Zeier, M., Handermann, M., Bahr, U., Rensch, B., Muller, S., Kehm, R., Muranyi, W., and Darai, G. (2005). New ecological aspects of hantavirus infection: A change of a paradigm and a challenge of prevention – A review. *Virus Genes 30*, 157–180.

Zeitz, P. S., Butler, J. C., Cheek, J. E., Samuel, M. C., Childs, J. E., Shands, L. A., Turner, R. E., Voorhees, R. E., Sarisky, J., Rollin, P. E., Ksiazek, T. G., Chapman, L., Reef, S. E., Komatsu, K. K., Dalton, C., Krebs, J. W., Maupin, G. O., Gage, K., Sewell, C. M., Brieman, R. F., and Peters, C. J. (1995). A case-control study of hantavirus pulmonary syndrome during an outbreak in the southwestern United States. *J Infect Dis 171*, 864–870.

3. Human Ehrlichioses and Anaplasmosis

JERE W. MCBRIDE AND DAVID H. WALKER

3.1. Human Ehrlichioses (Human Monocytotropic and Ehrlichiosis Ewingii)

3.1.1. Taxonomy

Historically, members of the genus *Ehrlichia* were classified on the basis of morphological, ecological, epidemiological, and clinical characteristics. However, recent application of contemporary molecular taxonomy has determined that previous criteria used for classification had resulted in incorrect placement of numerous organisms among several genera containing obligately intracellular bacteria. Hence, reorganization of the genus *Ehrlichia* has recently occurred and reflects a new molecularly based taxonomic classification using two highly conserved genes, *rrs* (16S ribosomal RNA genes) and *groESL* (Dumler et al., 2001). An amended and now smaller *Ehrlichia* genus consists of five formally named members (*E. canis, E. chaffeensis, E. muris, E. ruminantium* and *E. ewingii*) following the reassignment of six previously recognized members to the genera, *Anaplasma* (*E. phagocytophila, E. equi, E. platys,* and *E. bovis*) and *Neorickettsia* (*E. sennetsu* and *E. risticii*), and acquisition of one new member from the genus *Cowdria* (*C. ruminantium*). *E. chaffeensis* and *E. ewingii* are recognized as human pathogens and pathogens of veterinary importance in addition to *E. canis* and *E. ruminantium* (Table 3.1). The genus *Ehrlichia* is now assigned to the newly created family *Anaplasmataceae*, which also includes the genera *Anaplasma, Wolbachia,* and *Neorickettsia,* but remains in the order *Rickettsiales*.

3.1.2. Morphology

Ehrlichiae typically reside as microcolonies of bacteria in cytoplasmic vacuoles derived from early endosomes in immature and mature hemopoietic cells (monocytes/macrophages and neutrophils) (Barnewall

Table 3.1. Summary of tick-borne ehrlichioses of humans and animals

Disease	Agent	Hosts	Vector	Target cel	Geographic distribution	Diagnosis
Human monocy-totropic ehrlichiosis (HME)	*E. chaffeensis*	Humans, white-tailed deer, canids, goats	*A. americanum*	Monocyte/ macrophage	Southeastern, south-central United States	IFA, PCR
Human granulocytic ehrlichiosis (Ehrlichiosis ewingii)	*E. ewingii*	Canids, deer	*A. americanum*	Neutrophil	Southeastern, south-central United States	PCR, IFA
Canine monocytic ehrlichiosis (CME)	*E. canis*	Canids	*R. sangineus*	Monocyte/ macrophage	Worldwide	IFA/PCR
Heartwater	*E. ruminantium*	Cattle, sheep, goats, antelope	*Amblyomma* spp.	Endothelium	Africa/ Carribean Islands	IFA
Unnamed	*E. muris*	Voles, canids	*Haema-physalis flava*	Monocyte/ macrophage	Japan	IFA

et al., 1997). Morulae appear as dark-blue to purple intracytoplasmic inclusions by light microscopy using Romanovsky-type stains (Rikihisa, 1991) (Figs. 3.1 and 3.2). Examination of infected cells by electron microscopy demonstrates that numerous (1 to >400) morulae (1.0 to 6.0 µm) are usually present and contain as few as one, but more often numerous ehrichiae (>40). Individual ehrlichiae are coccoid and coccobacillary and exhibit two morphologic cell types, reticulate (0.4 to 0.6 µm by 0.7 to 1.9 µm) and dense-cored (0.4 to 0.6 µm in diameter) (Fig. 3.3). Both forms have a typical Gram-negative cell wall, characterized by a cytoplasmic membrane and outer membrane separated by a periplasmic space, but do not appear to have peptidoglycan. Reticulate cells are pleomorphic and have uniformly dispersed nucleoid filaments and ribosomes, and dense-cored cells are typically coccoid and have centrally condensed nucleoid filaments and ribosomes (Popov et al., 1995, 1998). Small and large morulae containing both reticulate and dense-cored cells or exclusively containing dense-cored cells usually in loosely packed clusters can be observed within a single infected cell (Popov et al., 1995, 1998). The intramorular space in some morulae contains a fibrillar matrix of ehrlichial origin (Popov et al., 1995).

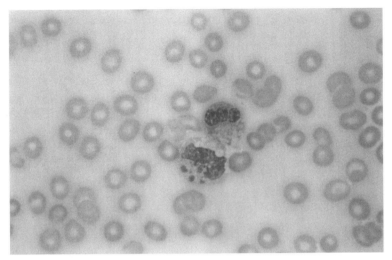

Figure 3.1. Peripheral blood smear from a patient with HME, demonstrating *E. chaffeensis* cytoplasmic inclusions (morulae) in a monocyte (lower cell). Each morula typically contains 40 to 100 ehrlichiae. Magnification, ×1000. (Photo courtesy of Christopher D. Paddock, Centers for Disease Control, Atlanta, GA; source *Clinical Microbiology Reviews*, 2003, American Society for Microbiology.)

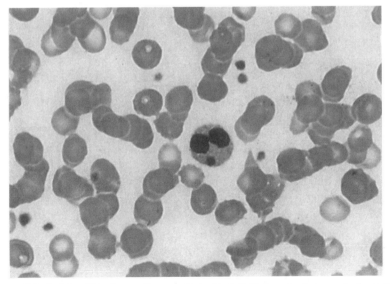

Figure 3.2. Peripheral blood smear from a patient with ehrlichiosis ewingii, demonstrating a cytoplasmic inclusion (morula) in a neutrophil (center).

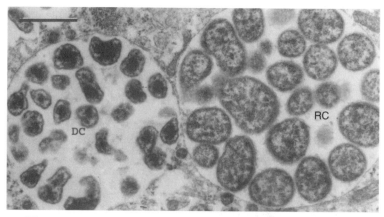

Figure 3.3. Electron photomicrograph of two adjacent *E. chaffeensis* cytoplasmic morulae containing the characteristic dense-cored (DC) and reticulate cell (RC) morphologic forms of the organism. Magnification, ×14,000; bar, 1 μm. (Reproduced with permission from V.L. Popov, University of Texas Medical Branch.)

3.1.3. Genetic, Antigenic, and Phenotypic Characteristics

⁃ The genomes of *E. chaffeensis, E. canis,* and *E. ruminantium* are small (1.2, 1.3, and 1.5 Mbp, respectively) containing approximately 900 protein-encoding genes with an average G + C content of only 27% (Collins et al., 2005). Substantially less is known about *E. ewingii* due to the failure to culture the organism *in vitro. E. chaffeensis* and *E. canis* are among the best characterized ehrlichiae at the molecular level. Functionally conserved genes, *rrs, rrl, rrf* (16S, 23S, and 5S rRNA, respectively) (Anderson et al., 1991; Massung et al., 2002), *groEL* and *groESL* (Sumner et al., 1993, 1997), thio-disulfide oxidoreductase (*dsb*) (McBride et al., 2002), ferric-ion binding protein (*fbp*) (Yu et al., 1999a; Doyle et al., 2005b), quinolate synthetase A (*nadA*) (Yu and Walker, 1997), and citrate synthase (*gltA*) (Inokuma et al., 2001), have been identified and characterized. A small group of major immunoreactive proteins of *E. chaffeensis* has been identified on the basis of immunoblot reactivity, but the functions of these proteins remain largely unknown. Major immunoreactive *E. chaffeensis* proteins are 200-, 120-, 88-, 55-, 47-, 40-, 28-, and 23-kDa (Chen et al., 1994b; Rikihisa et al., 1994), and major immunoreactive proteins identified in *E. canis* are 200-, 140-, 95-, 75-, 47-, 36-, 28-, and 19-kDa (McBride et al., 2003). Orthologs of five major immunoreactive proteins of *E. chaffeensis* (gp200, gp120, gp47, p42 [VLPT], and p28s [22 genes]) have been identified in *E. canis* (gp200, gp140, gp36, p19 [VLPT], and p28s [25 genes], respectively). Other *E. chaffeensis* immunoreactive proteins include *dsb* and *fbp* identified during antibody screening of genomic libraries, as well as the major antigenic protein 2 (MAP2) ortholog, identified first in *E. ruminantium*. These proteins are minor immunoreactive proteins by Western blot; however, the Fbp and the MAP2 orthologs of *E. chaffeensis* are substantially more immunoreactive in the native conformation (Alleman et al., 2000; Doyle et al., 2005b).

Four of the five recognized major immunoreactive *E. chaffeensis* proteins (gp200, gp120, gp47, gp28) that have been identified and characterized are glycoproteins, two of which (gp120 and gp47) have serine-rich tandem repeats (McBride et al., 2000, 2003; Singu et al., 2005). In addition, the immunoreactive variable length PCR target (VLPT) protein may also be a glycoprotein as it exhibits a mass two times larger than predicted by the amino acid sequence and has molecular characteristics (tandem repeats and serine-rich composition) found in other ehrlichial glycoproteins (Sumner et al., 1999). Strain-dependent sequence polymorphisms have been demonstrated in the number of serine/threonine-rich tandem repeats of gp120 (2 to 5) (Chen et al., 1997b; Yu et al., 1997; Yabsley et al., 2003) and VLPT (3 to 6) (Sumner et al., 1999) and in genes encoding the p28 multigene family (Yu et al., 1999b; Reddy and Streck, 2000). The observed molecular masses of these proteins vary depending on the number of repeat units (gp120, 80 to 130 kDa; VLPT, 35 to 55 kDa) (Chen et al., 1997a, 1997b; Sumner et al., 1999), and variation in sizes of other homologous proteins has been observed with monoclonal antibodies (MAb, 7C1-C, and 7C1-B) (Chen et al., 1997b). Antigenic heterogeneity has also been demonstrated with MAb 1A9 specific for p28 proteins, which does not react with all *E. chaffeensis* isolates (Chen et al., 1997b).

The first molecularly characterized major immunoreactive protein of *E. chaffeensis,* gp120, is a surface protein differentially expressed on dense-cored cells and is also a component of the fibrillar matrix found in some morulae. The molecular structure of the gp120 gene of the type strain (Arkansas) includes four 240-bp repeats, and human patient sera recognize the gp120 regardless of the number of repeats (Yu et al., 1997, 1999a). The serine-rich repeat regions appear to be heavily glycosylated by O-linked sugars, including glucose, galactose, and xylose (McBride et al., 2000). The gp120 is highly reactive with antibodies in convalescent sera from patients with human monocytotropic ehrlichiosis (HME) and is a strong candidate for development of recombinant serologic diagnostics (Yu et al., 1996, 1999a). The gp200 is the largest major immunoreactive protein identified in *E. chaffeensis* (1438 amino acids) by Western blot and has a predicted molecular mass of 156 kDa but exhibits a larger mass (~200 kDa) by gel electrophoresis. The gp200 contains numerous (at least 22) ankyrin repeats that likely mediate protein–protein interactions and therefore shares homology with numerous eukaryotic and prokaryotic ankyrin repeat–containing proteins including *A. phagocytophilum* AnkA (Caturegli et al., 2000). The gp200 is found primarily in the cytoplasm of ehrlichiae and in the nucleus (on condensed chromatin) of infected host cells. The gp200 does not have serine-rich tandem repeats, but glycans appear to be O-linked within the first 515 amino acids composing the N-terminal immunoreactive region of the protein. The gp47 is a glyco-protein that is differentially expressed on the surface of dense-cored cells and contains seven serine-rich 19-amino-acid tandem repeats. The gp47 appears to be secreted and is also observed in the fibrillar intramorular matrix. The *E. chaffeensis* VLPT is an immunoreactive protein that has 3 to 6 imperfect 30-amino-acid contiguous tandem repeats (Doyle et al., 2005). The VLPT has been used to determine genetic diversity of *E. chaffeensis* isolates based on the number of repeat units. VLPT patterns of *E. chaffeensis* amplified from patient blood predominantly contain 5 repeat units (Standaert et al., 2000). The *E. chaffeensis* p28 multigene family con-sists of 22 nonidentical paralogous genes (813 to 900 bp) found in a single 27-kb locus on the chromosome that encode mature surface-exposed major outer membrane proteins of 26 to 32 kDa with 20% to 80% amino acid sequence identity (Yu et al., 2000; Ohashi et al., 2001). The proteins contain three hypervarible regions, with a major B cell epitope located in the first hypervariable region (Li et al., 2002), and p28 proteins account for some antigenic cross-reactivity among the ehrlichiae. The potential for antigenic diversity by differential expression of p28 genes exists, but simultaneous transcription of all p28 genes does occur *in vitro* and in *E. chaffeensis*–infected dogs after needle inoculation (Long et al., 2002; Unver et al., 2002; Zhang et al., 2004a). The expression of only one paraolog (*omp-1B*) has been observed in ticks (Unver et al., 2002), but the p28 genes expressed in the mammalian host after tick inoculation are still unknown.

3.1.4. Pathogenesis and Immunity

Pathogenesis of HME begins with injection of *E. chaffeensis* by a feeding tick, hematogenous spread, and attachment to the target cell (monocyte/macrophage), entry, and intracellular survival. *E. chaffeensis* binding to the host cell receptors that include, but are not limited to, E- and L-selectin results in unconventional clathrin-independent recep-tor-mediated endocytosis (Barnewall et al., 1997; Zhang et al., 2003) involving caveolae and glycosylphosphatidylinositol-anchored proteins (Lin and Rikihisa, 2003a). Endocytosis of *E. chaffeensis* requires signaling events including protein cross-linking by transglutaminase, protein tyro-sine phosphorylation, phospholipase C (PLC)-γ2 activation, and calcium influx (Lin et al., 2002). After endocytosis, tyrosine phosphorylated proteins and PLC-γ2 colocalize with *E. chaffeensis* inclusions (Lin et al., 2002), suggesting their role in bacterial survival and proliferation in the macrophage. The unique endosomes containing *E. chaffeensis* express several early endosomal markers including an early endosomal antigen 1 (EEA1) and rab5 and do not fuse with lyosomes to form phagolysosomes (Barnewall et al., 1997; Mott et al., 1999), but colocal-ize with vesicle-associated membrane protein 2 (VAMP2), major histo-compatibility complex (MHC) class I and MHC class II molecules, β_2-microglobulin, and transferrin receptor (Barnewall et al., 1997, 1999; Mott et al., 1999). After entry, *E. chaffeensis* modulates the expression of various cytokines, toll-like receptors (TLR), transcription factors, apoptosis inhibitors, cell cyclins, membrane trafficking proteins, and transferrin receptor gene expression in the macrophage (Barnewall et al., 1999; Lin and Rikihisa, 2004; Zhang et al., 2004b). The inhibition of p38 MAPK by *E. chaffeensis* has been linked to the downregulation of tran-scription factor PU.1, which can also regulate the expression of TLRs and other genes (Lin and Rikihisa, 2004). Within 24 h of infection, *E. chaf-feensis* blocks tyrosine phosphorylation of Janus kinase (Jak) and signal transducer and activator of transcription (Stat) signaling, inhibiting the anti-ehrlichial effect of IFN-γ (Lee and Rikihisa, 1998). *E. chaffeensis* has eight genes encoding type IV secretion machinery that may be associated with intracellular survival and replication by delivering effector macro-molecules to the host cell and are transcribed in the blood of acutely ill patients (Ohashi et al., 2002). Some of these genes (*virB3, virB4* and *virB6*) are downstream of superoxide dismutase B (*sodB*) and are co-tran-scribed with *sodB* through a *sodB* promoter (Ohashi et al., 2002). Iron plays a critical role in the survival of *E. chaffeensis* in the host cell, and iron acquisition mechanisms in *E. chaffeensis* appear to be evolutionarily divergent from those of other Gram-negative bacteria (Doyle et al., 2005b). A structurally and functionally conserved ferric-ion binding protein (Fbp) has been identified in *E. chaffeensis* and *E. canis* that binds Fe(III), but not Fe(II), and Fbp is preferentially expressed on the surface of dense-cored ehrlichiae and is secreted extracellularly (Doyle et al., 2005b). The lack of iron availability prevents the survival of *E. chaffeensis,* which has been demonstrated with the intracellular iron chelator deferoxamine (Barnewall and Rikihisa, 1994). IFN-γ also appears to mediate killing of *E. chaffeensis* by downregulation of transferrin receptor, thus reducing the available labile cytoplasmic iron in human monocytes (Barnewall and Rikihisa, 1994). This anti-ehrlichial effect can be overcome by addition of iron-saturated transferrin, demonstrating the direct role for iron in ehrlichial survival. The role of the p28 multigene family in the pathogenesis of HME is unknown, but differential expression of p28 genes appears to occur in mammalian and tick hosts (Unver et al., 2002). *E. chaffeensis* demonstrates expression of 16 *p28* genes concurrently *in vitro* and *in vivo* (Long et al., 2002; Unver et al., 2002). These findings suggest that the p28s may play a role in ehrlichial adaptation in tick and mammalian hosts and are less likely to be involved in immune evasion by antigenic variation.

The role played by both innate and adaptive immune mechanisms in the elimination of *E. chaffeensis* from the host are not well understood. The innate immune response to *E. chaffeensis* is the least understood. Although new studies have not conclusively determined the adaptive immune mechanisms that are important, it appears that both humoral and cellular immunity plays a role in host defense against this pathogen. The primary host cell for *E. chaffeensis* is the monocyte/macrophage; thus an understanding of the role of innate immune recognition in immunity to *E. chaffeensis* is of considerable importance, yet little is known. *E. chaffeensis* lacks the genes for synthesis of two common Gram-negative bacterial cellular components, lipopolysaccharide (LPS) and peptidoglycan (PGN) (Lin and Rikihisa, 2003b), which are important pathogen-associated molecular patterns (PAMPs) recognized by the innate immune response. However, monocytes incubated with live and killed *E. chaffeensis* respond with strong production of IL-8 and minimal production of IL-1β and IL-10, while expression of TNF-α and IL-6 is absent (Lee and Rikihisa, 1996), which indicates that other uncharacterized ehrlichial PAMPs are involved. Induction of the innate immune response is linked to an *E. chaffeensis* carbohydrate component and is abrogated by periodate treatment (Lee and Rikihisa, 1996). More recent and extensive analysis of cytokine and chemokine induction in monocytes has demonstrated that the response to viable and killed *E. chaffeensis* is characterized by inflammatory chemokines including IL-8, MCP-1, and MIP-1β, while production of proinflammatory cytokines including TNF-α, IL-1β, or IL-10 is not observed (McBride, unpublished data). It appears that *E. chaffeensis* glycoproteins may be ehrlichial PAMPs as stimulation with *E. chaffeensis* recombinant glycoproteins gp120 and gp200 results in the same cytokine/chemokine profiles observed with the live organism, and periodate treatment of the glycoproteins abrogates the response (McBride, unpublished data). The TLRs involved in recognition of *E. chaffeensis* are not known, but *tlr4*-deficient mice have depressed nitric oxide and interleukin-6 production and have more prolonged infections with *E. chaffeensis* than wild-type mice (Ganta et al., 2002), suggesting a role for TLR4 recognition.

Understanding the adaptive immune mechanisms involved in immunity to *E. chaffeensis* has been hampered by resistance of inbred mice to infection with *E. chaffeensis* (Winslow et al., 1998). However, inbred mice deficient in various immune system components including MHC class II and TLR4 and mice with severe combined immunodeficiency (SCID) have been useful for identifying the role of specific immune system elements. Mice lacking functional MHC class II genes are unable to clear *E. chaffeensis* after infection, suggesting that CD4[+]T cells are essential for ehrlichial clearance (Ganta et al., 2002). *E. chaffeensis* infection of SCID mice (B- and T-cell deficient) results in an overwhelming infection, but passive transfer of anti–*E. chaffeensis* immune serum or MAbs directed against the first hypervariable domain of one (p28-19) of the p28 major outer membrane proteins before or during infection protects SCID mice from disease, but does not eliminate the organism (Winslow et al., 2000; Li et al., 2001, 2002). Futhermore, anti–*E. chaffeensis* antibody complexed with *E. chaffeensis* induces proinflammatory cytokine responses (IL-1, TNF-α, and IL-6) and prolonged degradation of IκB-α and activation of NF-κB (Lee and Rikihisa, 1997). This response is dependent on immune complex binding to the Fcγ receptor and may contribute to anti-ehrichial mechanisms. A role for CD1d and NK T-cells has recently been described in which glycolipid antigens of *Ehrlichia* activate NK T cells, and NK T-cell-deficient mice are unable to clear ehrlichial infection (Mattner et al., 2005).

Severe and fatal cases of HME in non-immunocompromised patients exhibit a relatively low bacterial burden in the blood and tissues, and the disease is often manifest as a toxic shock-like syndrome, suggesting that the host immune response may be involved (Maeda et al., 1987; Fichtenbaum et al., 1993). The first animal model of fatal human ehrlichiosis (Sotomayor et al., 2001) has been instrumental in understanding the mechanisms behind the toxic shock-like syndrome of severe and fatal human ehrlichiosis. In this model, mice inoculated with an ehrlichia (*Ixodes ovatus* ehrlichia; IOE) closely related to *E. chaffeensis* develop pathological lesions resembling those observed in HME and exhibit a similar disease course. This model has recently been used to investigate the basis of susceptibility to severe monocytotropic ehrlichiosis. Lethal infections with IOE are accompanied by extremely high levels of serum TNF-α, a high frequency of TNF-α producing CD8[+] splenic T cells, decreased *Ehrlichia*-specific CD4[+]T lymphocyte proliferation, low IL-12 levels in the spleen, and a 40-fold decrease in the number of antigen-specific IFN-γ-producing CD4[+] Th1 cells (Ismail et al., 2004). However, transfer of the combination of IOE-specific polyclonal antibody and IFN-γ-producing *Ehrlichia*-specific CD4[+] and CD8[+] type 1

cells protects naïve mice against lethal challenge (Ismail et al., 2004).
A second study also concluded that resistance to sublethal IOE infection
was dependent on CD4[+]T lymphocytes and required IFN-γ and TNF-α,
but not IL-4 (Bitsaktsis et al., 2004). Taken together, these studies provide
convincing evidence that classical cell-mediated immune mechanisms
involving CD4 cells and type 1 cytokines are responsible for macrophage
activation and elimination of *Ehrlichia*. Notably, similar conclusions
regarding the importance of MHC class I, CD4[+], and CD8[+] T cells, the
synergistic roles of IFN-γ and TNF-α, and role of antibody have been
observed in a mouse model of acute monocytotropic ehrlichiosis with
E. muris (Feng and Walker, 2004).

3.1.5. Emergence, Epidemiology, and Transmission

The emergence of *E. chaffeensis* in the United States is likely due to
many factors including increased *A. americanum* density (Ginsberg et al.,
1991), expanded vector geographic distribution (Means and White, 1997)
and vertebrate host populations of the tick vector *A. americanum* (Means
and White, 1997), increase in reservoir host populations for *E. chaffeensis*
(McCabe and McCabe, 1997), increased human contact with natural foci of
infection through recreational and occupational activities (Standaert et al.,
1995; Tal and Shannahan, 1995), increased size, longevity, and immunocompromised status of the human population (Palella, Jr. et al., 1998;
Paddock et al., 2001), the availability of diagnostic reagents, and improved
surveillance (Childs et al., 1999; McQuiston et al., 1999) (Fig. 3.4). The
most important factor in the emergence of *E. ewingii* appears to be
increased immunocompromised populations, because the infection has
been observed primarily in HIV-infected individuals and patients on
immunosuppressive therapies (Buller et al., 1999; Paddock et al., 2001).

The reported cases of HME are seasonal (peak incidence during
May through July) (Fishbein et al., 1994; Standaert et al., 1995) and occur
primarily within the geographic range of the tick vector *A. americanum*
(Lone star tick), that begins in west central Texas and east along the Gulf
Coast, north through Oklahoma and Missouri, eastward to the Atlantic
Coast and proceeds northeast through New Jersey, encompassing all the
south central, southeastern, and mid-Atlantic states. Human ehrlichioses
became nationally reportable in 1999, but passive surveillance of HME
underestimates the true incidence of disease due to inadequate clinical
and laboratory diagnosis and reporting (McQuiston et al., 1999).
Nevertheless, ehrlichiosis has similar infection rates as those reported for
Rocky Mountain spotted fever (Treadwell et al., 2000), with the highest
incidence reported in Arkansas, North Carolina, Missouri, Oklahoma,

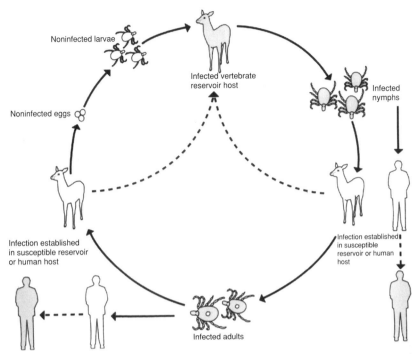

Figure 3.4. A life cycle of *E. chaffeensis*. *E. chaffeensis* is maintained in nature by persistently infected susceptible vertebrate reservoir hosts such as the white-tailed deer (shaded). Uninfected tick larvae (unshaded) feed on bacteremic vertebrate hosts and become infected (shaded). The infection is maintained transtadially in the tick, and nymphal and adult ticks can then transmit *E. chaffeensis* to other reservoir hosts or humans (shaded, incidental hosts). (Figure courtesy of Christopher D. Paddock, Centers for Disease Control, Atlanta, GA; source *Clinical Microbiology Reviews*, 2003, American Society for Microbiology.)

and New Jersey (McQuiston et al., 1999). Active surveillance in particular HME-endemic locations including southeastern Georgia and southeastern Missouri indicates an incidence that could be 10- to 100-times higher than those reported by individual states by passive surveillance (Fishbein et al., 1989; Olano et al., 2003). HME is more often diagnosed in male (>2:1) patients >40 years of age, the majority (>80%) report a tick bite (Fishbein et al., 1994; Olano et al., 2003), and HME outbreaks are associated with recreational or occupational activities (Petersen et al., 1989; Standaert et al., 1995). *E. chaffeensis* has been found in 5% to 15% of *A. americanum* ticks collected from endemic areas in the eastern United States (Ijdo et al., 2000b; Whitlock et al., 2000; Stromdahl et al., 2001) and has been detected in ticks collected from at least 15 states. *E. chaffeensis* has not been isolated outside the United States, and the only proven tick vector is restricted to North America, but *E. chaffeensis* or a closely related *Ehrlichia* sp. has been detected in other tick species located in other regions of the world, including Russia, Korea, Thailand, and China (Ravyn et al., 1999; Cao et al., 2000; Alekseev et al., 2001; Kim et al., 2003; Parola et al., 2003). Human infections with *E. chaffeensis* or antigenically related ehrlichiae have been reported in Europe (Nuti et al., 1998), Asia (Heppner et al., 1997), South America (Ripoll et al., 1999), and Africa (Uhaa et al., 1992). All stages of *A. americanum* readily feed on humans and white-tailed deer, which are considered to be the primary host for maintaining the *E. chaffeensis* transmission cycle (Lockhart et al., 1997). Antibodies reactive with *E. chaffeensis* have been detected in white-tailed deer (Lockhart et al., 1995), and laboratory-raised *A. americanum* ticks can acquire *E. chaffeensis* infection from deer (Ewing et al., 1995). Other potentially important reservoirs that are naturally infected with *E. chaffeensis* include goats, domestic dogs, and coyotes (Breitschwerdt et al., 1998; Dugan et al., 2000; Kocan et al., 2000).

3.1.6. Clinical Spectrum

HME and ehrlichiosis ewingii manifest as undifferentiated febrile illnesses 1 to 3 weeks after the bite of an infected tick, and infected individuals usually seek medical care within 4 days after onset of illness (Eng et al., 1990; Fishbein et al., 1994). For HME, the most frequent clinical findings reported anytime during acute illness are fever, malaise, headache, dizziness, chills, and myalgias (Fishbein et al., 1989, 1994; Eng et al., 1990; Olano et al., 2003). Other signs including respiratory or central nervous system involvement, lymphadenopathy, and rash are less frequent (Eng et al., 1990; Fishbein et al., 1994; Olano et al., 2003). Patients with ehrlichiosis ewingii present with a milder disease with few complications (Buller et al., 1999). A majority of these patients are immunocompromised, further suggesting that *E. ewingii* is less pathogenic. A large portion of HME patients (60–70%), including those that are immunocompromised, develop more serious manifestations or multisystem involvement including renal failure, disseminated intravascular coagulation, cardiomegaly, acute respiratory distress syndrome, spontaneous hemorrhage, and neurological manifestations requiring hospitalization (Eng et al., 1990; Fishbein et al., 1994; Paddock et al., 2001). Prevention of severe manifestions correlates well with diagnosis and treatment with tetracyclines within the first week of illness (Eng et al., 1990). Hematologic and biochemical abnormalities usually include leucopenia, thrombocytopenia, anemia, mildly elevated serum hepatic transaminase activities, and hyponatremia (Fishbein et al., 1994; Paddock et al., 2001; Olano et al., 2003). Lymphocytosis characterized by a predominance of γδ T cells is often seen in patients during recovery (Caldwell et al., 1995). A high proportion of immunocompetent (41% to 62%) and immunocompromised patients (86%) require hospitalization (Fishbein et al., 1994; Paddock et al., 2001; Olano et al., 2003). The case fatality rate is estimated to be 3% (McQuiston et al., 1999), and fatal disease is most often described in older patients and in patients debilitated by underlying disease or immunodeficiency (Eng et al., 1990; Paddock et al., 2001). Immunocompromised patients (human immunodeficiency virus–infected, transplant recipients, corticosteroid-treated) have a high risk of fatal infection associated with overwhelming infection not typically observed in immunocompetent patients (Paddock et al., 2001). No deaths have been reported as a result of infection with *E. ewingii* (Buller et al., 1999; Paddock et al., 2001).

3.1.7. Laboratory Diagnosis

Diagnosis of human ehrlichioses on the basis of clinical and epidemiologic findings is difficult, if not impossible, making laboratory testing necessary for a confirmed diagnosis (Walker, 2000). Laboratory diagnosis of HME and ehrlichiosis ewingii can be achieved by antibody detection with serologic tests, visualization of intracellular morulae in peripheral blood or CSF, detection of ehrlichial DNA by PCR, or detection of ehrlichiae in tissue by immunohistochemistry (*E. chaffeensis* only) (Paddock and Childs, 2003). Visualization of morulae in peripheral blood is the simplest but least sensitive diagnostic method (Childs et al., 1999). Serologic testing by immunofluorescence is considered to be the best choice at the current time (Walker, 2000), but serologic assays have limitations that can have a direct consequence on the outcome of the patient's illness due to delays in the administration of the appropriate therapy. Patients treated in the first week of illness, prior to the development of antibodies, have more favorable outcomes and less opportunity to develop severe disease manifestations (Eng et al., 1990). Unfortunately, because most patients seek medical attention 4 days after onset of illness, a large majority (67%) of those with HME may be missed because most patients do not have IgG antibodies during the first week, and IgM does not substantially improve clinical diagnostic sensitivity (Childs et al., 1999). In addition, it is difficult to determine the infecting agent based on serology due to the existence of closely related agents that induce cross-reactive antibodies. However, a fourfold or higher immunofluorescent antibody (IFA) end-point titer may be useful in discrimination between agents such as *E. chaffeensis* and *A. phagocytophilum* (Comer et al., 1999). *E. ewingii* has not been cultivated *in vitro,* and serologic diagnosis has been performed using surrogate antigens (*E. chaffeensis*) (Buller et al., 1999), but the reliability is not known. Protein immunoblotting can be useful in classifying indeterminant cases (Buller et al., 1999); however, lack of standardization remains a problem (Walker, 2000).

Molecular detection of *Ehrlichia* sp. in blood and CSF can provide earlier detection when antibodies are not present (Childs et al., 1999), is a valuable complement to serologic testing for *E. chaffeensis* (Walker, 2000), and provides the only definitive method for identification of *E. ewingii* in clinical samples. Several variations in PCR-based detection including nested PCR, reverse-transcriptase PCR, and real-time PCR for *Ehrlichia* sp. have been developed targeting numerous genes including *rrs*, VLPT, gp120, *dsb,* and p28 (Buller et al., 1999; Sumner et al., 1999; Gusa et al., 2001; Paddock et al., 2001; Loftis et al., 2003; Olano et al., 2003). Nested PCR using 16S rRNA as a target is the most widely used method and has the analytical sensitivity to detect low levels of ehrlichemia (Buller et al., 1999; Childs et al., 1999; Gusa et al., 2001; Paddock et al., 2001). Recently, a multicolor real-time PCR assay capable of detection of small quantities of ehrlichiae (comparable with nested PCR) and discrimination of ehrlichiae of medical and veterinary importance (*E. chaffeensis, E. ewingii,* and *E. canis*) in a single reaction has been developed and may be useful in clinical improvement of diagnostic capability and in surveillance to raise the level of diagnostic confirmation of HME and ehrlichiosis ewingii (Doyle et al., 2005a; Sirigireddy and Ganta, 2005).

3.1.8. Treatment and Prevention

Most patients with HME seek medical attention 4 days after onset of disease and usually before antibodies can be detected. Because therapeutic delay can result in the development of severe clinical manifestations and fatal outcome, patients suspected to have ehrlichiosis should be treated empirically with doxycycline or tetracycline (Fishbein et al., 1994; Olano et al., 2003). *E. chaffeensis* is resistant to most classes of antibiotics, but doxcycline and rifampin are highly active *in vitro* (Brouqui and Raoult, 1992; Branger et al., 2004). Tetracyclines are considered to be the drug of choice for treatment of human ehrlichioses, but rifampin may be preferred in pregnant women, and cases have been reported of successful treatment of closely related *Anaplasma phagocytophilum* infections with this antibiotic (Buitrago et al., 1998; Krause et al., 2003). *E. chaffeensis* is resistant to chloramphenicol *in vitro* (Brouqui and Raoult, 1992). Both treatment failures (Fichtenbaum et al., 1993) and successes with this antibiotic have been reported (Eng et al., 1990; Fishbein et al., 1994); thus it should not be considered a primary therapeutic option.

Disease prevention begins with reducing tick exposure through the use of tick repellents containing DEET (*N,N*-diethyl-*m*-toluamide), and barrier clothing when recreational or occupational activities will result in potential tick exposure. Early removal of any attached ticks will lower the risk of transmission, as it may require 24 or more hours for ehrlichiae to be inoculated.

3.2. Human Anaplasmosis

3.2.1. Taxonomy

Anaplasma phagocytophilum (formerly *Ehrlichia phagocytophilia, E. equi,* or the HGE agent), is the only *Anaplasma* species recognized for its ability to cause human infections. The clinical entity, formerly known as human granulocytotropic ehrlichiosis (HGE), is now recognized as human granulocytotropic anaplasmosis (HGA). Recent taxonomic reorganization of the family *Anaplasmataceae* based on genetic analysis of *rrs* and *groESL* genes has resulted in reorganization of the genus *Anaplasma* members, which now include the human and veterinary pathogen, *A. phagocytophilum*, and pathogens solely of veterinary importance, *A. marginale, A. centrale, A. platys* (formerly *E. platys*), *A. ovis,* and *A. bovis* (formerly *E. bovis*) (Dumler et al., 2001) (Table 3.2). The genus *Anaplasma* is a member of the order Rickettsiales.

3.2.2. Morphology

A. phagocytophilum reside within neutrophils as microcolonies of bacteria in cytoplasmic vacuoles that are not derived from early or late

Table 3.2. Summary of tick-borne anaplasmoses of humans and animals

Disease	Agent	Hosts	Vector	Target cell	Geographic distribution	Diagnosis
Human granulocytic anaplasmosis (HGA)	*A. phagocy-tophilum*	Humans, sheep, horses, deer, deer mice, canids	*Ixodes* spp.	Neutrophil	Upper Midwest, New England	IFA, PCR
Bovine anaplasmosis	*A.marginale, A. centrale, A. bovis*	Bovines	*Dermacentor, Boophilus, Ripicephalus*	Erythro-cyte	Worldwide	IFA, PCR
Canine cyclic thrombo-cytopenia	*A. platys*	Canids	*R. sanguineus*	Platelet	Worldwide	IFA/PCR

endosomes and are distinct from early endosomal vacuoles where *Ehrlichia* spp. reside (Rikihisa et al., 1997; Popov et al., 1998; Mott et al., 1999). *A. phagocytophilum* is a pleomorphic coccobacillus found in loosely packed clusters in membrane-lined vacuoles that are similar in appearance to ehrlichial inclusions but are typically smaller (1.5–2.5 μm in diameter) and do not contain the fibrillar matrix or have proximity with host cell mitochondria (Rikihisa et al., 1997; Popov et al., 1998). There are two morphologic cell types, reticulate (2.0 μm in diameter) and dense-cored (0.4 μm in diameter), and most morulae contain exclusively dense-cored or reticulate cells, and rarely both (Popov et al., 1998) (Fig. 3.5). *A. phagocytophilum* has a characteristic Gram-negative membrane structure, but notably has a very wavy and loose cell wall and expanded periplasmic space (Popov et al., 1998). Abnormal forms have been described manifesting protrusions of cytoplasmic membrane into the periplasmic space and long projections with inconsistent diameters that sometimes envelope the whole cell (Popov et al., 1998).

3.2.3. Genetic, Antigenic, and Phenotypic Characteristics

A. phagocytophilum (1.5 Mbp) and the closely related veterinary pathogen *A. marginale* (~1.2 Mbp) have relatively small bacterial genomes. Though the *A. phagocytophilum* genome has not been completely

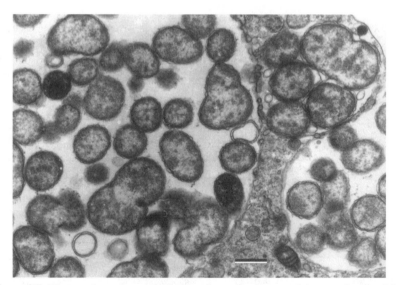

Figure 3.5. Electron photomicrograph of three adjacent *A. phagocytophilum* morulae containing mostly reticulate cell morphologic forms of the organism. Magnification, ×7200; bar, 1 μm. (Reproduced with permission from V.L. Popov, University of Texas Medical Branch.)

annotated, the complete *A. marginale* genome annotation has identified 949 coding sequences with an average gene length of 1077 bp and an usually high G + C content of 49% when compared with other obligately intracellular organisms within the order Rickettsiales (Brayton et al., 2005). Numerous pseudogenes have been identified in *A. phagocytophilum* encoding major outer membrane proteins.

Molecularly characterized genes of *A. phagocytophilum* include functionally conserved genes *rrs, rrl, rrf* (16S, 23S, and 5S rRNA, respectively) (Chen et al., 1994a; Massung et al., 2002), *groESL* heat shock operon (Kolbert et al., 1997; Sumner et al., 1997), *gltA* (Inokuma et al., 2001), *ftsZ* (Lee et al., 2003), and genes encoding type IV secretion machinery (Ohashi et al., 2002). Immunoblot analysis using sera from *A. phagcytophilum*–infected patients has identified numerous immunoreactive antigens including proteins with masses of 40-, 44-, 65-, 80-, 94-, 105-, 110-, 115-, and 125-kDa (Ijdo et al., 1997). The most frequently identified immunoreactive proteins are present within the ranges of 40- to 47-kDa and 65- to 80-kDa (Asanovich et al., 1997; Ijdo et al., 1997; Zhi et al., 1997). A family of *A. marginale* MSP-2 related immunodominant major outer membrane protein genes has been identified that encode the 44-kDa proteins of *A. phagocytophilum* (designated as P44) (Murphy et al., 1998; Zhi et al., 1998). This multigene family consists of more than 80 nonidentical polymorphic paralogs. Other dominant immunoreactive proteins including p100, p130, and p160 (Storey et al., 1998; Caturegli et al., 2000) have been molecularly characterized, but functions of these proteins are largely unknown. In addition, conserved single copy *msp2* and *msp4* gene orthologs of *A. marginale msp2* multigene family have been recently identified in *A. phagocytophilum* (Lin et al., 2004a; de la Fuente et al., 2005). The *p44* genes were considered orthologs of *msp2*, but the newly identified *msp2* gene appears to be distinct from *p44* genes, and this discovery supports the evolution of *msp2, p44,* and *omp1* (*Ehrlichia* spp.) genes from a common ancestral origin (Lin et al., 2004a).

The first molecularly characterized immunoreactive antigens of *A. phagocytophilum* were p100, p130, and p160, which reacted with sera from dogs and human patients recovering from the disease (Storey et al., 1998). Two of these proteins (p100 and p130) share amino acid homology with the gp120 of *E. chaffeensis*, presence of multiple tandem repeats, and larger than predicted masses, suggesting post-translational modification (Storey et al., 1998). The conserved 160-kDa protein (designated AnkA) located in the ehrlichial cytoplasm has been studied more extensively. AnkA has eight full-length (33 amino acids) and three partial ankyrin-like repeats, two 11- and two 27-amino-acid repeats, exhibits larger than predicted molecular mass, has sites for phosphorylation and glycosylation, and binds both host cell DNA and nuclear proteins (Storey et al., 1998; Caturegli et al., 2000; Park et al., 2004). AnkA gene is conserved, but geographic sequence polymophisms occur (Caturegli et al., 2000). Although the function of these proteins remains in question, the consistent presence of repeated regions suggests that these proteins may play roles in host cell binding, antigenic variation, or protein–protein interactions (Storey et al., 1998).

The 44-kDa major outer membrane of *A. phagocytophilum* is the immunodominant antigen most consistently recognized by patient sera (Asanovich et al., 1997; Ijdo et al., 1997; Zhi et al., 1997, 1998). The p44 outer membrane proteins are encoded by a polymorphic multigene family, the members of which are dispersed throughout the genome (Zhi et al., 1998; Murphy et al., 1998; Felek et al., 2004), and consist of more than 80 paralogs, many lacking start codons (Felek et al., 2004). The p44 is expressed through a polycistronic expression site (designated *p44-1/18*) where switching of *p44* hypervariable regions occurs through unidirectional conversion (nonsegmental gene conversion) of the expression site with sequences from pseudogenes (truncated copies of genes that are only expressed after recombinantion into an expression site) distributed throughout the chromosome (Lin et al., 2003) but may also be expressed at genomic loci distinct from the *p44-1/18* expression site (Zhi et al., 1999; Caspersen et al., 2002; Lin et al., 2003, 2004b). Genetic heterogeneity in the *p44-1/18* expression site locus has been reported among geographically divergent *A. phagocytophilum* strains from the northeastern United States compared with strains from the north-central and western United States, suggesting molecular evolution between strains, but *p44-18* and its chromosomal location are conserved in all United States strains (Lin et al., 2004b). P44 proteins each contain a central hypervariable region (range 23% to 80% identity) consisting of 94 amino acids and highly conserved N-(58-amino-acid) and C-terminal (65-amino-acid) flanking regions. Comparison of orthologous *p44* genes among different strains identifies greater variability in the flanking conserved regions than in hypervarible regions (Felek et al., 2004). The P44 appears to form dimer and oligomer complexes mediated by disulfide bonds and noncovalent bonds and may form complexes with other *A. phagocytophilum* proteins (Park et al., 2003b).

3.2.4. Pathogenesis and Immunity

A. phagocytophilum exhibits primary host cell tropism for neutrophils, and its infection of neutrophils results in impaired phagocytosis that may contribute to the development of opportunistic infections or exacerbation of disease (Garyu et al., 2005). Its affinity for the neutrophil is at least partially explained by the *A. phagocytophilum* receptor, P-selectin glycoprotein ligand-1 (PSGL-1) (Herron et al., 2000), and $\alpha2,3$-sialyated and $\alpha1,3$-fucosylated glycans (sialyl Lewis x) found on PSGL-1 and other neutrophil selectin ligands (Goodman et al., 1999; Herron et al., 2000). *A. phagocytophilum* binding to PSGL-1 appears to be less restricted than the binding requirements for P-selectin (Goodman et al., 1999; Yago et al., 2003). In addition to PSGL-1, *A. phagocytophilum* binding appears to involve a least two adhesins that bind cooperatively to two ligands (Carlyon et al., 2003; Yago et al., 2003). One *A. phagocytophilum* adhesin appears to be the major outer membrane protein P44 (Park et al., 2003a).

A. phagocytophilum enters the host cell and appears to reside in endocytic pathway vacuoles that do not fuse with lyosomes or colocalize with early endosomal markers (transferrin receptor, small GTPase, Rab5, early endosomal antigen 1) (Webster et al., 1998; Mott et al., 1999) and general endocytic pathway markers (clathrin heavy chain, annexin I, II, IV, or VI) (Mott et al., 1999). *A. phagocytophilum* inclusions do colocalize with MHC class I and class II molecules, but lack of localization with numerous endocytic markers indicates that the organism modifies the normal endocytic development of its inclusion (Carlyon and Fikrig, 2003). Neutrophils and HL-60 cells incubated with live or killed *A. phagocytophilum* produce chemokines (IL-8, MCP-1, MIP-1α, MIP-1β, and RANTES), which may play a role in recruitment of other susceptible cells (Klein et al., 2000). The outer membrane protein p44 also induces IL-8 secretion by HL-60 cells and appears to contribute partially to this response (Akkoyunlu et al., 2001). Antibodies to IL-8 and the IL-8 receptor, CXCR2, reduce the bacterial load (Akkoyunlu et al., 2001; Scorpio et al., 2004), suggesting that *A. phagocytophilum* exploits IL-8 induced chemotaxis to attract susceptible neutrophils to enhance the infection (Akkoyunlu et al., 2001).

The basis of intraneutrophil survival by *A. phagocytophilum* is partially explained by its ability to inhibit NADPH oxygen-dependent killing mechanisms (Banerjee et al., 2000b; Carlyon et al., 2002; Wang et al., 2002). The first reports of inhibition of preformed superoxide and rapid alteration of p22[phox] in human neutrophils after extracellular contact with *A. phagocytophilum* (Mott and Rikihisa, 2000; Mott et al., 2002) has come under considerable challenge by more recent studies (Carlyon et al., 2004; Ijdo and Mueller, 2004). The latter studies concluded that *A. phagocytophilum* binding stimulates respiratory burst (Choi and Dumler, 2003;

Carlyon et al., 2004) and membrane localization of at least two NADPH oxidase components (Carlyon et al., 2004). Others have reported that *A. phagocytophilum* binding does not inhibit the overall respiratory burst (Ijdo and Mueller, 2004). During binding and internalization, *A. phagocytophilum* avoids reactive oxygen species–mediated damage by directly detoxifying preformed superoxide (Carlyon et al., 2004; Ijdo and Mueller, 2004) via a heat-labile surface protein (Carlyon et al., 2004). A transcriptionally active superoxide dismutase B gene (*sodB*) has been demonstrated in *A. phagocytophilum* (Ohashi et al., 2002), but the role of *sodB,* or possibly *sodC,* in the superoxide detoxification mechanism and its location on the ehrlichial surface have not been demonstrated (Carlyon et al., 2004). Once internalized, *A. phagocytophilum* inhibits the respiratory burst by downregulating NADPH oxidase gene expression (*gp91^{phox}* and *rac2*), whereas other NADPH oxidase genes are unaffected (Banerjee et al., 2000b; Carlyon et al., 2002). Downregulation of gp91^{phox} is mediated by increased binding of repressor CCAAT displacement protein (CDP) to the promoter possibly through the reduced expression of activator proteins, including interferon regulatory factor (IRF-1) and PU.1 (Thomas et al., 2005). Furthermore, NADPH oxidase components, gp91^{phox} and p21^{phox}, are prevented from fusing with the vacuole where *A. phagocytophilum* resides by an undefined mechanism (Carlyon et al., 2004; Ijdo and Mueller, 2004). Although substantial evidence supports the ability of *A. phagocytophilum* to neutralize NADPH oxidase effects by a number of mechanisms, mice deficient in a NADPH oxidase component (gp91$^{phox-/-}$) can control and clear *A. phagocytophilum* infection, suggesting that NADPH oxidase is not required for eradication (Banerjee et al., 2000a; von Loewenich et al., 2004).

 A. phagocytophilum has a slow growth rate but establishes infection in neutrophils, which have a short life-span. One of the mechanisms used by this bacterium to effectively infect this host cell involves delaying apoptotic cell death in infected cells (Yoshiie et al., 2000; Scaife et al., 2003). The anti-apoptoic effect can be elicited by live or inactive bacteria and appears to be mediated by the interaction between an *A. phagocytophilum* surface protein with the host cell and subsequent cross-linking and/or internalization (Yoshiie et al., 2000). The anti-apoptotic mechanism does not involve bacterial new protein synthesis, host cell protein kinase A, nuclear translocation of NF-κB or IL-1β, which are known to be involved in inhibition of apoptosis by other agents (Yoshiie et al., 2000), but involves the upregulation of a *bcl-1* family anti-apoptotic gene *bfl-1*. Increased production of Bfl-1 likely sequesters truncated pro-apoptotic factor Bid (tBid) and inhibits its interaction with pro-apoptotic factor Bax in the mitochondrial membrane, preventing mitochondrial apoptotic protein release and activation of downstream caspase 3 (Ge et al., 2005).

Elimination of *A. phagocytophilum* is mediated in part by antibodies and T-cell-derived IFN-γ (Sun et al., 1997; Bunnell et al., 1999; Akkoyunlu and Fikrig, 2000; Wang et al., 2004), while the innate immune mechanisms important for the elimination of other intracellular pathogens (*Mycobacterium tuberculosis, Salmonella typhimurium, Leishmania major*, and *Toxoplasma gondii*) are dispensable for the control of *A. phagocytophilum* (von Loewenich et al., 2004). Mice deficient in pattern-recognition receptors (Toll-like receptors 2 and 4), intracellular signaling molecule (MyD88), tumor necrosis factor, and inducible nitric oxide synthase, or phagocytes' NADPH oxidase (gp91$^{phox-/-}$) are able to clear systemic infection with *A. phagocytophilum* (Banerjee et al., 2000a; von Loewenich et al., 2004). An atypical innate immune response is elicited by a heat-stable carbohydrate component(s) of *A. phagocytophilum* inducing inflammatory chemokine production by differentiated HL-60 cells consisting of MCP-1, MIP-1α, MIP-1β, RANTES, and IL-8, without production of proinflammatory cytokines IL-1, IL-6, and TNF-α (Klein et al., 2000). The lack of proinflammatory cytokine induction in response to *A. phagocytophilum* may be due to the absence of lipopolysaccharide and peptidoglycan (Lin and Rikihisa, 2003b). The pathogen-associated molecular patterns and host pathogen-recognition receptors (PRRs) involved in eliciting the inflammatory chemokine response are not known but may involve TLR2 or other unidentified PRRs, as *A. phagocytophilum* ligates TLR2 and not TLR4, and activates NF-κB nuclear translocation (Choi et al., 2004). The downstream effect of TLR2 ligation and NF-κB activation is not fully understood.

The role of an adaptive immune response in clearance of *A. phagocytophilum* has been appreciated by the fact that immune-deficient SCID mice become persistently infected with *A. phagocytophilum* (Bunnell et al., 1999), whereas immunocompetent mice control the infection (von Loewenich et al., 2004). Interestingly, adaptive immunity appears to be generated in the absence of a proinflammatory innate immune response (Ehlers, 2004). IFN-γ is important for clearance of *A. phagocytophilum* (Akkoyunlu and Fikrig, 2000; Martin et al., 2001; Wang et al., 2004) and has been observed early after infection (Martin et al., 2000), but also contributes to the histopathology associated with infection (Martin et al., 2001). Partial protection against challenge can be induced by vaccination, and passive transfer of *A phagocytophilum* antisera also provides partial protection against challenge, suggesting that antibodies also play a role in immunity to this organism (Barlough et al., 1995; Sun et al., 1997).

3.2.5. Emergence, Epidemiology, and Transmission

The factors contributing to the emergence of HGA in North America are not completely defined but coincide with those involved in the emergence of Lyme borreliosis. The primary vector for both is *Ixodes scapularis,* and ecological changes after reforestation of the New England area in recent times have contributed to increased *I. scapularis* density, increased tick hosts density and *A. phagocytophilum* reservoir populations (deer and white-footed mice), in addition to increased human populations and habitation of previously rural wooded areas where ticks and reservoir hosts are plentiful (Steere et al., 2004). Together these factors have resulted in increased contact between humans and *A. phagocytophilum*–infected ticks and the emergence of HGA. The first cases of HGA were identified in patients from Wisconsin and Minnesota who reported tick bites (Bakken et al., 1994; Chen et al., 1994a). The incidence of HGA is seasonal with a majority of cases (68%) reported between May and July (Bakken et al., 1996; Gardner et al., 2003), and geographic distribution of cases coincides with that of reported Lyme disease cases and within the range of the vectors *I. scapularis* and *I. pacificus* in the United States. Coinfections with *Borrelia burdorferi* and *A. phagocytophilum* have been noted (Nadelman et al., 1997; Steere et al., 2003). Human ehrlichioses (including HGA) became nationally reportable in 1999, but many states do not have a system for surveillance and do not test for ehrlichiosis in state diagnostic laboratories (McQuiston et al., 1999), thus the true incidence of the disease is likely to be much higher (McQuiston et al., 1999). The highest incidence of HGA reported through 1997 based on passive surveillance occurred in Connecticut (15.90/1 million population) and Wisconsin (8.79/1 million population) (McQuiston et al., 1999). Other studies have revealed incidences of 58 and 51 cases per 100,000 population in the upper Midwest and Connecticut (Bakken et al., 1996; Ijdo et al., 2000a; Gardner et al., 2003). HGA is most often diagnosed in males (78%) with a median age of 60 years, history of tick bite (78%), and frequent tick exposures (90%) associated with outdoor recreation or employment (Aguero-Rosenfeld et al., 1996; Bakken et al., 1996). Seroprevalance in North America and Europe indicates that the disease is widely distributed (Aguero-Rosenfeld et al., 2002; Walder et al., 2003; Grzeszczuk et al., 2004).

The major tick vectors of *A. phagocytophilum* are *I. scapularis* in the eastern United States, *I. pacficus* in the western United States (Richter, Jr. et al., 1996), and appears to be *I. ricinus* in Europe. The highest proportion of infected *I. scapularis* ticks (up to 50%) are found in the northeastern and upper Midwest United States (Chang et al., 1998; Courtney et al., 2003), and infected *I. pacificus* in California (7%) (Kramer et al., 1999), and high prevalences have been noted in *I. persulcatus* and

I. ricinus in Asia and Europe (Christova et al., 2001, 2003; Blanco and Oteo, 2002; Kim et al., 2003).

3.2.6. Clinical Spectrum

HGA manifests as an undifferentiated febrile illness 7 to 10 days after the bite of an infected tick. Patients most often exhibit high-grade fever, rigors, generalized myalgias, severe headache, and malaise but may also complain of anorexia, arthralgias, nausea, and a nonproductive cough (Bakken et al., 1994, 1996; Aguero-Rosenfeld et al., 1996). Very few patients present with a rash (10.9 %), which is not considered part of the HGA clinical presentation, except when patients are coinfected with Lyme borreliosis (Bakken and Dumler, 2000). Leukopenia, thrombocytopenia, and elevated hepatic transaminase activities are present in a majority of patients and suggest the diagnosis (Bakken et al., 1996, 2001). The illness may last a few days to weeks in the absence of appropriate antibiotic therapy. The severity of the illness is associated with increased age, and many patients require hospitalization (Bakken et al., 1996). Severe infections and poor outcomes have been observed in patients with preexisting immune dysfunction, advanced age, concomitant chronic illnesses (such as diabetes mellitus and collagen-vascular diseases), lack of diagnosis recognition or delayed onset of specific antibiotic therapy (Bakken et al., 1996; Bakken and Dumler, 2000). The case fatality rate based on numerous studies is estimated to be <1% (Bakken et al., 1994, 1996; Aguero-Rosenfeld et al., 1996; Wallace et al., 1998). Early consideration of the diagnosis and empirical therapy are important for providing the best prognosis and prevention of severe manifestations.

3.2.7. Laboratory Diagnosis

Diagnosis of HGA on the basis of clinical and epidemiologic findings is difficult, and laboratory testing demonstrating *A. phagocyotophilum* in peripheral blood neutrophils, immunohistochemical demonstration of the organism in tissues, culture of the organism from peripheral blood, demonstration of antibodies reactive with *A. phagcytophilum*, or detection of nucleic acids in peripheral blood are necessary to confirm the diagnosis (Aguero-Rosenfeld, 2002; Dumler and Brouqui, 2004). Visualization of morulae in peripheral blood neutrophils is the simplest test. Organisms can be detected in 25% to 80% of patients during active HGA, but specific identification of morulac can be challenging for inexperienced microscopists to differentiate from other similar appearing structures (Aguero-Rosenfeld, 2002; Dumler and Brouqui, 2004). Cell culture isolation of the agent from peripheral blood is possible but is performed routinely by only a few laboratories and usually requires 1 to 2 weeks for detection and identification (Aguero-Rosenfeld, 2002). Serologic diagnosis of HGA is the most frequently used method and is still considered the best indirect method to confirm a diagnosis, because of its sensitivity, specificity, and reliability (Walker, 2000; Dumler and Brouqui, 2004). A confirmed serologic diagnosis consists of a fourfold increase in antibodies between acute and convalescent samples or a single high titer in a patient with consistent clinical findings. However, antibodies are absent or develop in only a minority of patients 0 to 14 days after onset of symptoms (Dumler and Brouqui, 2004) and appear on average at 11 days (Aguero-Rosenfeld, 2002). Therefore, the necessity for early detection of *A. phagocytophilum* has defined the value of molecular diagnostics such as PCR. Several molecular targets have been utilized for detection of *A. phagocytophilum,* with *rrs* being the most widely used target (Dumler and Brouqui, 2004). Various levels of analytical and clinical sensitivity and specificity have been reported with primers designed to amplify *A. phagcytophilum rrs* (Massung and Slater, 2003). A study with relatively large numbers of patients demonstrated a sensitivity of 87% (Bakken et al., 1996), but technical proficiency and standardization of the technique are required for consistently reliable results. The diversity of PCR assays, protocols, reported sensitivity, specificity and potential for false positives have resulted in a general consensus among experts in the field that PCR alone is insufficient evidence of definite infection by *A. phagocytophilum* (Walker, 2000). Currently used criteria for the clinical diagnosis of HGA include fourfold or greater increase in antibody titer and successful isolation from blood or positive PCR result (Bakken and Dumler, 2000).

3.2.8. Prevention and Treatment

Most patients with HGA seek medical attention within 11 days after onset of disease and usually before antibodies can be detected, and because therapeutic delay can result in the development of severe clinical manifestations and fatal outcome, patients should be treated empirically with doxycycline or tetracycline (Dumler and Brouqui, 2004). *A. phagocytophilum* is resistant to most classes of antibiotics, but doxycycline and rifampin are highly active *in vitro* (Klein et al., 1997; Horowitz et al., 2001; Maurin et al., 2003). Tetracyclines are considered to be the drug of choice for treatment of HGA and also have the benefit of being effective against *Borrelia burgdorferi*, but rifampin may be preferred in pregnant women (Buitrago et al., 1998; Krause et al., 2003). Chloramphenicol does not appear to be effective based on treatment failures as well as *in vitro* resistance to this antibiotic (Bakken and Dumler, 2000; Horowitz et al., 2001; Maurin et al., 2003). Disease prevention begins with reducing tick exposure through the use of tick repellents containing DEET (*N,N*-diethyl-*m*-toluamide) and barrier clothing when recreational or occupational activities result in potential tick exposure. Early removal of attached ticks within 36 h lowers the risk of transmission (Hodzic et al., 1998; Katavolos et al., 1998). However, transmission has been reported within 24 h (Des and Fish, 1997).

3.3. Future Directions

HME is now recognized as one of the most prevalent life-threatening tick-borne diseases in North America. Many of the major immunoreactive proteins of *E. chaffeensis* have been molecularly characterized, which will help in the development of vaccines to protect those who are at increased risk through recreation, occupation, or elderly and immunocompromised individuals. Until recently, the lack of advanced diagnostics has resulted in underdiagnoses of human ehrlichoses and anaplasmosis, but improved diagnostics using new molecular and recombinant antigen serologic technologies are being developed, which will assist in the rapid and accurate diagnosis of these diseases in the future. Disease pathology is not well characterized, and the pathobiology of these rickettsial agents is not well understood. Future research to understand the spectrum of disease and the mechanisms involved in their ability to replicate in and manipulate phagocytes of the innate immune system will be facilitated by complete genomic sequence information and genome-wide studies. Future research to understand ehrlichial–host interactions will contribute to our broader understanding of pathogenic intracellular microbes.

References

Aguero-Rosenfeld, M.E., 2002. Diagnosis of human granulocytic ehrlichiosis: state of the art. *Vector Borne Zoonotic Dis. 2*, 233–239.

Aguero-Rosenfeld, M.E., Donnarumma, L., Zentmaier, L., Jacob, J., Frey, M., Noto, R., Carbonaro, C.A., Wormser, G.P., 2002. Seroprevalence of antibodies that react with *Anaplasma phagocytophila*, the agent of human granulocytic ehrlichiosis, in different populations in Westchester County, New York. *J. Clin. Microbiol. 40*, 2612–2615.

Aguero-Rosenfeld, M.E., Horowitz, H.W., Wormser, G.P., McKenna, D.F., Nowakowski, J., Munoz, J., Dumler, J.S., 1996. Human granulocytic ehrlichiosis: a case series from a medical center in New York State. *Ann. Intern. Med. 125*, 904–908.

Akkoyunlu, M., Fikrig, E., 2000. Gamma interferon dominates the murine cytokine response to the agent of human granulocytic ehrlichiosis and helps to control the degree of early rickettsemia. *Infect. Immun. 68*, 1827–1833.

Akkoyunlu, M., Malawista, S.E., Anguita, J., Fikrig, E., 2001. Exploitation of interleukin-8-induced neutrophil chemotaxis by the agent of human granulocytic ehrlichiosis. *Infect. Immun. 69*, 5577–5588.

Alekseev, A.N., Dubinina, H.V., Semenov, A.V., Bolshakov, C.V., 2001. Evidence of ehrlichiosis agents found in ticks (Acari: Ixodidae) collected from migratory birds. *J. Med. Entomol. 38*, 471–474.

Alleman, A.R., Barbet, A.F., Bowie, M.V., Sorenson, H.L., Wong, S.J., Belanger, M., 2000. Expression of a gene encoding the major antigenic protein 2 homolog of *Ehrlichia chaffeensis* and potential application for serodiagnosis. *J. Clin. Microbiol. 38*, 3705–3709.

Anderson, B.E., Dawson, J.E., Jones, D.C., Wilson, K.H., 1991. *Ehrlichia chaffeensis*, a new species associated with human ehrlichiosis. *J. Clin. Microbiol. 29*, 2838–2842.

Asanovich, K.M., Bakken, J.S., Madigan, J.E., Aguero-Rosenfeld, M., Wormser, G.P., Dumler, J.S., 1997. Antigenic diversity of granulocytic *Ehrlichia* isolates from humans in Wisconsin and New York and a horse in California. *J. Infect. Dis. 176*, 1029–1034.

Bakken, J.S., Dumler, J.S., 2000. Human granulocytic ehrlichiosis. *Clin. Infect. Dis. 31*, 554–560.

Bakken, J.S., Dumler, J.S., Chen, S.M., Eckman, M.R., Van, E.L., Walker, D.H., 1994. Human granulocytic ehrlichiosis in the upper Midwest United States. A new species emerging? *JAMA 272*, 212–218.

Bakken, J.S., Aguero-Rosenfeld, M.E., Tilden, R.L., Wormser, G.P., Horowitz, H.W., Raffalli, J.T., Baluch, M., Riddell, D., Walls, J.J., Dumler, J.S., 2001. Serial measurements of hematologic counts during the active phase of human granulocytic ehrlichiosis. *Clin. Infect. Dis. 32*, 862–870.

Bakken, J.S., Krueth, J., Wilson-Nordskog, C., Tilden, R.L., Asanovich, K., Dumler, J.S., 1996. Clinical and laboratory characteristics of human granulocytic ehrlichiosis. *JAMA 275*, 199–205.

Banerjee, R., Anguita, J., Fikrig, E., 2000a. Granulocytic ehrlichiosis in mice deficient in phagocyte oxidase or inducible nitric oxide synthase. *Infect. Immun. 68*, 4361–4362.

Banerjee, R., Anguita, J., Roos, D., Fikrig, E., 2000b. Cutting edge: infection by the agent of human granulocytic ehrlichiosis prevents the respiratory burst by down-regulating gp91phox. *J. Immunol. 15*, 3946–3949.

Barlough, J.E., Madigan, J.E., DeRock, E., Dumler, J.S., Bakken, J.S., 1995. Protection against *Ehrlichia equi* is conferred by prior infection with the human granulocytotropic *Ehrlichia* (HGE agent). *J. Clin. Microbiol. 33*, 3333–3334.

Barnewall, R.E., Ohashi, N., Rikihisa, Y., 1999. *Ehrlichia chaffeensis* and *E. sennetsu*, but not the human granulocytic ehrlichiosis agent, colocalize with transferrin receptor and up-regulate transferrin receptor mRNA by activating iron-responsive protein 1. *Infect. Immun. 67*, 2258–2265.

Barnewall, R.E., Rikihisa, Y., 1994. Abrogation of gamma interferon–induced inhibition of *Ehrlichia chaffeensis* infection in human monocytes with iron-transferrin. *Infect. Immun. 62*, 4804–4810.

Barnewall, R.E., Rikihisa, Y., Lee, E.H., 1997. *Ehrlichia chaffeensis* inclusions are early endosomes which selectively accumulate transferrin receptor. *Infect. Immun. 65*, 1455–1461.

Bitsaktsis, C., Huntington, J., Winslow, G., 2004. Production of IFN-gamma by CD4 T cells is essential for resolving ehrlichia infection. *J. Immunol. 172*, 6894–6901.

Blanco, J.R., Oteo, J.A., 2002. Human granulocytic ehrlichiosis in Europe. *Clin. Microbiol. Infect. 8*, 763–772.

Branger, S., Rolain, J.M., Raoult, D., 2004. Evaluation of antibiotic susceptibilities of *Ehrlichia canis*, *Ehrlichia chaffeensis*, and *Anaplasma phagocytophilum* by real-time PCR. *Antimicrob. Agents Chemother. 48*, 4822–4828.

Brayton, K.A., Kappmeyer, L.S., Herndon, D.R., Dark, M.J., Tibbals, D.L., Palmer, G.H., McGuire, T.C., Knowles, D.P., Jr., 2005. Complete genome sequencing of *Anaplasma marginale* reveals that the surface is skewed to two superfamilies of outer membrane proteins. *Proc. Natl. Acad. Sci. U. S. A. 102*, 844–849.

Breitschwerdt, E.B., Hegarty, B.C., Hancock, S.I., 1998. Sequential evaluation of dogs naturally infected with *Ehrlichia canis, Ehrlichia chaffeensis, Ehrlichia equi, Ehrlichia ewingii,* or *Bartonella vinsonii. J. Clin. Microbiol. 36*, 2645–2651.

Brouqui, P., Raoult, D., 1992. *In vitro* antibiotic susceptibility of the newly recognized agent of ehrlichiosis in humans, *Ehrlichia chaffeensis. Antimicrob. Agents Chemother. 36*, 2799–2803.

Buitrago, M.I., Ijdo, J.W., Rinaudo, P., Simon, H., Copel, J., Gadbaw, J., Heimer, R., Fikrig, E., Bia, F.J., 1998. Human granulocytic ehrlichiosis during pregnancy treated successfully with rifampin. *Clin. Infect. Dis. 27*, 213–215.

Buller, R.S., Arens, M., Hmiel, S.P., Paddock, C.D., Sumner, J.W., Rikhisa, Y., Unver, A., Gaudreault-Keener, M., Manian, F.A., Liddell, A.M., Schmulewitz, N., Storch, G.A., 1999. *Ehrlichia ewingii*, a newly recognized agent of human ehrlichiosis. *N. Eng. J. Med. 341*, 148–155.

Bunnell, J.E., Trigiani, E.R., Srinivas, S.R., Dumler, J.S., 1999. Development and distribution of pathologic lesions are related to immune status and tissue deposition of human granulocytic ehrlichiosis agent-infected cells in a murine model system. *J. Infect. Dis. 180*, 546–550.

Caldwell, C.W., Everett, E.D., McDonald, G., Yesus, Y.W., Roland, W.E., 1995. Lymphocytosis of gamma/delta T cells in human ehrlichiosis. *Am. J. Clin. Pathol. 103*, 761–766.

Cao, W.C., Gao, Y.M., Zhang, P.H., Zhang, X.T., Dai, Q.H., Dumler, J.S., Fang, L.Q., Yang, H., 2000. Identification of *Ehrlichia chaffeensis* by nested PCR in ticks from Southern China. *J. Clin. Microbiol. 38*, 2778–2780.

Carlyon, J.A., Abdel-Latif, D., Pypaert, M., Lacy, P., Fikrig, E., 2004. *Anaplasma phagocytophilum* utilizes multiple host evasion mechanisms to thwart NADPH oxidase-mediated killing during neutrophil infection. *Infect. Immun. 72*, 4772–4783.

Carlyon, J.A., Akkoyunlu, M., Xia, L., Yago, T., Wang, T., Cummings, R.D., McEver, R.P., Fikrig, E., 2003. Murine neutrophils require alpha1,3-fucosylation but not PSGL-1 for productive infection with *Anaplasma phagocytophilum*. *Blood 102*, 3387–3395.

Carlyon, J.A., Chan, W.T., Galan, J., Roos, D., Fikrig, E., 2002. Repression of rac2 mRNA expression by *Anaplasma phagocytophila* is essential to the inhibition of superoxide production and bacterial proliferation. *J. Immunol. 169*, 7009–7018.

Carlyon, J.A., Fikrig, E., 2003. Invasion and survival strategies of *Anaplasma phagocytophilum*. *Cell. Microbiol. 5*, 743–754.

Caspersen, K., Park, J.H., Patil, S., Dumler, J.S., 2002. Genetic variability and stability of *Anaplasma phagocytophila* msp2 (p44). *Infect. Immun. 70*, 1230–1234.

Caturegli, P., Asanovich, K.M., Walls, J.J., Bakken, J.S., Madigan, J.E., Popov, V.L., Dumler, J.S., 2000. ankA: an *Ehrlichia phagocytophila* group gene encoding a cytoplasmic protein antigen with ankyrin repeats. *Infect. Immun. 68*, 5277–5283.

Chang, Y.F., Novosel, V., Chang, C.F., Kim, J.B., Shin, S.J., Lein, D.H., 1998. Detection of human granulocytic ehrlichiosis agent and *Borrelia burgdorferi* in ticks by polymerase chain reaction. *J. Vet. Diagn. Invest. 10*, 56–59.

Chen, S.M., Cullman, L.C., Walker, D.H., 1997a. Western immunoblotting analysis of the antibody responses of patients with human monocytotropic ehrlichiosis to different strains of *Ehrlichia chaffeensis* and *Ehrlichia canis*. *Clin. Diag. Lab. Immunol. 4*, 731–735.

Chen, S.M., Dumler, J.S., Bakken, J.S., Walker, D.H., 1994a. Identification of a granulocytotropic *Ehrlichia* species as the etiologic agent of human disease. *J. Clin. Microbiol. 32*, 589–595.

Chen, S.M., Dumler, J.S., Feng, H.M., Walker, D.H., 1994b. Identification of the antigenic constituents of *Ehrlichia chaffeensis*. *Am. J. Trop. Med. Hyg. 50*, 52–58.

Chen, S.M., Yu, X.J., Popov, V.L., Westerman, E.L., Hamilton, F.G., Walker, D.H., 1997b. Genetic and antigenic diversity of *Ehrlichia chaffeensis*: comparative analysis of a novel human strain from Oklahoma and previously isolated strains. *J. Infect. Dis. 175*, 856–863.

Childs, J.E., Sumner, J.W., Nicholson, W.L., Massung, R.F., Standaert, S.M., Paddock, C.D., 1999. Outcome of diagnostic tests using samples from patients with culture-proven human monocytic ehrlichiosis: implications for surveillance. *J. Clin. Microbiol. 37*, 2997–3000.

Choi, K.S., Dumler, J.S., 2003. Early induction and late abrogation of respiratory burst in *A. phagocytophilum*-infected neutrophils. *Ann. N. Y. Acad. Sci. 990*, 488–493.

Choi, K.S., Scorpio, D.G., Dumler, J.S., 2004. *Anaplasma phagocytophilum* ligation to toll-like receptor (TLR) 2, but not to TLR4, activates macrophages for nuclear factor-kappa B nuclear translocation. *J. Infect. Dis. 189*, 1921–1925.

Christova, I., Schouls, L., van de Pol, I., Park, J., Panayotov, S., Lefterova, V., Kantardjiev, T., Dumler, J.S., 2001. High prevalence of granulocytic ehrlichiae and *Borrelia burgdorferi* sensu lato in *Ixodes ricinus* ticks from Bulgaria. *J. Clin. Microbiol. 39*, 4172–4174.

Christova, I., van de Pol, I., Yazar, S., Velo, E., Schouls, L., 2003. Identification of *Borrelia burgdorferi* sensu lato, *Anaplasma* and *Ehrlichia* species, and spotted fever group rickettsiae in ticks from Southeastern Europe. *Eur. J. Clin. Microbiol. Infect. Dis. 22*, 535–542.

Collins, N.E., Liebenberg, J., de Villiers, E.P., Brayton, K.A., Louw, E., Pretorius, A., Faber, F.E., van, H.H., Josemans, A., van Kleef, M., Steyn, H.C., van Strijp, M.F., Zweygarth, E., Jongejan, F., Maillard, J.C., Berthier, D., Botha, M., Joubert, F., Corton, C.H., Thomson, N.R., Allsopp, M.T., Allsopp, B.A., 2005. The genome of the heartwater agent *Ehrlichia ruminantium* contains multiple tandem repeats of actively variable copy number. *Proc. Natl. Acad. Sci. U. S. A. 102*, 838–843.

Comer, J.A., Nicholson, W.L., Olson, J.G., Childs, J.E., 1999. Serologic testing for human granulocytic ehrlichiosis at a national referral center. *J. Clin. Microbiol. 37*, 558–564.

Courtney, J.W., Dryden, R.L., Montgomery, J., Schneider, B.S., Smith, G., Massung, R.F., 2003. Molecular characterization of *Anaplasma phagocytophilum* and *Borrelia burgdorferi* in *Ixodes scapularis* ticks from Pennsylvania. *J. Clin. Microbiol. 41*, 1569–1573.

de la Fuente, J., Massung, R.F., Wong, S.J., Chu, F.K., Lutz, H., Meli, M., von Loewenich, F.D., Grzeszczuk, A., Torina, A., Caracappa, S., Mangold, A.J., Naranjo, V., Stuen, S., Kocan, K.M., 2005. Sequence analysis of the *msp4* gene of *Anaplasma phagocytophilum* strains. *J. Clin. Microbiol. 43*, 1309–1317.

Des Vignes, F., Fish, D., 1997. Transmission of the agent of human granulocytic ehrlichiosis by host-seeking *Ixodes scapularis* (Acari: Ixodidae) in southern New York state. *J. Med. Entomol. 34*, 379–382.

Doyle, C.K., Labruna, M.B., Breitschwerdt, E.B., Tang, Y.W., Corstvet, R.E., Hegarty, B.C., Bloch, K.C., Li, P., Walker D.H., McBride, J.W., 2005a. Detection of medically important *Ehrlichia* spp. by quantitative multicolor Taqman real-time PCR of the *dsb* gene. *J. Mol. Diagn. 7*, 504–510.

Doyle, C.K., Nethery, K.A., Popor, V.L., McBride, J.W., 2005. Differentially expressed and secreted major immunoreactive protein orthologs of *Ehrlichia canis* and *E. chaffeensis* elicit early antibody responses to epitopes on glycosylated tandem repeats. *Infect. immun. 74*, 711–720.

Doyle, C.K., Zhang, X., Popov, V.L., McBride, J.W., 2005b. An immunoreactive 38-kilodalton protein of *Ehrlichia canis* shares structural homology and iron-binding capacity with the ferric ion–binding protein family. *Infect. Immun. 73*, 62–69.

Dugan, V.G., Little, S.E., Stallknecht, D.E., Beall, A.D., 2000. Natural infection of domestic goats with *Ehrlichia chaffeensis*. *J. Clin. Microbiol. 38*, 448–449.

Dumler, J.S., Barbet, A.F., Bekker, C.P., Dasch, G.A., Palmer, G.H., Ray, S.C., Rikihisa, Y., Rurangirwa, F.R., 2001. Reorganization of genera in the families *Rickettsiaceae* and *Anaplasmataceae* in the order *Rickettsiales*: unification of some species of *Ehrlichia* with *Anaplasma*, *Cowdria* with *Ehrlichia* and *Ehrlichia* with *Neorickettsia*, descriptions of six new species combinations and designation of *Ehrlichia equi* and 'HGE agent' as subjective synonyms of *Ehrlichia phagocytophila*. *Int. J. Syst. Evol. Microbiol. 51*, 2145–2165.

Dumler, J.S., Brouqui, P., 2004. Molecular diagnosis of human granulocytic anaplasmosis. *Expert. Rev. Mol. Diagn. 4*, 559–569.

Ehlers, S., 2004. Commentary: adaptive immunity in the absence of innate immune responses? The un–Tolled truth of the silent invaders. *Eur. J. Immunol. 34*, 1783–1788.

Eng, T.R., Harkess, J.R., Fishbein, D.B., Dawson, J.E., Greene, C.N., Redus, M.A., Satalowich, F.T., 1990. Epidemiologic, clinical, and laboratory findings of human ehrlichiosis in the United States, 1988. *J. Am. Med. Assoc. 264*, 2251–2258.

Ewing, S.A., Dawson, J.E., Kocan, A.A., Barker, R.W., Warner, C.K., Panciera, R.J., Fox, J.C., Kocan, K.M., Blouin, E.F., 1995. Experimental transmission of *Ehrlichia chaffeensis* (Rickettsiales: Ehrlichieae) among white–tailed deer by *Amblyomma americanum* (Acari: Ixodidae). *J. Med. Entomol. 32*, 368–374.

Felek, S., Telford, S., III, Falco, R.C., Rikihisa, Y., 2004. Sequence analysis of p44 homologs expressed by *Anaplasma phagocytophilum* in infected ticks feeding on naive hosts and in mice infected by tick attachment. *Infect. Immun. 72*, 659–666.

Feng, H.M., Walker, D.H., 2004. Mechanisms of immunity to *Ehrlichia muris*: a model of monocytotropic ehrlichiosis. *Infect. Immun. 72*, 966–971.

Fichtenbaum, C.J., Peterson, L.R., Weil, G.J., 1993. Ehrlichiosis presenting as a life-threatening illness with features of the toxic shock syndrome. *Am. J. Med. 95*, 351–357.

Fishbein, D.B., Dawson, J.E., Robinson, L.E., 1994. Human ehrlichiosis in the United States, 1985 to 1990. *Ann. Intern. Med. 120*, 736–743.

Fishbein, D.B., Kemp, A., Dawson, J.E., Greene, N.R., Redus, M.A., Fields, D.H., 1989. Human ehrlichiosis: prospective active surveillance in febrile hospitalized patients. *J. Infect. Dis. 160*, 803–809.

Ganta, R.R., Wilkerson, M.J., Cheng, C., Rokey, A.M., Chapes, S.K., 2002. Persistent *Ehrlichia chaffeensis* infection occurs in the absence of functional major histocompatibility complex class II genes. *Infect. Immun. 70*, 380–388.

Gardner, S.L., Holman, R.C., Krebs, J.W., Berkelman, R., Childs, J.E., 2003. National surveillance for the human ehrlichioses in the United States, 1997–2001, and proposed methods for evaluation of data quality. *Ann. N. Y. Acad. Sci. 990*, 80–89.

Garyu, J.W., Choi, K.S., Grab, D.J., Dumler, J.S., 2005. Defective phagocytosis in *Anaplasma phagocytophilum*-infected neutrophils. *Infect. Immun. 73*, 1187–1190.

Ge, Y., Yoshiie, K., Kuribayashi, F., Lin, M., Rikihisa, Y., 2005. *Anaplasma phagocytophilum* inhibits human neutrophil apoptosis via upregulation of bfl-1, maintenance of mitochondrial membrane potential and prevention of caspase 3 activation. *Cell. Microbiol. 7*, 29–38.

Ginsberg, H.S., Ewing, C.P., O'Connell, A.F., Jr., Bosler, E.M., Daley, J.G., Sayre, M.W., 1991. Increased population densities of *Amblyomma americanum* (Acari: Ixodidae) on Long Island, New York. *J. Parasitol. 77*, 493–495.

Goodman, J.L., Nelson, C.M., Klein, M.B., Hayes, S.F., Weston, B.W., 1999. Leukocyte infection by the granulocytic ehrlichiosis agent is linked to expression of a selectin ligand. *J. Clin. Invest 103*, 407–412.

Grzeszczuk, A., Stanczak, J., Kubica-Biernat, B., Racewicz, M., Kruminis-Lozowska, W., Prokopowicz, D., 2004. Human anaplasmosis in north-eastern Poland: seroprevalence in humans and prevalence in *Ixodes ricinus* ticks. *Ann. Agric. Environ. Med 11*, 99–103.

Gusa, A.A., Buller, R.S., Storch, G.A., Huycke, M.M., Machado, L.J., Slater, L.N., Stockham, S.L., Massung, R.F., 2001. Identification of a *p28* gene in *Ehrlichia ewingii*: evaluation of gene for use as a target for a species-specific PCR diagnostic assay. *J. Clin. Microbiol. 39*, 3871–3876.

Heppner, D.G., Wongsrichanalai, C., Walsh, D.S., McDaniel, P., Eamsila, C., Hanson, B., Paxton, H., 1997. Human ehrlichiosis in Thailand. *Lancet 350*, 785–786.

Herron, M.J., Nelson, C.M., Larson, J., Snapp, K.R., Kansas, G.S., Goodman, J.L., 2000. Intracellular parasitism by the human granulocytic ehrlichiosis bacterium through the P-selectin ligand, PSGL-1. *Science 288*, 1653–1656.

Hodzic, E., Fish, D., Maretzki, C.M., De Silva, A.M., Feng, S., Barthold, S.W., 1998. Acquisition and transmission of the agent of human granulocytic ehrlichiosis by *Ixodes scapularis* ticks. *J. Clin. Microbiol. 36*, 3574–3578.

Horowitz, H.W., Hsieh, T.C., Aguero-Rosenfeld, M.E., Kalantarpour, F., Chowdhury, I., Wormser, G.P., Wu, J.M., 2001. Antimicrobial susceptibility of *Ehrlichia phagocytophila*. *Antimicrob. Agents Chemother. 45*, 786–788.

Ijdo, J.W., Meek, J.I., Cartter, M.L., Magnarelli, L.A., Wu, C., Tenuta, S.W., Fikrig, E., Ryder, R.W., 2000a. The emergence of another tickborne infection in the 12-town area around Lyme, Connecticut: human granulocytic ehrlichiosis. *J. Infect. Dis. 181*, 1388–1393.

Ijdo, J.W., Mueller, A.C., 2004. Neutrophil NADPH oxidase is reduced at the *Anaplasma phagocytophilum* phagosome. *Infect. Immun. 72*, 5392–5401.

Ijdo, J.W., Wu, C., Magnarelli, L.A., Stafford, K.C., III, Anderson, J.F., Fikrig, E., 2000b. Detection of *Ehrlichia chaffeensis* DNA in *Amblyomma americanum* ticks in Connecticut and Rhode Island. *J. Clin. Microbiol. 38*, 4655–4656.

Ijdo, J.W., Zhang, Y., Hodzic, E., Magnarelli, L.A., Wilson, M.L., Telford, S.R., III, Barthold, S.W., Fikrig, E., 1997. The early humoral response in human granulocytic ehrlichiosis. *J. Infect. Dis. 176*, 687–692.

Inokuma, H., Brouqui, P., Drancourt, M., Raoult, D., 2001. Citrate synthase gene sequence: a new tool for phylogenetic analysis and identification of *Ehrlichia*. *J. Clin. Microbiol. 39*, 3031–3039.

Ismail, N., Soong, L., McBride, J.W., Valbuena, G., Olano, J.P., Feng, H.M., Walker, D.H., 2004. Overproduction of TNF-alpha by CD8+ type 1 cells and down-regulation of IFN-gamma production by CD4+ Th1 cells contribute to toxic shock–like syndrome in an animal model of fatal monocytotropic ehrlichiosis. *J. Immunol. 172*, 1786–1800.

Katavolos, P., Armstrong, P.M., Dawson, J.E., Telford, S.R., III, 1998. Duration of tick attachment required for transmission of granulocytic ehrlichiosis. *J. Infect. Dis. 177*, 1422–1425.

Kim, C.M., Kim, M.S., Park, M.S., Park, J.H., Chae, J.S., 2003. Identification of *Ehrlichia chaffeensis*, *Anaplasma phagocytophilum*, and *A. bovis* in *Haemaphysalis longicornis* and *Ixodes persulcatus* ticks from Korea. *Vect. Borne Zoonotic Dis. 3*, 17–26.

Klein, M.B., Hu, S., Chao, C.C., Goodman, J.L., 2000. The agent of human granulocytic ehrlichiosis induces the production of myelosuppressing chemokines without induction of proinflammatory cytokines. *J. Infect. Dis. 182*, 200–205.

Klein, M.B., Nelson, C.M., Goodman, J.L., 1997. Antibiotic susceptibility of the newly cultivated agent of human granulocytic ehrlichiosis: promising activity of quinolones and rifamycins. *Antimicrob. Agents Chemother. 41*, 76–79.

Kocan, A.A., Levesque, G.C., Whitworth, L.C., Murphy, G.L., Ewing, S.A., Barker, R.W., 2000. Naturally occurring *Ehrlichia chaffeensis* infection in coyotes from Oklahoma. *Emerg. Infect. Dis. 6*, 477–480.

Kolbert, C.P., Bruinsma, E.S., Abdulkarim, A.S., Hofmeister, E.K., Tompkins, R.B., Telford, S.R., Mitchell, P.D., Adams-Stich, J., Persing, D.H., 1997. Characterization of an immunoreactive protein from the agent of human granulocytic ehrlichiosis. *J. Clin. Microbiol. 35*, 1172–1178.

Kramer, V.L., Randolph, M.P., Hui, L.T., Irwin, W.E., Gutierrez, A.G., Vugia, D.J., 1999. Detection of the agents of human ehrlichioses in ixodid ticks from California. *Am. J. Trop. Med. Hyg. 60*, 62–65.

Krause, P.J., Corrow, C.L., Bakken, J.S., 2003. Successful treatment of human granulocytic ehrlichiosis in children using rifampin. *Pediatrics 112*, e252–e253.

Lee, E.H., Rikihisa, Y., 1998. Protein kinase A–mediated inhibition of gamma interferon-induced tyrosine phosphorylation of Janus kinases and latent cytoplasmic transcription factors in human monocytes by *Ehrlichia chaffeensis*. *Infect. Immun. 66*, 2514–2520.

Lee, E.H., Rikihisa, Y., 1997. Anti-*Ehrlichia chaffeensis* antibody complexed with *E. chaffeensis* induces potent proinflammatory cytokine mRNA expression in human monocytes through sustained reduction of IkappaB–alpha and activation of NF-kappaB. *Infect. Immun. 65*, 2890–2897.

Lee, E.H., Rikihisa, Y., 1996. Absence of tumor necrosis factor alpha, interleukin-6 (IL-6), and granulocyte-macrophage colony–stimulating factor expression but presence of IL-1beta, IL-8, and IL-10 expression in human monocytes exposed to viable or killed *Ehrlichia chaffeensis*. *Infect. Immun. 64*, 4211–4219.

Lee, K.N., Padmalayam, I., Baumstark, B., Baker, S.L., Massung, R.F., 2003. Characterization of the *ftsZ* gene from *Ehrlichia chaffeensis*, *Anaplasma phagocytophilum*, and *Rickettsia rickettsii*, and use as a differential PCR target. *DNA Cell. Biol. 22*, 179–186.

Li, J.S., Chu, F., Reilly, A., Winslow, G.M., 2002. Antibodies highly effective in SCID mice during infection by the intracellular bacterium *Ehrlichia chaffeensis* are of picomolar affinity and exhibit preferential epitope and isotype utilization. *J. Immunol. 169*, 1419–1425.

Li, J.S., Yager, E., Reilly, M., Freeman, C., Reddy, G.R., Reilly, A.A., Chu, F.K., Winslow, G.M., 2001. Outer membrane protein-specific monoclonal antibodies protect SCID mice from fatal infection by the obligate intracellular bacterial pathogen *Ehrlichia chaffeensis*. *J. Immunol. 166*, 1855–1862.

Lin, M., Rikihisa, Y., 2004. *Ehrlichia chaffeensis* downregulates surface Toll-like receptors 2/4, CD14 and transcription factors PU.1 and inhibits lipopolysaccharide activation of NF-kappa B, ERK 1/2 and p38 MAPK in host monocytes. *Cell. Microbiol. 6*, 175–186.

Lin, M., Rikihisa, Y., 2003a. Obligatory intracellular parasitism by *Ehrlichia chaffeensis* and *Anaplasma phagocytophilum* involves caveolae and glycosylphosphatidylinositol-anchored proteins. *Cell. Microbiol. 5*, 809–820.

Lin, M., Rikihisa, Y., 2003b. *Ehrlichia chaffeensis* and *Anaplasma phagocytophilum* lack genes for lipid A biosynthesis and incorporate cholesterol for their survival. *Infect. Immun. 71*, 5324–5331.

Lin, M., Zhu, M.X., Rikihisa, Y., 2002. Rapid activation of protein tyrosine kinase and phospholipase C-gamma2 and increase in cytosolic free calcium are required by *Ehrlichia chaffeensis* for internalization and growth in THP-1 cells. *Infect. Immun. 70*, 889–898.

Lin, Q., Rikihisa, Y., Felek, S., Wang, X., Massung, R.F., Woldehiwet, Z., 2004a. *Anaplasma phagocytophilum* has a functional *msp2* gene that is distinct from *p44*. *Infect. Immun. 72*, 3883–3889.

Lin, Q., Rikihisa, Y., Massung, R.F., Woldehiwet, Z., Falco, R.C., 2004b. Polymorphism and transcription at the p44-1/p44-18 genomic locus in *Anaplasma phagocytophilum* strains from diverse geographic regions. *Infect. Immun. 72*, 5574–5581.

Lin, Q., Rikihisa, Y., Ohashi, N., Zhi, N., 2003. Mechanisms of variable *p44* expression by *Anaplasma phagocytophilum*. *Infect. Immun. 71*, 5650–5661.

Lockhart, J.M., Davidson, W.R., Dawson, J.E., Stallknecht, D.E., 1995. Temporal association of *Amblyomma americanum* with the presence of *Ehrlichia chaffeensis* reactive antibodies in white-tailed deer. *J. Wildlife Dis. 31*, 119–124.

Lockhart, J.M., Davidson, W.R., Stallknecht, D.E., Dawson, J.E., Howerth, E.W., 1997. Isolation of *Ehrlichia chaffeensis* from wild white-tailed deer (*Odocoileus virginianus*) confirms their role as natural reservoir hosts. *J. Clin. Microbiol. 35*, 1681–1686.

Loftis, A.D., Massung, R.F., Levin, M.L., 2003. Quantitative real-time PCR assay for detection of *Ehrlichia chaffeensis*. *J. Clin. Microbiol. 41*, 3870–3872.

Long, S.W., Zhang, X.F., Qi, H., Standaert, S., Walker, D.H., Yu, X.J., 2002. Antigenic variation of *Ehrlichia chaffeensis* resulting from differential expression of the 28-kilodalton protein gene family. *Infect. Immun. 70*, 1824–1831.

Maeda, K., Markowitz, N., Hawley, R.C., Ristic, M., Cox, D., McDade, J.E., 1987. Human infection with *Ehrlichia canis*, a leukocytic rickettsia. *N. Engl. J. Med. 316*, 853–856.

Martin, M.E., Bunnell, J.E., Dumler, J.S., 2000. Pathology, immunohistology, and cytokine responses in early phases of human granulocytic ehrlichiosis in a murine model. *J. Infect. Dis. 181*, 374–378.

Martin, M.E., Caspersen, K., Dumler, J.S., 2001. Immunopathology and ehrlichial propagation are regulated by interferon-gamma and interleukin-10 in a murine model of human granulocytic ehrlichiosis. *Am. J. Path. 158*, 1881–1888.

Massung, R.F., Lee, K., Mauel, M., Gusa, A., 2002. Characterization of the rRNA genes of *Ehrlichia chaffeensis* and *Anaplasma phagocytophila*. *DNA Cell Biol. 21*, 587–596.

Massung, R.F., Slater, K.G., 2003. Comparison of PCR assays for detection of the agent of human granulocytic ehrlichiosis, *Anaplasma phagocytophilum*. *J. Clin. Microbiol. 41*, 717–722.

Mattner, J., Debord, K.L., Ismail, N., Goff, R.D., Cantu, C., III, Zhou, D., Saint-Mezard, P., Wang, V., Gao, Y., Yin, N., Hoebe, K., Schneewind, O., Walker, D., Beutler, B., Teyton, L., Savage, P.B., Bendelac, A., 2005. Exogenous and endogenous glycolipid antigens activate NKT cells during microbial infections. *Nature 434*, 525–529.

Maurin, M., Bakken, J.S., Dumler, J.S., 2003. Antibiotic susceptibilities of *Anaplasma* (*Ehrlichia*) *phagocytophilum* strains from various geographic areas in the United States. *Antimicrob. Agents Chemother. 47*, 413–415.

McBride JW, Corstvet, R.E., Gaunt, S.D., Boudreaux, C., Guedry, T., Walker, D.H., 2003. Kinetics of antibody response to *Ehrlichia canis* immunoreactive proteins. *Infect. Immun. 71*, 2516–2524.

McBride, J.W., Comer, J.E., Walker, D.H., 2003. Novel immunoreactive glycoprotein orthologs of *Ehrlichia* spp. *Ann. N. Y. Acad. Sci. 990*, 678–684.

McBride, J.W., Ndip, L.M., Popov, V.L., Walker, D.H., 2002. Identification and functional analysis of an immunoreactive DsbA-like thio-disulfide oxidoreductase of *Ehrlichia* spp. *Infect. Immun. 70*, 2700–2703.

McBride, J.W., Yu, X.J., Walker, D.H., 2000. Glycosylation of homologous immunodominant proteins of *Ehrlichia chaffeensis* and *E. canis*. *Infect. Immun. 68*, 13–18.

McCabe TR, McCabe RE, 1997. Recounting whitetails past. In: McShea WJ, Underwood HB, Rappole JH (Eds.), *The Science of Over Abundance: Deer Ecology and Population Management*. Smithsonian Institution Press, Washington, D.C., pp. 11–26.

McQuiston, J.H., Paddock, C.D., Holman, R.C., Childs, J.E., 1999. Human ehrlichioses in the United States. *Emerg. Infect. Dis. 5*, 635–642.

Means, R.G., White, D.J., 1997. New distribution records of *Amblyomma americanum* (Acari: Ixodidae) in New York State. *J. Vect. Ecol. 22*, 133–145.

Mott, J., Barnewall, R.E., Rikihisa, Y., 1999. Human granulocytic ehrlichiosis agent and *Ehrlichia chaffeensis* reside in different cytoplasmic compartments in HL-60 cells. *Infect. Immun. 67*, 1368–1378.

Mott, J., Rikihisa, Y., 2000. Human granulocytic ehrlichiosis agent inhibits superoxide anion generation by human neutrophils. *Infect. Immun. 68*, 6697–6703.

Mott, J., Rikihisa, Y., Tsunawaki, S., 2002. Effects of *Anaplasma phagocytophila* on NADPH oxidase components in human neutrophils and HL-60 cells. *Infect. Immun. 70*, 1359–1366.

Murphy, C.I., Storey, J.R., Recchia, J., Doros-Richert, L.A., Gingrich-Baker, C., Munroe, K., Bakken, J.S., Coughlin, R.T., Beltz, G.A., 1998. Major antigenic proteins of the agent of human granulocytic ehrlichiosis are encoded by members of a multigene family. *Infect. Immun. 66*, 3711–3718.

Nadelman, R.B., Horowitz, H.W., Hsieh, T.C., Wu, J.M., Aguero-Rosenfeld, M.E., Schwartz, I., Nowakowski, J., Varde, S., Wormser, G.P., 1997. Simultaneous human granulocytic ehrlichiosis and Lyme borreliosis. *N. Engl. J. Med. 337*, 27–30.

Nuti, M., Serafini, D.A., Bassetti, D., Ghionni, A., Russino, F., Rombola, P., Macri, G., Lillini, E., 1998. *Ehrlichia* infection in Italy. *Emerg. Infect. Dis. 4*, 663–665.

Ohashi, N., Rikihisa, Y., Unver, A., 2001. Analysis of transcriptionally active gene clusters of major outer membrane protein multigene family in *Ehrlichia canis* and *E. chaffeensis*. *Infect. Immun. 69*, 2083–2091.

Ohashi, N., Zhi, N., Lin, Q., Rikihisa, Y., 2002. Characterization and transcriptional analysis of gene clusters for a type IV secretion machinery in human granulocytic and monocytic ehrlichiosis agents. *Infect. Immun. 70*, 2128–2138.

Olano, J.P., Masters, E., Hogrefe, W., Walker, D.H., 2003. Human monocytotropic ehrlichiosis, Missouri. *Emerg. Infect. Dis. 9*, 1579–1586.

Paddock, C.D., Childs, J.E., 2003. *Ehrlichia chaffeensis*: a prototypical emerging pathogen. *Clin. Microbiol. Rev. 16*, 37–64.

Paddock, C.D., Folk, S.M., Shore, G.M., Machado, L.J., Huycke, M.M., Slater, L.N., Liddell, A.M., Buller, R.S., Storch, G.A., Monson, T.P., Rimland, D., Sumner, J.W., Singleton, J., Bloch, K.C., Tang, Y.W., Standaert, S.M., Childs, J.E., 2001. Infections with *Ehrlichia chaffeensis* and *Ehrlichia ewingii* in persons coinfected with human immunodeficiency virus. *Clin. Infect. Dis. 33*, 1586–1594.

Palella, F.J., Jr., Delaney, K.M., Moorman, A.C., Loveless, M.O., Fuhrer, J., Satten, G.A., Aschman, D.J., Holmberg, S.D., 1998. Declining morbidity and mortality among patients with advanced human immunodeficiency virus infection. HIV Outpatient Study Investigators. *N. Engl. J. Med. 338*, 853–860.

Park, J., Choi, K.S., Dumler, J.S., 2003a. Major surface protein 2 of *Anaplasma phagocytophilum* facilitates adherence to granulocytes. *Infect. Immun. 71*, 4018–4025.

Park, J., Kim, K.J., Choi, K.S., Grab, D.J., Dumler, J.S., 2004. *Anaplasma phagocytophilum* AnkA binds to granulocyte DNA and nuclear proteins. *Cell. Microbiol. 6*, 743–751.

Park, J., Kim, K.J., Grab, D.J., Dumler, J.S., 2003b. *Anaplasma phagocytophilum* major surface protein-2 (Msp2) forms multimeric complexes in the bacterial membrane. *FEMS Microbiol. Lett. 227*, 243–247.

Parola, P., Cornet, J.P., Sanogo, Y.O., Miller, R.S., Thien, H.V., Gonzalez, J.P., Raoult, D., Telford, I.I.I., Sr., Wongsrichanalai, C., 2003. Detection of *Ehrlichia* spp., *Anaplasma* spp., *Rickettsia* spp., and other eubacteria in ticks from the Thai-Myanmar border and Vietnam. *J. Clin. Microbiol. 41*, 1600–1608.

Petersen, L.R., Sawyer, L.A., Fishbein, D.B., Kelley, P.W., Thomas, R.J., Magnarelli, L.A., Redus, M., Dawson, J.E., 1989. An outbreak of ehrlichiosis in members of an Army Reserve unit exposed to ticks. *J. Infect. Dis. 159*, 562–568.

Popov, V.L., Chen, S.M., Feng, H.M., Walker, D.H., 1995. Ultrastructural variation of cultured *Ehrlichia chaffeensis*. *J. Med. Microbiol. 43*, 411–421.

Popov, V.L., Han, V.C., Chen, S.M., Dumler, J.S., Feng, H.M., Andreadis, T.G., Tesh, R.B., Walker, D.H., 1998. Ultrastructural differentiation of the genogroups in the genus *Ehrlichia*. *J. Med. Microbiol. 47*, 235–251.

Ravyn, M.D., Korenberg, E.I., Oeding, J.A., Kovalevskii, Y.V., Johnson, R.C., 1999. Monocytic *Ehrlichia* in *Ixodes persulcatus* ticks from Perm, Russia [letter]. *Lancet 353*(9154), 722–723.

Reddy, G.R., Streck, C.P., 2000. Variability in the 28-kDa surface antigen protein multigene locus of isolates of the emerging disease agent *Ehrlichia chaffeensis* suggests that it plays a role in immune evasion. [Published erratum appears in *Mol. Cell. Biol. Res. Commun.* 2000;3(1):66] *Mol. Cell. Biol. Res. Commun. 1,* 167–175.

Richter, P.J., Jr., Kimsey, R.B., Madigan, J.E., Barlough, J.E., Dumler, J.S., Brooks, D.L., 1996. *Ixodes pacificus* (Acari: Ixodidae) as a vector of *Ehrlichia equi* (Rickettsiales: Ehrlichieae). *J. Med. Entomol. 33,* 1–5.

Rikihisa, Y., 1991. The tribe Ehrlichieae and ehrlichial diseases. *Clin. Microbiol. Rev. 4,* 286–308.

Rikihisa, Y., Ewing, S.A., Fox, J.C., 1994. Western immunoblot analysis of *Ehrlichia chaffeensis, E. canis,* or *E. ewingii* infections in dogs and humans. *J. Clin. Microbiol. 32,* 2107–2112.

Rikihisa, Y., Zhi, N., Wormser, G.P., Wen, B., Horowitz, H.W., Hechemy, K.E., 1997. Ultrastructural and antigenic characterization of a granulocytic ehrlichiosis agent directly isolated and stably cultivated from a patient in New York state. *J. Infect. Dis. 175,* 210–213.

Ripoll, C.M., Remondegui, C.E., Ordonez, G., Arazamendi, R., Fusaro, H., Hyman, M.J., Paddock, C.D., Zaki, S.R., Olson, J.G., Santos-Buch, C.A., 1999. Evidence of rickettsial spotted fever and ehrlichial infections in a subtropical territory of Jujuy, Argentina. *Am. J. Trop. Med. Hyg. 61,* 350–354.

Scaife, H., Woldehiwet, Z., Hart, C.A., Edwards, S.W., 2003. *Anaplasma phagocytophilum* reduces neutrophil apoptosis in vivo. *Infect. Immun. 71,* 1995–2001.

Scorpio, D.G., Akkoyunlu, M., Fikrig, E., Dumler, J.S., 2004. CXCR2 blockade influences *Anaplasma phagocytophilum* propagation but not histopathology in the mouse model of human granulocytic anaplasmosis. *Clin. Diag. Lab. Immunol. 11,* 963–968.

Singu, V., Liu, H., Cheng, C., Ganta, R.R., 2005. *Ehrlichia chaffeensis* expresses macrophage- and tick cell-specific 28-kilodalton outer membrane proteins. *Infect. Immun. 73,* 79–87.

Sirigireddy, K.R., Ganta, R.R., 2005. Multiplex detection of *Ehrlichia* and *Anaplasma* species pathogens in peripheral blood by real-time reverse transcriptase-polymerase chain reaction. *J. Mol. Diagn. 7,* 308–316.

Sotomayor, E., Popov, V.L., Feng, H.M., Walker, D.H., Olano, J.P., 2001. Animal model of fatal human monocytotropic ehrlichiosis. *Am. J. Pathol. 158,* 757–769.

Standaert, S.M., Dawson, J.E., Schaffner, W., Childs, J.E., Biggie, K.L., Singleton, J.J., Gerhardt, R.R., Knight, M.L., Hutcheson, R.H., 1995. Ehrlichiosis in a golf-oriented retirement community. *N. Engl. J. Med. 333,* 420–425.

Standaert, S.M., Yu, T., Scott, M.A., Childs, J.E., Paddock, C.D., Nicholson, W.L., Singleton, J., Jr., Blaser, M.J., 2000. Primary isolation of *Ehrlichia chaffeensis* from patients with febrile illnesses: clinical and molecular characteristics. *J. Infect. Dis. 181,* 1082–1088.

Steere, A.C., Coburn, J., Glickstein, L., 2004. The emergence of Lyme disease. *J. Clin. Invest. 113,* 1093–1101.

Steere, A.C., McHugh, G., Suarez, C., Hoitt, J., Damle, N., Sikand, V.K., 2003. Prospective study of coinfection in patients with erythema migrans. *Clin. Infect. Dis. 36,* 1078–1081.

Storey, J.R., Doros-Richert, L.A., Gingrich-Baker, C., Munroe, K., Mather, T.N., Coughlin, R.T., Beltz, G.A., Murphy, C.I., 1998. Molecular cloning and sequencing of three granulocytic *Ehrlichia* genes encoding high-molecular-weight immunoreactive proteins. *Infect. Immun. 66,* 1356–1363.

Stromdahl, E.Y., Evans, S.R., O'Brien, J.J., Gutierrez, A.G., 2001. Prevalence of infection in ticks submitted to the human tick test kit program of the U.S. Army Center for Health Promotion and Preventive Medicine. *J. Med. Entomol. 38,* 67–74.

Sumner, J.W., Childs, J.E., Paddock, C.D., 1999. Molecular cloning and characterization of the *Ehrlichia chaffeensis* variable-length PCR target: an antigen-expressing gene that exhibits interstrain variation. *J. Clin. Microbiol. 37,* 1447–1453.

Sumner, J.W., Nicholson, W.L., Massung, R.F., 1997. PCR amplification and comparison of nucleotide sequences from the groESL heat shock operon of *Ehrlichia* species. *J. Clin. Microbiol. 35,* 2087–2092.

Sumner, J.W., Sims, K.G., Jones, D.C., Anderson, B.E., 1993. *Ehrlichia chaffeensis* expresses an immunoreactive protein homologous to the *Escherichia coli* GroEL protein. *Infect. Immun. 61,* 3536–3539.

Sun, W., Ijdo, J.W., Telford, S.R., III, Hodzic, E., Zhang, Y., Barthold, S.W., Fikrig, E., 1997. Immunization against the agent of human granulocytic ehrlichiosis in a murine model. *J. Clin. Invest. 100,* 3014–3018.

Tal, A., Shannahan, D., 1995. Ehrlichiosis presenting as a life-threatening illness [letter; comment]. *Am. J. Med. 98*, 318–319.

Thomas, V., Samanta, S., Wu, C., Berliner, N., Fikrig, E., 2005. *Anaplasma phagocytophilum* modulates gp91phox gene expression through altered interferon regulatory factor 1 and PU.1 levels and binding of CCAAT displacement protein. *Infect. Immun. 73*, 208–218.

Treadwell, T.A., Holman, R.C., Clarke, M.J., Krebs, J.W., Paddock, C.D., Childs, J.E., 2000. Rocky Mountain spotted fever in the United States, 1993-1996. *Am. J. Trop. Med. Hyg. 63*, 21–26.

Uhaa, I.J., MacLean, J.D., Greene, C.R., Fishbein, D.B., 1992. A case of human ehrlichiosis acquired in Mali: clinical and laboratory findings. *Am. J. Trop. Med. Hyg. 46*, 161–164.

Unver, A., Rikihisa, Y., Stich, R.W., Ohashi, N., Felek, S., 2002. The omp-1 major outer membrane multigene family of *Ehrlichia chaffeensis* is differentially expressed in canine and tick hosts. *Infect. Immun. 70*, 4701–4704.

von Loewenich, F.D., Scorpio, D.G., Reischl, U., Dumler, J.S., Bogdan, C., 2004. Frontline: control of *Anaplasma phagocytophilum*, an obligate intracellular pathogen, in the absence of inducible nitric oxide synthase, phagocyte NADPH oxidase, tumor necrosis factor, Toll-like receptor (TLR)2 and TLR4, or the TLR adaptor molecule MyD88. *Eur. J. Immunol. 34*, 1789–1797.

Walder, G., Tiwald, G., Dierich, M.P., Wurzner, R., 2003. Serological evidence for human granulocytic ehrlichiosis in Western Austria. *Eur. J. Clin. Microbiol. Infect. Dis. 22*, 543–547.

Walker DH, 2000. Diagnosing human ehrlichiosis: Current status and recommendations. *ASM News 66*, 287–291.

Wallace, B.J., Brady, G., Ackman, D.M., Wong, S.J., Jacquette, G., Lloyd, E.E., Birkhead, G.S., 1998. Human granulocytic ehrlichiosis in New York. *Arch. Intern. Med. 158*, 769–773.

Wang, T., Akkoyunlu, M., Banerjee, R., Fikrig, E., 2004. Interferon-gamma deficiency reveals that 129Sv mice are inherently more susceptible to *Anaplasma phagocytophilum* than C57BL/6 mice. *FEMS Immunol. Med. Microbiol. 42*, 299–305.

Wang, T., Malawista, S.E., Pal, U., Grey, M., Meek, J., Akkoyunlu, M., Thomas, V., Fikrig, E., 2002. Superoxide anion production during *Anaplasma phagocytophila* infection. *J. Infect. Dis. 186*, 274–280.

Webster, P., Ijdo, J.W., Chicoine, L.M., Fikrig, E., 1998. The agent of human granulocytic ehrlichiosis resides in an endosomal compartment. *J. Clin. Invest. 101*, 1932–1941.

Whitlock, J.E., Fang, Q.Q., Durden, L.A., Oliver, J.H., Jr., 2000. Prevalence of *Ehrlichia chaffeensis* (Rickettsiales: Rickettsiaceae) in *Amblyomma americanum* (Acari: Ixodidae) from the Georgia coast and barrier islands. *J. Med. Entomol. 37*, 276–280.

Winslow, G.M., Yager, E., Shilo, K., Collins, D.N., Chu, F.K., 1998. Infection of the laboratory mouse with the intracellular pathogen *Ehrlichia chaffeensis*. *Infect. Immun. 66*, 3892–3899.

Winslow, G.M., Yager, E., Shilo, K., Volk, E., Reilly, A., Chu, F.K., 2000. Antibody-mediated elimination of the obligate intracellular bacterial pathogen *Ehrlichia chaffeensis* during active infection. *Infect. Immun. 68*, 2187–2195.

Yabsley, M.J., Little, S.E., Sims, E.J., Dugan, V.G., Stallknecht, D.E., Davidson, W.R., 2003. Molecular variation in the variable-length PCR target and 120-kilodalton antigen genes of *Ehrlichia chaffeensis* from white-tailed deer (*Odocoileus virginianus*). *J. Clin. Microbiol. 41*, 5202–5206.

Yago, T., Leppanen, A., Carlyon, J.A., Akkoyunlu, M., Karmakar, S., Fikrig, E., Cummings, R.D., McEver, R.P., 2003. Structurally distinct requirements for binding of P-selectin glycoprotein ligand-1 and sialyl Lewis x to *Anaplasma phagocytophilum* and P-selectin. *J. Biol. Chem. 278*, 37987–37997.

Yoshiie, K., Kim, H.Y., Mott, J., Rikihisa, Y., 2000. Intracellular infection by the human granulocytic ehrlichiosis agent inhibits human neutrophil apoptosis. *Infect. Immun. 68*, 1125–1133.

Yu, X.J., Crocquet-Valdes, P., Cullman, L.C., Walker, D.H., 1996. The recombinant 120-kilodalton protein of *Ehrlichia chaffeensis*, a potential diagnostic tool. *J. Clin. Microbiol. 34*, 2853–2855.

Yu, X.J., Crocquet-Valdes, P., Walker, D.H., 1997. Cloning and sequencing of the gene for a 120-kDa immunodominant protein of *Ehrlichia chaffeensis*. *Gene 184*, 149–154.

Yu, X.J., Crocquet-Valdes, P.A., Cullman, L.C., Popov, V.L., Walker, D.H., 1999a. Comparison of *Ehrlichia chaffeensis* recombinant proteins for serologic diagnosis of human monocytotropic ehrlichiosis. *J. Clin. Microbiol. 37*, 2568–2575.

Yu, X.J., McBride, J.W., Walker, D.H., 1999b. Genetic diversity of the 28-kilodalton outer membrane protein gene in human isolates of *Ehrlichia chaffeensis*. *J. Clin. Microbiol. 37*, 1137–1143.

Yu, X.J., McBride, J.W., Zhang, X.F., Walker, D.H., 2000. Characterization of the complete transcriptionally active *Ehrlichia chaffeensis* 28 kDa outer membrane protein multigene family. *Gene 248*, 59–68.

Yu, X.J., Walker, D.H., 1997. Sequence and characterization of an *Ehrlichia chaffeensis* gene encoding 314 amino acids highly homologous to the NAD A enzyme. *FEMS Microbiol. Lett. 154*, 53–58.

Zhang, J.Z., Guo, H., Winslow, G.M., Yu, X.J., 2004a. Expression of members of the 28-kilodalton major outer membrane protein family of *Ehrlichia chaffeensis* during persistent infection. *Infect. Immun. 72*, 4336–4343.

Zhang, J.Z., McBride, J.W., Yu, X.J., 2003. L-selectin and E-selectin expressed on monocytes mediating *Ehrlichia chaffeensis* attachment onto host cells. *FEMS Microbiol. Lett. 227*, 303–309.

Zhang, J.Z., Sinha, M., Luxon, B.A., Yu, X.J., 2004b. Survival strategy of obligately intracellular *Ehrlichia chaffeensis*: novel modulation of immune response and host cell cycles. *Infect. Immun. 72*, 498–507.

Zhi, N., Ohashi, N., Rikihisa, Y., 1999. Multiple p44 genes encoding major outer membrane proteins are expressed in the human granulocytic ehrlichiosis agent. *J. Biol. Chem. 274*, 17828–17836.

Zhi, N., Ohashi, N., Rikihisa, Y., Horowitz, H.W., Wormser, G.P., Hechemy, K., 1998. Cloning and expression of the 44-kilodalton major outer membrane protein gene of the human granulocytic ehrlichiosis agent and application of the recombinant protein to serodiagnosis. *J. Clin. Microbiol. 36*, 1666–1673.

Zhi, N., Rikihisa, Y., Kim, H.Y., Wormser, G.P., Horowitz, H.W., 1997. Comparison of major antigenic proteins of six strains of the human granulocytic ehrlichiosis agent by Western immunoblot analysis. *J. Clin. Microbiol. 35*, 2606–2611.

4. Cross-Species Transmission of Poxviruses

MIKE BRAY

4.1. Introduction: The Poxvirus Family

The poxviruses are an ancient group of intracellular pathogens whose "survival strategy" is based on the release of hardy virions from sites of replication on the external surface of the body. Their large size, complex genomes, and ability to replicate in the cytoplasm independent of the nucleus suggest that an ancestral agent was a free-living microbe that adapted to a lifestyle of intracellular parasitism by evolving a secure and efficient means of transmission to new hosts. The great age of the poxviruses is reflected in their division into two subfamilies, the entomopoxviruses that infect insects and the chordopoxviruses that infect vertebrates, indicating that an early progenitor parasitized creatures ancestral to both groups (Iyer et al., 2001; McLysaght et al., 2003; Gubser et al., 2004). The entomopoxviruses have become so highly adapted to their insect hosts over hundreds of millions of years of co-evolution that they are unable to cause productive infection in humans or other animals; they are therefore not considered further in this chapter.

The radiation of vertebrate animals into the myriad varieties that exist today has been accompanied by the differentiation of the chordopoxviruses that infect them, resulting in the existence of eight currently recognized viral genera and a large number of named species (Table 4.1; Fig. 4.1A). An additional candidate genus, Deerpoxvirus, has recently been described, and it seems certain that a large number of other poxviruses remain to be identified (Afonso et al., 2005). Division into genera is based principally on antigenic criteria, as determined by serologic assays and the ability of infection by one virus to induce resistance to subsequent infection by another. For example, although both orf virus and sheeppox virus cause disease in sheep, the former is assigned to the genus Parapoxvirus and the latter to the capripoxviruses, in part because the two agents do not cross-protect against each other. Within each genus,

Table 4.1. Genera of the poxvirus family, with some major recognized species

Genus	Species	Geographic range	Maintenance host	Other susceptible species
Orthopoxvirus	Variola	Eradicated	Humans	Non-human primates (laboratory experiments)
	Monkeypox	Sub-Saharan Africa	Squirrels, other rodents (?)	Non-human primates, prairie dogs, ground squirrels, other rodents
	Vaccinia	Unknown (smallpox vaccine virus)	Unknown	Cattle, camels, and other herd animals, rabbits, rodents, non-human primates
	Cowpox	Eurasia	Rodents	Domestic cats, large felines, cattle, elephants
	Ectromelia	Europe (?)	Wild mice (?)	None
	Camelpox	Southwest Asia, North Africa	Camels	None
	Raccoonpox	Eastern USA	Raccoons (?)	Unknown
	Skunkpox	Western USA	Skunks (?)	Unknown
	Volepox	Western USA	Voles	Unknown
	Taterapox	West Africa	Gerbils	Unknown
Yatapoxvirus	Tanapox	West Africa	Non-human primates (?)	Unknown
	Yaba monkey tumor virus	West Africa	Non-human primates (?)	Unknown
Parapoxvirus	Orf	Worldwide	Sheep, goats	Wild hoofed animals (mountain goats, reindeer)
	Pseudo-cowpox	Worldwide	Dairy cattle	Unknown
	Bovine papular stomatitis	Worldwide	Beef cattle	Unknown
	Ausdyk	SW Asia, Africa	Camels	Unknown
Mollus-cipoxvirus	Molluscum contagiosum	Worldwide	Humans	None
Leporipoxvirus	Myxoma	South America	Wild rabbits	Other rabbit/hare species
	Shope fibroma	Eastern North America	Wild rabbits	Other rabbit/hare species
Capripoxvirus	Sheeppox	India, Southwest Asia, North Africa	Sheep, goats	None
	Goatpox	India, Southwest Asia, North Africa	Sheep, goats	None
	Lumpy skin disease	East Africa	Wild and domestic cattle	None
Suipoxvirus	Swinepox	Worldwide	Pigs	None
Avipoxvirus	Fowlpox	Worldwide	Birds	None
	Canarypox	Worldwide	Birds	None
Deerpoxvirus	Deerpox	North America	Deer	Unknown

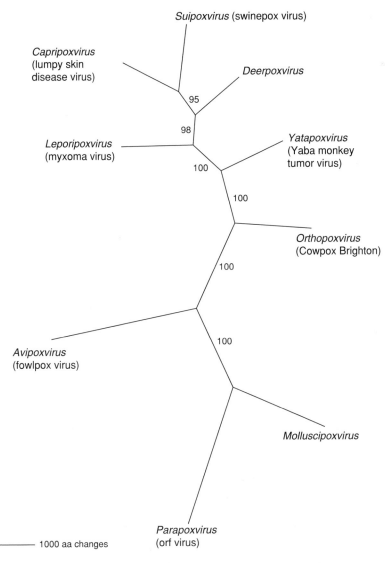

Figure 4.1. (A) Phylogenetic tree of eight genera and one proposed new genus (Deerpoxvirus) in the subfamily Chordopoxvirinae. Members of the most divergent genus, Avipoxvirus, are maintained in birds, whereas all others infect mammals. (Data courtesy of Chunlin Wang and Elliot Lefkowitz, University of Alabama, Birmingham.)

individual viral species are usually designated by the diseases they cause or the animals from which they were first isolated (Table 4.1; Fig. 4.1B). The ability of a poxvirus to induce resistance to other members of its genus is best illustrated by the orthopoxvirus vaccinia, which has been

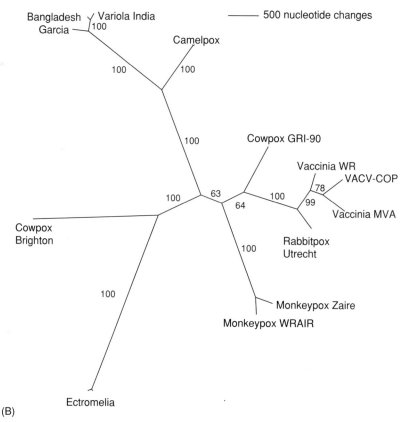

Figure 4.1. (*Continued*) (B) Phylogenetic tree of species in the genus Orthopoxvirus for which sequence data are available. As noted in the text, camelpox is the virus most closely related to variola, the agent of smallpox. Monkeypox virus, which also causes severe disease in humans, is only distantly related to variola. Two viruses currently classified as cowpox are genetically quite diverse and may in future be assigned to separate species. (Data courtesy of Chunlin Wang and Elliot Lefkowitz, University of Alabama, Birmingham.)

employed to vaccinate humans against smallpox, elephants against cowpox, and camels against camelpox.

The advent of full-length genomic sequencing is facilitating more refined classification of the poxviruses and helping to elucidate their evolutionary history. Two different approaches are employed to characterize genera and species, based on analysis of different portions of the genome (Gubser et al., 2004). Of the roughly 200 genes in a typical linear poxviral genome, those in the central region encode all enzymes, cofactors, and structural proteins required for transcription, genome replication, and virion formation. A core group of some 50 of these genes has been preserved in entomo- and chordopoxviruses, indicating that they were already possessed by a primordial ancester of all modern poxviruses (McLysaght et al., 2003). Even though the high replicative fidelity of the DNA polymerase has maintained the sequences of these essential genes, sufficient variation has accumulated to permit sequence comparisons that reflect the evolutionary history of the poxviral family (Fig. 4.1A). The flanking regions, by contrast, encode proteins that enable each virus to defend itself against its reservoir host; they therefore differ significantly among genera and somewhat less between species. These portions of the genome appear to have been assembled from host genetic material acquired through recombination during the more recent evolutionary history of the poxviruses and modified through mutation, rearrangement, duplication, and deletion as each agent adapted to its natural reservoir. Each currently existing poxviral species therefore possess a unique complement of functional genes in its flanking regions. In addition to differing in the number and order of genes, poxviral genera also vary in the relative percentage of A+T and G+C base pairs, ranging from an A+T content of 36% for the parapoxviruses to 75% for the capripoxviruses (Gubser et al., 2004). The analysis of full-length genomic sequences of a rapidly increasing number of poxviruses may lead to the development of a revised classification scheme that reflects their evolutionary history.

Examination of current poxviral transmission patterns indicates that the history of these agents has consisted of successful parasitism of a variety of maintenance hosts, with continuous chains of transmission spanning many millions of years, punctuated by innumerable episodes of virus transfer to other animal species, resulting from predation, sharing of living space, or other forms of direct or indirect contact. The possible outcomes of transferring a poxvirus from its reservoir host to another animal species range from the complete absence of visible evidence of viral replication through the formation of a localized skin lesion to the development of lethal disseminated disease. As discussed below, such outcomes appear to be determined principally by interactions between host innate and adaptive immune responses and viral countermeasures, in the form of a battery of virus-encoded immunomodulatory proteins. Even if a transferred virus is able to overcome host defenses and cause disease, that is no guarantee that infection will spread to other members of the new host population, because factors that include the mode and quantity of virus release and uptake, the stability of virions and the number, density, and contact rate of the host population will determine whether sustained transmission can occur.

The successful cross-species transfer of a poxvirus to a new reservoir host therefore tends to be a rare event but one that must nevertheless have occurred often over the vast evolutionary timescale. As discussed in this chapter, one such cross-species transmission was the spread of variola virus from an unknown animal reservoir to humans, which probably occurred some 5000 to 10,000 years ago (Bray and Buller, 2004). The establishment of camelpox virus and the capripoxviruses among animals herded by humans may have taken place in a similar manner. The summer of 2003 almost witnessed another such event, when monkeypox virus was introduced to captive prairie dogs and their human owners in the midwestern United States through the importation of virus-infected giant Gambian rats (Reed et al., 2004). If an infected prairie dog had been released or escaped into the wild, monkeypox virus might have accomplished a totally unexpected, transoceanic cross-species transfer by becoming established among local rodent populations.

4.1.1. The Poxvirus "Survival Strategy"

Three principal aspects of the poxviral replication cycle together constitute the highly effective "survival strategy" that has resulted in their continued existence for many hundreds of millions of years. First, replication results in the formation of large numbers of hardy virions that remain within necrotic cells and are released into the environment in shed debris or scabs or through mechanical transmission by skin-feeding arthropods. Once released, they remain capable of infecting new hosts for weeks to months by entering through breaks in the skin or the lining of the upper respiratory tract. Second, to accomplish such release, poxviruses establish foci of infection on the outer surface of the body (including the entrance to the respiratory tract), where replication and cell-to-cell spread are aided in many cases by the secretion of a virus-encoded epidermal growth factor from infected cells. Third, each focus of replication is sheltered against host innate and adaptive immune responses by an elaborate battery of virus-encoded immunomodulatory proteins, permitting infection to persist long enough to ensure production of large numbers of new virions (McFadden and Murphy, 2000; Turner and Moyer, 2002).

The early poxviral progenitor may have embarked on this evolutionary path soon after the development of multicellular organisms, which provided a new ecological niche based on infection of the external surface of the body. The subsequent co-evolution of these and other pathogens with their host species has presumably been characterized by the repeated development of new mechanisms of host resistance to cutaneous infection, followed in turn by the evolution of new viral countermeasures. Over hundreds of millions of years, this "struggle" has produced the complex, overlapping set of cutaneous immune responses possessed by humans and other mammals and the elaborate collection of immunomodulatory proteins by which the poxviruses defend themselves against them.

This sophisticated survival strategy, in which production of highly stable virions goes on beneath an "umbrella" provided by an array of virus-encoded countermeasures, reflects a basic division of labor within the poxviral genome. As previously described, a central core of highly conserved genes encodes all proteins needed to generate hardy virions. The flanking regions of the genome, by contrast, are responsible for defending foci of viral replication in each different reservoir host. These regions have been built up through random incorporation of host genetic material, but natural selection has presumably favored the retention only of those genes that favor virus survival. Most of these genes were apparently acquired millions of years ago, and there is no evidence that any of the orthopoxviruses has acquired new genetic material in the recent past. This suggests that an ancestral orthopoxvirus was already so well adapted to early mammals that the acquisition of additional genes did not provide a further survival advantage.

The high degree of evolutionary conservation of the complex poxviral replicative machinery has important implications for the development of effective antiviral therapy, because it implies the existence of critical steps in the production of new virions that could potentially be blocked by pharmacological agents. To date, the principal drug target has been the poxviral DNA polymerase, the sequence of which has been so highly conserved that the antiviral drug cidofovir, a cytidine analogue, is effective against members of the orthopox-, parapox-, and molluscipoxvirus genera (Neyts and Clercq, 2003). Attempts to develop cidofovir-resistant variants of vaccinia, cowpox, and other orthopoxviruses have shown that the proper functioning of this enzyme is so essential to rapid viral replication that drug-resistant mutants have a markedly reduced ability to cause disease in laboratory animals (Smee et al., 2002). A number of other highly conserved enzymes and structural proteins have been identified as potential drug targets, offering the prospect of combination chemotherapy that would be effective across the entire range of chordopoxviruses (Harrison et al., 2004).

4.1.2. Measures and Countermeasures

The co-evolution of poxviruses and other cutaneous pathogens with their vertebrate hosts has led to the development of a complex, overlapping set of innate antiviral responses. The primary defense against viral infection is programmed cell death, or apoptosis, in which virus entry into a cell triggers its rapid loss of function and breakup, preventing the completion of a full replication cycle. A second layer of defense triggered by viral infection consists of the synthesis and release of a variety of signal molecules that modify local blood flow, recruit inflammatory cells to the site of infection, and hasten the induction of antigen-specific immune responses. Specialized phagocytic cells recognize these signals, aided by the binding of circulating complement proteins to microbes and infected cells. In addition, the synthesis and release of type I interferon (interferon-α/β) acts at multiple sites to increase resistance to replication within the infected cell, induce an "antiviral state" in neighboring cells, and stimulate the activity of natural killer cells and the differentiation of antigen-presenting cells.

All of the chordopoxviruses appear to have acquired one or more countermeasures against each of these host responses (Table 4.2) (Bugert and Darai, 2000; McFadden and Murphy, 2000; Turner and Moyer, 2002). Virus-encoded proteins synthesized immediately after entry of the virion core into the cytoplasm act within the cell to block the induction of apoptosis, prevent the initiation of an interferon response, and inhibit the synthesis of the proinflammatory cytokine IL-1β and other mediators. At the same time, virus-encoded, truncated versions of host cytokine and chemokine receptors are synthesized and released into the extracellular fluid, where they serve as "decoys" to prevent the initiation of inflammatory responses and the action of type I and type II interferon. In most cases, virus and host remain fairly well matched, but the array of viral countermeasures can provide a poxvirus with a significant advantage over a host defective in some components of innate immunity. For example, persons with atopic dermatitis, who have impaired cutaneous responses to interferon-γ and appear to lack certain antimicrobial peptides, may develop rapidly progressive smallpox-like disease when inoculated with vaccinia virus or accidentally infected with cowpox virus (Engler et al., 2002; Bray, 2003; Howell et al., 2004).

Although the full array of innate antiviral responses possessed by humans is generally quite effective in slowing the pace of poxviral replication and spread to new cells, these measures may be incapable of eliminating a virus. Mechanisms have therefore evolved that supplement nonspecific antiviral responses by specifically identifying pathogens, blocking their infectivity, and destroying infected cells. Such antigen-specific or adaptive immune responses are required to control the "current generation" of poxviruses, but their role only becomes evident when they have been lost through inherited or acquired disease. Thus, immunocompetent persons are normally able to confine molluscum contagiosum virus (MCV) to a few small foci of infection and eliminate the agent altogether after several months, but in individuals with severe cell-mediated

Table 4.2. Host processes targetted by orthopoxviruses

Site of action	Virus-encoded protein	Host process targetted	Vaccinia	Variola	Cowpox
Intracellular	Serine proteinase inhibitor	Programmed cell death	crmA/ SPI2	+	+
	dsRNA BP	IFN response	E3L	+	+
	eIF2α homolog	Protein synthesis	K3L	+	+
Extracellular	Epidermal growth factor homolog	Keratinocyte proliferation	C11R	+	+
	TNF-α BP	Inflammatory response	–	+	+
	IFN-γ BP	Th1 response	B8R	+	+
	IFN-α/β BP	Type I IFN response	B18R	+	+
	IL-1-β BP	Inflammatory response	B15R	–	+
	IL-18 BP	Th1 response	B16R	+	+
	Chemokine BP	Recruitment of neutrophils and macrophages	P35	+	+
	Complement control protein	Lysis of virions and infected cells	C3L	+	+

Viral species differ in the number of functional immunomodulatory proteins encoded in their genomes; for example, cowpox virus encodes four different TNF-α-binding proteins, whereas variola has one and vaccinia none. Similarly, variola differs from the others in lacking a functional IL-1β-binding protein. Column 4 indicate the gene designations in vaccinia virus, the reference species. dsRNA, double-stranded RNA; TNF, tumor necrosis factor; IFN, interferon; SPI, serine proteinase inhibitor; IL, interleukin; BP, binding protein.

immunodeficiency secondary to human immunodeficiency virus (HIV) infection, the virus is able to cause progressive disseminated disease (Smith and Skelton, 2002). Similarly, experience during the universal vaccination campaigns of the mid-20th century showed that infants with severe, combined immunodeficiency invariably succumbed to the slow but relentless spread of vaccinia infection (Bray and Wright, 2003).

The response induced in an animal by a given poxvirus may provide visible evidence of the extent of its adaptation to that host, because it reflects the extent to which virus-encoded proteins inhibit mediators of apoptosis or acute inflammatory responses. For example, the ability of MCV to replicate quietly in the skin, unrecognized by the immune system, suggests that the virus has co-evolved with humans and their primate ancestors long enough to fashion an array of countermeasures that can effectively block all major components of innate antiviral immunity. By contrast, vaccinia virus evokes a strong innate response that leads to the rapid induction of antigen-specific immunity, and variola virus elicits such intense inflammation that the active disease course lasts for only a few weeks, ending either in elimination of the virus or death of the host. The development of an intense innate response to infection may thus be taken as evidence of cross-species transmission that has occurred too recently for the virus to have adapted to its new host.

4.1.3. Maintenance Hosts and Cross-Species Transmission

The survival of a poxvirus in nature requires both its successful replication in an individual host and its reliable transmission to other members of the host population. Chordopoxviral reservoir species therefore tend to be animals that exist in large numbers and live in close proximity to each other, ensuring the frequent transfer of virus to susceptible individuals. Examples include animals that aggregate in burrows (rodents and rabbits), in herds (sheep, cattle, and other grazing species), in flocks (chickens, turkeys, and many wild birds) and in cities (humans). This suggests that, even though some animals such as elephants and large felines have been found to be highly susceptible to cowpox virus (see below), their numbers and density may be insufficient for the agent to become established among those populations in the wild.

These considerations suggest that human activity has played a major role in the recent success of some poxviral species. By aggregating into cities, humans made possible the survival and spread of variola virus, and certain aspects of our behavior, such as a recent increase in multiple sexual contacts, have led to a higher prevalence of MCV infection. Human intervention has also generated novel virus:host combinations, such as cowpox virus infection of elephants, by bringing together geographically separated species of animals that would never have met under natural circumstances. Humans may also have supported the maintenance and spread of diseases such as goatpox, swinepox, camelpox, and fowlpox by gathering their host animals into large, dense aggregates that permit efficient virus transmission.

Information on the ability of various poxviruses to "jump species" and cause disease in animals other than their maintenance hosts has come both from observations in nature and from laboratory experiments. In some cases, the existence of a poxvirus species was first recognized when humans or animals entered an area inhabited by its reservoir host and came into contact with infected animals or contaminated materials. Cowpox virus provides the classic example of this phenomenon. The agent originally received its name from the pustular lesions it produced in occasional outbreaks in dairy cattle. The cause of the sporadic and unpredictable appearance of this disease remained unexplained until it was discovered that the virus is maintained among rodents and that cattle act as sentinels for its presence in the environment (Bennett et al., 1997). More recently, house cats have come to serve as the principal "detectors" of cowpox virus, because they may develop overwhelming illness when they acquire the agent from their rodent prey. They also act as amplifying hosts, because the development of systemic infection with numerous skin lesions facilitates the transfer of virus to humans (Bennett and Baxby, 1995; Hawranek et al., 2003).

Cross-species transmission can also occur when poxvirus-infected animals enter a new geographic area. Until recently, such movements occurred slowly, as changes in climate or topography caused host species gradually to alter their geographic range, but the advent of human activity now permits the abrupt transfer of pathogens from one part of the world to another. As mentioned, monkeypox virus unexpectedly crossed the Atlantic Ocean in summer 2003, when giant Gambian rats were imported into the United States. In this case, pet prairie dogs served as amplifying hosts by developing overwhelming infection and transferring the virus to their owners (Di Giulio and Eckburg, 2004). Humans may also introduce a poxvirus into a new region in the absence of an animal carrier, as occurred when vaccinia virus was accidentally transferred from recent vaccinees to their cattle in India and when myxoma virus was deliberately released among Australian feral rabbits.

Observations of viral host range from nature have been supplemented by laboratory studies. These have helped to confirm, for example, that variola virus has no natural host other than humans, by showing that the virus does not cause productive infection in rodents, rabbits, or other laboratory animals, and that large quantities of the agent must be introduced by aerosol or by intravenous injection to cause disease in nonhuman primates. Similarly, the strict host-range limitation of MCV has made it impossible to study the agent by cultivating it in cells of non-human origin or infecting captive primates. From a different point of view, the inability of avipoxviruses to cause disease in mammals has made them objects of interest as potential vaccine vectors.

4.1.4. Barriers to Cross-Species Transmission

Almost nothing is known about the specific factors that prevent a poxvirus from carrying out productive infection in a new host species (McFadden, 2005). The barrier evidently does not lie at the level of the cell membrane, because most poxviruses are able to infect a broad range of cells in culture. Instead, the existence of an elaborate array of virus-encoded immunomodulatory proteins indicates that these agents must be capable of blocking a variety of host responses in order to establish a focus of infection. The complete absence of a visible lesion, as occurs when variola virus is injected into rabbits, mice, and other non-primate species or when myxoma virus is inoculated into animals other than rabbits or hares, suggests that the agent is unable to prevent apoptosis or cannot block the induction of a type I interferon response (Wang et al., 2004; Johnston et al., 2005; McFadden, 2005).

By contrast, those chordopoxviruses that induce skin lesions are clearly capable of inhibiting some host responses, including apoptosis. As just described, the ability of MCV to establish a focus of infection that is virtually free of inflammation indicates that its immunomodulatory proteins effectively block innate responses, including the chemokines that would normally attract inflammatory cells to a site of viral infection. Vaccinia virus is also able to spread cell-to-cell, indicating that it can block apoptosis and perhaps type I interferon responses, but the resulting intense inflammatory response indicates that the virus is unable to block the induction of other innate antiviral mechanisms.

It is worth noting that the ability of MCV to block the innate responses of its host does not lead to widely disseminated infection, indicating that additional factors play a role in the systemic spread of viral infection. The means by which some chordopoxviruses, such as variola, camelpox, and monkeypox, are able to cause overwhelming illness in their hosts have not been characterized but may include inherent viral characteristics, such as the propensity of some agents to produce extracellular virions. Occasionally, both viral and host factors act together to increase the severity of systemic infection. Thus, defective innate responses in persons with atopic dermatitis allow vaccinia and cowpox viruses to cause rapidly progressive disseminated infection that closely resembles smallpox. It has also been postulated that a particularly aggressive, "flat" form of smallpox that occurred occasionally during the pre-eradication era may have resulted from the infection of persons with underlying atopic dermatitis (Bray and Buller, 2004).

4.2. Poxviruses That Cause Human Disease

Members of four chordopoxviral genera cause productive infection in humans, ranging from localized skin lesions to lethal disseminated disease (Table 4.3). Two members of the genus Orthopoxvirus, variola and monkeypox viruses, are the only poxviruses that cause systemic infection in immunocompetent individuals and the only ones transmitted by the respiratory route. The two known species in the genus Yatapoxvirus both cause no more than one or a few subcutaneous nodules, whereas several members of the genus Parapoxvirus produce cutaneous lesions at sites

Table 4.3. Poxviruses that are known to cause productive infection in humans

Genus	Species	Nature of illness	Mode of transmission
Orthopoxvirus	Variola	Diffuse vesiculopustular rash with severe systemic inflammatory syndrome	Saliva droplets containing virus released from oropharyngeal lesions
	Monkeypox	Similar to variola virus, but with lower case fatality rate	Same as variola
	Vaccinia	Localized skin lesion(s) in immunocompetent individuals	Vaccination or direct skin contact
	Cowpox	Same	Contact with infected animals
Yatapoxvirus	Tanapox	Same	Bite of infected arthropods
	Yaba monkey tumor virus	Same	Bite of infected arthropods
Parapoxvirus	Orf	Same	Contact with infected animals
	Pseudocowpox	Same	Contact with infected animals
	Bovine papular stomatitis	Same	Contact with infected animals
Molluscipoxvirus	Molluscum contagiosum	Same	Direct skin contact or spread via fomites

where virus penetrates the skin during direct contact with infected animals. The fourth genus, Molluscipoxvirus, contains only a single species, MCV, which evidently has become highly adapted to humans through lengthy co-evolution, as it is able to persist in the skin much longer than other poxviruses.

4.2.1. Orthopoxvirus

Members of this genus are maintained in a variety of mammals; they differ markedly in their capacity for cross-species transmission (Table 4.1). The adaptation of the orthopoxviruses to their maintenance hosts has apparently involved both the loss of some flanking-region genes from a large repertoire possessed by an early progenitor and the gradual mutation of the remainder in a manner favoring the survival of each virus in its reservoir species. The orthopoxviruses therefore share a highly conserved core of genes required for replication and virion structure but differ in the number and identity of complete open reading frames in the flanking regions that encode functional immunomodulatory proteins. Cowpox virus appears to be closest in genomic organization to an ancestral orthopoxvirus, as it possesses the largest number of intact open reading frames, many of which have been disrupted or deleted in other viruses

(Gubser et al., 2004). Interestingly, cowpox virus also has a very broad host range, whereas some other members of the Orthopoxvirus genus, such as variola and camelpox, are unable to replicate in animals other than their reservoir host and some closely related species.

4.2.1.1. Variola Virus

At the time of its eradication, variola virus was maintained only in humans. Although vaccination played a major role in the global eradication strategy, elimination of the virus was also greatly facilitated by the fact that it caused a brief infection that almost always required face-to-face contact for transmission and induced lifelong immunity in survivors. Even though shed scabs contained infectious virus, the spread of infection occurred almost exclusively by the respiratory route (Fenner et al., 1988). These characteristics placed variola in a precarious situation, because infection quickly died out in areas of low or dispersed population, such as islands or rural areas, and its continued survival ultimately depended on the existence of cities, which provided the agent with a constant supply of naïve hosts. More than any other human illness, smallpox was a true "disease of civilization" (Bray and Buller, 2004).

The requirement for large, densely aggregated human populations indicate that variola virus was originally an animal pathogen that succeeded in attaining continuous transmission among humans in the relatively recent past. Although the agent could presumably have spread to humans or their ancestors at any time in the past, sustained human-to-human spread only would have became possible some 5000 to 10,000 years ago, when the rise of cities in the ancient Near East for the first time provided sufficiently large populations to ensure a constant supply of new susceptible individuals (Fenner et al., 1988). Genetic analysis has shown that variola is most closely related to camelpox virus, which is found in the same region, suggesting that the two agents are descended from a virus maintained in an animal, such as a rodent, that has since become extinct. (Gubser and Smith, 2002).

Once variola virus had spread to humans, the high replicative fidelity of its DNA polymerase would have impaired its ability to adapt to its new host by preventing the genetic variation needed for the evolution of a more secure maintenance strategy. However, the eventual appearance of milder forms of smallpox, such as those caused by variola minor strains in Africa and alastrim in South America, can be seen as steps in this direction, in which natural selection favored the spread of viral variants that caused less severe disease, thereby permitting a higher contact rate with more opportunity for human-to-human transmission (Bray and Buller, 2004).

Although variola virus has been reported to cause systemic infection in newborn mice, it does not cause productive infection in animal species other than non-human primates (Fenner et al., 1988). On occasion, the agent was reported to produce disease in wild or tame non-human primates that came into contact with human smallpox patients. However, laboratory studies have indicated that macaques and other species are much less susceptible to infection than humans, so that large doses of virus are required to induce severe or lethal systemic disease. These animals are resistant to aerosolized virus, but intravenous inoculation can produce illness ranging from vesiculopustular skin lesions through overwhelming infection resembling the hemorrhagic variant of human smallpox (Jahrling et al., 2004).

4.2.1.2. Monkeypox Virus

With the eradication of smallpox, monkeypox became the only known poxvirus that is highly pathogenic for humans. The existence of this agent was first recognized in 1958, when it was accidentally transferred to Europe, causing an outbreak of smallpox-like disease among imported non-human primates in a laboratory in Copenhagen (Von Magnus, 1959). None of the personnel exposed to sick monkeys became ill, possibly reflecting a high level of vaccination coverage against smallpox. Despite extensive serologic surveys of captive primates from numerous sources, the origin of the virus could not be determined.

The natural reservoir of monkeypox virus was not discovered until 1970, when the elimination of smallpox from Zaire (now the Democratic Republic of Congo) revealed the continued sporadic occurrence of a smallpox-like illness among rural villagers, which was apparently acquired through contact with infected animals (Ladnyj et al., 1972). Human infections are now known to occur across a broad band of sub-Saharan Africa, principally among men and older children who hunt a variety of forest animals and in women who prepare the meat for cooking (Breman et al., 1980). Index cases apparently become infected by inhaling virus-containing material aerosolized during handling or butchering of an animal. Subsequent person-to-person spread is also believed to occur by the airborne route, in a manner similar to smallpox.

Despite field studies in the early 1980s, little is known about the identity of viral reservoirs and the mode of transmission from animals to humans. Monkeypox virus has to date been recovered from only two potential maintenance hosts: a rope squirrel and the giant Gambian rats in which it was imported into the United States. However, serologic studies suggest that a number of rodents and other species may act as maintenance hosts or be part of transmission chains (Khodakevich et al., 1986).

Detailed analysis of some 400 cases of human monkeypox in Central and West Africa, almost all of which occurred in Zaire, showed that the disease resembles the ordinary, discrete form of smallpox, characterized by the simultaneous formation of centrifugally distributed vesiculopustular skin lesions that are not sufficiently numerous to become confluent (Jezek and Fenner, 1988). Lymphadenopathy is more prominent than in smallpox. Monkeypox has a lower mortality rate than variola major and is less transmissible, as secondary cases are infrequent and chains of transmission rarely exceed four generations (Fine et al., 1988).

The monkeypox infections that occurred in the midwestern United States in 2003 were for the most part significantly milder than the disease typically reported from Central Africa, as the majority of cases were characterized by a small number of skin lesions, many of which were located at and adjacent to sites where patients had been bitten or scratched by pet prairie dogs (Di Giulio and Eckburg, 2004; Reed et al., 2004). Only a few cases of disseminated vesiculopustular disease occurred, and there was no clear evidence of human-to-human transmission. The most likely explanation of this reduced severity is that the virus was introduced in animals trapped in Ghana, where human monkeypox had never been reported, suggesting that the imported viral strain was of low virulence for humans. By contrast, the agent was highly pathogenic for prairie dogs, which served as amplifying hosts from which infection spread to humans (Guarner et al., 2004). The agent has also been found to cause rapidly lethal disease in American ground squirrels (Tesh et al., 2004). Monkeypox virus may therefore have the potential to become enzootic in wild rodents in the Western Hemisphere and other regions outside its ancestral homeland.

4.2.1.3. Vaccinia Virus

The natural host of vaccinia, the smallpox vaccine virus, has not been identified. Vaccinia was long assumed to be identical to Jenner's original cowpox virus, but genetic analysis has shown it to be a distinct species. It may actually be descended from the agent of horsepox or "grease," another zoonosis that was common in Britain in Jenner's time, but has since disappeared, possibly because the declining horse population deprived it of an adequate reservoir (Fenner et al., 1989). Although vaccinia virus can be found in nature, it exists only under circumstances consistent with accidental transfer from vaccinated humans to animals (see below).

Vaccinia virus is able to cause productive infection in a wide variety of mammals but is not highly pathogenic for any species. Deliberate inoculation of the virus into an immunocompetent human (vaccination) generally produces a single self-limited lesion, but in persons with atopic dermatitis, the virus may spread rapidly to cause a smallpox-like disease (Bray, 2003). By contrast, inadvertent vaccination of an individual with deficient cell-mediated immunity causes slowly progressive infection (Bray and Wright, 2003). A laboratory-derived mutant of vaccinia virus that arose in the course of passage among rabbits for vaccine production ("rabbitpox virus") causes rapidly overwhelming infection in that species, but it apparently does not differ from wild-type vaccinia in its virulence for other animals. The complete genomic sequence of rabbitpox virus has recently been determined, but the basis of its heightened pathogenicity for rabbits is still unknown.

The ability of vaccinia to replicate in the skin of cattle was long exploited for vaccine production. In a number of instances, this suscepti- bility to infection also permitted the accidental transfer of virus from recently vaccinated people to their dairy animals, resulting in sustained transmission among cattle and occasional transfer back to the humans tending them. In India, human vaccinia infection acquired from cattle is known as buffalopox, and a similar infection in Brazil is caused by a vac- cinia-like agent designated Cantagalo virus (Fenner and Marshall, 1957; Damaso et al., 2000; Kannangai et al., 2000). Sustained transmission has not been observed in other animal species.

4.2.1.4. Cowpox Virus

Cowpox virus has the widest geographic distribution and broadest host range of any orthopoxvirus. Initially recognized as a pathogen of dairy cattle, the agent is actually maintained in a variety of rodents found across Eurasia, from Britain to Turkmenistan (Baxby and Bennett, 1997; Bennett et al., 1997; Chantrey et al., 1999). All of these isolates are presently assigned to one species, but sequencing has revealed such marked genetic divergence between the Brighton strain, isolated in Great Britain, and the GRI-90 Russian isolate that these viruses should be con- sidered to be members of separate species (Fig. 4.1B) (Baxby et al., 1994; Gubser et al., 2004).

Bovine cowpox was sufficiently familiar to British farmers in the late 1700s to enable Edward Jenner to recognize its ability to protect milk- maids against smallpox, but it has never been a common disease. In both cattle and humans, cowpox virus usually causes only one or a few lesions at sites where it penetrates the skin. In recent years, the majority of human cowpox infections have been transmitted from domestic cats, which presumably acquire the agent by preying on wild rodents and act as amplifying hosts when they develop lethal systemic disease (Hawranek et al., 2003). Like vaccinia, cowpox virus can cause disseminated infection in persons with atopic dermatitis, and it poses a threat to individuals with cell-mediated immunodeficiency (Czerny et al., 1991).

The introduction of animals into regions where cowpox virus is maintained in rodents has shown that a wide range of species are susceptible to the agent. The virus causes fatal disseminated infection in felines, both in house cats and in cheetahs, lions, and other large felines in zoos and circuses (Baxby and Ghaboosi, 1977; Baxby et al., 1979, 1982; Pilaski, 1988). Lethal disease has also occurred in captive elephants and other animals, but such outbreaks have always "burned out" quickly when the virus could not be transmitted to new hosts (Pilaski, 1988; Meyer et al., 1999). Cowpox virus has also been introduced into colonies of rats and mice in Russia, presumably through the entry of infected animals or contaminated bedding. There is no record that the agent has ever been exported to regions outside Eurasia. As discussed above, although the virus is capable of causing self-limited epizootics among susceptible wild animals such as elephants, their populations may not be sufficiently large and dense to support sustained transmission.

4.2.1.5. Ectromelia Virus

Ectromelia, or mousepox, virus has been studied extensively in the laboratory, but almost nothing is known about its maintenance in nature (Chen et al., 2003). The virus was first discovered in 1930, when it caused an outbreak of severe, acute disease in a mouse colony in Hampstead, England. The viral species acquired its name from its propensity to enter through footpad skin, leading to intense local inflammation that frequently led to limb amputation (ectromelia) (Fenner et al., 1989). Despite extensive laboratory exposure, the virus has never caused illness in humans, and it has not been found to cause productive infection in other animal species.

Because ectromelia virus causes rapidly lethal disease in some strains of mice, whereas other strains are solidly resistant, it has been suggested that the agent's natural host is a species of mouse that undergoes limited infection (Buller et al., 1986). Studies employing inbred, transgenic, and knockout mice have been especially useful for studying the basis of susceptibility and resistance to poxviral infection and identifying viral genes critical for virulence. Some data suggest that the enhanced virulence of ectromelia virus for mice, compared with vaccinia, reflects a greater affinity of the ectromelia virus–encoded interferon-gamma receptor for the murine cytokine, but this is only one of many virus:host interactions that influence disease outcome (Mossman et al., 1995).

4.2.1.6. Camelpox Virus

Camelpox virus is found in regions of North Africa and Southwest Asia where camels are kept in large numbers as beasts of burden. No reservoir host other than these animals has been identified. The agent causes a smallpox-like illness in both bactrian and dromedary camels that is most severe in young animals (Jezek et al., 1983). Despite frequent exposure, there is no evidence that camelpox virus has ever been transmitted to humans. Vaccination with vaccinia virus has been used to protect young animals, especially valuable racing camels.

As noted, camelpox virus is most closely related to variola, suggesting that both agents are descended from an ancestral species whose host is now extinct (Gubser and Smith, 2002; Afonso et al., 2002b). Like smallpox, camelpox is a relatively brief illness that induces lifelong immunity to reinfection in survivors. Conditions essential for the continued maintenance and transmission of camelpox virus in nature therefore resemble those required for the survival of variola virus before its eradication, with large herds of camels playing the role of cities, and the movement of infected animals between herds simulating the role of human travellers in periodically reintroducing the virus to vulnerable populations. The dependence of virus survival on human activity suggests that camelpox could readily be eradicated through a program of case identification, isolation of sick animals, and ring vaccination.

4.2.1.7. Other Orthopoxviruses

A number of agents currently classified as members of the Orthopoxvirus genus have been isolated from animals in Eurasia and the Western Hemisphere (Table 4.1) (Fenner et al., 1989). The former include Uasin Gishu virus, recovered from horses in East Africa, and taterapoxvirus, isolated from West African gerbils. Orthopoxviruses recovered from raccoons, skunks, and voles in North America have not unexpectedly been found to be genetically distant from the Old World orthopoxviruses. In some cases, it is not known with certainty whether the animals from which these viruses were isolated, such as raccoons, represent the true reservoir host. None of these agents have been reported to cause disease in humans or other animals, but few or no laboratory investigations have been performed. Because poxviruses may cause innocuous infections in their reservoir species, which might easily be missed on cursory inspection, it is highly probable that the great majority of ortho-poxviruses remain unidentified.

4.2.2. Yatapoxvirus

The genus Yatapoxvirus contains two known species, tanapoxvirus and Yaba monkey tumor virus. Both cause disease in humans and non-human primates that is limited to the formation of one or a cluster of sub-cutaneous lesions. No reservoir species (other than non-human primates) has been identified, and the natural history of these agents remains obscure (Dhar et al., 2004).

Tanapoxvirus was first isolated during an outbreak of acute illness associated with extensive flooding of the Tana River in Kenya in 1957 and 1962. Most reported cases since that time have occurred in areas adjacent to rivers, suggesting that the agent is transmitted by mosqui-toes or other biting arthropods that proliferate under wet conditions (Manson-Bahr and Downie, 1973). An essentially indistinguishable virus caused similar lesions in imported macaques in the United States in the 1960s, from which infection spread to animal caretakers. When it occurs in non-human primates, tanapoxvirus infection is known as Yaba-like disease.

Persons infected with tanapoxvirus develop fever and malaise, fol-lowed by the appearance of a single subcutaneous nodule or a closely grouped cluster of such lesions. Disseminated infection has not been reported. Tanapox lesions differ in their structure and time course from those caused by vaccinia and other orthopoxviruses. Each begins as a small, itchy papule, then enlarges to form a subcutaneous nodule that reaches a diameter of 1–2 cm by the end of the second week, accompa-nied by inflammation and swelling of surrounding tissues and tender enlargement of regional lymph nodes. The nodules persist for several weeks, sometimes with ulceration of overlying skin, then gradually resolve. Person-to-person transmission may occur through direct contact.

Human tanapox has been recognized in Kenya and the Democratic Republic of Congo, and the virus presumably circulates in other countries in the region. Even though HIV infection is increasingly prevalent in this area, severe tanapoxvirus infection in immunodeficient persons has not been reported. The agent is capable of causing lesions in a variety of monkey species, but serologic tests have found no evidence of infection of wild primates outside equatorial Africa. If non-human primates are actually the reservoir of these viruses, their comparatively small popula-tions would imply that infection is able to persist for a prolonged period in those animals, possibly in a manner similar to human MCV infection. Some investigators have postulated that yatapoxviruses are maintained in wild rodents, but appropriate serologic or virologic studies have not been performed.

The other Yatapoxvirus species, Yaba monkey tumor virus (YMTV), was first recognized when rhesus macaques in a research facility in Nigeria developed subcutaneous tumors. The agent has not been linked to any naturally occurring human illness. Accidental transmission to animal caretakers has not been reported, but deliberate inoculation of the virus into volunteers resulted in the formation of subcutaneous nodules similar to those seen in macaques (Grace and Mirand, 1963).

4.2.3. Parapoxvirus

Parapoxviruses are worldwide in distribution, infecting many different species of wild and domestic hoofed animals (Buttner and Rziha, 2002; Delhon et al., 2004). Parapoxviruses have also been isolated from a few other mammalian species, such as seals, in which infection has generally been recognized when humans have become infected through direct contact with the animals. Parapoxvirus infections of humans are almost invariably an occupational disease of farmers and veterinarians, usually taking the form of lesions on the hands after direct contact with infected animals.

In contrast with cowpox virus, which affects cattle only when introduced to their living area by infected rodents, parapoxviruses are able to persist among fairly small herds of cattle, sheep, or camels. The persistence of viral transmission is aided by the prolonged survival of hardy virions in scabs shed into pastures or animal bedding. Disease outbreaks are often observed in the spring, when infection of the udders of nursing mothers leads to transfer of virus to the face and mouth of their offspring and further contact spread through the herd.

The parapoxviruses that most commonly infect humans cause similar syndromes in their animal hosts, consisting of a cluster of skin lesions that do not disseminate to the entire body or cause severe illness. Orf, the prototype agent, causes contagious pustular dermatitis, or "scabby mouth," in sheep, and the agents of bovine papular stomatitis and pseudocowpox produce similar syndromes in beef cattle and in dairy animals, respectively. Farm workers who handle sick animals may develop one or a few lesions on the hands or face. Interestingly, Jenner was able to differentiate between orthopoxvirus and parapoxvirus infection in dairy cattle, as he cautioned that pseudocowpox, which causes "milker's nodule" in milkmaids, failed to protect against smallpox.

In contrast with other members of the poxvirus family, parapox virions are ovoid, rather than brick-shaped. Parapoxviruses differ markedly from the orthopoxviruses in the A:T/G:C ratio of their DNA but share a group of core genes, and their overall genomic organization is similar. The agents show some degree of serologic cross-reactivity with the orthopoxviruses and some other agents but induce cross-protection only against other members of their genus. In contrast with other poxviruses, the parapoxviruses induce fairly short-lived immunity that permits frequent reinfection, though secondary cases tend to be milder than the initial illness.

4.2.4. Molluscipoxvirus

Since the eradication of smallpox, MCV is the only poxvirus maintained exclusively in humans (Bugert and Darai, 1997). The agent is worldwide in distribution. Sequencing has revealed the existence of four distinct subtypes, but because all of them produce a similar disease, they are considered to be members of a single species. Lengthy adaptation to humans and their primate ancestors has rendered MCV incapable of replicating in other animals, including non-human primates, and the infection therefore provides the best characterized example of the co-evolution of a poxvirus with its reservoir host.

Even though MCV has followed a unique evolutionary path, natural selection has resulted in its adoption of a survival strategy similar to that of the orthopoxviruses, based on the acquisition of a large collection of host genes encoding a variety of immunomodulatory proteins (Moss et al., 2000). These countermeasures are highly effective in concealing molluscum lesions from the immune system, permitting them to shed virus into the environment for as long as 1–2 years. MCV can therefore be maintained among relatively small groups of humans, giving reason to believe that it infected our remote primate ancestors.

Molluscum lesions occur most often at sites in the skin where humans come into direct contact with each other or with contaminated fomites. In children, they are seen most commonly on the face and limbs, whereas in adults, sexual transmission leads to their occurrence in the anogenital area. Lesions tend to develop in crops, either because of multiple simultaneous inoculations or because scratching leads to local mechanical spread of virus. Consistent with the transmission of virus through direct inoculation, molluscum lesions develop within the epidermis and do not penetrate the dermis until trauma or bacterial superinfection disrupts the dermal–epidermal junction. Histologically, they are characterized by a central core of virus-infected cells surrounded by a volcano-shaped mass of proliferating keratinocytes. Because MCV does not encode a homolog of epidermal growth factor, some other virus-encoded product apparently stimulates these cells to enter the growth cycle. Each focus of infection may enlarge slowly for weeks or months without eliciting an inflammatory response, until trauma or bacterial superinfection exposes viral antigens to the immune system, often resulting in the simultaneous elimination of all existing lesions.

Molluscum contagiosum demonstrates the relative role of innate and adaptive immune responses in the control of poxviral infection. In persons with atopic dermatitis, defective innate responses may permit the spread of infection over a considerable area, but dissemination is eventually reined in by the development of antigen-specific immunity. The virus is a much more serious problem for persons with defective cell-mediated immunity, who may develop relentlessly progressive infection that eventually covers large areas of skin, particularly on the face and in the anogenital region. Vaccination with vaccinia virus does not provide cross-protection, but the DNA polymerase inhibitor cidofovir has been used successfully to treat MCV infection in both immunocompetent and immunodeficient individuals (Smith and Skelton, 2002).

4.3. Genera that have not Caused Human Disease

4.3.1. Leporipoxvirus

Leporipoxviruses are maintained in rabbits, hares, and squirrels, principally in species native to the Western Hemisphere (Kerr and Best, 1998). The members of this genus provide a vivid example of the potential of cross-species transmission to cause severe disease and to result in rapid co-evolution of virus and host.

As has often been the case with poxviruses, the existence of the leporipoxviruses was first recognized when poxvirus-naïve animals were transported from one geographic region to another, bringing them into contact with a reservoir host. In this instance, European rabbits (*Oryctolagus cuniculus*) brought to a research laboratory in Brazil in 1896 unexpectedly developed a rapidly fatal illness, characterized by the formation of multiple subcutaneous nodules (myxomatosis). The source of infection was found to be a native rabbit species (the tapeti, *Sylvilagus brasiliensis*), which develops a milder, localized form of the same illness. The recovered virus, now designated myxoma, was one of the first animal pathogens to be identified as a "filterable agent." The dramatic difference in virulence of this virus for two geographically separated species of rabbits demonstrates how prolonged co-evolution of an animal and its attendant poxvirus can lead to remarkably tight host restriction. Recent studies indicate that the narrow host range of myxoma virus is determined at least in part by its ability to suppress the type I interferon response in different animal species (Wang et al., 2004; McFadden, 2005).

Myxoma virus is maintained in wild rabbits in Brazil and other regions of South and Central America. Mosquitoes and other biting arthropods play a major role in spreading the virus, but transmission may also occur through direct contact between animals. The introduction of rabbit farming into California revealed the existence of another highly virulent leporipoxvirus species carried by local brush rabbits (*Sylvilagus bachmani*). Other viruses found in eastern North America are much less virulent for European rabbits and can be employed as natural vaccines.

As early as 1918, it was suggested that myxoma virus could be used as a pest-control agent in regions where the absence of natural predators had allowed imported rabbits to multiply without limit and become a major hindrance to agriculture. Such "biological warfare" was put to the test in 1950, when virus imported from Brazil was released among feral European rabbits in Australia (Best and Kerr, 2000; Saint et al., 2001). The agent spread like wildfire, infecting millions of animals within the first year, with a mortality rate exceeding 99%. However, major evolutionary changes in both host and pathogen soon took place as transmission continued over succeeding decades. Genetic diversity in the immense rabbit population was sufficient to favor the survival of the small percentage of naturally resistant animals, leading within a few years to a measurably lower case fatality rate. Natural selection also initially favored the emergence of less virulent strains of virus that caused more prolonged disease, thereby providing greater opportunity for animal-to-animal spread. However, the increasing resistance of the rabbit population reversed this process, so that circulating strains of myxoma are now more virulent for laboratory rabbits than the originally introduced virus. One-half century after its deliberate release, the transmission of myxoma virus among feral Australian rabbits continues to provide a laboratory of evolution in action.

4.3.2. Capripoxvirus

This genus consists of three closely related species that cause severe disease in sheep, goats, and cattle. Sheeppox and goatpox virus are found across a broad region extending from India across southern Asia to North Africa, and lumpy skin disease virus causes illness in cattle in the eastern half of Africa, in a band extending to the southern tip of the continent. Some strains of sheeppox and goatpox virus cause disease in both species, whereas others are more host-specific. The three agents cross-react serologically and induce resistance to each other in animals but can be distinguished by sequencing (Tulman et al., 2001, 2002, 2004).

Outbreaks of sheeppox and goatpox are associated with airborne dissemination of virus, causing the rapid spread of infection and high mortality. The disease is most severe in young animals. Initial signs include nasal discharge, conjunctivitis, swelling about the eyes, increased respiratory rate, and fever. Multiple subcutaneous nodules appear a few days later, in a distribution consistent with blood-borne dissemination, and persist for several weeks before forming scabs and resolving. As in human smallpox, lesions in the squamous epithelial lining of the mouth and upper pharynx ulcerate and release virus into saliva, which becomes the vehicle of respiratory transmission. Infection is also spread through shedding of scabs into bedding or paddocks and through mechanical transmission by biting arthopods.

No reservoir host of sheeppox or goatpox has been identified. As in the case of camelpox, human activity appears to have contributed to the ongoing transmission of the capripoxviruses by providing these agents with large herds of animals and with frequent opportunities for infected animals to be introduced into naïve populations through trade. The ability of these agents to persist among herds of sheep or goats is also aided by the hardiness of the virions, which remain infectious for months in contaminated pasturage or bedding.

Lumpy skin disease virus causes a febrile illness in cattle characterized by multiple cutaneous lesions, but in contrast with goatpox and sheeppox, infection does not involve the respiratory tract. The agent is spread principally by biting arthropods. Lumpy skin disease was first recognized when it affected European species of cattle introduced into Zambia in the late 1920s. It has since spread progressively northward, presumably through the movement of infected animals, eventually reaching Egypt and Israel. The virus also infects native species, such as Cape buffalo, which may be its original maintenance host. Lumpy skin disease may thus be a "man-made" poxviral disease that began with the transfer of virus from native to introduced cattle species and has been aided in its persistence by modern farming methods.

4.3.3. Suipoxvirus

This genus has only one species, the agent of swinepox (De Boer, 1975; Afonso et al., 2002a). The disease occurs in pig herds throughout the world but is found predominantly in impoverished regions with poor animal hygiene. Infection presumably also occurs in wild swine species. Swinepox virus is transmitted among pigs by lice and other biting arthropods. Individual skin lesions mature from papule to vesicle to pustule over the course of about a week. Multiple inoculations may result in the formation of a large number of lesions, with systemic illness and fever, but true disseminated infection does not occur. Swinepox does not involve the respiratory tract and is never fatal. Natural transmission of the virus to other species has not been described, and experimental inoculation has not caused disease in laboratory animals.

4.3.4. Avipoxvirus

The evolutionary radiation of birds into multiple genera and a vast number of species has been accompanied by the differentiation of the poxviruses that infect them (Tripathy and Reed, 2003). Individual named species have now been recovered from more than 60 species of wild and domestic birds. All of them are currently classified in a single genus, Avipoxvirus, but a number of studies have revealed marked genetic differences among these agents that may lead to a revised classification system.

Naturally occurring cross-species transmission of avipoxviruses among wild and domestic birds has not been well characterized, but the experimental inoculation of viruses into various species leads to a variety of outcomes, ranging from complete absence of visible infection to rapidly lethal disease. Individual isolates also differ markedly in their ability to induce resistance against other avipoxviruses, providing evidence of distant evolutionary relationships that may support the division of these agents into separate genera. Sequencing has provided additional evidence of marked heterogeneity among the avipoxviruses, as the genome of canarypoxvirus is some 25% longer than that of the prototype species, fowlpox virus, and contains 39 more open reading frames (Afonso et al., 2000; Tulman et al., 2004).

Prolonged adaptation has rendered the avipoxviruses incapable of causing productive infection in animals other than birds, possibly because they are unable to prevent cells of other species from undergoing apoptosis. These agents are therefore of principal concern as threats to agriculture, with fowlpox of chickens and turkeys imposing the greatest economic burden. Although fowlpox shares certain features with poxviral infections of mammals, true systemic viral dissemination does not occur. In its most common form, virus inoculation by biting arthropods results in multiple cutaneous lesions that may interfere with feeding and growth if tissues around the eyes or beak become secondarily infected. A more severe form of illness involves the mucosa of the upper respiratory tract, where infection may result in the formation of a diphtheritic pseudomembrane that blocks breathing. The occurrence of this form of disease may lead to the rapid spread of infection through a flock by means of contaminated saliva droplets.

4.4. Newly Identified Poxviral Genera

Viruses now classified as deerpox have been isolated from North American mule deer, in which they cause mucocutaneous lesions. The prevalence of infection among these animals is not known, nor has it been determined whether they are actually the viral reservoir host. Sequencing has shown deerpoxvirus to be sufficiently divergent from other chordopoxviruses to warrant its designation as a new genus (Fig. 4.1A) (Afonso et al., 2005). Its potential for spread to humans or other animal species is not known.

4.5. Conclusion

The chordopoxviruses have co-evolved with vertebrate animals over hundreds of millions of years, and many have become so closely adapted to their reservoir hosts that they are unable to cause disease in other species. Extensive experience of exposure to sick animals has shown that the leporipox-, capripox-, suipox-, and avipoxviruses are unable to cause productive infection in humans. However, many members of these genera have the potential to cause disease in domestic animals if accidentally or deliberately introduced to new geographic areas. Some members of two other genera, the parapox- and yatapoxviruses, can cause illness in humans, but evidence to date shows that they produce only localized, self-limited lesions in immunocompetent individuals.

The major threat of cross-species transmission of the known poxviruses to humans resides with the Orthopoxvirus genus, which includes monkeypox virus, the only agent that causes severe disease in immunocompetent persons. Even though it was first identified nearly 50 years ago, this pathogen remains poorly characterized, and research is urgently needed to identify its natural reservoir species and other animals in which it is capable of productive infection and to determine routes of animal-to-human and human-to-human transmission. In addition to their direct threat to humans, a particular concern with monkeypox and some other orthopoxviruses is the possibility that an agent could become established in new maintenance hosts if transferred to a new region, as might occur if monkeypox virus were introduced to prairie dogs or ground squirrels in North America or to rodent species in other areas. Cowpox virus may also be capable of spreading outside its current geographic range to become enzootic in other rodents, from which it could potentially spread to a variety of large animal species.

In addition to the threat of these known poxviruses, the possibility exists that as yet unidentified members of the poxvirus family may be capable of spreading from their unknown reservoir hosts to cause disease in humans or domestic animals. As noted, several Old and New World orthopoxviruses isolated in recent decades remain poorly characterized in terms of their potential for cross-species transmission. Although the absence of a demonstrated ability to spread to humans may indicate a high degree of adaptation of these agents to their reservoir hosts, it could also simply reflect infrequent opportunities for transmission. Fortunately, the high conservation of core genes across the genus, including those encoding virion structural proteins, means that vaccinia-derived vaccines should provide protection against these and other orthopoxviruses.

The remarkable degree of evolutionary conservation of the poxviral replication strategy also provides some assurance that antiviral compounds that target essential enzymatic mechanisms will prove effective against all poxviruses, both known and unknown. As cited above, for example, the cytidine analogue cidofovir inhibits the DNA polymerase of members of the orthopox-, parapox-, and molluscipoxvirus genera and is probably active against other poxviruses as well. To ensure that drugs will be available to defend against even highly virulent agents, additional licensed medications that inhibit different steps in the replication pathway may be needed as an "insurance policy" against future cross-species transmission of poxviruses.

References

Afonso, C. L., Delhon, G., Tulman, E. R., Lu, Z., Zsak, A., Becerra, V. M., Zsak, L., Kutish, G. F., and Rock, D. L. (2005). Genome of deerpox virus. *J Virol 79*, 966–77.

Afonso, C. L., Tulman, E. R., Lu, Z., Zsak, L., Kutish, G. F., and Rock, D. L. (2000). The genome of fowlpox virus. *J Virol 74*, 3815–31.

Afonso, C. L., Tulman, E. R., Lu, Z., Zsak, L., Osorio, F. A., Balinsky, C., Kutish, G. F., and Rock, D. L. (2002a). The genome of swinepox virus. *J Virol 76*, 783–90.

Afonso, C. L., Tulman, E. R., Lu, Z., Zsak, L., Sandybaev, N. T., Kerembekova, U. Z., Zaitsev, V. L., Kutish, G. F., and Rock, D. L. (2002b). The genome of camelpox virus. *Virology 295*, 1–9.

Baxby, D., Ashton, D. G., Jones, D., Thomsett, L. R., and Denham, E. M. (1979). Cowpox virus infection in unusual hosts. *Vet Rec 104*, 175.

Baxby, D., Ashton, D. G., Jones, D. M., and Thomsett, L. R. (1982). An outbreak of cowpox in captive cheetahs: virological and epidemiological studies. *J Hyg (Lond) 89*, 365–72.

Baxby, D., and Bennett, M. (1997). Cowpox: a re–evaluation of the risks of human cowpox based on new epidemiological information. *Arch Virol Suppl 13*, 1–12.

Baxby, D., Bennett, M., and Getty, B. (1994). Human cowpox 1969-93: a review based on 54 cases. *Br J Dermatol 131*, 598–607.

Baxby, D., and Ghaboosi, B. (1977). Laboratory characteristics of poxviruses isolated from captive elephants in Germany. *J Gen Virol 37*, 407–14.

Bennett, M., Crouch, A. J., Begon, M., Duffy, B., Feore, S., Gaskell, R. M., Kelly, D. F., McCracken, C. M., Vicary, L., and Baxby, D. (1997). Cowpox in British voles and mice. *J Comp Pathol 116*, 35–44.

Best, S. M., and Kerr, P. J. (2000). Coevolution of host and virus: the pathogenesis of virulent and attenuated strains of myxoma virus in resistant and susceptible European rabbits. *Virology 267*, 36–48.

Bray, M. (2003). Pathogenesis and potential antiviral therapy of complications of smallpox vaccination. *Antiviral Res 58*, 101–14.

Bray, M., and Buller, M. (2004). Looking back at smallpox. *Clin Infect Dis 38*, 882–9.

Bray, M., and Wright, M. E. (2003). Progressive vaccinia. *Clin Infect Dis 36*, 766–74.

Breman, J. G., Kalisa, R., Steniowski, M. V., Zanotto, E., Gromyko, A. I., and Arita, I. (1980). Human monkeypox, 1970-79. *Bull World Health Organ 58*, 165–82.

Bugert, J. J., and Darai, G. (1997). Recent advances in molluscum contagiosum virus research. *Arch Virol Suppl 13*, 35–47.

Bugert, J. J., and Darai, G. (2000). Poxvirus homologues of cellular genes. *Virus Genes 21*, 111–33.

Buller, R. M., Potter, M., and Wallace, G. D. (1986). Variable resistance to ectromelia (mousepox) virus among genera of Mus. *Curr Top Microbiol Immunol 127*, 319–22.

Buttner, M., and Rziha, H. J. (2002). Parapoxviruses: from the lesion to the viral genome. *J Vet Med B Infect Dis Vet Public Health 49*, 7–16.

Chantrey, J., Meyer, H., Baxby, D., Begon, M., Bown, K. J., Hazel, S. M., Jones, T., Montgomery, W. I., and Bennett, M. (1999). Cowpox: reservoir hosts and geographic range. *Epidemiol Infect 122*, 455–60.

Chen, N., Danila, M. I., Feng, Z., Buller, R. M., Wang, C., Han, X., Lefkowitz, E. J., and Upton, C. (2003). The genomic sequence of ectromelia virus, the causative agent of mousepox. *Virology 317*, 165–86.

Czerny, C. P., Eis–Hubinger, A. M., Mayr, A., Schneweis, K. E., and Pfeiff, B. (1991). Animal poxviruses transmitted from cat to man: current event with lethal end. *Zentralbl Veterinarmed B 38*, 421–31.

Damaso, C. R., Esposito, J. J., Condit, R. C., and Moussatche, N. (2000). An emergent poxvirus from humans and cattle in Rio de Janeiro State: Cantagalo virus may derive from Brazilian smallpox vaccine. *Virology 277*, 439–49.

De Boer, G. F. (1975). Swinepox. Virus isolation, experimental infections and the differentiation from vaccinia virus infections. *Arch Virol 49*, 141–50.

Delhon, G., Tulman, E. R., Afonso, C. L., Lu, Z., de la Concha-Bermejillo, A., Lehmkuhl, H. D., Piccone, M. E., Kutish, G. F., and Rock, D. L. (2004). Genomes of the parapoxviruses ORF virus and bovine papular stomatitis virus. *J Virol 78*, 168–77.

Dhar, A. D., Werchniak, A. E., Li, Y., Brennick, J. B., Goldsmith, C. S., Kline, R., Damon, I., and Klaus, S. N. (2004). Tanapox infection in a college student. *N Engl J Med 350*, 361–6.

Di Giulio, D. B., and Eckburg, P. B. (2004). Human monkeypox. *Lancet Infect Dis 4*, 15–25.

Engler, R. J., Kenner, J., and Leung, D. Y. (2002). Smallpox vaccination: Risk considerations for patients with atopic dermatitis. *J Allergy Clin Immunol 110*, 357–65.

Fenner, F., Henderson, D.A., Arita, I., Jezek, Z., Ladnyi, I.D. (1988). *Smallpox and Its Eradication*. World Health Organization, Geneva, Switzerland.

Fenner, F., and Marshall, I. D. (1957). A comparison of the virulence for European rabbits (Oryctolagus cuniculus) of strains of myxoma virus recovered in the field in Australia, Europe and America. *J Hyg (Lond) 55*, 149–91.

Fenner, F., Wittek, R., Dumbell, K. (1989). *The Orthopoxviruses*. Academic Press, San Diego, CA.

Fine, P. E., Jezek, Z., Grab, B., and Dixon, H. (1988). The transmission potential of monkeypox virus in human populations. *Int J Epidemiol 17*(3), 643–50.

Grace, J. T., Mirand, E.A. (1963). Human susceptibility to a simian tumor virus. *Ann N Y Acad Sci*, 1123–1128.

Guarner, J., Johnson, B. J., Paddock, C. D., Shieh, W. J., Goldsmith, C. S., Reynolds, M. G., Damon, I. K., Regnery, R. L., and Zaki, S. R. (2004). Monkeypox transmission and pathogenesis in prairie dogs. *Emerg Infect Dis 10*, 426–31.

Gubser, C., Hue, S., Kellam, P., and Smith, G. L. (2004). Poxvirus genomes: a phylogenetic analysis. *J Gen Virol 85*, 105–17.

Gubser, C., and Smith, G. L. (2002). The sequence of camelpox virus shows it is most closely related to variola virus, the cause of smallpox. *J Gen Virol 83*, 855–72.

Harrison, S. C., Alberts, B., Ehrenfeld, E., Enquist, L., Fineberg, H., McKnight, S. L., Moss, B., O'Donnell, M., Ploegh, H., Schmid, S. L., Walter, K. P., and Theriot, J. (2004). Discovery of antivirals against smallpox. *Proc Natl Acad Sci U S A 101*, 11178–92.

Hawranek, T., Tritscher, M., Muss, W. H., Jecel, J., Nowotny, N., Kolodziejek, J., Emberger, M., Schaeppi, H., and Hintner, H. (2003). Feline orthopoxvirus infection transmitted from cat to human. *J Am Acad Dermatol 49*, 513–8.

Howell, M. D., Jones, J. F., Kisich, K. O., Streib, J. E., Gallo, R. L., and Leung, D. Y. (2004). Selective killing of vaccinia virus by LL-37: implications for eczema vaccinatum. *J Immunol 172*, 1763–7.

Iyer, L. M., Aravind, L., and Koonin, E. V. (2001). Common origin of four diverse families of large eukaryotic DNA viruses. *J Virol 75*, 11720–34.

Jahrling, P. B., Hensley, L. E., Martinez, M. J., Leduc, J. W., Rubins, K. H., Relman, D. A., and Huggins, J. W. (2004). Exploring the potential of variola virus infection of cynomolgus macaques as a model for human smallpox. *Proc Natl Acad Sci U S A 101*, 15196–200.

Jezek, Z., Fenner, F. (1988). Human monkeypox. *Monogr Virol 17*, 1–140.

Jezek, Z., Kriz, B., and Rothbauer, V. (1983). Camelpox and its risk to the human population. *J Hyg Epidemiol Microbiol Immunol 27*, 29–42.

Johnston, J. B., Nazarian, S. H., Natale, R., and McFadden, G. (2005). Myxoma virus infection of primary human fibroblasts varies with cellular age and is regulated by host interferon responses. *Virology 332*, 235–48.

Kannangai, R., Finny, G. J., John, T. J., Sridharan, G., and Gopal, R. (2000). Vaccinia reactive antibodies in a south Indian population. *J Med Virol 62*, 293–7.

Kerr, P. J., and Best, S. M. (1998). Myxoma virus in rabbits. *Rev Sci Tech 17*, 256–68.

Khodakevich, L., Jezek, Z., and Kinzanzka, K. (1986). Isolation of monkeypox virus from wild squirrel infected in nature. *Lancet 1*, 98–9.

Ladnyj, I. D., Ziegler, P., and Kima, E. (1972). A human infection caused by monkeypox virus in Basankusu Territory, Democratic Republic of the Congo. *Bull World Health Organ 46*, 593–7.

Manson-Bahr, P. E., and Downie, A. W. (1973). Persistence of tanapox in Tana River valley. *Br Med J 2*, 151–3.

McFadden, G. (2005). Poxvirus tropism. *Nat Rev Microbiol 3*, 201–13.

McFadden, G., and Murphy, P. M. (2000). Host-related immunomodulators encoded by poxviruses and herpesviruses. *Curr Opin Microbiol 3*, 371–8.

McLysaght, A., Baldi, P. F., and Gaut, B. S. (2003). Extensive gene gain associated with adaptive evolution of poxviruses. *Proc Natl Acad Sci USA 100*, 15655–60.

Meyer, H., Schay, C., Mahnel, H., and Pfeffer, M. (1999). Characterization of orthopoxviruses isolated from man and animals in Germany. *Arch Virol 144*, 491–501.

Moss, B., Shisler, J. L., Xiang, Y., and Senkevich, T. G. (2000). Immune-defense molecules of molluscum contagiosum virus, a human poxvirus. *Trends Microbiol 8*, 473–7.

Mossman, K., Upton, C., Buller, R. M., and McFadden, G. (1995). Species specificity of ectromelia virus and vaccinia virus interferon-gamma binding proteins. *Virology 208*, 762–9.

Neyts, J., and Clercq, E. D. (2003). Therapy and short-term prophylaxis of poxvirus infections: historical background and perspectives. *Antiviral Res 57*, 25–33.

Pilaski, J., Rosen-Wolff, A. (1988). Poxvirus infection in zoo-kept mammals. In: *Virus Diseases in Laboratory and Captive Animals* (G. Darai, Ed.). Nijhoff Publishers, Boston, MA 83–100.

Reed, K. D., Melski, J. W., Graham, M. B., Regnery, R. L., Sotir, M. J., Wegner, M. V., Kazmierczak, J. J., Stratman, E. J., Li, Y., Fairley, J. A., Swain, G. R., Olson, V. A., Sargent, E. K., Kehl, S. C., Frace, M. A., Kline, R., Foldy, S. L., Davis, J. P., and Damon, I. K. (2004). The detection of monkeypox in humans in the Western Hemisphere. *N Engl J Med 350*, 342–50.

Saint, K. M., French, N., and Kerr, P. (2001). Genetic variation in Australian isolates of myxoma virus: an evolutionary and epidemiological study. *Arch Virol 146*, 1105–23.

Smee, D. F., Sidwell, R. W., Kefauver, D., Bray, M., and Huggins, J. W. (2002). Characterization of wild-type and cidofovir-resistant strains of camelpox, cowpox, monkeypox, and vaccinia viruses. *Antimicrob Agents Chemother 46*, 1329–35.

Smith, K. J., and Skelton, H. (2002). Molluscum contagiosum: recent advances in pathogenic mechanisms, and new therapies. *Am J Clin Dermatol 3*, 535–45.

Tesh, R. B., Watts, D. M., Sbrana, E., Siirin, M., Popov, V. L., and Xiao, S. Y. (2004). Experimental infection of ground squirrels (Spermophilus tridecemlineatus) with monkeypox virus. *Emerg Infect Dis 10*, 1563–7.

Tripathy, D. N., Reed, W.M. (2003). Pox. In: *Diseases of Poultry* (Y. M. Saif, et al., Eds.), pp. 253–265. Iowa State Press, Ames, IA.

Tulman, E. R., Afonso, C. L., Lu, Z., Zsak, L., Kutish, G. F., and Rock, D. L. (2001). Genome of lumpy skin disease virus. *J Virol 75*, 7122–30.

Tulman, E. R., Afonso, C. L., Lu, Z., Zsak, L., Kutish, G. F., and Rock, D. L. (2004). The genome of canarypox virus. *J Virol 78*, 353–66.

Tulman, E. R., Afonso, C. L., Lu, Z., Zsak, L., Sur, J. H., Sandybaev, N. T., Kerembekova, U. Z., Zaitsev, V. L., Kutish, G. F., and Rock, D. L. (2002). The genomes of sheeppox and goatpox viruses. *J Virol 76*, 6054–61.

Turner, P. C., and Moyer, R. W. (2002). Poxvirus immune modulators: functional insights from animal models. *Virus Res 88*, 35–53.

Von Magnus, P., Anderson, E., Peterson, K., Birch-Anderson, A. (1959). A pox-like disease in cynomolgus monkeys. *Acta Pathol Microbiol Scand 46*, 156–176.

Wang, F., Ma, Y., Barrett, J. W., Gao, X., Loh, J., Barton, E., Virgin, H. W., and McFadden, G. (2004). Disruption of Erk-dependent type I interferon induction breaks the myxoma virus species barrier. *Nat Immunol 5*, 1266–74.

Section II: Newly Recognized Human Viruses

5. The Severe Acute Respiratory Syndrome

Kwok-Yung Yuen, Samson S.Y. Wong, and J.S. Malik Peiris

5.1. Introduction

Severe acute respiratory syndrome (SARS) was the first major pandemic of the new millennium. It had dramatic impact on the health care systems, economies, and societies of countries directly affected. Since its emergence in 2002–2003, much has been learned about the disease and the causative agent, and this chapter summarizes the current understanding of the SARS coronavirus and the disease it causes.

5.2. Sequence of Events

In the past century, Southern China has been the epicenter for emergence of some notable infectious diseases. The Hong Kong Special Administrative Region (HKSAR), being part of southern China, which has enjoyed a relatively more advanced public health infrastructure and international connectivity, often became the first place where such emerging infectious diseases were discovered and from where they disseminated globally. The first such example occurred in 1894 when an outbreak of plague started in Canton (now the Guangdong Province) of China. A similar outbreak, this time an acute community-acquired atypical pneumonia syndrome, occurred in the Guangdong Province in late 2002. Retrospective investigations showed that severe cases of atypical pneumonia had been recorded in five cities around Guangzhou over a period of 2 months. The index case was reported on 16 November 2002 in Foshan, a city 24 km away from Guangzhou. The second case appeared in December 2002 when a chef from Heyuan who worked in a restaurant in Shenzhen was affected. He had an occupational history of regular contact with wild-game food animals. He transmitted the disease to his wife, two sisters, and seven hospital staff who had contact with him. From 16 November 2002 to 9 February 2003, 305 cases of atypical pneumonia were reported in mainland China with 105 of them being health care workers. The link between the outbreak in mainland China and the devastating epidemics in HKSAR and the rest of the world was a professor of nephrology from a teaching hospital in Guangzhou, China. He had contact with patients suffering from this unusual atypical pneumonia between 11 and 13 February 2003, then developed flu-like symptoms, including a fever and cough, before coming to Hong Kong. He arrived in Hong Kong on 21 February and within a day transmitted infection to 16 other people in the hotel that he stayed in. Thorough investigation of this patient failed to reveal any significant pathogens. One of the secondary cases, his brother-in-law who subsequently became infected, underwent an open lung biopsy that was pivotal in the discovery of the etiology this disease. The virus was a novel coronavirus, subsequently called the severe acute respiratory syndrome (SARS) coronavirus.

Infected contacts in the hotels unknowingly carried the disease to other hospitals in the HKSAR and to other countries and continents including Vietnam, Canada, Singapore, the Philippines, the United Kingdom, the United States, and back again to China. Dr. Carlo Urbani, a physician stationed at the World Health Organization (WHO) office in Hanoi, was the first to notify the WHO of the occurrence of this disease outside Guangdong after witnessing an explosive nosocomial outbreak in a hospital in Hanoi. The index case of this outbreak was one of those who acquired infection on 21–22 February in the hotel in Hong Kong. The WHO named this "atypical pneumonia" as severe acute respiratory syndrome (SARS). Dr Urbani's description of the disease, to which he later succumbed, alerted health authorities throughout the world and started an unprecedented collaboration of 11 research laboratories in 9 countries to identify the etiological agent responsible.

5.3. Epidemiologic Characteristics

SARS is essentially an acute community-acquired or nosocomial pneumonia that does not respond to conventional antimicrobial therapy for known pneumonia pathogens. As of mid-2003, 8096 cases with 774 deaths occurred on five continents (World Health Organization, 2003a). Interpersonal transmission has occurred in health care facilities, workplaces, homes, and public transports (World Health Organization, 2003b). From September 2003 to May 2004, three laboratory-associated outbreaks were reported (Lim et al., 2004; Orellana, 2004). The laboratory-acquired cases in Singapore and Taiwan were each limited to one affected person, whereas that in Beijing was associated with secondary and tertiary cases (World Health Organization, 2004).

SARS-coronavirus (SARS-CoV) is most likely zoonotic in origin and then transmitted to humans. The virus may have been circulating among wild game animals in the wet markets of southern China. The palm civet is now considered to be the most likely amplification host and one of the likely candidates for introduction to humans (Guan et al., 2003). A seroprevalence of about 80% was recently reported for civets in animal markets in Guangzhou (Tu et al., 2004). The initial human cases of the 2003 pandemic and those of the 2004 Guangdong outbreak were epidemiologically linked to game animals either because of occupational contact or eating (Zhong et al., 2003). The most important route of inter-personal spread appears to be direct or indirect contact of the mucosae with infectious respiratory droplets or fomites (World Health Organization, 2003b). SARS-CoV has been detected in respiratory secretions, feces, urine, and tears (Chan et al., 2004a; Loon et al., 2004). Nosocomial transmission of SARS could be facilitated by the use of nebulizers, suction, intubation, bronchoscopy, or cardiopulmonary resuscitation on SARS patients by generation of large numbers of infectious droplets (Lee et al., 2003b; Varia et al., 2003; World Health Organization 2003b; Christian et al., 2004). Almost half of the SARS cases in Hong Kong acquired the infection within health care facilities and institutions (Leung et al., 2004a). The overall attack rate among hospital workers is 1.2% and the attack rate was correlated with the number of SARS patients admitted (Lau et al., 2004c). Airborne transmission is considered uncommon given the relatively low attack rates. A unique form of airborne transmission was considered the likely explanation for a large community outbreak in a private housing estate: Negative pressure generated by exhaust fans coupled with dry U traps of sewage drains was thought to facilitate the dissemination of contaminated aerosols between toilets. It is suggested that the plume of contaminated warm air along the light well was then carried by wind to other blocks of the housing complex (Yu et al., 2004). The finding of culturable viruses in stool and the high fecal viral load shown by quantitative reverse transcriptase polymerase chain reaction (RT-PCR) (Peiris et al., 2003a) suggested the possibility of fecal-oral transmission though this has not been proved conclusively.

The incubation period is estimated to be 2 to 14 days. Epidemiologic control measures based on the World Health Organization recommended maximal incubation period of 10 days was effective in most cases to interrupt transmission, though there had been occasionally cases in which the incubation period was found to be longer (Chan et al., 2004b). The average number of secondary cases resulting from a single case is two to four (World Health Organization, 2003b). Most of the transmissions resulted from contacts with patients with overt disease rather than asymptomatic or mildly symptomatic cases. Seroprevalence appeared to be low (0%, 0.43%, 1.2%) for normal individuals and about 1% for health care workers, around 1% for asymptomatic family contacts under quarantine, and 0.19% for asymptomatic contacts overall (Lee et al., 2003a; Peiris et al., 2003a; Leung et al., 2004b; Woo et al., 2004; Zheng et al., 2004a; Chen et al., 2005). Transmission from symptomatic patients tended to occur on or after the fifth day of onset of disease, which could be explained by the rising viral load in the nasopharyngeal secretion, which peaked at around day 10. The median time for RT-PCR to convert to negative is 30 days after onset of illness and 13 days after discharge from hospital (Chu et al., 2005).

A definite seasonality of SARS could not be documented at this stage, though there have been correlations between the incidence of the disease and ambient temperature (Tan et al., 2005). There was also definite geographic clustering of cases upon retrospective analysis by the geographic information system (Lai et al., 2004).

5.4. General Virology

The family Coronaviridae consists of a group of large, enveloped, positive-sense, single-stranded RNA viruses that are of human and veterinary importance (Table 5.1). They have the largest genome of all the RNA viruses. The SARS-CoV is one of the newly described members of the genus Coronavirus (Drosten et al., 2003; Ksiazek et al., 2003; Peiris et al., 2003b). Primary viral isolation can be achieved by inoculating embryonal monkey cell lines such as Vero E6 and FRhK-4 cells. Subcultures can be made on other Vero cells, Huh-7 (a liver cancer cell line; Simmons et al., 2004) and CACO-2 (a colonic carcinoma cell line), and two pig cell lines (POEK, PS) (Hattermann et al., 2005). In contrast with other human coronaviruses, SARS-CoV can be maintained in cell culture easily and it produces obvious cytopathetic effects in Vero E6 within 48 h. SARS-CoV has a higher degree of stability in the environment as compared with other known human coronaviruses (Duan et al., 2003; World Health Organization 2003c; Rabenau et al., 2005): it survives for at least 2 to 3 days on dry surfaces at room temperature and 2 to 4 days in stool (Rabeneu et al., 2005).

Electron microscopy appearance and genome order (Fig. 5.1) of 5'-replicase-structural (spike-envelope-membrane-nucleocapsid)-polyT-3' on complete genomic sequencing are similar to other members of Coronaviridae. SARS-CoV is phylogenetically distinct from any of the three groups of known coronaviruses. Human coronaviruses 229E and NL63 belong to group 1 (Fouchier et al., 2004; van der Hoek et al., 2004); human coronavirus OC43 belongs to group 2, and group 3 consists of all

Table 5.1. Classification of coronaviruses

Order	Family	Genus	Species
Nidovirales	Arteriviridae	Arterivirus	Equine arteritis virus
			Lactate dehydrogenase–elevating virus
			Porcine respiratory and reproductive syndrome virus
			Simian hemorrhagic fever virus
	Coronaviridae	Coronavirus	
		Group 1	Canine coronavirus
			Feline coronavirus
			Human coronavirus 229E
			Human coronavirus NL63
			Porcine epidemic diarrhea virus
			(Porcine) Transmissible gastroenteritis coronavirus
		Group 2	Bovine coronavirus
			Canine respiratory coronavirus
			Human coronavirus HKU1
			Human coronavirus OC43
			Murine hepatitis virus
			Porcine hemagglutinating encephalomyelitis virus
			Puffinosis virus
			Rat coronavirus
		Group 3	Turkey coronavirus
			(Avian) Infectious bronchitis virus
		Group 4	SARS coronavirus
		Torovirus	Bovine torovirus
			Equine torovirus
			Human torovirus
			Porcine torovirus
	Roniviridae	Okavirus	Gill-associated virus
			Yellow head virus

From the Universal Virus Database of the International Committee on Taxonomy of Viruses. Available at http://www.ncbi.nlm.nih.gov/ICTVdb/Ictv/index.htm.

the avian coronaviruses. Phylogenetic analysis of the spike protein of 139 SARS-CoV isolates in the Hong Kong outbreak showed that several introductions had occurred but only one of them was associated with the major outbreak in Hong Kong and the rest of the world (Guan et al., 2004). Some of the strains found in the early stages of the outbreak were phylogenetically distinct from the major cluster and were closer to some of the Guangdong and Beijing strains. This concurred with the fact that the index patient of the Hong Kong outbreak was a Guangzhou medical doctor who had traveled to Hong Kong. Another molecular epidemiological study of a Guangdong outbreak suggested that the disease spread from Guangdong to Hong Kong and the rest of the world, and the index case

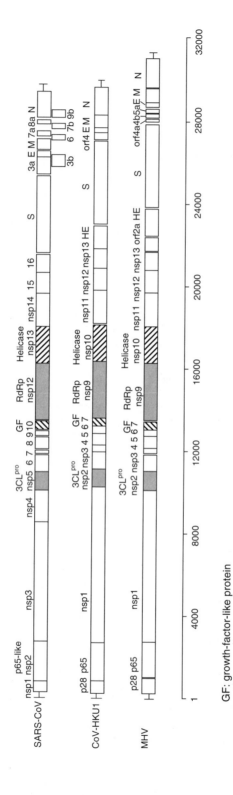

GF: growth-factor-like protein
RdRp: RNA-dependent RNA polymerase

Figure 5.1. Comparison of the gene order of selected group 2 coronavirus genomes.

was a chef who handled game animals (Zhong et al., 2003). Subsequent animal surveillance in China recovered coronavirus isolates that have a nucleotide homology of 99.8% with the SARS-CoV (Guan et al., 2003). A characteristic 29-base insertion between open reading frames (ORF) 10 to 11 (also named as ORF8a and 8b) was found in these animal isolates (Guan et al., 2003; Snijder et al., 2003). This 29-nucleotide segment was deleted after or before crossing the species barrier to humans. The biological effect of this deletion remains elusive. A number of SARS-CoV in the later stages of the epidemic showed larger deletions around this site (The Chinese SARS Molecular Epidemiology Consortium, 2004). Two independent molecular epidemiological studies comparing the complete genome of 12 and 63 virus isolates also found evidence of a strong positive selection at the beginning of the epidemic that is followed by a purifying selection, as indicated by the amino acid substitution rate at the spike, Orf3a, and nsp3 (The Chinese SARS Molecular Epidemiology Consortium, 2004; Yeh et al., 2004; Song et al., 2005). Both studies suggested that molecular adaptation of the virus had occurred after interspecies transmission from animals to humans. In the small outbreak of Guangzhou in 2004, all four human isolates belonged to a separate sublineage with the concurrent animal, predominantly civet cat, isolates that are distinct from the human pandemic or animal virus of the 2003. Though the SARS-CoV is distinct from the three existing groups of coronaviruses, it may be closer to group 2 because 19 out of 20 cysteines found in the S1 domain of the spike protein are spatially conserved when compared with the group 2 consensus sequence, whereas only 5 cysteine residues are conserved when compared with that of the groups 1 and 3 (Eickmann et al., 2003; Snijder et al., 2003). Because coronaviruses are believed to have co-evolved with their animal hosts, it was possible that rats, mice, and cattle harboring group 2 coronaviruses are more likely to be the animal host for SARS-CoV than cats, which harbor group 1 coronavirus. However when a comparison of the phylogenetic trees for 11 known host-species and nucleocapsid sequences of 36 coronaviruses was done using an interference approach with sliding window analysis, there is statistical incongruence that indicates multiple host-species shifts between the coronaviruses of many animals that are phylogenetically distant (Rest and Mindell, 2003). Thus, even if the civet cats or other related mammals are the true animal reservoir rather than mice and rats, it would not be too big a surprise. Moreover, the civet cats and other related mammals had at least served as a major amplification mechanism in the markets of southern China irrespective of the original animal reservoir. The control of these animals and the markets plays a pivotal role in the epidemiological control of SARS. Genomic evidence of another animal-to-human interspecies transmission events was demonstrated in a small outbreak of four cases in early 2004 in Guangzhou (Song et al., 2005).

A metalloprotease angiotensin-converting enzyme 2 (ACE2) from Vero E6 cells was found to bind the S1 domain of the spike protein of the SARS-CoV (Li et al., 2003c). The 293T cells transfected with ACE2 can form multinucleated syncytia with cells expressing the spike. ACE2 expression is detected by immunohistochemical staining on enterocytes, pneumocytes, vascular endothelial and smooth muscle cells. (Leung et al., 2003; Hamming et al., 2004). This is compatible with the clinical and histopathological manifestations of SARS, which include diffuse alveolar damage, colonic mucosal presence of abundant viral particles in a patient with diarrhea, and pulmonary vasculitis and thrombosis. The lack of virus infection in some cell lines that express ACE2 has led to a rush for finding coreceptors for cell entry (To and Lo, 2004a). Recently, a C-type lectin called L-SIGN was shown to be an alternative receptor for binding and cell entry (Jeffers et al., 2004), although it is not clear whether this is a functional receptor for the virus that can lead to productive virus replication. Murine ACE2 binds less efficiently with the S1 domain of SARS-CoV, and even less well with rat ACE2, which suggests that efficient replication in the mouse or rat is limited by their ACE2 type (Greenough et al., 2005).

Pseudotyped retroviral vector carrying the S, M, or E proteins revealed that the S protein is both necessary and sufficient for virus attachment on susceptible cells (Simmons et al., 2004; Wang et al., 2004a). Virus entry occurred via a pH-dependent receptor-mediated endocytic pathway (Yang et al., 2004). Pseudotyped virus carrying the S protein binds to DC-SIGN on dendritic cells, without causing cell death or replication, but this dendritic cell may serve as a conduit for infection of susceptible host cells as in the case of human immunodeficiency virus (HIV) infection. The fragment of S1-containing amino acids 270 to 510 of the S1 domain was localized to be the minimal receptor-binding region found by truncation and binding assays (Babcock et al., 2004).

The helicase and 3CL proteinase were cloned and characterized (Anand et al., 2003; Chou et al., 2003; Tanner et al., 2003; Yang et al., 2003).The E (envelope) protein was found to form cation-selective ion channel in planar lipid bilayer (Wilson et al., 2004). A molecular model of the RNA-dependent RNA polymerase has also been published (Xu et al., 2003), which provides clues to the functional aspect of the enzyme and therefore may facilitate the design of new antivirals in the future. Other putative targets such as the helicase (nsp13), a putative mRNA cap-1 methyltransferase (nsp16), a manganese-dependent endoribonulcease (nsp 15) (Bhardwaj et al., 2004), and a single-stranded RNA binding protein (nsp9) are being investigated intensively by bioinformatics and crystal structure studies (Campanacci et al., 2003; von Grotthuss et al., 2003; Egloff et al., 2004). The nomenclature of these nonstructural proteins is summarized in Table 5.3. A full-length cDNA of the viral genome was shown to cause lytic infection in cell line with good viral titer and antigen expression (Yount et al., 2003). This would provide the tool to study function of many nonstructural proteins by reverse genetics.

Table 5.2. Putative genes and annotation of SARS coronavirus[*]

Open reading frames	Proteins	Function	Number of amino acids
Orf1a	nsp1	Unknown	180
	nsp2	Unknown	638
	nsp3	Papain-like cysteine protease/ adenosinediphosphate ribose phosphatase	1922
	nsp4	Unknown	500
	nsp5	3C-like cysteine protease(main)	306
	nsp6	Unknown (many transmembrane domain)	290
	nsp7	Unknown	83
	nsp8	Unknown	198
	nsp9	Single-strand RNA-binding protein	113
	nsp10	Unknown (growth factor-like domain present)	139
	nsp11	Unknown	13
Orf1b	nsp12	RNA-dependent RNA polymerase	932
	nsp13	Helicase (dNTPase and RNA 5′-triphosphatase activities)	601
	nsp14	Unknown. ?Exonuclease (homolog of ExoN)	527
	nsp15	Manganese dependent RNA endonuclease (homologue of XendoU)	346
	nsp16	?mRNA cap1 2′-O-ribose methyltransferase	298
Orf2		Spike protein	1255
Orf3a (X1/U274/Orf3)		Accessory protein associated with plasma membrane and trafficking of intracellular viral particles	274
Orf3b (Orf4)		Unknown	154
Orf4(X2)		Envelope (forms cation-selective ion channel)	76
Orf5(X3)		Membrane	221
Orf6 (X3/Orf7)		Unknown	63
Orf7a (X4/Orf8)		Unknown (antigenic protein expressed in infected cells)	122
Orf7b (Orf9)		Unknown	44
Orf8a (Orf10)		Unknown	39
Orf8b (X5/Orf11)		Unknown	84
Orf9a		Nucleocapsid	422
Orf9b (Orf13)		Unknown	98

[*]Mara et al. (2003); Rota et al. (2003); Thiel et al. (2003).

5.5. Clinical Findings

The typical manifestation of SARS in two-thirds of the cases is that of a viral pneumonia with rapid respiratory deterioration (World Health Organization, 2003b). The presenting symptoms are generally fever, chills, myalgia, malaise, and nonproductive cough (Tsang et al., 2003). Rhinorrhea and sore throat are less frequently seen. Clinical deterioration often occurs 1 week after the onset of illness and may be accompanied by watery diarrhea. Physical signs on chest examination are mild when compared with the radiographical abnormalities. The chest radiograph may show ground-glass opacities and focal consolidations, typically over the periphery and often in the subpleural regions of the lower zones. Progressive involvement of both lungs may occur, as may shifting radiographic shadows and pneumomediastinum without previous use of positive pressure ventilation.

Diarrhea is the commonest extrapulmonary manifestation (Cheng et al., 2004a), followed by hepatic dysfunction (Chau et al., 2004), dizziness that may be related to diastolic cardiac impairment (Li et al., 2003b), abnormal urinalysis, petechiae (Wu et al., 2003), myositis (Wang et al., 2003b), and epileptic fits (Lau et al., 2004a). The neuromuscular abnormalities are likely to be related to critical-illness polyneuropathy and/or myopathy (Tsai et al., 2004). The elderly patient may merely be admitted for a fall and fracture in the absence of fever or other symptoms and signs suggestive of SARS (Wong et al., 2003; Chow et al., 2004). Infections in children appear to be milder than in adults (Kwan et al., 2004), whereas pregnant women infected by SARS could pose a significant management problem and carries a high case-fatality rate, although no transmission to the neonate has been documented (Wong et al., 2004; Yudin et al., 2005). Viral replication at different sites appears to account for the various clinical and laboratory abnormalities of SARS (Hung et al., 2004; Farcas et al., 2005). Nasopharyngeal and serum viral load were associated with oxygen desaturation, mechanical ventilation, and mortality (Chu et al., 2004b); stool viral load with diarrhea; and urine viral load with abnormal urinalysis.

Peripheral lymphocytopenia is common with or without thrombocytopenia, increases in D-dimers, and activated partial thromboplastin time. Elevated hepatic parenchymal enzymes, muscle enzymes, and lactate dehydrogenase may be seen. About 20% to 30% of the patients will deteriorate and require mechanical ventilation and the overall mortality is 15%. Death is usually related to respiratory failure, concurrent sepsis, or deterioration of underlying medical illness. Age, presence of comorbidities such as cardiac problems and diabetes mellitus, increased lactate dehydrogenase level, hypouricemia (Wu et al., 2005), acute renal failure (Chu et al., 2005), more extensive pulmonary radiological involvement at presentation (Hui et al., 2004), and a high neutrophil count at the time of admission are poor prognostic indicators. Most survivors have residual ground-glass opacifications on follow-up chest x-rays probably due to fibrosis. The radiological abnormalities improve with time, but advanced age, previous intensive care unit admission, mechanical ventilation, alternative treatment, higher peak lactate dehydrogenase, and the peak radiographic involvement during treatment have a positive correlation with overall reticulation and total parenchymal involvement at 6 months (Wong et al., 2004). Restrictive lung function abnormalities attributed to residual lung fibrosis and muscle weakness is commonly seen in the convalescent phase with an incidence of at least 20% in some studies (Chan et al., 2003b; Ng et al., 2004; Ong et al., 2004). Depression and post-traumatic stress disorder are especially common in patients with affected family members and among health care workers; psychosis could be related to the use of corticosteroids and underlying predispositions (Lee et al., 2004). As a result of treatment with corticosteroids, a patient may have biochemical evidence of adrenal insufficiency after recovery. There is also a cumulative dose-related risk of osteonecrosis, ranging from 0.6% to 13% (Griffith at al., 2005).

5.6. Laboratory Diagnostics

There are no pathognomonic signs or symptoms of SARS. Etiological diagnosis and differentiation from other causes of atypical pneumonia can only be made by laboratory confirmation. A positive viral culture from the respiratory, fecal, and occasionally urine specimens, a fourfold rise of neutralizing antibody titer in the serum taken on admission and 28 days afterwards are the most definitive evidence of infection. Of these methods, real-time quantitative RT-PCR of the nasopharyngeal aspirate is most practicable in aiding clinical diagnosis and can achieve a sensitivity of 80% with good specificity if it is collected within the first 3 days of illness (Poon et al., 2003). For antibody testing, the indirect immunofluorescent antibody test is more commonly performed than the neutralizing antibody test since the former does not involve manipulation of infectious virus and therefore carries less biohazard risk. Recombinant nucleocapsid enzyme immunoassay (EIA) can be used as a rapid screening test and possesses high sensitivity as early as 5 days after onset of illness (Che, 2004). EIA against the nucleocapsid antigen of SARS-CoV may occasionally yield false-positive results with HCoV-OC43 and HCoV-229E and may require confirmation by Western blot against the

spike polypepetide of SARS-CoV (Woo et al., 2004). A new immunofluorescence assay using recombinant nucleocapsid-spike fusion protein as
antigen has been described (He et al., 2005). Viral load determination of
nasopharyngeal specimens or serum on presentation might have clinical
value as it is an important prognostic factor (Cheng et al., 2004a).

The three laboratory outbreaks of SARS have prompted the use of
pseudotype viruses for research and neutralization antibody testing.

5.7. Pathology and Immunology

Acute diffuse alveolar damage with airspace edema were the most
prominent features in patients who died before the tenth day after onset of
illness (Franks et al., 2003; Nicholls et al., 2003). Hyaline membranes,
interstitial edema, interstitial infiltrates of inflammatory cells, bronchiolar injury with loss of cilia, bronchiolar epithelial denudation, and focal
deposition of fibrin on the exposed basement membranes were other
observed features. Patients who died after the tenth day of illness exhibited a mixture of acute changes and the organizing phase of diffuse alveolar damage. There were interstitial and airspace fibroblast proliferation,
type II pneumocyte hyperplasia, and squamous metaplasia of bronchial
epithelium. The alveolar spaces contained a combination of macrophages,
desquamated pneumocytes, and multinucleated cells. Hemophagocytosis
in the alveolar exudates and thrombosis of venules were noted in some
cases. Other pulmonary complications might include secondary bacterial
bronchopneumonia and invasive aspergillosis (Wang et al., 2003a).
Systemic vasculitis involving the walls of small veins with edema, fibrinoid necrosis, and infiltration by monocytes, lymphocytes and plasma
cells were noted in one report (Ding et al., 2003).

No tissue destruction or inflammatory process in association with
viral infection were noted in other organs or tissues. Viral particles can be
detected by *in situ* hybridization in pneumocytes and enterocytes of the
small intestine (To et al., 2004b). However, inflammation, cellular apoptosis, or microvilli atrophy are not found in the intestinal mucosa to
account for the watery diarrhea. Immunohistochemical staining showed
the presence of viral proteins in pneumocytes and occasional macrophages. Necrosis or atrophy in the lymphoid tissue of lymph nodes and
white pulp of the spleen is a commonly observed extrapulmonary pathology. Flow cytometry examination of the peripheral blood at the time of
admission before the use of steroid had shown decreases in levels of dendritic cell subsets, natural killer cells, CD4+ and CD8+ T lymphocytes
and B lymphocytes (Cui et al., 2003; Li et al., 2004; Zhang et al., 2004b).
A study of three SARS patients suggested that a self-limiting or abortive

infection of peripheral blood mononuclear cells can occur as evident by the presence of the minus-RNA, the replicative intermediate of the virus during the initial week of the illness (Li et al., 2003a). Study of the cytokine profile of SARS patients showed significant elevation of the plasma chemokines interleukin (IL)-8, monocyte chemotactic protein 1 (MCP-1), and interferon-gamma-inducible protein 10 (IP-10), Th1-related cytokine interferon-gamma and IL-12, and inflammatory cytokines IL-1β and IL-6, which can induce an intense inflammatory response (Jones et al., 2004; Wong et al., 2004; Huang et al., 2005; Jiang et al., 2005). This may account for the recruitment and accumulation of alveolar macro-phages and polymorphs and the activation of Th1 cell-mediated immunity by the stimulation of natural killer and cytotoxic T lymphocytes. In con-trast, SARS-CoV appears to evade triggering an alpha and beta interferon response in human macrophages (Cheung et al., 2005). The lack of this antiviral innate immune response may permit uncontrolled viral replica-tion with progressive increase in viral load continuing into the second week of illness until the appearance of the adaptive immune response brings the virus replication under control. Moreover, comparative transcriptomal microarray analysis showed that the SARS-CoV rather than the HCoV-229E markedly upregulates genes associated with apop-tosis, inflammation, stress response, and procoagulation during the early phase of infection of a human liver cancer cell line (Huh7). Both findings help to explain the clinical severity of SARS in relation to the high viral load up to 2 weeks of illness and the intense inflammatory response as evident from the serum cytokine profile and the histopathology (Tang et al., 2005).

In general, specific serum antibody by indirect immunofluorescence or neutralization test starts to appear at around day 10, plateaus at around the second month, and is maintained for more than 12 months. IgM and IgG appeared at around the same time, but the former is not detected after 2 to 3 months. Serum testing by recombinant nucleocapsid EIA can detect antibody as early as the fifth day after the onset of symptoms.

Some studies have suggested a possible association of HLA-B*4601 with susceptibility to and severity of SARS among the Chinese population in Taiwan (Lin et al., 2003). Among the Hong Kong Chinese population, similar associations have been found with HLA-B*0703 (Ng et al., 2004).

5.8. Animal Models and Koch's Postulates

The Koch's postulates for SARS-CoV as a causative agent of SARS was fulfilled by a primate model using cynomolgus macaques (*Macaca fascicularis*), which demonstrated clinical and pathological features similar to those found in humans (Kuiken et al., 2003). On the contrary, African green monkeys (*Cercopithecus aethiops*) did not develop significant lung pathology after inoculation with the SARS-CoV (Bukreyev et al., 2004). The lack of consistency in primate animal models (rhesus, cynomolgus, and African green monkey) for experimental SARS disease was noted in a recent study (McAuliffe et al., 2004). Ferrets (*Mustela furo*) and domestic cats (*Felis domesticus*) are also susceptible to infection by SARS-CoV (Martina et al., 2003). The cats remained asymptomatic, but some of the infected ferrets died from the disease. BALB/c mice demonstrated asymptomatic infections in lungs and nasal turbinates by intranasal inoculation, in contrast with golden Syrian hamsters in which high levels of viral replication can be seen (Roberts et al., 2005). Recently, palm civets (*Paguma larvata*) were shown to be susceptible to symptomatic infection by SARS coronavirus with or without the 29-bp signature sequence (Wu et al., 2005). Experimental infection of SARS-CoV has also been demonstrated in pigs (Weingartl et al., 2004a). Because different SARS-CoV isolates were used by each of the groups, it is therefore uncertain whether one particular animal would be better than others as a model for SARS-CoV. However, the diverse range of mammalian species that are susceptible to experimental infection by SARS-CoV is a cause for concern. Indeed, our first report on animal SARS coronavirus showed that Chinese ferret badgers (*Melogale moschata*) and raccoon dogs (*Nyctereutes procyonoides*) could also be infected with SARS-CoV (Guan et al., 2003).

5.9. Clinical Management

Clinical management of SARS relies on respiratory support and intensive care because there are no randomized clinical trials on the value of potential antiviral agents. Oxygen delivery by low-flow nasal cannula rather than the high-flow facemask should be used to minimize the risk of nosocomial airborne spread. Other modes of noninvasive ventilation such as continuous positive airway pressure (CPAP) and bilevel positive airway pressure (BIPAP) should only be performed in negative-pressure isolation rooms with adequate personal protective equipment for the health care workers (Cheung et al., 2004). Broad-spectrum antimicrobial coverage for community-acquired pneumonia should be given at presentation while pending virological confirmation. Nosocomial infections are important complications after prolonged intubation, hospitalization, and the use of corticosteroids.

5.9.1. Antivirals and Immunomodulators

The association between viral loads and clinical outcome raises the possibility that effective suppression of viral replication may be beneficial. *In vitro* susceptibility testing results were conflicting, which may partly be due to the use of different assay conditions and end-point determination. There have been contradictory results on the *in vitro* activities of interferon β-1a (Cinatl et al., 2003b; Hensley et al., 2004; Tan et al., 2004) and interferon α-2b (Stroher et al., 2004; Tan et al., 2004). The antiviral effects of interferon β appeared to be mediated by mechanisms other than MxA protein (Spiegel et al., 2004). Overall, it appears that interferon β, interferon α-n1, interferon α-n3, and leukocytic interferon α do have some activity and could be considered for further studies in clinical trials (Chen et al., 2004; Spiegel et al., 2004; Zheng et al., 2004b).

Some reports noted the sensitivity to ribavirin at a concentration of 200 to 1000 mg/L is related to cellular toxicity (Tan et al., 2004), whereas another reported that the 50% cytotoxic concentration of ribavirin exceeds 1000 mg/L (Cinatl et al., 2003a). It is interesting to see that the same group reported good activity of ribavirin in other human and animal cell lines despite their initial report of the lack of activity of ribavirin in Vero cells (Morgenstern et al., 2005).

Glycyrrhizin, baicalin (Cinatl et al., 2003a), reserpine (Wu et al., 2004b), niclosamide (Wu et al., 2004a), aurintricarboxylic acid (He et al., 2004), chloroquine (Keyaerts et al., 2004), and the protease inhibitors, especially nelfinavir (Xiong et al., 2003; Yamamoto et al., 2004), were found to have antiviral acitivity against SARS-CoV. It is also interesting to find that an organic nitric oxide donor, *S*-nitro-*N*-acetylpenicillamine, also appeared to have inhibitory activity against SARS-CoV (Akerstrom et al., 2005), which provides a rationale for the use of nitric oxide inhalation as a rescue therapy for SARS (Chen et al., 2004). Good *in vitro* antiviral activities have also been observed for ACE2 analogues (Towler et al., 2004), helicase inhibitor, and nucleoside analogues screened from combinatorial chemical libraries. Synergistic activities have been seen with combinations of interferons or the above compounds with ribavirin (Cinatl et al., 2003b; Chen et al., 2004) The SARS-CoV spike protein uses a mechanism similar to that of class 1 fusion proteins in mediating membrane fusion and hence cell entry (Bosch et al., 2004). Antiviral peptides designed to inhibit this claw mechanics of the spike protein might be useful *in vitro* (Kliger and Levanon, 2003; Liu et al., 2004). Peptides derived from the heptad repeat 2 region of the SARS-CoV S protein were able to block viral infections (Xu et al., 2004; Yuan et al., 2004; Zhu et al., 2004a). siRNA designed for sequence-specific degradation of viral RNA generated during transcription demonstrated activities in reducing cytopathic effects, viral replication, and viral protein expression in cell lines. (He et al., 2003; Zhang et al., 2003; Lu et al., 2004; Wang et al., 2004b; Zhang et al., 2004a; Zheng et al., 2004c). Screening of combinatorial chemical libraries have identified inhibitors for protease, helicase, and spike-mediated cell entry (Kao et al., 2004).

Immunodulators have been empirically used in the treatment of SARS during the initial epidemic (Cheng et al., 2004b). These include corticosteroids, intravenous immunoglobulins, pentaglobin (Ho et al., 2004), thymosin, thalidomide, and anti-tumor necrosis factor. Corticosteroids have previously been used in the management of viral pneumonias due to varicella-zoster virus, influenza virus, and other viruses (Greaves et al., 1981; Ahmed et al., 2002). Mortality in the first two infections appeared to be lower with corticosteroids than supportive treatment alone. High-dose hydrocortisone can reduce the expression of the proinflammatory chemokines CXCL8 and CXCL 10 in coronavirus-infected CACO-2 cell lines (Cinatl et al., 2005). However, unless an effective antiviral agent is available, early use of high doses of corticosteroids for prolonged period could be detrimental and may increase the risks of nosocomial infections and avasuclar bone necrosis. One study has shown that the early use of corticosteroid actually increased the plasma viral load (Lee et al., 2004). Pegylated interferon α-2a was shown to be useful for prophylaxis and reducing respiratory viral shedding and lung pathology when used as an early treatment in a monkey model (Haagmans et al., 2004). Combinations of steroid with either alfacon-1 (a recombinant consensus interferon-α) (Loutfy et al., 2003) or protease inhibitors and ribavirin improved outcomes in two different treatment trials using historical controls (Chan et al., 2003a; Chu et al., 2004a).

5.9.2. Passive and Active Immunization

Passive immunization using convalescent plasma with high titers of neutralizing antibody had been used for SARS patients who continued to deteriorate. No significant adverse reactions were noted, although this did not appear to be beneficial, either. Currently, only hyperimmune globulin produced from convalescent patients' plasma and the equine plasma immunized by inactivated SARS-CoV are available for prophylactic trials in human. A human monoclonal IgG1 produced from a single-chain variable region fragment against the S1 domain from two nonimmune human antibody libraries has also been produced (Sui et al., 2004). One of the single-chain variable region fragments 80R blocks the spike–ACE2 receptor interaction through binding to the S1 domain. In a murine model of asymptomatic SARS infection, passive immunization by high titers of

Table 5.3. Studies on active and passive immunization for SARS

Type of vaccine	Target	Animal model	Response	References
Protein fragment	S protein	Rabbits, BALB/c mice	Neutralizing antibodies	Zhang et al., 2004c
Inactivated whole virus	Inactivated SARS-CoV	BALB/c mice	Neutralizing antibodies	Tang et al., 2004
Inactivated whole virus	Inactivated SARS-CoV	BALB/c mice (intranasal)	Neutralizing antibodies; specific IgA in tracheal/lung wash fluid with adjuvant-added or PEG-precipitated vaccine only	Qu et al., 2005
Inactivated whole virus	Inactivated SARS-CoV	BALB/c mice, rabbits	Specific antibodies recognizing RBD of S1; blocked binding of RBD to ACE2; significant decrease in S protein–mediated cell entry in pseudo-typed virus assay	He et al., 2004
Adenoviral vector	S, M, and N proteins	Rhesus macaques	Neutralizing antibodies, T-cell responses	Gao et al., 2003
Modified vaccinia Ankara	S protein	BALB/c mice	Neutralizing antibodies; decrease in lung/nasal viral titers, passive serum transfer protective	Bisht et al., 2004
Modified vaccinia Ankara	S protein	BALB/c mice, rabbits, Chinese rhesus monkeys	Neutralizing antibodies; decrease in lung/nasal viral titers	Chen et al., 2005
Modified vaccinia Ankara	S protein	Ferrets	Neutralizing antibodies; enhanced hepatitis in vaccinated ferrets when challenged with SARS-CoV	Weingartl et al., 2004b
Recombinant attenuated HPIF3	S protein	African green monkey	Neutralizing antibodies, decrease in viral shedding	Bukreyev et al., 2004
DNA vaccine	S protein	BALB/c mice	Neutralizing antibodies, T-cell responses; decrease in lung/nasal viral titers; serum transfer protective	Yang et al., 2004

(Continued)

Table 5.3. Studies on active and passive immunization for SARS—Cont'd

Type of vaccine	Target	Animal model	Response	References
DNA vaccine	S protein	C57BL/6 mice	T-cell responses; decrease in surrogate viral titer in lungs	Kim et al., 2004
DNA vaccine	S protein	BALB/c mice	Neutralizing antibodies, T-cell responses	Zeng et al., 2004
DNA vaccine	N protein	C3H/He mice	Specific antibodies, T-cell responses	Zhu et al., 2004
DNA vaccine	S protein	Rabbits	Neutralizing antibodies	Wang et al., 2005
DNA vaccine	N protein	Mice	Specific antibodies, N-specific splenocytes proliferation responses, DTH and CD8+ CTL responses	Zhao et al., 2005
Human monoclonal antibody	S protein	Ferret	Decrease in lung viral titer, decrease in viral shedding, prevention of viral-induced tissue pathology	ter Meulen et al., 2004
Human monoclonal antibody	S protein	BALB/c mice	Decrease in lung/nasal viral titers	Traggiai et al., 2004
Human monoclonal antibody from transgenic (HuMantibody) mice	S protein	BALB/c mice	Decrease in lung/nasal viral titers	Greenough et al., 2005
Human monoclonal antibody from phage display library	S, N proteins		Decrease in binding of recombinant S fragment and neutralized SARS-CoV in Vero cell assay	van den Brink et al., 2005

ACE, angiotensin-converting enzyme; CTL, cytotoxic T cell; DTH, delayed-type hypersensitivity; M, SARS-CoV membrane protein; N, SARS-CoV nucleoprotein; RBD, receptor-binding domain; S, SARS-CoV spike protein.

neutralizing antibody prevented virus replication in the lungs but not as effectively in the nasal turbinates (Subbarao et al., 2004). Similarly, passive immunization of mice and ferrets with a human IgG1 monoclonal antibody CR3014 was effective in preventing the development of lung pathology but less effective in reducing pharyngeal excretion (ter Meulen et al., 2004). Currently, there are no randomized placebo control trials on the role of antibody therapy for pre- or postexposure prophylaxis in at-risk groups during the SARS epidemic. Retrospective analysis of outcome in a human study using SARS convalescent plasma suggested that passive immunization had no major side effects and perhaps some clinical benefits (Soo et al., 2004).

It appears that the antibody response against the viral spike antigen is the key factor for protection against infection. Similar findings were found in the murine model using either intramuscular or intranasal administration of the highly attenuated modified vaccinia virus Ankara carrying the spike protein (Bisht et al., 2004). Mucosal immunization of African green monkeys with the recombinant attenuated parainfluenza virus–SARS-CoV spike protein chimeric virus resulted in a good neutralizing antibody response and protection from viral replication in the upper and lower respiratory tracts after live SARS-CoV challenge (Bukreyev et al., 2004). Other approaches to active immunization involved the use of an adenoviral vector (carrying S, M, and N proteins) in rhesus macaques (Gao et al., 2003), inactivated whole virus vaccine in mice (Tang et al., 2004), S protein fragments in rabbits and mice (Zhang et al., 2004c), DNA vaccination with the nucleocapsid gene in mice (Zhu et al., 2004b); adenoviral vector carrying the S1 domain, membrane and nucleoprotein or a DNA vaccine linking nucleocapsid protein to calreticulin (Kim et al., 2004). A plasmid DNA vaccine carrying the spike protein encoded by humanized codons was highly protective in a mouse model (Zeng et al., 2004). Furthermore, T-cell depletion with specific monoclonal antibodies against CD4 or CD8, alone or in combination with CD90 did not affect the protective immunity, which was confirmed by adoptive T-cell transfer. Donor T cells alone did not inhibit pulmonary viral replication in recipient mice, whereas passive transfer of purified IgG from immunized mice achieved similar protection. In summary (Table 5.3), all vaccines based on the spike protein appeared to be capable of inducing neutralizing antibody responses, and those carrying nucleoprotein induced nucleoprotein-specific cell-mediated immunity.

The relative importance of systemic or mucosal immunity in terms of neutralizing antibody or cytotoxic T lymphocyte response against spike, nucleocapsid, or other targets in terms of recovery from SARS is unknown. Nevertheless, neutralizing antibody against spike appears to be crucial for prophylactic immunity. Live-attenuated virus is unlikely to be useful owing to the concern for reversion to virulence or recombination with wild strains to form new wild types. An inactivated SARS-CoV is the most likely candidate for clinical trials. Recombinant proteins expressed in mammalian cells can also be used to induce good neutralizing antibody response. Irrespective of the approach to immunization, one should bear in mind the phenomenon of immune enhancement of disease has occurred in feline peritonitis coronavirus infection. SARS-CoV vaccine may indeed lead to increased derangement in the liver function of challenged ferrets that had previously been vaccinated (Weingartl et al., 2004b). Atypical or a more severe form of disease had occurred after the use of inactivated measles and respiratory syncytial virus vaccination. The economic viability of SARS vaccine depends very much on the risk of having another SARS epidemic and future major antigenic variations that might appear.

5.10. Laboratory Safety, Community and Hospital Infection Control

Infection control against SARS is of paramount importance within health care facilities given the relative stability of SARS-CoV in the environment, absence of protective immunity in the general population, and the lack of effective antivirals or vaccines. Triage of suspected cases, early case detection, and prompt isolation of suspected cases are the principal measures against nosocomial transmission (Ho et al., 2003). Respiratory droplet and contact precautions are effective under most circumstances (Seto et al., 2003). Airborne precautions must be considered in situations where droplet nuclei are likely to be generated. Strict hand hygiene, preferably with a patrol nurse overseeing all gowning and degowning procedures, in a SARS ward are critically important. Contact tracing, quarantine of contacts to prevent community spread, temperature checks at borders, health declarations for travelers, public education and effective risk communication with public media were all used in the 2003 pandemic for effective control. All SARS laboratories must strictly comply with the World Health Organization standards, and live viruses should only be cultivated and handled in accredited biosafety level 3 laboratories. Daily checking of temperature and reporting of sickness should be part of the monitoring protocol for laboratory workers handling live viruses.

Although screenings at international borders and airports were widely practiced during the epidemic, the value of such screening has recently been questioned (St John et al., 2005). Nevertheless, travelers during the epidemic may be less vigilant on preventive measures against the disease, and they remain an important target in the prevention of cross-border spread of the infection (Lau et al., 2004b).

References

Ahmed R, Ahmed QA, Adhami NA, Memish ZA (2002). Varicella pneumonia: another "steroid responsive" pneumonia? *J Chemother* 14: 220–222.

Akerstrom S, Mousavi-Jazi M, Klingstrom J, Leijon M, Lundkvist A, Mirazimi A (2005). Nitric oxide inhibits the replication cycle of severe acute respiratory syndrome coronavirus. *J Virol* 79: 1966–1969.

Anand K, Ziebuhr J, Wadhwani P, Mesters JR, Hilgenfeld R (2003). Coronavirus main proteinase (3CLpro) structure: basis for design of anti-SARS drugs. *Science* 300: 1763–1767.

Babcock GJ, Esshaki DJ, Thomas WD Jr, Ambrosino DM (2004). Amino acids 270 to 510 of the severe acute respiratory syndrome coronavirus spike protein are required for interaction with receptor. *J Virol* 78: 4552–4560.

Bhardwaj K, Guarino L, Kao CC (2004). The severe acute respiratory syndrome coronavirus Nsp15 protein is an endoribonuclease that prefers manganese as a cofactor. *J Virol* 78: 12218–12224.

Bisht H, Roberts A, Vogel L, Bukreyev A, Collins PL, Murphy BR, Subbarao K, Moss B (2004). Severe acute respiratory syndrome coronavirus spike protein expressed by attenuated vaccinia virus protectively immunizes mice. *Proc Natl Acad Sci U S A* 101: 6641–6646.

Bosch BJ, Martina BE, Van Der Zee R, Lepault J, Haijema BJ, Versluis C, Heck AJ, De Groot R, Osterhaus AD, Rottier PJ (2004). Severe acute respiratory syndrome coronavirus (SARS-CoV) infection inhibition using spike protein heptad repeat-derived peptides. *Proc Natl Acad Sci U S A* 101: 8455–8460.

Bukreyev A, Lamirande EW, Buchholz UJ, Vogel LN, Elkins WR, St Claire M, Murphy BR, Subbarao K, Collins PL (2004). Mucosal immunisation of African green monkeys (*Cercopithecus aethiops*) with an attenuated parainfluenza virus expressing the SARS coronavirus spike protein for the prevention of SARS. *Lancet* 363: 2122–2127.

Campanacci V, Egloff MP, Longhi S, Ferron F, Rancurel C, Salomoni A, Durousseau C, Tocque F, Bremond N, Dobbe JC, Snijder EJ, Canard B, Cambillau C (2003). Structural genomics of the SARS coronavirus: cloning, expression, crystallization and preliminary crystallographic study of the Nsp9 protein. *Acta Crystallogr D Biol Crystallogr* 59: 1628–1631.

Chan KS, Lai ST, Chu CM, Tsui E, Tam CY, Wong MM, Tse MW, Que TL, Peiris JS, Sung J, Wong VC, Yuen KY (2003a). Treatment of severe acute respiratory syndrome with lopinavir/ritonavir: a multicentre retrospective matched cohort study. *Hong Kong Med J* 9: 399–406.

Chan KS, Zheng JP, Mok YW, Li YM, Liu YN, Chu CM, Ip MS (2003b). SARS: prognosis, outcome and sequelae. *Respirology* 8(Suppl): S36–40.

Chan WM, Yuen KS, Fan DS, Lam DS, Chan PK, Sung JJ (2004a). Tears and conjunctival scrapings for coronavirus in patients with SARS. *Br J Ophthalmol* 88: 968–969.

Chan WM, Kwan YW, Wan HS, Leung CW, Chiu MC (2004b). Epidemiologic linkage and public health implication of a cluster of severe acute respiratory syndrome in an extended family. *Pediatr Infect Dis J* 23: 1156–1159.

Chau TN, Lee KC, Yao H, Tsang TY, Chow TC, Yeung YC, Choi KW, Tso YK, Lau T, Lai ST, Lai CL (2004). SARS-associated viral hepatitis caused by a novel coronavirus: report of three cases. *Hepatology* 39: 302–310.

Che XY (2004). Nucleocapsid protein as early diagnostic marker for SARS. *Emerg Infect Dis* 10: 1947–1949.

Chen F, Chan KH, Jiang Y, Kao RY, Lu HT, Fan KW, Cheng VC, Tsui WH, Hung IF, Lee TS, Guan Y, Peiris JS, Yuen KY (2004). In vitro susceptibility of 10 clinical isolates of SARS coronavirus to selected antiviral compounds. *J Clin Virol* 31: 69–75.

Chen L, Liu P, Gao H, Sun B, Chao D, Wang F, Zhu Y, Hedenstierna G, Wang CG (2004). Inhalation of nitric oxide in the treatment of severe acute respiratory syndrome: a rescue trial in Beijing. *Clin Infect Dis* 39: 1531–1535.

Chen WQ, Lu CY, Wong TW, Ling WH, Lin ZN, Hao YT, Liu Q, Fang JQ, He Y, Luo FT, Jing J, Ling L, Ma X, Liu YM, Chen GH, Huang J, Jiang YS, Jiang WQ, Zou HQ, Yan GM (2005). Anti-SARS-CoV immunoglobulin G in health care workers, Guangzhou, China. *Emerg Infect Dis* 11: 89–94.

Chen Z, Zhang L, Qin C, Ba L, Yi CE, Zhang F, Wei Q, He T, Yu W, Yu J, Gao H, Tu X, Gettie A, Farzan M, Yuen KY, Ho DD (2005). Recombinant modified vaccinia virus Ankara expressing the spike glycoprotein of severe acute respiratory syndrome coronavirus induces protective neutralizing antibodies primarily targeting the receptor binding region. *J Virol* 79: 2678–2688.

Cheng VC, Hung IF, Tang BS, Chu CM, Wong MM, Chan KH, Wu AK, Tse DM, Chan KS, Zheng BJ, Peiris JS, Sung JJ, Yuen KY (2004a). Viral replication in the nasopharynx is associated with diarrhea in patients with severe acute respiratory syndrome. *Clin Infect Dis* 38: 467–475.

Cheng VC, Tang BS, Wu AK, Chu CM, Yuen KY (2004b). Medical treatment of viral pneumonia including SARS in immunocompetent adult. *J Infect* 49: 262–273.

Cheung CY, Poon LL, Ng IH, Luk W, Sia SF, Wu MH, Chan KH, Yuen KY, Gordon S, Guan Y, Peiris JS (2005). Cytokine responses in severe acute respiratory syndrome coronavirus-infected macrophages in vitro: possible relevance to pathogenesis. *J Virol* 79: 7819–7826.

Cheung TM, Yam LY, So LK, Lau AC, Poon E, Kong BM, Yung RW (2004). Effectiveness of noninvasive positive pressure ventilation in the treatment of acute respiratory failure in severe acute respiratory syndrome. *Chest* 126: 845–850.

The Chinese SARS Molecular Epidemiology Consortium (2004). Molecular evolution of the SARS coronavirus during the course of the SARS epidemic in China. *Science* 303: 1666–1669.

Chou KC, Wei DQ, Zhong WZ (2003). Binding mechanism of coronavirus main proteinase with ligands and its implication to drug design against SARS. *Biochem Biophys Res Commun* 308: 148–151.

Chow KY, Lee CE, Ling ML, Heng DM, Yap SG (2004). Outbreak of severe acute respiratory syndrome in a tertiary hospital in Singapore, linked to an index patient with atypical presentation: epidemiological study. *Br Med J* 328: 195.

Christian MD, Loutfy M, McDonald LC, Martinez KF, Ofner M, Wong T, Wallington T, Gold WL, Mederski B, Green K, Low DE; SARS Investigation Team (2004). Possible SARS coronavirus transmission during cardiopulmonary resuscitation. *Emerg Infect Dis* 10: 287–293.

Chu CM, Cheng VC, Hung IF, Wong MM, Chan KH, Kao RY, Poon LL, Wong CL, Guan Y, Peiris JS, Yuen KY; HKU/UCH SARS Study Group (2004a). Role of lopinavir/ritonavir in the treatment of SARS: initial virological and clinical findings. *Thorax* 59: 252–256.

Chu CM, Poon LL, Cheng VC, Chan KS, Hung IF, Wong MM, Chan KH, Leung WS, Tang BS, Chan VL, Ng WL, Sim TC, Ng PW, Law KI, Tse DM, Peiris JS, Yuen KY (2004b). Initial viral load and the outcomes of SARS. *CMAJ* 171: 1349–1352.

Chu CM, Leung WS, Cheng VC, Chan KH, Lin AW, Chan VL, Lam JY, Chan KS, Yuen KY (2005). Duration of RT-PCR positivity in severe acute respiratory syndrome. *Eur Respir J* 25:12–14.

Chu KH, Tsang WK, Tang CS, Lam MF, Lai FM, To KF, Fung KS, Tang HL, Yan WW, Chan HW, Lai TS, Tong KL, Lai KN (2005). Acute renal impairment in coronavirus-associated severe acute respiratory syndrome. *Kidney Int* 67: 698–705.

Cinatl J, Morgenstern B, Bauer G, Chandra P, Rabenau H, Doerr HW (2003a). Glycyrrhizin, an active component of liquorice roots, and replication of SARS-associated coronavirus. *Lancet* 361: 2045–2046.

Cinatl J, Morgenstern B, Bauer G, Chandra P, Rabenau H, Doerr HW (2003b). Treatment of SARS with human interferons. *Lancet* 362: 293–294.

Cinatl J Jr, Michaelis M, Morgenstern B, Doerr HW (2005). High-dose hydrocortisone reduces expression of the pro-inflammatory chemokines CXCL8 and CXCL10 in SARS coronavirus-infected intestinal cells. *Int J Mol Med* 15: 323–327.

Cui W, Fan Y, Wu W, Zhang F, Wang JY, Ni AP (2003). Expression of lymphocytes and lymphocyte subsets in patients with severe acute respiratory syndrome. *Clin Infect Dis* 37: 857–859.

Ding Y, Wang H, Shen H, Li Z, Geng J, Han H, Cai J, Li X, Kang W, Weng D, Lu Y, Wu D, He L, Yao K (2003). The clinical pathology of severe acute respiratory syndrome (SARS): a report from China. *J Pathol* 200: 282–289.

Drosten C, Gunther S, Preiser W, van der Werf S, Brodt HR, Becker S, Rabenau H, Panning M, Kolesnikova L, Fouchier RA, Berger A, Burguiere AM, Cinatl J, Eickmann M, Escriou N, Grywna K, Kramme S, Manuguerra JC, Muller S, Rickerts V, Sturmer M, Vieth S, Klenk HD, Osterhaus AD, Schmitz H, Doerr HW (2003). Identification of a novel coronavirus in patients with severe acute respiratory syndrome. *N Engl J Med* 348: 1967–1976.

Duan SM, Zhao XS, Wen RF, Huang JJ, Pi GH, Zhang SX, Han J, Bi SL, Ruan L, Dong XP; SARS Research Team (2003). Stability of SARS coronavirus in human specimens and environment and its sensitivity to heating and UV irradiation. *Biomed Environ Sci* 16: 246–255.

Egloff MP, Ferron F, Campanacci V, Longhi S, Rancurel C, Dutartre H, Snijder EJ, Gorbalenya AE, Cambillau C, Canard B (2004). The severe acute respiratory syndrome-coronavirus replicative protein nsp9 is a single-stranded RNA-binding subunit unique in the RNA virus world. *Proc Natl Acad Sci U S A* 101: 3792–3796.

Eickmann M, Becker S, Klenk HD, Doerr HW, Stadler K, Censini S, Guidotti S, Masignani V, Scarselli M, Mora M, Donati C, Han JH, Song HC, Abrignani S, Covacci A, Rappuoli R (2003). Phylogeny of the SARS coronavirus. *Science* 302: 1504–1505.

Farcas GA, Poutanen SM, Mazzulli T, Willey BM, Butany J, Asa SL, Faure P, Akhavan P, Low DE, Kain KC (2005). Fatal severe acute respiratory syndrome is associated with multiorgan involvement by coronavirus. *J Infect Dis* 191: 193–197.

Fouchier RA, Hartwig NG, Bestebroer TM, Niemeyer B, De Jong JC, Simon JH, Osterhaus AD (2004). A previously undescribed coronavirus associated with respiratory disease in humans. *Proc Natl Acad Sci U S A* 101: 6212–6216.

Franks TJ, Chong PY, Chui P, Galvin JR, Lourens RM, Reid AH, Selbs E, McEvoy CP, Hayden CD, Fukuoka J, Taubenberger JK, Travis WD (2003). Lung pathology of severe acute respiratory syndrome (SARS): a study of 8 autopsy cases from Singapore. *Hum Pathol* 34: 743–748.

Gao W, Tamin A, Soloff A, D'Aiuto L, Nwanegbo E, Robbins PD, Bellini WJ, Barratt-Boyes S, Gambotto A (2003). Effects of a SARS-associated coronavirus vaccine in monkeys. *Lancet* 362: 1895–1896.

Greaves IA, Colebatch HJ, Torda TA (1981). A possible role for corticosteroids in the treatment of influenzal pneumonia. *Aust N Z J Med* 11: 271–276.

Greenough TC, Babcock GJ, Roberts A, Hernandez HJ, Thomas WD Jr, Coccia JA, Graziano RF, Srinivasan M, Lowy I, Finberg RW, Subbarao K, Vogel L, Somasundaran M, Luzuriaga K, Sullivan JL, Ambrosino DM (2005). Development and characterization of a severe acute respiratory syndrome-associated coronavirus-neutralizing human monoclonal antibody that provides effective immunoprophylaxis in mice. *J Infect Dis* 191: 507–514.

Griffith JF, Antonio GE, Kumta SM, Cheong Hui DS, Tak Wong JK, Joynt GM, Lun Wu AK, Kiu Cheung AY, Chiu KH, Chan KM, Leung PC, Ahuja AT (2005). Osteonecrosis of hip and knee in patients with severe acute respiratory syndrome treated with steroids. *Radiology* 235: 168–175.

Guan Y, Zheng BJ, He YQ, Liu XL, Zhuang ZX, Cheung CL, Luo SW, Li PH, Zhang LJ, Guan YJ, Butt KM, Wong KL, Chan KW, Lim W, Shortridge KF, Yuen KY, Peiris JS, Poon LL (2003). Isolation and characterization of viruses related to the SARS coronavirus from animals in southern China. *Science* 302: 276–278.

Guan Y, Peiris JS, Zheng B, Poon LL, Chan KH, Zeng FY, Chan CW, Chan MN, Chen JD, Chow KY, Hon CC, Hui KH, Li J, Li VY, Wang Y, Leung SW, Yuen KY, Leung FC (2004). Molecular epidemiology of the novel coronavirus that causes severe acute respiratory syndrome. *Lancet* 363: 99–104.

Haagmans BL, Kuiken T, Martina BE, Fouchier RA, Rimmelzwaan GF, van Amerongen G, van Riel D, de Jong T, Itamura S, Chan KH, Tashiro M, Osterhaus AD (2004). Pegylated interferon-alpha protects type 1 pneumocytes against SARS coronavirus infection in macaques. *Nat Med* 10: 290–293.

Hamming I, Timens W, Bulthuis ML, Lely AT, Navis GJ, van Goor H (2004). Tissue distribution of ACE2 protein, the functional receptor for SARS coronavirus. A first step in understanding SARS pathogenesis. *J Pathol* 203: 631–637.

Hattermann K, Muller MA, Nitsche A, Wendt S, Donoso Mantke O, Niedrig M (2005). Susceptibility of different eukaryotic cell lines to SARS-coronavirus. *Arch Virol* 150: 1023–1031.

He ML, Zheng B, Peng Y, Peiris JS, Poon LL, Yuen KY, Lin MC, Kung HF, Guan Y (2003). Inhibition of SARS-associated coronavirus infection and replication by RNA interference. *JAMA* 290: 2665–2666.

He R, Adonov A, Traykova-Adonova M, Cao J, Cutts T, Grudesky E, Deschambaul Y, Berry J, Drebot M, Li X (2004). Potent and selective inhibition of SARS coronavirus replication by aurintricarboxylic acid. *Biochem Biophys Res Commun* 320: 1199–1203.

He Q, Manopo I, Lu L, Leung BP, Chng HH, Ling AE, Chee LL, Chan SW, Ooi EE, Sin YL, Ang B, Kwang J (2005). Novel immunofluorescence assay using recombinant nucleocapsid-spike fusion protein as antigen to detect antibodies against severe acute respiratory syndrome coronavirus. *Clin Diagn Lab Immunol* 12: 321–328.

He Y, Zhou Y, Siddiqui P, Jiang S (2004). Inactivated SARS-CoV vaccine elicits high titers of spike protein-specific antibodies that block receptor binding and virus entry. *Biochem Biophys Res Commun* 325: 445–452.

Hensley LE, Fritz LE, Jahrling PB, Karp CL, Huggins JW, Geisbert TW (2004). Interferon-beta 1a and SARS coronavirus replication. *Emerg Infect Dis* 10: 317–319.

Ho JC, Wu AY, Lam B, Ooi GC, Khong PL, Ho PL, Chan-Yeung M, Zhong NS, Ko C, Lam WK, Tsang KW (2004). Pentaglobin in steroid-resistant severe acute respiratory syndrome. *Int J Tuberc Lung Dis* 8: 1173–1179.

Ho PL, Tang XP, Seto WH (2003). SARS: hospital infection control and admission strategies. *Respirology* 8(Suppl):S41–45.

Holmes KV (2001). Coronaviruses. In Knipe DM, Howley PM (eds) *Fields Virology*. Lippincott Williams & Wilkins, Philadelphia, pp. 1187–1203.

Huang KJ, Su IJ, Theron M, Wu YC, Lai SK, Liu CC, Lei HY (2005). An interferon-gamma-related cytokine storm in SARS patients. *J Med Virol* 75: 185–194.

Hui DS, Wong KT, Antonio GE, Lee N, Wu A, Wong V, Lau W, Wu JC, Tam LS, Yu LM, Joynt GM, Chung SS, Ahuja AT, Sung JJ (2004). Severe acute respiratory syndrome: correlation between clinical outcome and radiologic features. *Radiology* 233: 579–585.

Hung IFN, Cheng VCC, Wu AKL, Tang BSF, Chan KH, Chu CM, Wong MML, Hui WT, Poon LLM, Tse DMW, Chan KS, Woo PCY, Lau SKP, Peiris JSM, Yuen KY (2004). Viral loads in clinical specimens and SARS manifestations. *Emerg Infect Dis* 10: 1550–1557.

Jackwood MW, Hilt DA, Callison SA, Lee CW, Plaza H, Wade E. (2001). Spike glycoprotein cleavage recognition site analysis of infectious bronchitis virus. *Avian Dis* 45: 366–372.

Jeffers SA, Tusell SM, Gillim-Ross L, Hemmila EM, Achenbach JE, Babcock GJ, Thomas WD Jr, Thackray LB, Young MD, Mason RJ, Ambrosino DM, Wentworth DE, Demartini JC, Holmes KV (2004). CD209L (L-SIGN) is a receptor for severe acute respiratory syndrome coronavirus. *Proc Natl Acad Sci U S A* 101: 15748–15753.

Jiang Y, Xu J, Zhou C, Wu Z, Zhong S, Liu J, Luo W, Chen T, Qin Q, Deng P (2005). Characterization of cytokine and chemokine profiles of severe acute respiratory syndrome. *Am J Respir Crit Care Med*

Jones BM, Ma ES, Peiris JS, Wong PC, Ho JC, Lam B, Lai KN, Tsang KW (2004). Prolonged disturbances of in vitro cytokine production in patients with severe acute respiratory syndrome (SARS) treated with ribavirin and steroids. *Clin Exp Immunol* 135: 467–473.

Kao RY, Tsui WHW, Lee TSW, Tanner JA, Watt RM, Hung JD, Hu LH, Chen GH, Chen ZW, Zhang LQ, He T, Chan KH, Tse H, To APC, Ng LWY, Wong BCW, Tsoi HW, Yang D, Ho DD, Yuen KY (2004). Identification of novel small molecule inhibitors of severe acute respiratory syndrome-associated coronavirus by chemical genetics. *Chem Biol* 11: 1293–1299.

Keyaerts E, Vijgen L, Maes P, Neyts J, Ranst MV (2004). In vitro inhibition of severe acute respiratory syndrome coronavirus by chloroquine. *Biochem Biophys Res Commun* 323: 264–268.

Kim TW, Lee JH, Hung CF, Peng S, Roden R, Wang MC, Viscidi R, Tsai YC, He L, Chen PJ, Boyd DA, Wu TC (2004). Generation and characterization of DNA vaccines targeting the nucleocapsid protein of severe acute respiratory syndrome coronavirus. *J Virol* 78: 4638–4645.

Kliger Y, Levanon EY (2003). Cloaked similarity between HIV-1 and SARS-CoV suggests an anti-SARS strategy. *BMC Microbiol* 3: 20.

Krempl C, Schultze B, Herrler G. (1995). Analysis of cellular receptors for human coronavirus OC43. *Adv Exp Med Biol* 380: 371–374.

Ksiazek TG, Erdman D, Goldsmith CS, Zaki SR, Peret T, Emery S, Tong S, Urbani C, Comer JA, Lim W, Rollin PE, Dowell SF, Ling AE, Humphrey CD, Shieh WJ, Guarner J, Paddock CD, Rota P, Fields B, DeRisi J, Yang JY, Cox N, Hughes JM, LeDuc JW, Bellini WJ, Anderson LJ; SARS Working Group (2003). A novel coronavirus associated with severe acute respiratory syndrome. *N Engl J Med* 348: 1953–1966.

Kuiken T, Fouchier RA, Schutten M, Rimmelzwaan GF, van Amerongen G, van Riel D, Laman JD, de Jong T, van Doornum G, Lim W, Ling AE, Chan PK, Tam JS, Zambon MC, Gopal R, Drosten C, van der Werf S, Escriou N, Manuguerra JC, Stohr K, Peiris JS, Osterhaus AD (2003). Newly discovered coronavirus as the primary cause of severe acute respiratory syndrome. *Lancet* 362: 263–270.

Kwan MY, Chan WM, Ko PW, Leung CW, Chiu MC (2004). Severe acute respiratory syndrome can be mild in children. *Pediatr Infect Dis J* 23: 1172–1174.

Lai PC, Wong CM, Hedley AJ, Lo SV, Leung PY, Kong J, Leung GM (2004). Understanding the spatial clustering of severe acute respiratory syndrome (SARS) in Hong Kong. *Environ Health Perspect* 112: 1550–1556.

Lau KK, Yu WC, Chu CM, Lau ST, Sheng B, Yuen KY (2004a). Possible central nervous system infection by SARS coronavirus. *Emerg Infect Dis* 10: 342–344.

Lau JT, Yang X, Tsui HY, Pang E (2004b). SARS related preventive and risk behaviours practised by Hong Kong-Mainland China cross border travellers during the outbreak of the SARS epidemic in Hong Kong. *J Epidemiol Community Health* 58: 988–996.

Lau JT, Yang X, Leung PC, Chan L, Wong E, Fong C, Tsui HY (2004c). SARS in three categories of hospital workers, Hong Kong. *Emerg Infect Dis* 10: 1399–1404.

Lee DT, Wing YK, Leung HC, Sung JJ, Ng YK, Yiu GC, Chen RY, Chiu HF (2004). Factors associated with psychosis among patients with severe acute respiratory syndrome: a case-control study. *Clin Infect Dis* 39: 1247–1249.

Lee HK, Tso EY, Chau TN, Tsang OT, Choi KW, Lai TS (2003a). Asymptomatic severe acute respiratory syndrome-associated coronavirus infection. *Emerg Infect Dis* 9: 1491–1492.

Lee N, Hui D, Wu A, Chan P, Cameron P, Joynt GM, Ahuja A, Yung MY, Leung CB, To KF, Lui SF, Szeto CC, Chung S, Sung JJ (2003b). A major outbreak of severe acute respiratory syndrome in Hong Kong. *N Engl J Med* 348: 1986–1994.

Lee N, Allen Chan KC, Hui DS, Ng EK, Wu A, Chiu RW, Wong VW, Chan PK, Wong KT, Wong E, Cockram CS, Tam JS, Sung JJ, Lo YM (2004). Effects of early corticosteroid treatment on plasma SARS-associated Coronavirus RNA concentrations in adult patients. *J Clin Virol* 31: 304–309.

Leung WK, To KF, Chan PK, Chan HL, Wu AK, Lee N, Yuen KY, Sung JJ (2003). Enteric involvement of severe acute respiratory syndrome-associated coronavirus infection. *Gastroenterology* 125: 1011–1017.

Leung GM, Hedley AJ, Ho LM, Chau P, Wong IO, Thach TQ, Ghani AC, Donnelly CA, Fraser C, Riley S, Ferguson NM, Anderson RM, Tsang T, Leung PY, Wong V, Chan JC, Tsui E, Lo SV, Lam TH (2004a). The epidemiology of severe acute respiratory syndrome in the 2003 Hong Kong epidemic: an analysis of all 1755 patients. *Ann Intern Med* 141: 662–673.

Leung GM, Chung PH, Tsang T, Lim W, Chan SK, Chau P, Donnelly CA, Ghani AC, Fraser C, Riley S, Ferguson NM, Anderson RM, Law YL, Mok T, Ng T, Fu A, Leung PY, Peiris JS, Lam TH, Hedley AJ (2004b). SARS-CoV antibody prevalence in all Hong Kong patient contacts. *Emerg Infect Dis* 10: 1653–1656.

Li L, Wo J, Shao J, Zhu H, Wu N, Li M, Yao H, Hu M, Dennin RH (2003a). SARS-coronavirus replicates in mononuclear cells of peripheral blood (PBMCs) from SARS patients. *J Clin Virol* 28: 239–244.

Li SS, Cheng CW, Fu CL, Chan YH, Lee MP, Chan JW, Yiu SF (2003b). Left ventricular performance in patients with severe acute respiratory syndrome: a 30-day echocardiographic follow-up study. *Circulation* 108: 1798–1803.

Li W, Moore MJ, Vasilieva N, Sui J, Wong SK, Berne MA, Somasundaran M, Sullivan JL, Luzuriaga K, Greenough TC, Choe H, Farzan M (2003c). Angiotensin-converting enzyme 2 is a functional receptor for the SARS coronavirus. *Nature* 426: 450–454.

Li T, Qiu Z, Zhang L, Han Y, He W, Liu Z, Ma X, Fan H, Lu W, Xie J, Wang H, Deng G, Wang A (2004). Significant changes of peripheral T lymphocyte subsets in patients with severe acute respiratory syndrome. *J Infect Dis* 189: 648–651.

Lim PL, Kurup A, Gopalakrishna G, Chan KP, Wong CW, Ng LC, Se-Thoe SY, Oon L, Bai X, Stanton LW, Ruan Y, Miller LD, Vega VB, James L, Ooi PL, Kai CS, Olsen SJ, Ang B, Leo YS (2004). Laboratory-acquired severe acute respiratory syndrome. *N Engl J Med* 350: 1740–1745.

Lin M, Tseng HK, Trejaut JA, Lee HL, Loo JH, Chu CC, Chen PJ, Su YW, Lim KH, Tsai ZU, Lin RY, Lin RS, Huang CH (2003). Association of HLA class I with severe acute respiratory syndrome coronavirus infection. *BMC Med Genet* 4: 9.

Liu S, Xiao G, Chen Y, He Y, Niu J, Escalante CR, Xiong H, Farmar J, Debnath AK, Tien P, Jiang S (2004). Interaction between heptad repeat 1 and 2 regions in spike protein of SARS-associated coronavirus: implications for virus fusogenic mechanism and identification of fusion inhibitors. *Lancet* 363: 938–947.

Loon SC, Teoh SC, Oon LL, Se-Thoe SY, Ling AE, Leo YS, Leong HN (2004). The severe acute respiratory syndrome coronavirus in tears. *Br J Ophthalmol* 88: 861–863.

Loutfy MR, Blatt LM, Siminovitch KA, Ward S, Wolff B, Lho H, Pham DH, Deif H, LaMere EA, Chang M, Kain KC, Farcas GA, Ferguson P, Latchford M, Levy G, Dennis JW, Lai EK, Fish EN (2003). Interferon alfacon-1 plus corticosteroids in severe acute respiratory syndrome: a preliminary study. *JAMA* 290: 3222–3228.

Lu A, Zhang H, Zhang X, Wang H, Hu Q, Shen L, Schaffhausen BS, Hou W, Li L (2004). Attenuation of SARS coronavirus by a short hairpin RNA expression plasmid targeting RNA-dependent RNA polymerase. *Virology* 324: 84–89.

McAuliffe J, Vogel L, Roberts A, Fahle G, Fischer S, Shieh WJ, Butler E, Zaki S, St Claire M, Murphy B, Subbarao K (2004). Replication of SARS coronavirus administered into the respiratory tract of African Green, rhesus and cynomolgus monkeys. *Virology* 330: 8–15.

Martina BE, Haagmans BL, Kuiken T, Fouchier RA, Rimmelzwaan GF, Van Amerongen G, Peiris JS, Lim W, Osterhaus AD (2003). SARS virus infection of cats and ferrets. *Nature* 425: 915.

Morgenstern B, Michaelis M, Baer PC, Doerr HW, Cinatl J Jr (2005). Ribavirin and interferon-beta synergistically inhibit SARS-associated coronavirus replication in animal and human cell lines. *Biochem Biophys Res Commun* 326: 905–908.

Ng MH, Lau KM, Li L, Cheng SH, Chan WY, Hui PK, Zee B, Leung CB, Sung JJ (2004). Association of human-leukocyte-antigen class I (B*0703) and class II (DRB1*0301) genotypes with susceptibility and resistance to the development of severe acute respiratory syndrome. *J Infect Dis* 190: 515–518.

Ng CK, Chan JW, Kwan TL, To TS, Chan YH, Ng FY, Mok TY (2004). Six month radiological and physiological outcomes in severe acute respiratory syndrome (SARS) survivors. *Thorax* 59: 889–891.

Nicholls JM, Poon LL, Lee KC, Ng WF, Lai ST, Leung CY, Chu CM, Hui PK, Mak KL, Lim W, Yan KW, Chan KH, Tsang NC, Guan Y, Yuen KY, Peiris JS (2003). Lung pathology of fatal severe acute respiratory syndrome. *Lancet* 361: 1773–1778.

Ong KC, Ng AW, Lee LS, Kaw G, Kwek SK, Leow MK, Earnest A (2004). Pulmonary function and exercise capacity in survivors of severe acute respiratory syndrome. *Eur Respir J* 24: 436–442.

Orellana C (2004). Laboratory-acquired SARS raises worries on biosafety. *Lancet Infect Dis* 4: 64.

Otsuki K, Noro K, Yamamoto H, Tsubokura M (1979). Studies on avian infectious bronchitis virus (IBV). II. Propagation of IBV in several cultured cells. *Arch Virol* 60: 115–122.

Peiris JS, Chu CM, Cheng VC, Chan KS, Hung IF, Poon LL, Law KI, Tang BS, Hon TY, Chan CS, Chan KH, Ng JS, Zheng BJ, Ng WL, Lai RW, Guan Y, Yuen KY; HKU/UCH SARS Study Group (2003a). Clinical progression and viral load in a community outbreak of coronavirus-associated SARS pneumonia: a prospective study. *Lancet* 361: 1767–1772.

Peiris JS, Lai ST, Poon LL, Guan Y, Yam LY, Lim W, Nicholls J, Yee WK, Yan WW, Cheung MT, Cheng VC, Chan KH, Tsang DN, Yung RW, Ng TK, Yuen KY; SARS study group (2003b). Coronavirus as a possible cause of severe acute respiratory syndrome. *Lancet* 361: 1319–1325.

Poon LL, Chan KH, Wong OK, Yam WC, Yuen KY, Guan Y, Lo YM, Peiris JS (2003). Early diagnosis of SARS coronavirus infection by real time RT-PCR. *J Clin Virol* 28: 233–238.

Qu D, Zheng B, Yao X, Guan Y, Yuan ZH, Zhong NS, Lu LW, Xie JP, Wen YM (2005). Intranasal immunization with inactivated SARS-CoV (SARS-associated coronavirus) induced local and serum antibodies in mice. *Vaccine* 23: 924–931.

Rabenau HF, Cinatl J, Morgenstern B, Bauer G, Preiser W, Doerr HW (2005). Stability and inactivation of SARS coronavirus. *Med Microbiol Immunol (Berl)* 194: 1–6.

Rest JS, Mindell DP (2003). SARS associated coronavirus has a recombinant polymerase and coronaviruses have a history of host-shifting. *Infect Genet Evol* 3: 219–225.

Roberts A, Vogel L, Guarner J, Hayes N, Murphy B, Zaki S, Subbarao K (2005). Severe acute respiratory syndrome coronavirus infection of golden Syrian hamsters. *J Virol* 79: 503–511.

Rota PA, Oberste MS, Monroe SS, Nix WA, Campagnoli R, Icenogle JP, Penaranda S, Bankamp B, Maher K, Chen MH, Tong S, Tamin A, Lowe L, Frace M, DeRisi JL, Chen Q, Wang D, Erdman DD, Peret TC, Burns C, Ksiazek TG, Rollin PE, Sanchez A, Liffick S, Holloway B, Limor J, McCaustland K, Olsen-Rasmussen M, Fouchier R, Gunther S, Osterhaus AD, Drosten C, Pallansch MA, Anderson LJ, Bellini WJ (2003). Characterization of a novel coronavirus associated with severe acute respiratory syndrome. *Science* 300: 1394–1399.

Seto WH, Tsang D, Yung RW, Ching TY, Ng TK, Ho M, Ho LM, Peiris JS; Advisors of Expert SARS group of Hospital Authority (2003). Effectiveness of precautions against droplets and contact in prevention of nosocomial transmission of severe acute respiratory syndrome (SARS). *Lancet* 361: 1519–1520.

Simmons G, Reeves JD, Rennekamp AJ, Amberg SM, Piefer AJ, Bates P (2004). Characterization of severe acute respiratory syndrome-associated coronavirus (SARS-CoV) spike glycoprotein-mediated viral entry. *Proc Natl Acad Sci U S A* 101: 4240–4245.

Snijder EJ, Bredenbeek PJ, Dobbe JC, Thiel V, Ziebuhr J, Poon LL, Guan Y, Rozanov M, Spaan WJ, Gorbalenya AE (2003). Unique and conserved features of genome and proteome of SARS-coronavirus, an early split-off from the coronavirus group 2 lineage. *J Mol Biol* 331: 991–1004.

Song HD, Tu CC, Zhang GW, Wang SY, Zheng K, Lei LC, Chen QX, Gao YW, Zhou HQ, Xiang H, Zheng HJ, Chern SW, Cheng F, Pan CM, Xuan H, Chen SJ, Luo HM, Zhou DH, Liu YF, He JF, Qin PZ, Li LH, Ren YQ, Liang WJ, Yu YD, Anderson L, Wang M, Xu RH, Wu XW, Zheng HY, Chen JD, Liang G, Gao Y, Liao M, Fang L, Jiang LY, Li H, Chen F, Di B, He LJ, Lin JY, Tong S, Kong X, Du L, Hao P, Tang H, Bernini A, Yu XJ, Spiga O, Guo ZM, Pan HY, He WZ, Manuguerra JC, Fontanet A, Danchin A, Niccolai N, Li YX, Wu CI, Zhao GP (2005). Cross-host evolution of severe acute respiratory syndrome coronavirus in palm civet and human. *Proc Natl Acad Sci U S A* 102: 2430–2435.

Soo YO, Cheng Y, Wong R, Hui DS, Lee CK, Tsang KK, Ng MH, Chan P, Cheng G, Sung JJ (2004). Retrospective comparison of convalescent plasma with continuing high-dose methylprednisolone treatment in SARS patients. *Clin Microbiol Infect* 10: 676–678.

Spiegel M, Pichlmair A, Muhlberger E, Haller O, Weber F (2004). The antiviral effect of interferon-beta against SARS-coronavirus is not mediated by MxA protein. *J Clin Virol* 30: 211–213.

St John RK, King A, de Jong D, Bodie-Collins M, Squires SG, Tam TW (2005). Border screening for SARS. *Emerg Infect Dis* 11: 6–10.

Stroher U, DiCaro A, Li Y, Strong JE, Aoki F, Plummer F, Jones SM, Feldmann H (2004). Severe acute respiratory syndrome-related coronavirus is inhibited by interferon-alpha. *J Infect Dis* 189: 1164–1167.

Subbarao K, McAuliffe J, Vogel L, Fahle G, Fischer S, Tatti K, Packard M, Shieh WJ, Zaki S, Murphy B (2004). Prior infection and passive transfer of neutralizing antibody prevent replication of severe acute respiratory syndrome coronavirus in the respiratory tract of mice. *J Virol* 78: 3572–3577.

Sui J, Li W, Murakami A, Tamin A, Matthews LJ, Wong SK, Moore MJ, Tallarico AS, Olurinde M, Choe H, Anderson LJ, Bellini WJ, Farzan M, Marasco WA (2004). Potent neutralization of severe acute respiratory syndrome (SARS) coronavirus by a human mAb to S1 protein that blocks receptor association. *Proc Natl Acad Sci U S A* 101: 2536–2541.

Tan ELC, Ooi EE, Lin CY, Tan HC, Ling AE, Lim B, Stanton LW (2004). Inhibition of SARS coronavirus infection in vitro with clinically approved antiviral drugs. *Emerg Infect Dis* 10: 581–586.

Tan J, Mu L, Huang J, Yu S, Chen B, Yin J (2005). An initial investigation of the association between the SARS outbreak and weather: with the view of the environmental temperature and its variation. *J Epidemiol Community Health* 59: 186–192.

Tang L, Zhu Q, Qin E, Yu M, Ding Z, Shi H, Cheng X, Wang C, Chang G, Zhu Q, Fang F, Chang H, Li S, Zhang X, Chen X, Yu J, Wang J, Chen Z (2004). Inactivated SARS-CoV vaccine prepared from whole virus induces a high level of neutralizing antibodies in BALB/c mice. *DNA Cell Biol* 23: 391–394.

Tang BS, Chan KH, Cheng VC, Woo PC, Lau SK, Lam CC, Chan TL, Wu AK, Hung IF, Leung SY, Yuen KY (2005). Comparative host gene transcription by microarray analysis early after infection of the Huh7 cell line by severe acute respiratory syndrome coronavirus and human coronavirus 229E. *J Virol* 79: 6180–6193.

Tanner JA, Watt RM, Chai YB, Lu LY, Lin MC, Peiris JS, Poon LL, Kung HF, Huang JD (2003). The severe acute respiratory syndrome (SARS) coronavirus NTPase/helicase belongs to a distinct class of 5′ to 3′ viral helicases. *J Biol Chem* 278: 39578–39582.

ter Meulen J, Bakker AB, van den Brink EN, Weverling GJ, Martina BE, Haagmans BL, Kuiken T, de Kruif J, Preiser W, Spaan W, Gelderblom HR, Goudsmit J, Osterhaus AD (2004). Human monoclonal antibody as prophylaxis for SARS coronavirus infection in ferrets. *Lancet* 363: 2139–2141.

Thiel V, Ivanov KA, Putics A, Hertzig T, Schelle B, Bayer S, Weissbrich B, Snijder EJ, Rabenau H, Doerr HW, Gorbalenya AE, Ziebuhr J (2003). Mechanisms and enzymes involved in SARS coronavirus genome expression. *J Gen Virol* 84: 2305–2315.

To KF, Lo AW (2004a). Exploring the pathogenesis of severe acute respiratory syndrome (SARS): the tissue distribution of the coronavirus (SARS-CoV) and its putative receptor, angiotensin-converting enzyme 2 (ACE2). *J Pathol* 203: 740–743.

To KF, Tong JH, Chan PK, Au FW, Chim SS, Chan KC, Cheung JL, Liu EY, Tse GM, Lo AW, Lo YM, Ng HK (2004b). Tissue and cellular tropism of the coronavirus associated with severe acute respiratory syndrome: an in-situ hybridization study of fatal cases. *J Pathol* 202: 157–163.

Towler P, Staker B, Prasad SG, Menon S, Tang J, Parsons T, Ryan D, Fisher M, Williams D, Dales NA, Patane MA, Pantoliano MW (2004). ACE2 X-ray structures reveal a large hinge-bending motion important for inhibitor binding and catalysis. *J Biol Chem* 279: 17996–18007.

Traggiai E, Becker S, Subbarao K, Kolesnikova L, Uematsu Y, Gismondo MR, Murphy BR, Rappuoli R, Lanzavecchia A (2004). An efficient method to make human monoclonal antibodies from memory B cells: potent neutralization of SARS coronavirus. *Nat Med* 10: 871–875.

Tsai LK, Hsieh ST, Chao CC, Chen YC, Lin YH, Chang SC, Chang YC (2004). Neuromuscular disorders in severe acute respiratory syndrome. *Arch Neurol* 61: 1669–1673.

Tsang KW, Ho PL, Ooi GC, Yee WK, Wang T, Chan-Yeung M, Lam WK, Seto WH, Yam LY, Cheung TM, Wong PC, Lam B, Ip MS, Chan J, Yuen KY, Lai KN (2003). A cluster of cases of severe acute respiratory syndrome in Hong Kong. *N Engl J Med* 348: 1977–1985.

Tu C, Crameri G, Kong X, Chen J, Sun Y, Yu M, Xiang H, Xia X, Liu S, Ren T, Yu Y, Eaton BT, Xuan H, Wang LF (2004). Antibodies to SARS coronavirus in civets. *Emerg Infect Dis* 10: 2244–2248.

van den Brink EN, Ter Meulen J, Cox F, Jongeneelen MA, Thijsse A, Throsby M, Marissen WE, Rood PM, Bakker AB, Gelderblom HR, Martina BE, Osterhaus AD, Preiser W, Doerr HW, de Kruif J, Goudsmit J (2005). Molecular and biological characterization of human monoclonal antibodies binding to the spike and nucleocapsid proteins of severe acute respiratory syndrome coronavirus. *J Virol* 79: 1635–1644.

van der Hoek L, Pyrc K, Jebbink MF, Vermeulen-Oost W, Berkhout RJ, Wolthers KC, Wertheim-Van Dillen PM, Kaandorp J, Spaargaren J, Berkhout B (2004). Identification of a new human coronavirus. *Nat Med* 10: 368–373.

Varia M, Wilson S, Sarwal S, McGeer A, Gournis E, Galanis E, Henry B; Hospital Outbreak Investigation Team (2003). Investigation of a nosocomial outbreak of severe acute respiratory syndrome (SARS) in Toronto, Canada. *CMAJ* 19: 285–292.

von Grotthuss M, Wyrwicz LS, Rychlewski L (2003). mRNA cap-1 methyltransferase in the SARS genome. *Cell* 113: 701–702.

Wang H, Ding Y, Li X, Yang L, Zhang W, Kang W (2003a). Fatal aspergillosis in a patient with SARS who was treated with corticosteroids. *N Engl J Med* 349: 507–508.

Wang JL, Wang JT, Yu CJ, Chen YC, Hsueh PR, Hsiao CH, Kao CL, Chang SC, Yang PC (2003b). Rhabdomyolysis associated with probable SARS. *Am J Med* 15: 421–422.

Wang P, Chen J, Zheng A, Nie Y, Shi X, Wang W, Wang G, Luo M, Liu H, Tan L, Song X, Wang Z, Yin X, Qu X, Wang X, Qing T, Ding M, Deng H (2004a). Expression cloning of functional receptor used by SARS coronavirus. *Biochem Biophys Res Commun* 315: 439–444.

Wang S, Chou TH, Sakhatskyy PV, Huang S, Lawrence JM, Cao H, Huang X, Lu S (2005). Identification of two neutralizing regions on the severe acute respiratory syndrome coronavirus spike glycoprotein produced from the mammalian expression system. *J Virol* 79: 1906–1910.

Wang Z, Ren L, Zhao X, Hung T, Meng A, Wang J, Chen YG (2004b). Inhibition of severe acute respiratory syndrome virus replication by small interfering RNAs in mammalian cells. *J Virol* 78: 7523–7527.

Weingartl HM, Copps J, Drebot MA, Marszal P, Smith G, Gren J, Andova M, Pasick J, Kitching P, Czub M (2004a). Susceptibility of pigs and chickens to SARS coronavirus. *Emerg Infect Dis* 10: 179–184.

Weingartl H, Czub M, Czub S, Neufeld J, Marszal P, Gren J, Smith G, Jones S, Proulx R, Deschambault Y, Grudeski E, Andonov A, He R, Li Y, Copps J, Grolla A, Dick D, Berry J, Ganske S, Manning L, Cao J (2004b). Immunization with modified vaccinia virus Ankara-based recombinant vaccine against severe acute respiratory syndrome is associated with enhanced hepatitis in ferrets. *J Virol* 78: 12672–12676.

Wilson L, McKinlay C, Gage P, Ewart G (2004). SARS coronavirus E protein forms cation-selective ion channels. *Virology* 330: 322–331.

Wong CK, Lam CW, Wu AK, Ip WK, Lee NL, Chan IH, Lit LC, Hui DS, Chan MH, Chung SS, Sung JJ (2004). Plasma inflammatory cytokines and chemokines in severe acute respiratory syndrome. *Clin Exp Immunol* 136: 95–103.

Wong KC, Leung KS, Hui M (2003). Severe acute respiratory syndrome (SARS) in a geriatric patient with a hip fracture. A case report. *J Bone Joint Surg Am* 85A: 1339–1342.

Wong SF, Chow KM, Leung TN, Ng WF, Ng TK, Shek CC, Ng PC, Lam PW, Ho LC, To WW, Lai ST, Yan WW, Tan PY (2004). Pregnancy and perinatal outcomes of women with severe acute respiratory syndrome. *Am J Obstet Gynecol* 191: 292–297.

Woo PC, Lau SK, Tsoi HW, Chan KH, Wong BH, Che XY, Tam VK, Tam SC, Cheng VC, Hung IF, Wong SS, Zheng BJ, Guan Y, Yuen KY (2004). Relative rates of non-pneumonic SARS coronavirus infection and SARS coronavirus pneumonia. *Lancet* 363: 841–845.

Woo PC, Lau SK, Wong BH, Chan KH, Hui WT, Kwan GS, Peiris JS, Couch RB, Yuen KY (2004). False-positive results in a recombinant severe acute respiratory syndrome-associated coronavirus (SARS-CoV) nucleocapsid enzyme-linked immunosorbent assay due to HCoV-OC43 and HCoV-229E rectified by Western blotting with recombinant SARS-CoV spike polypeptide. *J Clin Microbiol* 42: 5885–5888.

World Health Organization (2003a). Summary of probable SARS cases with onset of illness from 1 November 2002 to 31 July 2003. Available at http://www.who.int/csr/sars/country/table2004_04_21/en/.

World Health Organization (2003b). Consensus document on the epidemiology of severe acute respiratory syndrome (SARS). Available at www.who.int/csr/sars/en/WHOconsensus.pdf.

World Health Organization (2003c). First data on stability and resistance of SARS coronavirus compiled by members of WHO laboratory network. Available at http://www.who.int/csr/sars/survival_2003_05_04/en/.

World Health Organization (2004). SARS situation update 5. Available at httptp://www.who.int/csr/don/2004_04_30/en/.

Wu CJ, Jan JT, Chen CM, Hsieh HP, Hwang DR, Liu HW, Liu CY, Huang HW, Chen SC, Hong CF, Lin RK, Chao YS, Hsu JT (2004a). Inhibition of severe acute respiratory syndrome coronavirus replication by niclosamide. *Antimicrob Agents Chemother* 48: 2693–2696.

Wu CY, Jan JT, Ma SH, Kuo CJ, Juan HF, Cheng YS, Hsu HH, Huang HC, Wu D, Brik A, Liang FS, Liu RS, Fang JM, Chen ST, Liang PH, Wong CH (2004b). Small molecules targeting severe acute respiratory syndrome human coronavirus. *Proc Natl Acad Sci U S A* 101: 10012–10017.

Wu D, Tu C, Xin C, Xuan H, Meng Q, Liu Y, Yu Y, Guan Y, Jiang Y, Yin X, Crameri G, Wang M, Li C, Liu S, Liao M, Feng L, Xiang H, Sun J, Chen J, Sun Y, Gu S, Liu N, Fu D, Eaton BT, Wang LF, Kong X (2005). Civets are equally susceptible to experimental infection by two different severe acute respiratory syndrome coronavirus isolates. *J Virol* 79: 2620–2625.

Wu EB, Sung JJ (2003). Haemorrhagic-fever-like changes and normal chest radiograph in a doctor with SARS. *Lancet* 361: 1520–1521.

Wu VC, Huang JW, Hsueh PR, Yang YF, Tsai HB, Kan WC, Chang HW, Wu KD (2005). Renal hypouricemia is an ominous sign in patients with severe acute respiratory syndrome. *Am J Kidney Dis* 45: 88–95.

Xiong B, Gui CS, Xu XY, Luo C, Chen J, Luo HB, Chen LL, Li GW, Sun T, Yu CY, Yue LD, Duan WH, Shen JK, Qin L, Shi TL, Li YX, Chen KX, Luo XM, Shen X, Shen JH, Jiang HL (2003). A 3D model of SARS-CoV 3CL proteinase and its inhibitors design by virtual screening. *Acta Pharmacol Sin* 24: 497–504.

Xu X, Liu Y, Weiss S, Arnold E, Sarafianos SG, Ding J (2003). Molecular model of SARS coronavirus polymerase: implications for biochemical functions and drug design. *Nucleic Acids Res* 31: 7117–7130.

Xu Y, Lou Z, Liu Y, Pang H, Tien P, Gao GF, Rao Z (2004). Crystal structure of SARS-CoV spike protein fusion core. *J Biol Chem* 279: 49414–49419.

Yamamoto N, Yang R, Yoshinaka Y, Amari S, Nakano T, Cinatl J, Rabenau H, Doerr HW, Hunsmann G, Otaka A, Tamamura H, Fujii N, Yamamoto N (2004). HIV protease inhibitor nelfinavir inhibits replication of SARS-associated coronavirus. *Biochem Biophys Res Commun* 318: 719–725.

Yang H, Yang M, Ding Y, Liu Y, Lou Z, Zhou Z, Sun L, Mo L, Ye S, Pang H, Gao GF, Anand K, Bartlam M, Hilgenfeld R, Rao Z (2003). The crystal structures of severe acute respiratory syndrome virus main protease and its complex with an inhibitor. *Proc Natl Acad Sci U S A* 100: 13190–13195.

Yang ZY, Huang Y, Ganesh L, Leung K, Kong WP, Schwartz O, Subbarao K, Nabel GJ (2004). pH-dependent entry of severe acute respiratory syndrome coronavirus is mediated by the spike glycoprotein and enhanced by dendritic cell transfer through DC-SIGN. *J Virol* 78: 5642–5650.

Yang ZY, Kong WP, Huang Y, Roberts A, Murphy BR, Subbarao K, Nabel GJ (2004). A DNA vaccine induces SARS coronavirus neutralization and protective immunity in mice. *Nature* 428: 561– 564.

Yeh SH, Wang HY, Tsai CY, Kao CL, Yang JY, Liu HW, Su IJ, Tsai SF, Chen DS, Chen PJ; National Taiwan University SARS Research Team (2004). Characterization of severe acute respiratory syndrome coronavirus genomes in Taiwan: molecular epidemiology and genome evolution. *Proc Natl Acad Sci U S A* 101: 2542–2547.

Yount B, Curtis KM, Fritz EA, Hensley LE, Jahrling PB, Prentice E, Denison MR, Geisbert TW, Baric RS (2003). Reverse genetics with a full-length infectious cDNA of severe acute respiratory syndrome coronavirus. *Proc Natl Acad Sci U S A* 100: 12995–13000.

Yu IT, Li Y, Wong TW, Tam W, Chan AT, Lee JH, Leung DY, Ho T (2004). Evidence of airborne transmission of the severe acute respiratory syndrome virus. *N Engl J Med* 350: 1731–1739.

Yuan K, Yi L, Chen J, Qu X, Qing T, Rao X, Jiang P, Hu J, Xiong Z, Nie Y, Shi X, Wang W, Ling C, Yin X, Fan K, Lai L, Ding M, Deng H (2004). Suppression of SARS-CoV entry by peptides corresponding to heptad regions on spike glycoprotein. *Biochem Biophys Res Commun* 319: 746–752.

Yudin MH, Steele DM, Sgro MD, Read SE, Kopplin P, Gough KA (2005). Severe acute respiratory syndrome in pregnancy. *Obstet Gynecol* 105: 124–127.

Zeng F, Chow KY, Hon CC, Law KM, Yip CW, Chan KH, Peiris JS, Leung FC (2004). Characterization of humoral responses in mice immunized with plasmid DNAs encoding SARS-CoV spike gene fragments. *Biochem Biophys Res Commun* 315: 1134–1139.

Zhang R, Guo Z, Lu J, Meng J, Zhou C, Zhan X, Huang B, Yu X, Huang M, Pan X, Ling W, Chen X, Wan Z, Zheng H, Yan X, Wang Y, Ran Y, Liu X, Ma J, Wang C, Zhang B (2003). Inhibiting severe acute respiratory syndrome-associated coronavirus by small interfering RNA. *Chin Med J (Engl)* 116: 1262–1264.

Zhang Y, Li T, Fu L, Yu C, Li Y, Xu X, Wang Y, Ning H, Zhang S, Chen W, Babiuk LA, Chang Z (2004a). Silencing SARS-CoV Spike protein expression in cultured cells by RNA interference. *FEBS Lett* 560: 141–146.

Zhang Z, Wang FS, Zhao M, Liu JC, Xu DP, Jin L, Chen JM, Wang M, Chu FL (2004b). Characterization of peripheral dendritic cell subsets and its implication in patients infected with severe acute respiratory syndrome. *Zhonghua Yi Xue Za Zhi* 84: 22–26.

Zhang H, Wang G, Li J, Nie Y, Shi X, Lian G, Wang W, Yin X, Zhao Y, Qu X, Ding M, Deng H (2004c). Identification of an antigenic determinant on the S2 domain of the severe acute respiratory syndrome coronavirus spike glycoprotein capable of inducing neutralizing antibodies. *J Virol* 78: 6938–6945.

Zhao P, Cao J, Zhao LJ, Qin ZL, Ke JS, Pan W, Ren H, Yu JG, Qi ZT (2005). Immune responses against SARS-coronavirus nucleocapsid protein induced by DNA vaccine. *Virology* 331: 128–135.

Zheng BJ, Wong KH, Zhou J, Wong KL, Young BW, Lu LW, Lee SS (2004a). SARS-related virus pre-dating SARS outbreak, Hong Kong. *Emerg Infect Dis* 10: 176–178.

Zheng B, He ML, Wong KL, Lum CT, Poon LL, Peng Y, Guan Y, Lin MC, Kung HF (2004b). Potent inhibition of SARS-associated coronavirus (SCOV) infection and replication by type I interferons (IFN-alpha/beta) but not by type II interferon (IFN-gamma). *J Interferon Cytokine Res* 24: 388–390.

Zheng BJ, Guan Y, Tang Q, Du C, Xie FY, He ML, Chan KW, Wong KL, Lader E, Woodle MC, Lu PY, Li B, Zhong N (2004c). Prophylactic and therapeutic effects of small interfering RNA targeting SARS-coronavirus. *Antivir Ther* 9: 365–374.

Zhong NS, Zheng BJ, Li YM, Poon, Xie ZH, Chan KH, Li PH, Tan SY, Chang Q, Xie JP, Liu XQ, Xu J, Li DX, Yuen KY, Peiris, Guan Y (2003). Epidemiology and cause of severe acute respiratory syndrome (SARS) in Guangdong, People's Republic of China, in February, 2003. *Lancet* 362: 1353–1358.

Zhu J, Xiao G, Xu Y, Yuan F, Zheng C, Liu Y, Yan H, Cole DK, Bell JI, Rao Z, Tien P, Gao GF (2004a). Following the rule: formation of the 6-helix bundle of the fusion core from severe acute respiratory syndrome coronavirus spike protein and identification of potent peptide inhibitors. *Biochem Biophys Res Commun* 319: 283–288.

Zhu MS, Pan Y, Chen HQ, Shen Y, Wang XC, Sun YJ, Tao KH (2004b). Induction of SARS-nucleoprotein-specific immune response by use of DNA vaccine. *Immunol Lett* 92: 237–243.

6. Newly Identified Human Herpesviruses: HHV-6, HHV-7, and HHV-8

LAURIE T. KRUG, CHONG-GEE TEO, KEIKO TANAKA-TAYA, AND NAOKI INOUE

Herpesviruses are enveloped, double-stranded DNA viruses that undergo DNA replication in the nucleus. The unique feature of the herpesviruses is the establishment of life-long latency after primary infection coupled with intermittent reactivation from latency in response to various stimuli and under certain immunological conditions. Subfamilies, designation, and disease associations of eight known human herpesviruses (HHVs) are summarized in Table 6.1. In this chapter, we describe three of these viruses, HHV-6, HHV-7, and HHV-8, all of which were identified in the past 20 years. These are not newly emerged viruses; rather, they have evolved with humans, stemming from a common herpesvirus ancestor approximately 200 million years ago (McGeoch et al., 2000). The three viruses share many properties with other herpesviruses with respect to virion structure, genetic contents, and the temporal pattern of gene expression during the productive replication cycle, and yet each has novel strategies for persisting in particular niches of the host. The NCBI website (www.ncbi.nlm.nih.gov/ genomes/ VIRUSES/10292.html) provides the details of their genome structures and coding contents. The betaherpesviruses HHV-6 and -7 are prevalent in normal populations. HHV-6 is classified into two variants, HHV-6A and -6B, which are closely related but show distinct biological and genetic characteristics (Ablashi et al., 1993). HHV-7 and HHV-6B but not HHV-6A cause roseola infantum (exanthem subitum; ES), a mild childhood illness (Fig. 6.1A). In contrast, the gammaherpesvirus member HHV-8, also known as Kaposi's sarcoma–associated herpesvirus (KSHV), is less prevalent in immunocompetent individuals. It is known as the etiologic agent of Kaposi's sarcoma (KS)

Table 6.1. Pathogenic profiles of human herpesviruses (HHVs)

Subfamily	Genus	ICTV name	Commonly used	Primary infection	Reactivation/ chronic infection
				Disease association	
Alpha	Simplexvirus	HHV-1	HSV-1	Neonatal infections, oral lesion, encephalitis	
		HHV-2	HSV-2	Genital lesions, encephalitis	
	Varicellovirus	HHV-3	VZV	Varicella	Zoster
Beta	Cytomegalovirus	HHV-5	HCMV	Congenital diseases	Multisystem diseases
	Roseolovirus	HHV-6		Exanthem subitum	Encephalitis
		HHV-7		Exanthem subitum	
Gamma	Lympho-cryptovirus	HHV-4	EBV	IM	BL, NPC, gastric carcinoma
	Rhadinovirus	HHV-8	HHV-8/ KSHV		KS, PEL, MCD

IM, infectious mononucleosis; BL, Burkitt lymphoma; NPC, nasopharyngeal carcinoma; KS, Kaposi's sarcoma; PEL, primary effusion lymphoma; MCD, multicentric Castleman's disease.

(Fig. 6.1B–1D) and primary effusion lymphoma (PEL). Here we focus mainly on their novel biological properties and relate them to the epidemiology, the pathogenesis, and the clinical manifestations of the diseases they cause.

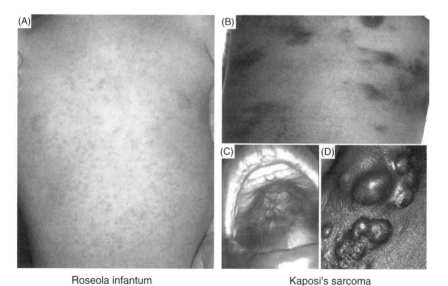

Roseola infantum   Kaposi's sarcoma

Figure 6.1. Roseola infantum in a child (A). Kaposi's sarcoma (KS) on the trunk (B), on the palate (C), and behind the ear (D). (Courtesy of Dr. Clifford J. Gunthel, Emory University, Atlanta, Georgia [B, D], and Dr. Tim Hodgson, Eastman Institute of Oral Health Care Sciences, London [C]).

6.1. HHV-6 and HHV-7

6.1.1. Biology

6.1.1.1. Cell Tropism and Viral Entry

HHV-6 and -7 grow well in stimulated primary T cells *in vitro,* and several isolates have been adapted for growth in T-cell lines. HHV-6 can also infect fibroblasts, endothelial cells, epithelial cells, and immune cell types, including natural killer (NK) cells, monocyte/macrophages, and dendritic cells (DCs). Reports of HHV-6 infection of neural cell types, including astrocytes, glial precursor cells, and oligodendrocytes are intriguing, because oligodendrocytes are the neural cells responsible for myelin production and are the primary target cells in demyelinating diseases such as multiple sclerosis (Lusso et al., 1993; He et al., 1996; Albright et al., 1998; Pauk et al., 2001; Dietrich et al., 2004). HHV-6A is more neurovirulent than HHV-6B (Hall et al., 1998), and it replicates more efficiently in primary oligodendrocytes (De Bolle et al., 2005).

HHV-6 and -7 may persist in a wide range of tissues in infected individuals. HHV-6 has been detected in CD4+ lymphocytes (Takahashi et al., 1989) and in monocytes/macrophages (Kondo et al., 2002a) obtained from ES patients. Other tissues include brain, liver, salivary glands, and endothelium. HHV-6 and -7 latently infect early bone marrow progenitor cells to be transmitted longitudinally to cells that differentiate along the committed pathways (Luppi et al., 1999; Mirandola et al., 2000). HHV-7 structural antigens are detectable in the lungs, skin, mammary glands, liver, kidney, and tonsils (Kempf et al., 1998). HHV-6 and -7 are likely transmitted via saliva as they can be isolated from saliva of normal adult individuals (Black et al., 1993; Harnett et al., 1990).

The entry of most herpesviruses proceeds in two phases: (i) binding of the virion to the cell surface, mainly to glycosaminoglycans on the plasma membrane, and (ii) membrane fusion between the virion envelope and cell membrane via interactions between viral glycoproteins and cellular receptors. Heparin and heparan sulfate inhibit HHV-6 binding to the cell surface less efficiently than herpes simplex virus type 1 (HSV-1) binding, and treatment of cells with heparitinase and heparinase has little effect on HHV-6 binding (Conti et al., 2000). HHV-7 glycoprotein B (gB) binds to heparin and heparan sulfate on the cell surface (Secchiero et al., 1997).

Both variants of HHV-6 utilize the complement regulator CD46 (membrane cofactor protein) as a receptor for cell–cell fusion and entry into cells (Santoro et al., 1999). All four CD46 isoforms can be used as a receptor. In contrast with measles virus glycoproteins that depend strictly on the short consensus repeat (SCR) regions 1 and 2 in the extracellular portion of CD46, HHV-6 glycoproteins interact with SCRs 2 and 3 but not SCRs 1 or 4 (Greenstone et al., 2002). Like other herpesviruses, HHV-6 encodes multiple glycoproteins that often form complexes with other viral glycoproteins. gH forms a complex with gL and binds to CD46 (Santoro et al., 2003). The gH–gL complex associates with a third component, gQ or gO (Mori et al., 2003, 2004). gO is encoded by U47, a positional homolog of human cytomegalovirus (HCMV) gO. gQ, which is unique to HHV-6, is encoded by U100. The U100 products of HHV-6A have been reported to form the gp82–105 complex, which is a major virion component and a target for neutralizing antibodies (Pfeiffer et al., 1995). The HHV-6A gH–gL–gQ complex but not the gH–gL–gO complex binds to CD46 (Mori et al., 2004). There are two forms of gQ, gQ1 and gQ2, and the gH–gL–gQ complex contains both forms of gQ to generate a tetrameric complex (Akkapaiboon et al., 2004). The HHV-6A and -6B gO and gQ gene products have much lower intravariant identity than the other glycoproteins, suggesting that gO and gQ may account for the difference in cell tropism. The cellular receptor for HHV-6A and -6B gH–gL–gO complexes has yet to be identified.

HHV-7 utilizes CD4 as a component of the receptor for entry and interferes with infection by HIV, which also uses CD4 as a receptor (Lusso et al., 1994). HHV-7 gp65, a positional homolog of HHV-6 gp105 (gQ), binds to heparan sulfate proteoglycans. Antiserum against gp65 neutralizes HHV-7 infection, suggesting that gp65 is involved in the viral entry process (Skrincosky et al., 2000). The HHV-7 glycoprotein that mediates CD4-dependent entry remains unknown. Because some of the cell lines expressing surface CD4 by adenovirus gene transfer do not support HHV-7 replication (Yasukawa et al., 1997) and because the chemokine receptors CXCR4 and CCR5 are the main coreceptors for T lymphocyte–tropic and macrophage-tropic HIV-1, respectively, the possibility of these molecules being used as coreceptors for HHV-7 has been analyzed. Although HHV-7 downregulates surface expression of CXCR4, anti-CXCR4 treatment does not block infection (Yasukawa et al., 1999a; Zhang et al., 2000). This indicates that HHV-7 infection does not require CXCR4. HHV-7 infects CCR5-deficient cells, indicating that CCR5 is also not required for entry (Yasukawa et al., 1999a). Therefore, additional cellular factors for HHV-7 entry remain to be identified.

6.1.1.2. Gene Expression and Replication

HHV-6 and -7 share the common features of the herpesvirus lytic replication cycle after entry: (i) HHV-6 and -7 nucleocapsids are transported to nuclear pore complexes, (ii) the viral genomes are released into the nucleoplasm, (iii) the genomes circularize (Severini et al., 2003), (iv) viral genes are expressed in a regulated, temporal cascade (Oster and Hollsberg, 2002), (v) viral genomes replicate, leading to (vi) encapsidation, maturation, and egress of progeny virions. Figure 6.2 shows the ultrastructual characteristics of HHV-6B–infected cells and HHV-6B virions.

There are two unusual features of HHV-6 and -7 replication. Unlike HCMV, HHV-6 and -7 share a feature of alphaherpesviruses by their encoding of an origin-binding protein (OBP) that plays a key role in recognition of the viral lytic origin and initiation of DNA replication processes (Dewhurst et al., 1993; Inoue et al., 1994; Krug et al., 2001b). There is a slight difference in the consensus origin sequence and affinity for binding OBP among HSV-1, HHV-6, and HHV-7 (Inoue and Pellett, 1995; Krug et al., 2001a) but the mechanisms for initiating DNA replication are likely conserved. Another unique feature is that HHV-6 glycoproteins are not detected on the plasma membrane (Cirone et al., 1994; Torrisi et al., 1999), suggesting that the intracellular maturation pathway of HHV-6 is different from other herpesviruses. This absence of the viral glycoproteins on the cell surface may represent an immune evasion strategy by HHV-6.

6.1.1.3. Latency and Reactivation

HHV-6 and -7 establish latency in monocytes/macrophages *in vitro* (Kondo et al., 1991; Kempf et al., 1997). Treatment of latently-infected cells with phorbol ester (Kondo et al., 1991) or by superinfection with

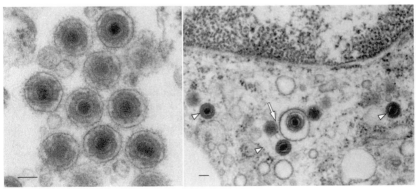

Bar=100nm

⇒ A virion in a vacuole of the cytoplasm

▷ Immature virus particles in the cytoplasm

Figure 6.2. Ultrastructual characteristics of HHV-6 virions and infected cells. (Courtesy of Drs. Mariko Yoshida and Masao Yamada, Okayama University, Japan.)

HHV-7 (Katsafanas et al., 1996) reactivates HHV-6 from latency. Four latency-associated transcripts (LTs) of HHV-6 have been identified. Although the transcripts are in the same orientation as the immediate-early 1 and 2 (IE1/IE2) genes and share their protein-coding region with IE1/IE2, their transcription start sites and exon(s) differ from lytic transcripts (Kondo et al., 2002b). LTs are maximally expressed at a fairly stable intermediate stage between latency and reactivation both *in vitro* and *in vivo*. Products encoded by the abundantly expressed LTs can have an ability to reactivate latently-infected virus (Kondo et al., 2003). The regulation of LT expression and other features of HHV-6 latency are similar to what has been described for HCMV. HHV-6B but not -6A has established latency in two novel Philadelphia chromosome–positive myeloid cell lines that manifest different hematologic characteristics. Phorbol ester treatment reactivates HHV-6 from one of the latently-infected cells (Yasukawa et al., 1999b). These novel cell lines can serve as useful models of HHV-6 latency and reactivation.

The site of latent HHV-6 and -7 infections *in vivo* is not completely clear. HHV-7 is readily isolated from lymph nodes but not the spleens of AIDS patients, suggesting the lymph nodes as a site of latency (Kempf et al., 2000). HHV-7 is reactivated from latently-infected peripheral blood mononuclear cells (PBMCs) by T-cell activation; however, HHV-6B cannot be reactivated under similar conditions (Katsafanas et al., 1996). Because monocytes have a short life span, reactivation may play a critical role in virus persistence. Alternatively, latently-infected early bone marrow progenitors may support HHV-6 growth upon differentiation. CD34+ cells obtained from peripheral blood under conditions that permit differentiation toward the myeloid lineage lead to cell expansion and HHV-6 reactivation (Andre-Garnier et al., 2004).

Generally, herpesvirus genomes are maintained as extrachromosomal episomes during latency. The HHV-6 genome has been found to integrate into host cell chromosomes preferentially at the telomeric regions of chromosome 1, 17, and 22, but integration is an uncommon event (Luppi et al., 1994; Torelli et al., 1995; Daibata et al., 1998, 1999; Tanaka-Taya et al., 2004). A few familial cases containing the HHV-6 genome integrated at the same chromosomal locations suggest germline transmission of the genome (Daibata et al., 1999; Tanaka-Taya et al., 2004). Treatment of a cell line containing chromosomally integrated HHV-6 with phorbol ester, sodium *n*-butyrate, or a calcium ionophore can induce HHV-6 gene expression (Daibata et al., 1998), but the production of progeny virus has not been demonstrated. HHV-6, but not HHV-7, encodes U94, a homolog of the adeno-associated virus (AAV) *rep* product that functions to mediate site-specific DNA integration of AAV into chromosomes. It is an intriguing possibility that U94 mediates the integration. U94 is expressed at low levels during lytic replication (Mori et al., 2000; Rapp et al., 2000). Overexpression of the HHV-6 U94 product in T cells represses HHV-6 replication, pointing to a potential role in HHV-6 latency (Rotola et al., 1998). Although U94 has ssDNA-binding activity, it does not specifically bind to AAV terminal repeats, to which the AAV2 rep products bind (Dhepakson et al., 2002), nor does it exhibit an increased efficiency of transduction of AAV vectors (Inoue, Krug, and Pellett, unpublished).

6.1.1.4. Immune Responses and Immune Evasion

Cell-mediated immune responses against HHV-6 are generally present in healthy individuals (Wang et al., 1999a), and T-cell clones against HHV-6 have been isolated (Yasukawa et al., 1993). During the acute febrile phase of HHV-6 infection, there is a significant increase in interferon (IFN)-α levels and NK cytotoxicity as compared with the convalescent stage (Takahashi et al., 1992). Upregulated IL-15 expression in HHV-6–infected cells increases NK activity (Flamand et al., 1996). Studies of the immune response against HHV-7 have been very limited.

Expression of viral homologs of cytokines, chemokines, and their receptors constitutes an important strategy for host immune evasion. HHV-6 U83 encodes a CC chemokine ligand (CCL) (Zou et al., 1999), which functions as a highly selective and efficacious agonist for the human CC chemokine receptor 2 (CCR2), driving signal transduction and inducing chemotaxis (Luttichau et al., 2003). Because macrophages and lymphocytes express CCR2, the U83 product might attract these cells as targets for HHV-6 infection and establishment of latency. HHV-6 and HHV-7 U12 and U51 are positional homologs of HCMV UL33 and UL78, respectively, and encode seven transmembrane glycoproteins with similarity to G protein–coupled chemokine receptors (GPCR). The HHV-6 U51 product expressed in epithelial cells binds specifically to CCL5 (RANTES) and induces morphological alteration of the cells (Milne et al., 2000). It is likely that the cell surface expression of U51 requires a T-cell specific function (Menotti et al., 1999). HHV-6 and HHV-7 U12 encode functional β-chemokine receptors with a significant similarity to CCR-3 and CCR-7 (EBI1), respectively. HHV-6 U12 is activated by CCL-5, macrophage inflammatory protein 1α (MIP-1α), MIP-1β, and monocyte chemoattractant protein 1 (MCP-1), but not by the α-chemokine interleukin-8 (IL-8) (Isegawa et al., 1998). HHV-7 U12 specifically responds to the EBI1 ligand chemokine, MIP-3β. The biological roles of these CCL and CCR homologs of HHV-6 and HHV-7 in their replication and pathological effects *in vivo* are not yet fully elucidated.

Modulation of MHC class I (MHC-I) antigen presentation is another mechanism for immune evasion exploited by HHV-6 and -7 that is also employed by HCMV (reviewed in Hewitt, 2003). The HHV-7 glycoprotein encoded by U21 binds to and diverts properly folded MHC-I molecules to a lysosomal compartment (Hudson et al., 2001). The suppression of *de novo* synthesis of MHC-I reported for HHV-6A but not for HHV-6B requires the expression of HHV-6 IE or early genes (Hirata et al., 2001).

Activation or suppression of host gene expression for cytokines, chemokine, and immunomodulatory molecules is a third mechanism that HHV-6 and -7 employ to modulate the immune response and to create an environment suitable for viral replication and survival. HHV-6A and -6B increase the expression of proinflammatory and chemokine genes in T cells and in endothelial cells and decrease expression of anti-inflammatory genes (Hasegawa et al., 1994; Mayne et al., 2001; Caruso et al., 2002, 2003). HHV-6 infection also induces the expression of cyclooxygenase-2 (COX-2), a cellular enzyme critical for the inflammatory response (Janelle et al., 2002); however, its biological consequence remains to be determined.

6.1.1.5. Pathogenesis

HHV-6 infection has been associated with bone marrow suppression (Drobyski et al., 1993; Carrigan and Knox, 1994). Several *in vitro* infection experiments have demonstrated the effects of HHV-6 infection in lymphoid cells and bone marrow hematopoietic cells (Knox and Carrigan, 1992; Burd et al., 1993; Isomura et al., 1997, 2000, 2003). Both HHV-6A and -6B can infect human tonsil tissue fragments productively in the absence of exogenous stimulation. The majority of cells expressing viral antigens are CD4+ T lymphocytes of a non-naive phenotype, while CD8+ T cells are efficiently infected with HHV-6A but not with HHV-6B (Grivel et al., 2003). HHV-6B suppresses colony formation of granulocyte/macrophage colony-forming units (CFU-GM), erythroid burst-forming units (BFU-E), and megakaryocyte colony-forming units (CFU-Meg) *in vitro* in a dose-dependent manner. HHV-6A suppresses the formation of CFU-Meg and BFU-E colonies but not CFU-GM as efficiently as HHV-6B. However, HHV-7 has no effect on hematopoietic colony formation. The more differentiated CD34+ cells are more susceptible to the suppressive effects of HHV-6 on their growth (Isomura et al., 1997, 2000, 2003). HHV-6 infection of monocyte-derived immature DCs, which are professional antigen-presenting cells, also induces maturation of DCs as well as impairs their capacity for the presentation of alloantigens and exogenous virus antigens but not HLA class II–binding peptides to T lymphocytes (Kakimoto et al., 2002). Exposure of human macrophages to HHV-6A or -6B profoundly impairs their ability to produce IL-12 upon stimulation with IFN-γ and lipopolysaccharide (LPS), representing a novel potential mechanism of HHV-6–mediated immunosuppression (Smith et al., 2003).

6.1.1.6. Animal Models

The lack of a reliable and simple animal model has hampered studies of HHV-6 pathogenesis. Using a degenerate consensus primer PCR method for amplifying the herpesvirus DNA polymerase gene, the presence of a simian HHV-6 homolog, MndHVβ, has been found in mandrill monkeys (Lacoste et al., 2000), but isolation of the virus has not been reported yet. Experimental infection of African green monkeys with HHV-6 has resulted in appearance of a rash in one monkey but asymptomatic infection in other monkeys (Yalcin et al., 1992).

HHV-6 infection destroys human thymic tissue implanted in SCID-hu Thy/Liv mice. The depletion of thymocytes by HHV-6 may be due to infection and destruction of immature T cell precursors (Gobbi et al., 1999).

6.1.2. Epidemiology

6.1.2.1. Primary Infection

Clinical manifestations of primary HHV-6B and HHV-7 infections include roseola infantum (exanthem subitum; ES) (Yamanishi et al., 1988; Tanaka et al., 1994) (Fig. 6.1A) and non-specific febrile illnesses (Pruksananonda et al., 1992; Hall et al., 1994; Torigoe et al., 1995). An illness caused by HHV-6A has yet to be clearly identified.

HHV-6 and HHV-7 infections are widespread and common throughout the world (e.g., Saxinger et al., 1988; Okuno et al., 1989; Black et al., 1996; Nielsen and Vestergaard, 1996). Seroepidemiological investigations show that most children have antibody to HHV-6 before 2 years of age (Okuno et al., 1989; Yoshikawa et al., 1989; Huang et al., 1992; Hall et al., 1994). In contrast, HHV-7 infects children somewhat later in childhood (Wyatt et al., 1991; Tanaka-Taya et al., 1996; Caserta et al., 1998). When HHV-7 infection occurs in patients seropositive for HHV-6, an increase in HHV-6 antibody can be observed (Tanaka-Taya et al., 2000), which is consistent with HHV-7 reactivation of HHV-6 *in vitro* described in Section 6.1.1.3.

In a large prospective study in the United States (US), the number of febrile children who presented to the emergency department of a hospital due to primary HHV-6 infection peaked at 6–8 months of age (Pruksananonda et al., 1992). The National Epidemiological Surveillance of Infectious Diseases (NESID) in Japan shows that >95% of ES, reflecting HHV-6 or HHV-7 primary infection, occurs in the first year of life (Fig. 6.3). Monthly reports of NESID reveal that ES is not seasonal or cyclical. In Japan, there has been a gradual shift in age of primary infection during the past 20 years.

6.1.2.2. Transmission

Although the modes of transmission of HHV-6 remain unclear, saliva is most likely the major vehicle for transmission. HHV-6B and -7 have been found frequently in the secretions of asymptomatic individuals, including parents and siblings, suggesting horizontal infection from people living closely with infants (Tanaka-Taya et al., 1996; Zerr et al., 2005b). Occasional outbreaks of HHV-6 infection have also been observed in institutions for children (Okuno et al., 1991).

HHV-6 DNA can be detected in the cervix and in the female genital tract, suggesting perinatal transmission (Leach et al., 1994; Okuno et al., 1995). Congenital HHV-6, but not HHV-7, infection occurs asymptomatically in about 1% of births, similar to the rate for HCMV infection (Hall et al., 2004). Follow-up studies are required to see whether asymptomatic infants have any subsequent developmental deficits, like congenital HCMV infection. Breast-feeding has been ruled out as a major source of HHV-6 during infancy (Kusuhara et al., 1997; Fujisaki et al., 1998).

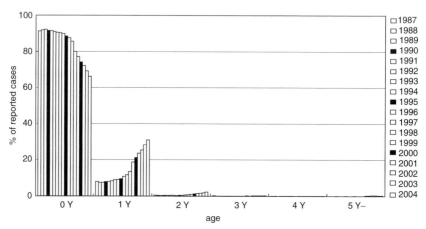

Figure 6.3. Yearly incidence of exanthem subitum by age group, 1987–2004, Japan. (Source: National Epidemiological Surveillance of Infectious Diseases [NESID] in Japan.)

6.1.2.3. *Proposed Disease Associations*

6.1.2.3.1. Multiple Sclerosis (MS). MS is a chronic progressive neurological disorder that results from an interaction of genetic and environmental factors. Several herpesviruses have been proposed as triggers of MS, with HHV-6 identified as a leading candidate (Challoner et al., 1995). Nonetheless, findings from studies of the association between HHV-6 and MS have been contradictory. A more rigorous standardization of methodology and case definition is required to establish a definitive link between HHV-6 and MS (reviewed in Clark, 2004).

6.1.2.3.2. Chronic Fatigue Syndrome (CFS). CFS is characterized by persistent debilitating fatigue and is accompanied by symptoms that include neurocognitive problems, musculoskeletal pain, sore throat, and lymphadenitis (Fukuda et al., 1994). The pathophysiology of CFS involves a cytokine imbalance in the central nervous system and in the circulation. Many patients with CFS report having influenza-like illnesses prior to the onset of disease, suggesting that CFS, or at least a subset of cases of CFS, may be associated with viral infection (Komaroff, 1988). However, a vigorous case control study did not support an etiological role for HHV-6 or -7 in CFS (Reeves et al., 2000).

6.1.2.3.3. Pityriasis Rosea (PR). PR is an acute exanthematous inflammatory skin disease long suspected to be due to viral infection. Although some reports have proposed an association of HHV-6 or -7 with PR (Drago et al., 1997; Watanabe et al., 2002), it remains controversial (reviewed in Chuh et al., 2004).

6.1.3. Clinical Spectrum

6.1.3.1. *Exanthem Subitum (Roseola)*

Patients with ES (Fig. 6.1A) typically develop a high fever at onset (38–40°C) that lasts for about 2–3 days, which then defervesces abruptly. The defervescence is accompanied by a maculopapular rash. The rash consists of bright-red spotted papulae without pigmentation, appearing on the face, trunk, and limbs, and lasts for several days. Accompanying symptoms include swelling of the eyelid, lymph node enlargement, diarrhea, and bulging of the anterior fontanel. Prognosis is generally good, although febrile convulsions frequently result (Suga et al., 2000). Occasionally, severe complications such as encephalitis/encephalopathy, fulminant hepatitis, and thrombocytopenic purpura can occur.

6.1.3.2. Encephalitis

As described in Section 6.1.1.1., HHV-6 is neurotropic. HHV-6 DNA can be detected in the CSF for up to 5 days after onset of ES, suggesting that HHV-6 invades the CNS during the acute phase. It has also been suggested that febrile convulsions may reactivate HHV-6 (Kondo et al., 1993). HHV-6 is present in the brain tissue of healthy individuals and is associated with the development of neurological complications in many patient groups, including bone marrow transplant (BMT) recipients, liver transplant recipients, and immunocompetent hosts of all ages. These manifestations include febrile seizures and encephalitis.

HHV-7 infection in childhood can lead to a febrile illness complicated by seizures (Caserta et al., 1998). Infection may also be associated with febrile convulsions and encephalitis (Pohl-Koppe et al., 2001; Chan et al., 2004).

6.1.3.3. Post-transplantation Disease

Reactivation of latent HHV-6 mainly occurs in immunocompromised hosts, such as transplant recipients and patients with AIDS. The importance of HHV-6 as a pathogen or co-pathogen in viral syndromes after solid organ and bone marrow transplantation has become increasingly apparent. Besides leading to encephalitis and bone marrow suppression in these patients, HHV-6 upon reactivation or reinfection can also interact with other herpesviruses such as HCMV and HHV-7 to exert indirect immunologic effects that may lead to allograft rejection or facilitate bacterial or fungal infections (reviewed in Clark, 2002).

6.1.3.3.1. Stem Cell Transplantation (SCT). HHV-6 infection is frequently observed after allogeneic SCT (Wang et al., 1996; Imbert-Marcille et al., 2000; Ljungman et al., 2000; Yoshikawa et al., 2002), which can lead to the following outcomes: delayed monocyte and platelet engraftment, increased platelet transfusion requirements, all-cause mortality, graft-versus-host disease (GVHD), and neurological dysfunction (Zerr et al., 2005a). Reactivation in the recipients and infection from the seropositive donor bone marrow are two likely sources of the infection (Cone et al., 1999). Allogenic peripheral blood SCT may be preferred to allogenic BMT to avoid HHV-6 reactivation and subsequent complications (Maeda et al., 1999). Although cord blood SCT (CBSCT) has become a popular treatment modality, HHV-6 infection has been identified more frequently, and associated with a higher circulating viral load in CBSCT as compared with BMT and peripheral blood SCT. Because CBSCT recipients are mainly infants and children, many of whom may be experiencing primary HHV-6 infection shortly before transplantation, monitoring for active HHV-6 infection in these patients has been advocated (Sashihara et al., 2002). Administration of anti-CD3 monoclonal antibody for prophylaxis of acute GVHD increases the risk of HHV-6 reactivation (Jacobs et al., 1994; Zerr et al., 2001).

Similar to HHV-6, HHV-7 has been detected at a significantly higher frequency in allogeneic as compared with autologous SCT (Miyoshi et al., 2001) and in umbilical cord or marrow compared with peripheral blood transplants (Chan et al., 2004). Treatment with acyclovir has not been observed to exert an effect on the rate of HHV-7 reactivation, but treatment with ganciclovir may be associated with a lower rate (Chan et al., 2004). One patient succumbed to HHV-7–associated brain-stem encephalitis, and another developed HHV-7–associated meningitis and optic neuritis, both after allogeneic SCT (Yoshikawa et al., 2003; Chan et al., 2004).

6.1.3.3.2. Solid Organ Transplantation. HHV-6 and -7 infections are important causes of morbidity after solid organ transplantation. HHV-6 infection occurs frequently in liver and renal transplant recipients usually within 2–4 weeks after the procedure (Okuno et al., 1990; Yoshikawa et al., 1992; Yalcin et al., 1994; Hoshino et al., 1995; Dockrell et al., 1997; Griffiths et al., 1999; Rossi et al., 2001; Humar et al., 2002; Deborska et al., 2003). Invasive HHV-6 infection after transplantation may be associated with fever (Yoshikawa et al., 2000), encephalitis or encephalopathy (Paterson et al., 1999; Montejo et al., 2002; Feldstein et al., 2003), bone marrow suppression (Singh et al., 1997), and graft dysfunction and rejection (Lautenschlager et al., 2000; Feldstein et al., 2003; Hoshino et al., 1995). More severe disease has been noted after primary HHV-6 infection, rather than reactivation, in pediatric liver transplant patients, and, in one study, none of the recipients were observed to develop a rash during primary HHV-6 infection (Yoshikawa et al., 2001). An association between HHV-6 or HHV-7 infection and severe CMV diseases has been observed in both renal and liver transplant recipients (Dockrell et al., 1997; Osman et al., 1996; Ratnamohan et al., 1998; DesJardin et al., 1998, 2001; Kidd et al., 2000; Tong et al., 2000).

HHV-6 infection should be differentiated from graft rejection, as recipients with primary HHV-6 infection or reactivation may present with sustained fever of unknown origin and transient allograft dysfunction. HHV-6 infection has been associated with increased expression of adhesion molecules and lymphocyte infiltration in liver allografts (Lautenschlager et al., 2002), which suggests that the persistent immunological response in the graft impairs the liver functions and triggers the rejection. HHV-6 infection of renal tissues may predispose grafts for rejection (Okuno et al., 1990).

6.1.4. Management and Prevention

6.1.4.1. Antivirals

Ganciclovir, foscarnet, and cidofovir but not acyclovir are effective against HHV-6 and HHV-7 infection *in vitro* (Yoshida et al., 1998; Manichanh et al., 2000; De Clercq et al., 2001). Ganciclovir and foscarnet, either alone or in combination, may be used for the management of HHV-6–related neurological disease. Foscarnet, unlike ganciclovir, may be effective against HHV-7–related CNS disease but this requires further evaluation through prospective clinical trials. Recently, cidofovir has been found to be useful for the treatment of HHV-6 encephalitis among immunocompetent adults (Denes et al., 2004).

6.1.4.2. Transplantation Management

Among children, determination of the preoperative HHV-6 antibody status in potential recipients as well as their donors is useful to evaluate the risk of primary infection. Post-transplantation diagnosis of HHV-6 infection is based on the detection of plasma HHV-6 DNA, isolation of HHV-6, and/or detection of HHV-6 IgM antibody.

The occurrence of HHV-6 infection should be monitored for up to 4 weeks, especially during the 2- to 3-week period after transplantation. Ganciclovir or foscarnet has been used for the treatment of HHV-6–related neurological diseases in transplant recipients (Mookerjee and Vogelsang, 1997; Cole et al., 1998; Bethge et al., 1999; Paterson et al., 1999; Tokimasa et al., 2002; Yoshida et al., 2002; Zerr et al., 2002; Nash et al., 2004). Prophylactic treatment of BMT recipients with ganciclovir was found more effective against HHV-6 reactivation than the treatment with acyclovir (Rapaport et al., 2002). However, the prophylactic administration of ganciclovir to prevent HHV-6 reactivation may only be appropriate for patients at high risk for HHV-6–related manifestations, because ganciclovir can cause bone marrow suppression. Treatment with ganciclovir was associated with a lower rate of HHV-7 reactivation, whereas acyclovir had no effect (Chan et al., 2004). Rational strategies for prophylaxis of HHV-6 and -7 infections in transplant recipients require further studies.

6.2. HHV-8

6.2.1. Biology

6.2.1.1. Cell Tropism and Viral Entry

Multiple cell types, including B cells, endothelial cells, epithelial cells, fibroblast cells, and keratinocytes, are susceptible to HHV-8 infection *in vitro* (Mesri et al., 1996; Moore et al., 1996b; Foreman et al., 1997; Flore et al., 1998; Kliche et al., 1998; Renne et al., 1998; Moses et al., 1999; Cerimele et al., 2001; Ciufo et al., 2001). Infection is predominantly latent with a low level of lytic infection. HHV-8 infection of endothelial cells *in vitro* induces a change in morphology from a cobblestone to spindle-shaped cell pattern (Fig. 6.4). Treatment with phorbol ester as well as infection with HCMV and with HHV-6 activates lytic replication in the latently-infected cells (Vieira et al., 2001; Vieira and O'Hearn, 2004; Lu et al., 2005). The generation of infectious virus for in vitro studies depends on PEL cell lines (Arvanitakis et al., 1996; Mesri et al., 1996; Renne et al., 1996).

HHV-8 gB and K8.1 mediate the initial binding of virions to glycosaminoglycans, such as heparan sulfate, on cell surfaces (Akula et al., 2001; Birkmann et al., 2001; Wang et al., 2001a). However, K8.1 is dispensable for virus entry (Luna et al., 2004). HHV-8 gB, gH, and gL can mediate cell fusion, suggesting their involvement in the entry process (Pertel, 2002). Integrin $\alpha3\beta1$ functions as a cellular receptor for entry (Akula et al., 2002). HHV-8 gB interacts with integrin $\alpha3\beta1$ and induces the integrin-dependent focal adhesion kinase (FAK)-Src-phosphatidylinositol 3-kinase-Rho GTPase signal pathways and cytoskeletal rearrangements (Sharma-Walia et al., 2004). HHV-8 enters fibroblasts and epithelial cells by a pH-dependent endocytosis pathway (Akula et al., 2003; Inoue et al., 2003). Infection in the presence of polybrene may bypass the integrin $\alpha3\beta1$ receptor usage (Inoue et al., 2003). The expression of HIV Tat and the oncogene Raf enhances the early phase of infection (Akula et al., 2004; Aoki and Tosato, 2004).

6.2.1.2. Latency and Reactivation

In contrast with other herpesviruses, HHV-8 infection *in vitro* is characterized by the concurrent expression of latent and a limited number

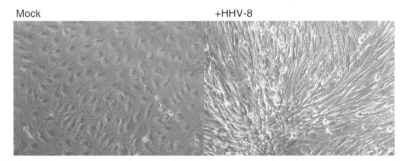

Figure 6.4. Morphologic changes in primary human dermal microvascular endothelial cells 14 days after infection with HHV-8. Magnification, ×100. (Courtesy of Dr. Margaret K. Offermann, Emory University, Atlanta, Georgia.)

of lytic genes immediately after infection and a subsequent decline or absence of lytic gene expression. Restricted expression of lytic cycle genes during the initial phases of infection may contribute to immune evasion (Krishnan et al., 2004). Latently-infected cells maintain HHV-8 genome as an episome and express latency-associated nuclear antigen (LANA) encoded by ORF73 and a few other latent gene products. LANA is essential for maintenance of the latent episome through tethering of the viral genome to host chromosomes (Ballestas et al., 1999; Cotter and Robertson, 1999; Ye et al., 2004). The importance of LANA for establishment of latency *in vivo* is demonstrated in an animal model using a mutant of murine gammaherpesvirus 68 (γHV68) (Fowler et al., 2003; Moorman et al., 2003b).

Under certain cell culture conditions, HHV-8 can be induced to undergo lytic replication. The replication and transcription activator (RTA), encoded by ORF50, plays a critical role in switching from latent to lytic replication. Overexpression of RTA is sufficient for the initiation of lytic replication and the production of viral progeny (Lukac et al., 1998; Sun et al., 1998; Xu et al., 2005). RTA binds to several viral promoters in a sequence-specific fashion (Lukac et al., 2001; Song et al., 2001; Chang et al., 2002). In addition, it interacts with RBP-Jκ, a transcriptional repressor that is the target of the Notch-signaling pathway, and the interaction targets RTA to RBP-Jκ recognition sites in viral promoters, resulting in the replacement of RBP-Jκ's intrinsic repressive action with activation mediated by the transactivation domain of RTA (Liang et al., 2002). Interaction of RTA with many other viral and cellular proteins also modulates RTA-dependent transactivation (Gwack et al., 2001, 2003a, 2003b; Wang et al., 2001b). RTA is also required for DNA replication (AuCoin et al., 2004).

γHV68 RTA and herpesvirus saimiri (HVS) ORF50 have largely conserved the transactivation and replication functions of HHV-8 RTA (Wu et al., 2000, 2001; Goodwin et al., 2001; Pavlova et al., 2003). γHV68 recombinants that constitutively express RTA achieve higher acute titers *in vivo,* yet are unable to establish splenic latency (May et al., 2004; Rickabaugh et al., 2004).

LANA physically associates with RBP-Jκ and downmodulates RTA's promoter activity through RBP-Jκ binding sites within the RTA promoter, suggesting that LANA may play a critical role in maintaining latency by targeting a major downstream effector of the Notch signaling pathway (Lan et al., 2004).

6.2.1.3. *Immune Response and Immune Evasion*

HHV-8 and other rhadinoviruses carry many ORFs that encode homologs to cellular proteins involved in immune evasion, signal transduction, cell cycle regulation, and the inhibition of apoptosis (Table 6.2). Sections 6.2.1.3, 6.2.1.4, and 6.2.1.5 explain the functions of these homologs from the aspects of immune responses, pathogenesis, and animal models, respectively.

6.2.1.3.1. Viral Modulation of Innate Immunity. The innate arm of the immune system is the first line of defense that the virus encounters upon infecting a cell. Innate immunity involves the activation of interferon regulatory factors (IRFs) including IRF3 and IRF7 transcription factors that drive the expression and subsequent secretion of IFN-α/β from infected cells (Malmgaard, 2004). IFNs induce the expression and activation of IRF-1 and IRF-7, resulting in upregulation of MHC class I expression and thereby the recruitment and activation of immune effecter cells. IFNs induce the expression of the protein synthesis inhibitor PKR and arrest the cell cycle through the induction of cyclin-dependent kinase inhibitors.

IFNs have the potent antiviral effects against HHV-8 infection in PEL and endothelial cells *in vitro*. IFN-α treatment upregulates PKR and the death receptor tumor necrosis factor–related apoptosis inducing ligand (TRAIL), inhibits the reactivation of HHV-8 from PEL cells, and leads to apoptosis (Toomey et al., 2001; Pozharskaya et al., 2004a, 2004b). IFN-α blocks *de novo* infection of DEVECs by HHV-8 (Krug et al., 2004). In addition, IFN-α and IFN-γ interfere with lytic gene expression and virus production in endothelial cells (Krug et al., 2004; Milligan et al., 2004). These are biologically relevant because IFN-α can induce KS lesion regression in HIV-infected patients with adequate CD4+ T-cell counts (Krown et al., 1992; Fischl et al., 1996;). IFN-γ, in addition to other inflammatory cytokines, has been detected in KS tissues (Milligan et al., 2004), suggesting that the virus in the infected cells must counteract the effect of the cytokines in order to persist.

HHV-8 counteracts the IFN-mediated antiviral response by inhibiting cellular IRF function and by blocking IFN signaling (reviewed in Weber et al., 2004). Four viral IRF proteins, vIRFs 1–4, are encoded by HHV-8 (Table 6.2) (reviewed in Dourmishev et al., 2003). Except for vIRF3 (also referred to as LANA2), the vIRFs are classified as early lytic genes in PEL cells (Wang et al., 2001c; Cunningham et al., 2003). vIRF1 is detected with LANA in some KS tissues (Yen-Moore et al., 2000), but only vIRF2 is expressed upon *de novo* infection of endothelial cells (Krishnan et al., 2004). vIRF2 interacts with PKR to inhibit downstream phosphorylation of the eukaryotic translation initiation factor 2α (Burysek and Pitha, 2001) and can also modulate gene expression through interactions with IRF-1, IRF-2, p65, and p300 to inhibit IRF-1 and -3 transcriptional activation (Burysek et al., 1999b). The latency-associated vIRF3 and

Table 6.2. Rhadinovirus-encoded genes that relate to immune evasion and oncogenesis

Protein	ORF			Cellular target	Properties and function	Expression
	HHV-8	γHV68	HVS			
Immune modulation/evasion						
vIRF-1	K9	—	—	IRF-1	Inhibits IFN signaling, CBP/p300, p53	Lytic, latent
vIRF-2	K11	—	—	IRF-1,-2, PKR	Inhibits IFN signaling, CBP/p300	Lytic
vIRF-3	K10.5	—	—	IRF	Inhibits IFN signaling, p53	Latent
vIRF-4	K10	—	—	IRF	Inhibits IFN signaling?	Lytic
ORF45	ORF45	ORF45	—	IRF 7	Promotes IRF-7 ubiquitination/degradation, inhibits IFN expression	Lytic
vIL-6	K2	—	—	IL-6R, gp130	Activates lymphocyte signaling, induces VEGF, inhibits IFN signaling	Lytic
CCP	ORF4 (KCP)	ORF4 (RCA)	ORF4	Complement system	Inhibits C3b deposition on cell surface, inactivation of C3b and C4b	Lytic
vCCL-1(vMIP-I)	K6	—	—	CCR-5,-8 agonist	Induces angiogenesis, induces Th2 chemotaxis	Lytic
vCCL-2(vMIP-II)	K4	—	—	CCR-3,-5 agonist	Induces angiogenesis, induces Th2 chemotaxis	Lytic
vCCL-3(vMIP-III)	K4.1	—	—	CCR4 agonist	Induces angiogenesis, induces Th2 chemotaxis	Lytic
vOX-2	K14	—	—	OX-2 receptor	Modulation of monocyte-lineage cell activation	Lytic
vMIR1	K3	mK3	—	MHCI	Downregulation of MHCI via ubiquitination	Lytic
vMIR2	K5	—	—	MHCI, ICAM, B7.2	Downregulation of MHCI via ubiquitination	Lytic
Oncogenesis						
LANA	ORF73	ORF73	ORF73		Latent replication, binds p53, pRB	Latent
v-cyclin	ORF72	ORF72	ORF72	Cyclin-dependent kinase	Cell cycle progression, reactivation	Latent
vGPCR	ORF74	ORF74	ORF74		Tumor progression by paracrine mechanism	Lytic

K1	K1	—	STP		Syk signaling via ITAM, transform rodent fibroblasts	Latent
K15	K15	—	TIP	TRAF	Syk activation via SH2-binding motif	Latent
vFLIP	K13		ORF71	FLICE, IKK	Inhibitor of Fas-mediated apoptosis, induces tumors in mice	Latent
vBcl2	ORF16	M11	ORF16		Anti-apoptotic	Lytic
vIAP	K7	—			Anti-apoptotic	Lytic
Kaposin	K12	—	—		Transforms fibroblasts	Latent

IRF, interferon regulatory factor; IFN, interferon; IL, interleukin; CCP, complement control protein; CCL, CC-chemokine ligand; MIP, macrophage inflammatory protein; MIR, modulator of immune response protein; GPCR, G protein–coupled receptor; IAP, inhibitor of apoptosis protein.

lytic-cycle associated vIRF1 both inhibit p53-mediated transcription and apoptosis (Nakamura et al., 2001; Seo et al., 2001).

vIRF1 is the best characterized vIRF and has been found to inhibit apoptosis in response to numerous stimuli including IFN-α and IFN-β, TNF-α, and activation-induced cell death (Kirchhoff et al., 2002). While vIRF1 functions as a transactivator (Li et al., 1998; Roan et al., 1999), it inhibits the transcription of a broad range of genes by interacting with the coactivators CBP/p300 (Seo et al., 2000) and by interfering with p300 histone acetyltransferase activity (Li et al., 2000). The sequestration of CBP/p300 in addition to direct interaction with IRF-1 and -3 blocks the expression of IFN-responsive antiviral genes including IFN, p21^{waf} cell cycle inhibitor, CCL-5, and CXCL-10 (Flowers et al., 1998; Zimring et al., 1998; Burysek et al., 1999a; Lin et al., 2001). vIRF1 is necessary for efficient reactivation from latency in PEL cells (Li et al., 1998). Gross alterations in gene expression and apoptotic inhibition by vIRF1 likely relates to its ability to transform rodent fibroblasts (Li et al., 1998) and induce tumors in nude mice (Gao et al., 1997).

Activation of the cellular IRF7 transcription factor is inhibited during an HHV-8 infection by two immediate early lytic genes. ORF45 encodes a virion tegument protein that interacts with IRF7 to prevent its phosphorylation and nuclear translocation, thereby blocking IFN-α/β expression at the earliest stages of infection (Zhu et al., 2002). HHV-8 RTA acts as an ubiqutin E3 ligase by promoting the ubiquitination of IRF7 and its subsequent proteosome-mediated degradation (Yu et al., 2005).

Viral subversion of the IFN response is not complete and may be overcome by exogenous addition of IFN (Pozharskaya et al., 2004b). In addition, treatment of HHV-8+ PEL-engrafted NOD/SCID mice using a combination of azidothymidine and IFN-α has been shown to improve their mean survival time (Wu et al., 2005).

HHV-8 K2 encodes a viral IL-6 (vIL-6) homolog that has conserved nearly all of the biological activities of the cellular IL-6 (hIL-6) (Moore et al., 1996a; Nicholas et al., 1997). vIL-6 activates the signal transducers and activators of transcription (STATs) and the Ras/mitogen-activated protein kinase (MAPK) pathways, induces vascular endothelial growth factor (VEGF) expression, and drives the proliferation of B lymphocytes (Burger et al., 1998; Osborne et al., 1999; Hideshima et al., 2000; Liu et al., 2001). vIL-6 is detected in KS lesions (Cannon et al., 1999; Brousset et al., 2001), and PEL cells express and depend on vIL-6 as an autocrine growth factor (Yu et al., 2005). In contrast with hIL-6, vIL-6 can directly activate the gp130 membrane signaling protein in addition to interacting with the IL-6 receptor (gp80) (Molden et al., 1997; Li et al., 2001; Boulanger et al., 2004b). Although upon IFN-α stimulation of latently-infected PEL cells the IL-6 receptor is downregulated and the cyclin-dependent kinase inhibitor p21CIP is induced to arrest the cell cycle, vIL-6 expression is upregulated by IFN-α to drive gp130-mediated signaling and cell proliferation, suggesting a novel feedback mechanism to counteract IFN-mediated cell growth arrest (Chatterjee et al., 2002). The induction of VEGF and inhibition of IFN signaling by the vIL-6 cytokine likely plays a critical role in the genesis of KS-associated malignancies.

ORF4 of rhadinoviruses encodes a complement control protein (CCP) (Russo et al., 1996). CCP blocks both alternative and classical complement pathways; it prevents the deposition of C3b, the proteolytic active form of C3, on the cell surface and drives factor I cleavage and inactivation of the C3 convertase subunits C3b and C4b (Mullick et al., 2003; Spiller et al., 2003). γHV68 CCP was found important for viral persistence and lethality in IFN-γR-/-mice (Kapadia et al., 2002). Thus, it is likely that interference of the complement pathway enhances virus replication and spread in the host.

6.2.1.3.2. Viral Modulation of the Adaptive Immune Response. HHV-8 encodes three secreted chemokines with a broad range of immune modulatory activities: viral CCL homologs, vCCL-1, -2, and –3 (previously known as viral macrophage inflammatory proteins vMIP-I, -II, and –III) (Table 6.2). The vCCLs are antagonistic to a broad range of CC and CXC lymphocyte receptors that likely enhance T helper cell subtype 2 (Th2) recruitment (Kledal et al., 1997; Chen et al., 1998; Luttichau et al., 2001) and thereby direct the host response away from cell-mediated clearance toward a less effective, antibody-dependent immune response. There is also accumulating evidence to support a model in which the vCCLs play a role in viral dissemination in the host, perhaps by recruiting monocytes to KS tissues. Depending on the experimental approach, each viral chemokine is reported to function as an agonist for at least one CCR molecule on monocytes or Th2-type T cells as evidenced by Ca^{2+} signaling and target cell chemotaxis (CCR-5 and -8 for vCCL-1, CCR-3 and -5 for vCCL-2, and CCR4 for vCCL-3) (Boshoff et al., 1997; Dairaghi et al., 1999; Endres et al., 1999; Stine et al., 2000; Nakano et al., 2003). An additional function of vCCLs is their ability to drive angiogenesis in a chick chorioallantoic membrane assay (Boshoff et al., 1997; Stine et al., 2000). This property likely involves the induction of VEGF secretion as observed after treatment of PEL cells with vCCL-1 and vCCL-2 (Liu et al., 2001). vCCL-1 and -2 are expressed in PEL cell cultures, and vCCL-3 is detected in KS lesions (Moore et al., 1996a; Stine et al., 2000).

K14 encodes a homolog of the cellular OX-2, a glycoprotein that provides negative signals to limit the activation of T cells and monocyte-lineage cells (reviewed in Barclay et al., 2002). vOX-2 is a viral glyco-protein that is expressed on the surface of lytically infected cells (Chung et al., 2002; Foster-Cuevas et al., 2004). The role of this protein in the activation of macrophages is not clear, but it is worth noting that K14 is transcribed with ORF74 as a lytic cycle bicistronic transcript (Talbot et al., 1999) and is likely not expressed in the majority of infected cells of a KS lesion.

Escape from CTL-mediated killing by downregulation of MHC-I is a common strategy of herpesviruses. K3 and K5 of HHV-8 encode mod-ulators of immune response proteins (vMIR1 and vMIR2, respectively) that downregulate cell surface expression of MHC-I (Coscoy and Ganem, 2000; Ishido et al., 2000b; Stevenson et al., 2000). vMIR2 primarily downregulates HLA-A and -B (Ishido et al., 2000b). vMIR1 targets HLA-A, -B, -C, and -E in addition to the NK cell-mediated cytotoxicity recep-tors intercellular adhesion molecules (ICAMs) and B7-2 (Coscoy and Ganem, 2000; Ishido et al., 2000a, 2000b). The N-terminal C_4HC_3 zinc-finger motifs of vMIR1 and vMIR2 are similar to RING domains of E3 ubiquitin ligases. The ubiquitination of MHC-I by vMIR1 and vMIR2 is believed to drive its endocytosis and targeting to the trans-Golgi network (Lorenzo et al., 2002; Means et al., 2002). The diacidic clusters in the C-terminal region of K3 are responsible for targeting MHC-I to lysosomal compartments for destruction (Means et al., 2002). The γHV68 counter-part of HHV-8 K3, mK3, mediates ubiquitination and degradation of MHC-I and transporter associated with antigen processing (TAP)-1 and TAP-2 molecules through its N- and C-terminal domains, respectively (Boname and Stevenson, 2001; Wang et al., 2004; Boname et al., 2004, 2005; Wang et al., 2005b). MHC-I degradation is dependent on TAP-1, TAP-2, and tapasin components of the peptide loading complex (Lybarger et al., 2003; Boname et al., 2004, 2005). A γHV68 mutant lacking mK3 has a CTL-dependent decrease in splenic latency (Stevenson et al., 2002), demonstrating the *in vivo* importance of this immune evasion molecule.

6.2.1.4. Pathogenesis

6.2.1.4.1. Transformation. HHV-8 DNA and viral products can be detected in all KS lesions. However, cells cultured from KS tumors do not main-tain the HHV-8 genome, so the early consequences of cellular transfor-mation are not possible to study. Because endothelial cells are the likely precursors of KS spindle cells, *in vitro* endothelial cell models of HHV-8 infection are utilized to dissect the role of HHV-8 in KS spindle cell development and growth. Flore et al. (1998) demonstrated that HHV-8 infection causes long-term proliferation and survival of primary bone marrow–derived endothelial cells, which are associated with the acquisition of telomerase activity and anchorage-independent growth. Because HHV-8 was present only in a subset of cells, it is thought that paracrine mechanisms may play a role in the survival of uninfected cells. Establishment of immortalized human DMVECs has allowed the extended maintenance of age- and passage-matched mock-infected controls for the evaluation of virus-induced cellular changes. Infection of HPV E6/7–immortalized DMVECs is followed primarily by latent infection with a small percentage of cells spontaneously entering the lytic cycle. The infected cells develop a spindle shape with a transformed phenotype including loss of contact inhibition and acquisition of anchorage-independent growth (Moses et al., 1999). Several proto-oncogenes, particularly the receptor tyrosine kinase c-kit, are induced in the infected cells. Expression of the c-kit ligand, stem cell factor (SCF), leads to cellular proliferation, and c-kit inhibitors reversed SCF-dependent proliferation and HHV-8–induced morphological transformation (Moses et al., 2002). After HHV-8 infection of TIME cells, a telomerase-immortalized DMVEC line, expression of many genes specific to lymphatic endothelium, including VEGFR3, podoplanin, LYVE-1, and Prox-1, is significantly increased. HHV-8 infection also induces hIL-6 while strongly inhibiting secretion of IL-8, a gene product that is decreased by differentiation of blood to lymphatic endothelial cells, suggesting that latent HHV-8 infection of blood endothelial cells drives their differentiation to lymphatic endothelial cells (Carroll et al., 2004). Similar observations have been made in DMVECs (Hong et al., 2004).

NF-κB, a potent inducer of genes involved in the proliferative and survival responses of lymphocytes, is constitutively activated in all HHV-8–infected PEL cell lines and patient primary PEL specimens. NF-κB inhibitors downregulate the NF-κB–inducible cytokines and induce apoptosis, suggesting that NF-κB activity is necessary for survival of HHV-8–infected lymphoma cells (Keller et al., 2000).

The following subsections describe several HHV-8 homologs of cellular oncogenes and viral products with *in vitro* transforming capability (Table 6.2).

6.2.1.4.2. LANA. LANA (ORF73) promotes cell survival by the targeting and alteration of p53 function, interaction with the retinoblastoma (Rb) protein and glycogen synthase kinase-3ß, and activation of the telomerase promoter (Friborg, Jr., et al., 1999; Krithivas et al., 2000; Lim et al., 2000; Knight et al., 2001; Fujimuro and Hayward, 2003). LANA also protects lymphoid cells from cell cycle arrest induced by p16 INK4a, a CDK4/6 inhibitor (An et al., 2005). In cooperation with the cellular oncogene H-ras, LANA transforms primary rat embryo fibroblasts and renders them tumorigenic, indicating that LANA acts as a transcription cofactor that may contribute to oncogenesis by targeting the RB-E2F transcriptional regulatory pathway (Radkov et al., 2000). LANA is capable of inducing a prolonged life span and growth advantage, but not transformation, in primary human endothelial cells (Watanabe et al., 2003; Krug et al., 2004).

6.2.1.4.3. v-Cyclin. The ORF72 gene of HHV-8 and HVS encodes a functional cyclin D homolog, v-cyclin. These cyclin homologs are functional cyclins that predominantly associate with CDK6, induce phosphorylation of Rb and histone H1, and overcome Rb-mediated cell cycle arrest (Nicholas et al., 1992; Jung et al., 1994; Godden-Kent et al., 1997; Li et al., 1997; Swanton et al., 1997; Schulze-Gahmen and Kim, 2002). Compared with cellular cyclin D-CDK4/6, the HHV-8 and HVS v-cyclin-CDK6 complexes have a broader substrate range *in vitro*. They interact with, and phosphorylate, components of the replication machinery, such as Orc1, and mimic cyclin A-cdk2 complexes to directly drive the initiation of nuclear DNA replication *in vitro* (Laman et al., 2001). HHV-8 v-cyclin interacts with the activation domain of STAT3, inhibits its DNA-binding and transcriptional activities, and overcomes growth-suppressive signals (Lundquist et al., 2003). In addition, the v-cyclin–CDK6 complexes induce degradation of the CDK inhibitor p27Kip (Ellis et al., 1999; Mann et al., 1999).

Expression of HHV-8 v-cyclin transgenically targeted to the B- and T-lymphocyte compartments leads to the development of lymphoma, and the loss of p53 accelerates the frequency of v-cyclin–induced lymphoma-genesis (Verschuren et al., 2004). Similarly, expression of γHV68 v-cyclin under the *lck* proximal promoter in transgenic mice promotes cell cycle progression of thymocytes and leads to a high rate of lymphoma (van Dyk et al., 1999). γHV68 virus mutants that do not express v-cyclin are defective in reactivation from latently-infected splenocytes and peritoneal cells (Hoge et al., 2000; van Dyk et al., 2000) and are unable to persistently replicate in the peritoneal cells of immunodeficient IFN-γ-/ mice (Gangappa et al., 2002b). In B-cell-deficient mice, v-cyclin is required for maintenance of latency and γHV68-induced mortality (van Dyk et al., 2003). HVS lacking v-cyclin retains transformation properties *in vitro* and has led to disseminated T-cell lymphoma in cotton-top tamarins (Ensser et al., 2001).

6.2.1.4.4. vGPCR, K1, K15 (Proteins for Cellular Activation Signaling). HHV-8, HVS, and γHV68 ORF74 encode viral GPCR (vGPCR) homologs, which is a seven-transmembrane receptor protein with the greatest sequence similarity to the cellular IL-8 receptor. Although vGPCRs of HHV-8 but not γHV68 are constitutively active, they retain the ability to bind to various chemokines that result in up- or downregulation of signaling (Arvanitakis et al., 1997; Geras-Raaka et al., 1998a, 1998b; Gershengorn et al., 1998; Verzijl et al., 2004). HVS vGPCR is more restricted than its HHV-8 counterpart in the classes of G proteins through which it constitutively signals, and it generates strong signaling and activation of transcription factors CREB, NFAT, and NF-κB via ligand-mediated G protein–coupled signaling (Rosenkilde et al., 2004). HHV-8 vGPCR can activate p38MAPK and Akt/PKB pathways (Sodhi et al., 2000, 2004; Montaner et al., 2001). HHV-8 and γHV68 vGPCRs induce cell transformation and tumorigenicity with an angiogenic phenotype mediated by vascular endothelial growth factor (Bais et al., 1998; Wakeling et al., 2001). Endothelial cells expressing HHV-8 vGPCR promote the tumorigenic potential of cells expressing latent KSHV genes through a paracrine mechanism (Montaner et al., 2003). Expression of HHV-8 vGPCR in transgenic mice leads to angioproliferative lesions that exhibit most of the characteristics of KS (Yang et al., 2000; Guo et al., 2003). Pharmacological inhibition of the Akt pathway prevents proliferation of vGPCR-expressing endothelial cells *in vitro* and inhibits their tumorigenic potential *in vivo* (Sodhi et al., 2004). Inhibition of the small G protein Rac1, through which NF-κB, AP-1, and NFAT are stimulated, blocks vGPCR-induced transcription and secretion of KS cytokines *in vitro* and reduces vGPCR-mediated tumorigenesis *in vivo*. Moreover, endothelial-specific infection with the constitutively active Rac1QL induces vascular lesions in mice similar to early vGPCR experimental lesions, indicating Rac1 as a key mediator of vGPCR-induced neoplasia (Montaner et al., 2004). γHV68 lacking ORF74 has a reduced ability to reactivate from latency in splenocytes and peritoneal cells after intraperitoneal infection (Lee et al., 2003; Moorman et al., 2003a), indicative of a critical role of vGPCR in virus persistence.

At a genome position equivalent to EBV latent membrane protein (LMP)-1 and HVS transformation-associated protein (Stp), HHV-8 encodes a transmembrane glycoprotein, K1. While the N-terminal extracellular domain of K1 is extremely variable among isolates, the C-terminal short cytoplasmic tail that contains a functional immunoreceptor tyrosine-based activation motif (ITAM) is relatively well conserved. The ITAM is capable of transducing signals to induce cellular activation, calcium mobilization, and tyrosine phosphorylation, which are all indicative of lymphocyte activation (Lagunoff et al., 1999; Lee et al., 1998a). K1 signaling, similar to EBV LMP-1 signaling, is constitutive and interacts with several cellular signal transduction proteins, including Vav, p85 subunit of phosphatidylinositol-3 kinase (PI3K), and Syk kinase. K1 inhibits intracellular transport of B-cell receptor (BCR) complexes and has effects on viral lytic reactivation and replication (Lee et al., 2000; Lagunoff et al., 2001). K1 transforms rodent fibroblasts *in vitro* and common marmoset T lymphocytes *in vivo* (Lee et al., 1998b). Transgenic expression of K1 enhances NF-κB activity in nonmalignant lymphocytes; a spindle-cell sarcomatoid tumor and a malignant plasmablastic lymphoma have been observed in K1-transgenic mice (Prakash et al., 2002).

The K15 gene is composed of eight alternatively spliced exons that encode membrane proteins with a variable number of transmembrane regions and a common C-terminal cytoplasmic domain. The cytoplasmic domain contains signaling motifs, such as SH2- and SH3-binding motifs, and like LMP-1, the C-terminal region of K15 associates with TRAFs 1, 2, and 3 (Glenn et al., 1999; Choi et al., 2000b). These motifs are conserved in both P and M alleles of K15 (Poole et al., 1999). K15 can activate a number of intracellular signaling pathways, including MAPK, NF-κB, and c-Jun N-terminal kinase/SAPK pathways (Brinkmann et al., 2003). K15 protein interacts with the Bcl-2–related protein HAX-1 and colocalizes in the endoplasmic reticulum and mitochondria (Sharp et al., 2002). There is as yet no evidence that K15 association with HAX-1 affects cell survival, but such a function could be important both to lytic and latent infection.

Stp and the tyrosine kinase interacting protein (Tip), functional HVS homologs of HHV-8 K1 and K15, are described in Section 6.2.1.5.2.

6.2.1.4.5. vBcl2, vFLIP, K7 (Anti-apoptotic Proteins). The HHV-8 viral Bcl-2 encoded by ORF16 can block apoptosis as efficiently as cellular Bcl-2 or the EBV Bcl-2 homolog and may contribute to the development of KS (Cheng et al., 1997; Boshoff and Chang, 2001). The overall polypeptide fold of vBcl-2 is the same, but there are key differences in the lengths of the helices and loops between vBcl-2 and the other Bcl-2 family members. HHV-8 vBcl-2 cannot homodimerize or heterodimerize with other Bcl-2 family members, and the specificity of the viral protein is very different from those of Bcl-x$_L$ and Bcl-2 (Huang et al., 2002).

M11 of γHV68 encodes a Bcl-2 homolog that inhibits Fas- and TNF-induced apoptosis (Wang et al., 1999b; Roy et al., 2000). γHV68 vBcl-2 is cleaved by caspases, yet does not convert to a proapoptotic molecule as found for the cleavage products of cellular Bcl-2, Bcl-x$_L$, and Bid (Bellows et al., 2000). M11 is detected during lytic infection *in vitro* and *in vivo* (Virgin et al., 1999; Roy et al., 2000; Marques et al., 2003; Martinez-Guzman et al., 2003). Recombinant viruses containing stop codons early in the M11 gene show no lytic replication defect *in vitro* or *in vivo* and can establish latency at a normal frequency. However, M11 mutants are unable to reactivate and persistently replicate in IFN-γ-/-mice, resulting in decreased mortality in IFN-γR-/-mice (Weck et al., 1997; Dal Canto et al., 2000; Gangappa et al., 2002b).

HHV-8 K13 encodes a viral FLICE-inhibitory protein (vFLIP) that contains two death effector domains that bind and inhibit the Fas-associated death domain protein and activation of FLICE/caspase 8 (Thome et al., 1997). vFLIP also interacts with the IκB kinase (IKK) to activate IKK, leading to NF-κB activation through the classical pathway (Liu et al., 2002; Field et al., 2003; Matta et al., 2003). vFLIP drives NF-kB2/p100 processing to p52 in an IKK1-dependent manner (Matta and Chaudhary, 2004). Inhibition of vFLIP by RNA interference in PEL cells results in decreased NF-κB activation and induction of apoptosis (Guasparri et al., 2004). Expression of vFLIP in a growth factor–dependent TF-1 leukemia cell line upregulates the expression of Bcl-x_L, which is a known target of the NF-κB pathway, and protects against growth factor withdrawal–induced apoptosis (Sun et al., 2003). These anti-apoptotic functions likely play a role in the development of tumors upon the transfer of A20 murine B cells transfected with vFLIP into mice (Djerbi et al., 1999). vFLIP is expressed in latently-infected B cells, endothelial cells, and KS lesions (Sarid et al., 1998; Dittmer, 2003; Krishnan et al., 2004). HVS lacking vFLIP is replication competent, and the anti-apoptotic effect is lost. However, HVS vFLIP is dispensable for pathogenicity in cotton-top tamarins in vivo (Glykofrydes et al., 2000).

HHV-8 K7 is a membrane protein structurally related to survivin-DeltaEx3, a splice variant of human survivin that protects cells from apoptosis by an undefined mechanism. K7 apparently targets multiple cellular factors to allow escape from host antiviral destruction (Feng et al., 2002; Wang et al., 2002). Its interaction with calcium-modulating cyclophilin ligand (CAML) alters the kinetics and amplitudes of intracellular Ca^{2+} responses on stress stimulation, thereby inhibiting apoptosis (Feng et al., 2002). K7 binds to Bcl-2 via its putative Bcl-2 homology domain and to caspase 3 via its baculovirus inhibitor-of-apoptosis repeat domain and thus inhibits the activity of caspase-3 (Wang et al., 2002). In addition, K7 interacts with protein-linking integrin-associated protein and cytoskeleton 1 (PLIC1), through its central hydrophobic region. K7 interaction inhibits PLIC1 activity, resulting in rapid degradation of IκB and p53 and inhibition of p53-dependent apoptosis (Feng et al., 2004).

6.2.1.4.6. Kaposin. Kaposin A encoded by K12 is a type II membrane protein and has been detected in KS lesions and in PEL cells. Its expression in Rat-3 cells induces tumorigenic transformation (Muralidhar et al., 1998). Kaposin A interacts with cytohesin-1, a guanine nucleotide exchange factor for ADP-ribosylation factor (ARF) GTPases and regulator of integrin-mediated cell adhesion, and activates cytohesin-1 by recruiting it to the cell membrane, resulting in the stimulation of ARF-GTPase (Kliche et al., 2001).

6.2.1.4.7. Host Gene Shutoff. Host gene expression is strongly inhibited by 10–12 h after HHV-8 lytic reactivation. Expression of most vGPCR target genes is drastically curtailed by this host shutoff. However, rare cellular genes, particularly hIL-6, escape the host shutoff and are potently upregulated during lytic HHV-8 growth (Glaunsinger and Ganem, 2004).

6.2.1.5. Animal Models

6.2.1.5.1. Infection by Murine Gammaherpesvirus 68 (γHV68). Although a wealth of data has been gathered from the study of the human gammaherpesviruses and their individual proteins in cell culture, validating the biological relevance of cell culture phenotypes and mechanisms of infection is not possible *in vivo* due to strict species-specific tropisms. γHV68 is being increasingly used for studies of gammaherpesvirus latency, reactivation, virus-associated pathologies, and host immunity (reviewed in Doherty et al., 2001; Nash et al., 2001). γHV68 infects rodent species including bank voles and wood mice. γHV68 is easily propagated in tissue culture and infects inbred mice to generate a clinical course that parallels an infection by EBV. The genetic and biologic properties that γHV68 shares with its human counterparts, in addition to its ease of generating recombinant viruses utilizing bacterial artificial chromosome cloning systems (Adler et al., 2003) coupled with an ever-expanding library of knockout and transgenic mouse systems, has made it an ideal tractable model system for human gammaherpesviruses (Speck and Virgin, 1999; Nash et al., 2001). Lessons learned from this potent mouse model system will be valuable for understanding virus–host interactions of its human gammaherpesvirus counterparts.

Intranasal infection with γHV68 leads to an acute phase of lytic replication in the lung epithelium and a rapid expansion of lymphocytes that approximates the course of infectious mononucleosis (Sunil-Chandra et al., 1992a, 1992b, 1994; Usherwood et al., 1996). Within several weeks, in a CD8 and CD4 T-cell-dependent manner, actively replicating virus is cleared and becomes undetectable in the lung and spleen (Doherty et al., 2001; Sparks-Thissen et al., 2004; Braaten et al., 2005). The virus establishes a predominantly latent infection with a probable low level of persistent replication that requires immunosurveillance to prevent reactivation (Doherty et al., 2001; Tibbetts et al., 2002; Sparks-Thissen et al., 2004). Its predominant long-term latency reservoir is memory B cells (Flano et al., 2002; Kim et al., 2003; Willer and Speck, 2003). This suggests that γHV68 utilizes a post–germinal center (GC) B-cell type as its long-lived latency reservoir as found for EBV (Babcock et al., 1998; Hochberg et al., 2004) and HHV-8 (Said et al., 2001; Jenner et al., 2003).

The classical paradigm for B-cell development entails that peripheral naive B-cell exposure to specific antigen, appropriate CD40-dependent T-cell interactions, and co-stimulatory molecules drive B-cell expansion, affinity maturation, and immunoglobulin isotype switching. Proper specificity and affinity of the B-cell receptor for its cognate antigen permits cell survival and exit from GC reactions as either memory B cells or plasma cells. γHV68 is detected in 1 of 1500 germinal center, memory B cells in the spleen (Willer and Speck, 2003) and is present at 100-fold greater levels in the CD40+ isotype-switched B cells over CD40-B cells (Kim et al., 2003), supporting a model in which virus-infected B cells participate in and possibly drive GC reactions. The next challenge in this field is delineating the latent viral gene expression program and virus–host interactions required for GC transit.

The prolific expansion and activation of infected B cells by latent gene products is postulated to put cells at risk for acquiring oncogenic mutations while bypassing normal cell cycle checkpoints (Thompson and Kurzrock, 2004). EBV and HVS can directly transform primary lymphocytes, while infection by HHV-8 and γHV68 leads to cell proliferation and enhanced survival (Flore et al., 1998; Dutia et al., 1999). γHV68 is associated with a 10% incidence of B-cell lymphoma after an extended period of infection in mice (Sunil-Chandra et al., 1994). γHV68 also encodes homologs to cellular proteins, many in common with HHV-8 and HVS (Table 6.2). These genes subvert cell signaling and cell cycle control mechanisms, block apoptosis, and function as immunomodulatory and immunoevasion molecules, as described in Sections 6.2.1.3. and 6.2.1.4.

In vivo analyses of the function of viral genes involved in latent and lytic stages of the γHV68 life cycle have led to the design of vaccines. Vaccination with single lytic antigens inhibited acute replication and early latent infection upon challenge yet did not prevent long-term latency (reviewed in Doherty et al., 2001). Infection with viruses that are unable to establish latency due to a deletion in ORF73 (Fowler and Efstathiou, 2004) or overexpression of RTA (Rickabaugh et al., 2004) or with viruses that are unable to reactivate due to a LacZ insertion in v-cyclin (γHV68. v-cyclin.LacZ) (Tibbetts et al., 2003) reduce the ability of challenge virus to establish splenic latency at early and late times after infection to levels at or below the limit of detection. Vaccination with γHV68.v-cylin.LacZ is dependent on CD4 T cells or CD8 T cells and independent of B cells for preventing latency in the spleen (McClellan et al., 2004), although passive transfer of antibody to a lytic cycle protein can reduce latency (Gangappa et al., 2002a).

6.2.1.5.2. Infection by Herpesvirus Saimiri (HVS). *Saimiriine herpesvirus-2* (SaHV-2), more commonly referred to as herpesvirus saimiri (HVS), is a highly prevalent, natural pathogen of squirrel monkeys (*Saimiri sci-ureus*), which are New World primates that inhabit South America. Natural transmission via saliva and experimental infection of squirrel monkeys is asymptomatic (Melendez et al., 1968), whereas HVS infec-tion of other New World primates results in the rapid development of fatal leukemia, lymphoma, and lymphoproliferative disorders (Fleckenstein and Desrosiers, 1982). HVS is a potent model system for tumorigenesis by gammaherpesviruses. HVS can be isolated from infected animals by cocultivation of peripheral blood lymphocytes with owl monkey kidneys cells (Falk et al., 1972). HVS is amenable to genetic manipulation because it is easily propagated in fibroblasts to high titer. This permits an examination of the role of distinct viral genes in transformation *in vitro* and lymphomagenesis in animals.

HVS clinical isolates can be classified into subgroups A, B, and C based on sequence variability at the left end of the genome and their differing abilities to induce lymphoma development in animals and immortalize primary lymphocytes in cell culture. Overall, subgroup C is more oncogenic than the other subgroups, and subgroup B has the weakest transforming capacity. Infection with HVS subgroups A and C can induce tumors in numerous New World primates and immortalize their lymphocytes *in vitro* without the addition of exogenous IL-2, although HVS subgroup B can only induce lymphomas in cottontop tamarins and only infrequently immortalizes common marmoset lym-phocytes with the constant supplementation of IL-2 (Szomolanyi et al., 1987; Varnell et al., 1995; Reiss et al., 2002). HVS subgroup C also can induce lymphomas in Old World monkeys (Fickenscher and Fleckenstein, 2001) and New Zealand white rabbits (Ablashi et al., 1985). In addition, infection with HVS subgroup C strain 488 can immortalize both CD4+CD8- and CD4-CD8+ primary human T lymphocytes (Biesinger et al., 1992).

A small percentage of cells in transformed T lymphocyte cultures from New World primates spontaneously undergo lytic virus production as found with many PEL cell lines latently-infected with HHV-8, although human T-cell lines derived from HVS C488-immortalization are not permissive for virus production even upon treatment with phorbol esters (Biesinger et al., 1992; Fickenscher et al., 1996).

HVS encodes many of the same homologs of cellular genes found in HHV-8 (Table 6.2). Stp and Tip, however, are the major proteins of interest in relation to the transforming properties of HVS (reviewed in Tsygankov, 2004). The oncogenic properties of the HVS subgroups directly relate to the transformation potential of Stp. Stp of subgroup C (StpC) can transform fibroblasts and generate tumors in nude mice to a greater degree than StpA (Jung et al., 1991). While not essential for viral replication, StpA is essential for immortalization of marmoset T lymphocytes and induction of lymphomas *in vivo* (Desrosiers et al., 1985, 1986; Murthy et al., 1989). HVS C488 lacking StpC is unable to transform cotton marmoset T lymphocytes *in vitro* or *in vivo* (Duboise et al., 1998a). StpA transgenic mice develop T-cell lymphomas (Kretschmer et al., 1996). In contrast, transgenic mice expressing StpC develop invasive epithelial tumors (Murphy et al., 1994), suggesting an additional role for other viral factors such as Tip in the transformation of T lymphocytes. StpC activates NF-κB via a TRAF/NIK/IκB kinase pathway similar to EBV LMP-1 (Sorokina et al., 2004). A recombinant HVS C488 that contains this TRAF binding mutant form of StpC in place of the wild-type version retains its ability to transform common marmoset T lymphocytes *in vitro* and *in vivo* but is unable to transform primary human lymphocytes or rodent fibroblasts (Lee et al., 1999). StpC also binds to Ras to activate downstream signaling, and the interactions coincide with the ability of those mutants to transform fibroblasts (Jung and Desrosiers, 1995). Furthermore, the introduction of c-ras or v-ras into Stp-deficient HVS C488 rescues its ability to transform primary common marmoset T lymphocytes (Guo et al., 1998). StpA interacts with TRAF yet fails to activate NF-κB (Lee et al., 1999). In addition, StpA binds the SH2 domain of Src kinase and leads to StpA tyrosine phosphorylation and its interaction with Lck and Fyn, and activation of STAT3 (Lee et al., 1997; Hor et al., 2001; Chung et al., 2004; Park et al., 2004). Constitutive activation of STAT3 by StpA drives cell survival and proliferation upon serum deprivation (Chung et al., 2004). Stp B also interacts with TRAF, Src, and Stat3 (Choi et al., 2000a; Hor et al., 2001). StpB has conserved most motifs found in StpA and StpC, yet it lacks the collagen repeat sequence and an optimal SH2 domain. The introduction of collagen repeat sequences into StpB results in oligomerization and NF-κB activation, and imparts the ability to transform rat fibroblast cells onto the nontransforming StpB (Choi et al., 2000a). K1 can functionally replace Stp for immortalization and lymphomagenesis by HVS (Lee et al., 1998b).

Tip, the homolog of HHV-8 K15, is encoded only by subgroup C and is essential for HVS C488 oncogenesis (Duboise et al., 1998a). Stp and

Tip synergistically upregulate IL-2 in immortalized T cells upon mito-genic stimulation (Merlo and Tsygankov, 2001). Although Tip does not directly transform fibroblasts *in vitro* as found for Stp (Jung and Desrosiers, 1991), conditional transgenic expression of Tip in mice leads to the development of T-cell lymphomas (Wehner et al., 2001). Tip inter-acts with Lck, a Src-family protein tyrosine-kinase of T cells, and induces STAT1 and STAT3 and NFAT-dependent gene expression (Jung et al., 1995; Lund et al., 1997, 1999; Hartley et al., 2000; Kjellen et al., 2002). The biological relevance of the Tip–Lck interaction is not clear because a mutation in the SH3 binding domain essential for Lck interaction retains its oncogenicity *in vivo* (Duboise et al., 1998b). Tip modulates lympho-cyte receptor signaling pathways that likely play a critical role in the maintenance of latency in the host. Tip downregulates the surface expres-sion of the TCR, analogous to EBV LMP2A downregulation of the BCR (Dykstra et al., 2001; Park et al., 2003).

6.2.2. Epidemiology

6.2.2.1. Seroepidemiology

6.2.2.1.1. Assay Development. The epidemiology of HHV-8 infection has been much clarified by the availability and wide application of tests for anti HHV-8 antibodies (reviewed in Martin, 2003). The first-generation assays included indirect immunofluorescence assay (IFA) and immunoblot-ting using PEL cell lines that express the latency-associated nuclear antigen (LANA) under standard culture conditions. After phorbol ester treatment, 10% to 30% of the cells produce cytoplasmic antigens that correspond with structural proteins and replication enzymes associated with HHV-8 lytic infection. Findings from PEL-based assays can be con-founded by nonspecific reactions against cellular components because matched HHV-8–negative PEL cell lines are not available for use as negative control and because of cross-reaction with antibodies against EBV. Adsorption with EBV antigens, isolation of nuclei from PEL cells, and use of higher serum dilutions may minimize the problem. The current generation of assays includes enzyme-linked immunosorbent assays (ELISAs) using defined antigens such as purified whole virions, and recombinant vp19/ORF 65 and ORF26 proteins. Although assays using lytic-phase PEL cell lines and recombinant proteins have achieved better sensitivity than those based on testing for antibodies to latent antigens, the problem of cross-reactivity to other herpesvirus antibodies remains. This consideration has prompted the development of assays using HHV-8–specific antigens, for example, such as IFA using recombinant ORF K8.1

antigen expressed by Semliki Forest virus (Inoue et al., 2000) and an ELISA based on a four-branch, multiple antigenic peptide derived from the K8.1 protein (Lam et al., 2002).

Comparative evaluations have led to proposals of applying assay combinations to achieve satisfactory results in terms of sensitivity and specificity (Rabkin et al., 1998; Spira et al., 2000; Schatz et al., 2001). Use of well-defined subjects and existing assays in combination with appropriate statistical analyses allows calibration of new assays and - provides relatively reliable estimation of anti-HHV-8 seroprevalences (Martin et al., 2000;Corchero et al., 2001). Although most current generation of assays are satisfactory for studying high-risk populations, use of these assays to determine more precise seroprevalences in low-prevalence populations and to evaluate risks associated with HHV-8 transmission, for example, via transfusions or organ transplantation, and diagnosis of HHV-8 infection requires more careful consideration. A comparison of the performance of six laboratories testing a large serum panel of American blood donors indicates that standardization and comparison of assays is still essential to warrant good specificity (Pellett et al., 2003).

6.2.2.1.2. Geographical Variation. Antibodies to HHV-8 are found in most, if not all, patients with KS and are also more common in individuals at risk for this disease than in the general population (Kedes et al., 1996; Simpson et al., 1996; Melbye et al., 1998). The HHV-8 seropositivity rates in general populations are less clear, with wide variability reported from different geographic areas. In Africa, HHV-8 seroprevalences are very high (de The et al., 1999), particularly in sub-Saharan Africa, where endemic KS has been reported. In this region, the seroprevalence of antibodies against lytic antigens among children ranges from 13% to 47% (Mayama et al., 1998; Olsen et al., 1998; Gessain et al., 1999; Nuvor et al., 2001). The rates among adults range from 22% in Central Africa to 48% in Zambia (Belec et al., 1998; He et al., 1998). Very high rates, between 76% and 87%, have been reported in the Congo and in Botswana (Engels et al., 2000) and among older adults in Ghana (43%) and Zambia (71%) (Olsen et al., 1998; Nuvor et al., 2001). The anti-lytic antibody prevalence among prepubescent children from Central Africa ranges between 40% to 50% and shows positive correlation with age (Kasolo et al., 1997; Mayama et al., 1998; Nuvor et al., 2001).

In Europe, HHV-8 infection in the general population is more common in regions reporting high KS incidence rates. Particularly high rates (>20%) have been reported in southern Italy, Sardinia, and Sicily (Gao et al., 1996b; Calabro et al., 1998; Whitby et al., 1998; Ascoli et al.,

2001; Santarelli et al., 2001). Much lower HHV-8 seroprevalences (0–5%) are found in the general populations of non-Mediterranean European countries and North America (Simpson et al., 1996; Pellett et al., 2003). In Texas, however, the overall anti-latent and anti-lytic antibody prevalences seem to be substantially higher (15%) than other parts of North America (Baillargeon et al., 2001; Hudnall et al., 2003).

Reports from other parts of the world are more limited. The prevalence rates in the Caribbean and Central America have been found to be between 0% as determined by serologic assays using latent antigens and up to 30% by serologic assays using lytic antigens (Lennette et al., 1996). The use of a lytic antigen assay in blood donors from Central and South America has yielded a rate between 2% and 7% (Perez et al., 2004). In Brazil, anti-latent antibody seroprevalence was found to be particularly high among Amerindians (53%) (Biggar et al., 2000). In Asia, the seropositivity rate of the general population is very variable: <2% in Japan (Satoh et al., 2001), 20% in Taiwan (Huang et al., 2000), and 45% in the Xinjiang area of China (Dilnur et al., 2001). In Northern Thailand, the anti-lytic antibody seroprevalence was 30% among HIV-seropositive and 20% among HIV-seronegative attendees of a sexually transmitted disease clinic (Chen et al., 2004).

6.2.2.1.3. Subpopulations. Most studies show that HHV-8 seroprevalence in the general population of various countries is equally distributed between men and women but is positively correlated with increasing age (Calabro et al., 1998; Huang et al., 2000; Hudnall et al., 2003). However, one study of American blood donors found that there were no significant relationships between HHV-8 seropositivity and demographic characteristics (Pellett et al., 2003).

In Europe and North America, the highest HHV-8 seroprevalence rates are found among HIV-seropositive men who have sex with men (MSM). A study of MSM in the San Francisco area, from samples dating back to 1984, reported a seroprevalence of 48% among homosexual or bisexual men who were HIV-seropositive without KS (Martin et al., 1998). A similar study conducted in Amsterdam between 1984 and 1996 reported a baseline HHV-8 incidence of 30% among HIV-seropositive MSM without KS (Dukers et al., 2000). Similar anti-HHV-8 seroprevalence values for HIV-1–seropositive MSM (30–60%) have been described elsewhere in North America and Western Europe (Gao et al., 1996b; Kedes et al., 1996; Simpson et al., 1996). HIV-1–uninfected MSM consistently show a lower seroprevalence of HHV-8 infection (10–30%) than HIV-1–infected MSM (Kedes et al., 1996; Martin et al., 1998; Melbye et al., 1998).

In Africa, although some correlation between number of sexual partners and HHV-8 infection has been found (Sitas et al., 1999a), the high HHV-8 prevalence in children is indicative of a significant nonsexual route of transmission. In Cameroon, the seroprevalence was observed to increase to 39% among 12- to 14-year olds rising to 48% in children over 15 years of age, which approaches the level reported in adults (Gessain et al., 1999). A Zambian study confirmed that the pattern of HHV-8 infection is different from that of a sexually transmitted infection; thus, the HHV-8 seroprevalence was already high (47%) in adolescents between the ages of 14 and 19 years, thereafter increasing with age (Olsen et al., 1998). This pattern of HHV-8 infection is consistent with the coexistence of childhood nonsexual transmission with sexual transmission throughout adulthood.

In Mediterranean and Middle Eastern countries, the evidence also supports nonsexual transmission among children, although the route of transmission is less clear than that for equatorial and Southern Africa. In Egyptian children, the HHV-8 seroprevalence is as high as 45%, with a steady increase up to 10 years of age (Andreoni et al., 1999).

In Italy, ~5% of children tested were found to carry HHV-8 antibodies, with no significant variation noted between children living in the north and south of Italy (Whitby et al., 2000). In a Sardinian study sample, clustering of HHV-8 seroprevalence among spouses, children, and siblings could be demonstrated with no an apparent mother–child predominance, indicating horizontal HHV-8 transmission in the family along broader, nonsexual routes (Angeloni et al., 1998).

The emerging picture, from these various seroepidemiological studies conducted in African and Mediterranean HHV-8–endemic regions, is that of significant nonsexual horizontal HHV-8 transmission in subpopulations not at or at little risk of sexually-transmitted infection and of such transmission occurring principally within the household.

6.2.2.2. HHV-8 Genotypes

Studies comparing HHV-8 genome sequences from both KS biopsies and PEL cell lines show that the genome is highly conserved, with only 0.1% nucleotide variation between sequences, except for a locus of increased polymorphism at each of the far ends of the genome. Initial investigations into the molecular epidemiology of HHV-8 exploited sequence variations in the prototypic sequence within ORF 26 (Di Alberti et al., 1997a). More extensive analysis of the ORF 26 and ORF 75 have shown the existence of three main genotypes (subtypes) (Zong et al., 1997).

A locus of hypervariability at the far left-hand side of the genome in ORF K1 provides a more discriminatory basis for genotyping. The sequence polymorphism in the extracellular domain of K1 is at minimum 16% at the nucleotide level and 32% at the amino acid level (Meng et al., 1999). Two blocks of the greatest polymorphism, designated variable region (VR) 1 and VR2, are located within the variable amino acid positions 20 to 226 region (Zong et al., 1999). The K1 sequences have been assigned to one of four genotypes, I–IV (Meng et al., 1999). Genotype I may be further divided into four subsections, A–F. Four main genotypes, assigned A–D, from which 13 clades or subtypes could be further discriminated (e.g., A1–A5, C1, etc.), have been independently identified (Zong et al., 1999). A later evaluation has identified up to 24 ORF K1 genotypic variants (Zong et al., 2002).

The distribution of K1 subtypes correlates with ethnicity and geography. The B subtype is predominant in sub-Saharan Africa or in persons of African heritage. Study of B-subtype sequences, which are very divergent in K1 and show little phylogenetic clustering, allows subgroups to be clearly distinguished (B1, B2, and B3). Less frequently, African samples carry A5 type. The A and C subtypes are widely distributed throughout Europe, the United States, Asia, and the Middle East. AIDS KS patients in the United States are predominantly infected with subtypes A1, A4, and C3 (Zong et al., 1999). These subtypes reflect reactivation of endogenous HHV-8 variants, originally introduced by immigrants as well as from horizontal transmission occurring locally. The rare D subtypes have been characterized from persons of Pacific Island heritage only (Poole et al., 1999). Another divergent subtype, E, was reported in an isolated group of Brazilian Amerindians (Biggar et al., 2000). Geographically prevalent subtypes often display a high degree of sequence similarity despite frequent population movements, suggesting that HHV-8 is transmitted in a familial fashion (between family members).

Genotypes at three major loci, ORF 26, T0.7/K12, and ORF 75 confirm that a linkage exists across the genome with the K1 subtype patterns. There is, however, evidence that recombination can occur between loci. ORF K15 contains two highly divergent alleles P (predominant) and M (minority) (Poole et al., 1999), and the divergent M allele is thought to be the result of a recombination event with an exogenous primate virus, followed by recombination events, first with K1 subtype C viruses of the P form and then with A and B types (Poole et al., 1999). Differences in intraperson genotypes and subgenotypes suggest HHV-8 superinfection (Beyari et al., 2003).

6.2.2.3. Transmission

6.2.2.3.1. Sexual Transmission. Cross-sectional (Melbye et al., 1998; Dukers et al., 2000) and longitudinal studies (Martin et al., 1998; Casper et al., 2002) have pointed to sexual transmission in the MSM populations. Seminal transmission of HHV-8 seems to contribute little to sexual transmission, however. Whereas HHV-8 DNA has been detected in prostate tissue biopsies (Staskus et al., 1997; Diamond et al., 1998), indicating a potential of HHV-8 shedding from the prostate into the semen, it is rarely detected in the semen of patients with KS and almost never in healthy semen donors (reviewed in Boshoff and Weiss, 2001).

There are possible linkages between sexual behavior and HHV-8 infection. Among MSM, the increased seroprevalence correlates with the extent of homosexual activity and the number of sexual partners (Martin et al., 1998; Blackbourn et al., 1999). Various sexual practices are associated with increased risk for HHV-8 infection among MSM: anal–genital sexual contact (Melbye et al., 1998), insertive oral–anal sexual contact (Grulich et al., 1999), and insertive and receptive orogenital contact (Dukers et al., 2000). Despite the findings of some of these studies that implicate anal contact as a high-risk factor, there is no evidence to suggest infection from fecal transmission. Thus, although HHV-8 genomic DNA had been sought by PCR techniques from gastrointestinal tissues of MSMs with KS, and, in one study, found detectable in a substantial proportion (46%) of rectal tissues (Thomas et al., 1996), HHV-8 DNA has not been amplified from fecal samples of patients with AIDS-associated KS (Whitby et al., 1995; LaDuca et al., 1998).

Oral sex among MSM is a more important predictor of HHV-8 infection than the number of sexual partners (Dukers et al., 2000). Such findings, and the identification of deep kissing as also being a risk factor for HHV-8 infection (Pauk et al., 2000), posit saliva as the vehicle of transmission. HHV-8 DNA is frequently detected in tissue biopsies taken at various sites from the mouth of HIV-infected patients (Di Alberti et al., 1997a). Epithelial cells of the buccal mucosa of HHV-8–seropositive MSM frequently carry HHV-8 DNA and RNA (Pauk et al., 2000). Furthermore, salivary HHV-8 DNA can be detected from HIV-infected/KS-positive, HIV-infected/KS-negative, and HIV-uninfected/KS-positive persons in the United States (Koelle et al., 1997; Blackbourn et al., 1998; LaDuca et al., 1998) and from AIDS-associated and classic KS patients in Italy (Cattani et al., 1998; Vitale et al., 2000). HHV-8 DNA and infectious HHV-8, or both, have been detected in large amounts in the saliva of HHV-8–seropositive individuals (Koelle et al., 1997; Vieira et al., 1997; Blackbourn et al., 1998; Pauk et al., 2000), and HHV-8 in the cell-free fraction of saliva of these individuals is infectious (Vieira et al., 1997). Some men shed virus into saliva at consistently high titers despite showing no signs of clinical KS disease (LaDuca et al., 1998; Pauk et al., 2000). The high extent of oral shedding of HHV-8 among MSMs is now well confirmed (Gandhi et al., 2004; Marcelin et al., 2004). Primary and immortalized oral epithelial cells, even derived from healthy donors, are indeed susceptible to infection by laboratory-adapted and wild-type HHV-8 (Duus et al., 2004). These various findings provide clear evidence that oral epithelial cells constitute a reservoir of HHV-8 infection and provide the basis for the consideration that saliva is a significant vehicle of HHV-8. Salivary IgA and IgG specific to HHV-8 have been identified (Mbopi-Keou et al., 2004), and it would be important to study how such antibodies influence infection.

Among heterosexuals, correlations with sexual transmission have not been consistently maintained (Smith et al., 1999; Wawer et al., 2001). Heterosexual transmission is not likely to be a major route and seems to require frequent sexual exposures for infection to take place. When HHV-8 seroprevalence is found elevated in heterosexuals, these individuals tend to be those who have had a high number of sexual partners (Bestetti et al., 1998; Tedeschi et al., 2000; de Sanjose et al., 2002).

6.2.2.3.2. Vertical Transmission. The extent to which HHV-8 infection may be transmitted from mother to child is unclear. A study in South Africa suggested a rate of vertical transmission as high as 30% (Bourboulia et al., 1998). Another study showed that the risk of transmission increases with increasing maternal antibody titers (Sitas et al., 1999b). Most children born to HHV-8–seropositive mothers possess passively transmitted antibodies and then serorevert by 2 years of age (Calabro et al., 2000). *In utero* infections are rare (Sarmati et al., 2004). Whether breast milk is a vehicle of mother-to-infant transmission is being clarified. A study conducted in South Africa revealed the presence of HHV-8 DNA in a substantial proportion of breast milk samples (Dedicoat et al., 2004), but a Zambian study (Brayfield et al., 2004) did not provide confirmatory findings.

6.2.2.3.3. Nonsexual Transmission. In developed countries, nonsexual transmission appears rare. Thus, transmission before puberty very seldom occurs in the United States (Blauvelt et al., 1997). In contrast, findings from HHV-8–hyperendemic countries suggest widespread transmission. In Africa, HHV-8 infection is very common among children. Correlation with hepatitis B infection suggests that HHV-8 is transmitted horizontally in conditions of close contact and crowding (Mayama et al., 1998). A population of villagers in French Guiana shows HHV-8 seroprevalences of

15% by the age of 15 years rising sharply to about 30% after 40 years; there was evidence of horizontal familial transmission between children and their mothers but not their fathers, and between children and their siblings (Plancoulaine et al., 2000). A more recent similar study conducted in rural Tanzania also found associations between the HHV-8 serostatus of spouses and between the serostatus of the father and that of his children (Mbulaiteye et al., 2003). In South Africa, transmission between mothers and their children has been estimated to occur at a rate of 30% or more, and the probability of HHV-8 transmission is increased in mothers with a high HHV-8 antibody titer (Sitas et al., 1999a). In that population, very few children of HHV-8–seronegative mothers under the age of 10 years are found HHV-8–seropositive, implicating the mother as the source of most transmissions. In a molecular epidemiological study of KS patients and their first-degree relatives in Malawi, both identical and nonidentical HHV-8 subgenomic sequences were observed between family members, suggesting transmission of HHV-8 along intrafamilial as well as extrafamilial transmission routes (Cook et al., 2002). In Middle Eastern countries, studies of HHV-8 infection in children also support nonsexual transmission and contact within the household (Andreoni et al., 1999, 2002). In Sardinia, which has the highest incidence of classic KS in Italy, a study of HHV-8 prevalence within families reported equally high rates among individuals with classic KS and their relatives; these rates were considerably higher than those among a sample of individuals from the general population who were matched by sex and age. Clustering of HHV-8 seroprevalence between spouses, children, and siblings has been observed (Angeloni et al., 1998).

The importance of saliva as a source of HHV-8, even in people unaffected by KS, is emerging. A study of Egyptian children with primary HHV-8 infection showed that children preferentially carry HHV-8 in saliva than blood (Andreoni et al., 2002). Another study, conducted in Malawi of asymptomatic family members of patients with KS, found HHV-8 DNA in mouth-rinses of 27% of the study individuals but not in any of their blood samples (Cook et al., 2002). Moreover, orally-shed HHV-8 was found to originate from the buccal mucosa, palatal mucosa, and parotid glands (Beyari et al., 2003). Subsequent studies conducted in other African communities have confirmed the relatively high rate of oral HHV-8 shedding (Brayfield et al., 2004; Mbulaiteye et al., 2004; Taylor et al., 2004).

Fecal-oral transmission is unlikely to explain HHV-8 endemicity, given the poor detection rates of HHV-8 DNA in fecal samples (Whitby et al., 1995; Thomas et al., 1996; LaDuca et al., 1998). Urinary shedding of HHV-8 has been reported (Cattani et al., 1999; Cannon et al., 2003;

Beyari et al., 2004), and the frequency of shedding is consistently low (~5%) across the different geographical regions studied so far and independent of the HIV serostatus of the subjects sampled. Although objects contaminated with HHV-8–carrying urine might plausibly act as vehicles of transmission if licked or ingested, it seems unlikely that HHV-8 endemicity would be much enhanced by such practices.

6.2.2.3.4. Organ Transplantion. Seroconversion to HHV-8 has been observed after heart (Emond et al., 2002) and kidney transplantation (Luppi et al., 2002). Few organ donation recipients develop KS in areas of low seroprevalence, but a higher incidence may be found in areas of higher KS incidence. In most cases, transplant patients are infected with HHV-8 prior to transplantation (Parravicini et al., 1997), and KS may develop as a result of viral reactivation due to drug-induced immunosuppression.

6.2.2.3.5. Parenteral Transmission. HHV-8 is transmissible by blood or blood products (Blackbourn et al., 1997; Engels et al., 1999; Cannon et al., 2001). In a study of persons who received blood products from HIV-1- and HHV-8-coinfected donors, seroconversions to HIV-1 but not to HHV-8 were noted (Operskalski et al., 1997). Among injecting drug users (IDUs) in the West, injecting behavior does not appear to promote the spread of HHV-8 (Renwick et al., 2002). Some studies performed in more highly endemic populations have shown that the prevalence may be somewhat higher among IDUs compared with the general population and that there is a higher degree of association between HHV-8 infection and injecting behavior (Sosa et al., 2001; Parisi et al., 2002).

6.2.3. Clinical Spectrum

6.2.3.1. Primary Infection

Clinical manifestations of primary HHV-8 infection have been described in immunocompetent children. It may be associated with fever presenting with or without rash (Kasolo et al., 1997; Andreoni et al., 2002); rashes, if observed, are maculopapular (Andreoni et al., 2002). The outcome of primary HHV-8 infection in the immunosuppressed host is variable. In two HHV-8 seronegative adults who were transplanted with kidneys derived from a single cadaveric HHV-8–seropositive donor, one developed fever followed by bone marrow failure and the other developed KS (Luppi et al., 2000). HIV-1–infected people who seroconvert to HHV-8 after HIV infection have been observed to show a greater relative risk for progression to KS than those who seroconvert prior to HIV infection (Goudsmit et al., 2000). Hence, it appears that primary HHV-8 infection is associated with a higher morbidity in those who are HIV-1–infected than in those who reactivate latent HHV-8 infection. Primary HHV-8 infection during post-transplant immunosuppression carries a lower risk for KS than does reactivation of a previous infection (Jenkins et al., 2002). An active role of HIV-1 in the development of HHV-8–associated diseases has been proposed (e.g., Aoki et al., 2004).

6.2.3.2. Kaposi's Sarcoma

Four epidemiological forms of KS (Fig. 1B–1D), based on clinical and epidemiological differences, are recognized: classic KS, endemic or African KS, iatrogenic KS, and epidemic or AIDS-associated KS. All forms of KS have indistinguishable histological features. KS is a complex multifocal vascular lesion. At the early stage, "the patch stage," the histological picture is that of endothelial-lined spaces surrounding normal blood vessels; there is often a variable degree of inflammatory infiltrate. The "plaque" stage is characterized by an increased growth of spindle-shaped vascular processes in the dermis, along with the formation of slit-like vascular spaces filled with erythrocytes. In the late, "nodular" stage, the lesion is composed primarily of spindle-shaped cells arranged in large sheets, some of which are undergoing mitosis, with slit-like vascular spaces and hemosiderin pigmentation (Cockerell, 1991).

Classic KS occurs most frequently in elderly patients of Mediterranean (mainly Italian and Greek), Jewish, or Arabic decent and is more common in men than women (Iscovich et al., 2000). The incidence peaks after the sixth decade of life. It is an indolent cutaneous disease, rarely metastasizes, and preferentially afflicts men rather than women. Nodules, firm and purple-blue or reddish-brown in appearance, remain confined to the lower extremities, slowly increasing in size over years or decades.

Iatrogenic KS is directly related to drug-induced immunosuppression and was first identified among organ transplant patients (Penn, 1995). Removal of immunosuppression often leads to remission of KS disease. It can present either chronically or with rapid progression, and both cutaneous and visceral forms of the disease may be encountered. People belonging to ethnic groups at risk of classic KS are at an increased risk of acquiring post-transplantation KS and do continue to be at risk even if they are born in or have emigrated to a region of lower incidence. It occurs in <1% of transplant patients in the United States and Western Europe (Penn, 1995) but up to 5% of renal transplant patients in Saudi Arabia (Qunibi et al., 1988).

Endemic KS was rarely encountered in Africa prior to the AIDS era (Oettle, 1962; Maclean, 1963). A band of endemicity stretches across equatorial Africa, with particularly high rates noted in northeastern Zaire, western Uganda, and Tanzania (Cook-Mozaffari et al., 1998). This form of KS may present as benign nodular cutaneous disease predominantly in young adults; plaques and nodules on one to four limbs may be evident, accompanied by local lymphadenopathy and peripheral edema, and the nodules may ulcerate. Localized cutaneous disease have been observed to progress rapidly to invade adjacent tissues or disseminate. A florid muco-cutaneous and visceral disease may also be seen on presentation. Young children are prone to adopt a fulminant lymphadenopathic course (Bayley, 1991).

The epidemic form of KS heralded the AIDS epidemic (Friedman-Kien, 1981; Hymes et al., 1981). It later became recognized as an AIDS-defining condition in HIV-infected individuals. The overall risk of KS in AIDS patients was 20,000 times greater than that of the general popula-tion and 300 times that of other immunosuppressed patients (Beral et al., 1990). In the West, MSM who were more sexually active and engaged sexual partners from the epicenters of the AIDS epidemic were found to be at greatest risk of developing KS. The median age of KS-affected indi-viduals was the late thirties (Goedert, 2000). The elevated risk was observed even among men aged 13–24 years, suggesting a rapid increase in risk after homosexual contact. Striking differences in risks of acquiring AIDS-KS were observed between different HIV transmission groups, with the risk in homosexual men being more than men with hemophilia and the risk in women acquiring HIV from bisexual men higher than het-erosexual intravenous drug users (Beral et al., 1990; Serraino et al., 1995). The disease is typically lymphoadenopathic, tending to involve the viscera and mucosa as well as the skin. It is commonly multifocal and symmetrical at presentation, frequently over the upper body, head, and neck, with the mouth, particularly at the hard palate, as the site of predilection (Hengge et al., 2002). Lesions evolve quickly, both in terms of the local progression and of visceral dissemination. HIV-1 probably promotes the pathogenesis of KS other than by immunosuppression. The priming of target cells and the tissue microenvironment by HIV-infected T cells that favor HHV-8 infection and replication (Mercader et al., 2000), the direct effects of HIV-1 encoded products on HHV-8 gene expression and viral replication (Huang et al., 2001), and the angiogenic effect of the HIV-1 tat protein (Barillari and Ensoli, 2002) may contribute to the patho-genesis. The incidence of AIDS-KS in the West is declining, in the wake of the widespread therapeutic use of anti-retroviral agents (Jones et al.,

2000). In Africa, however, AIDS-KS continues to be widespread, its prevalence varying according to geographic region (Cook-Mozaffari et al., 1998) but affecting men more often than women (Parkin et al., 1999; Chokunonga et al., 2000). The AIDS epidemic has resulted in dramatic increases in the incidence of childhood KS (Chintu et al., 1995; Ziegler and Katongole-Mbidde, 1996).

It has not been established whether KS is a true cancer or a reactive hyperplasia. Although the spindle-shaped cells are thought to be neoplastic, they lack aneuploidy. Furthermore, very few spindle-like cells are present in early patch/plaque stage. The remission of disease observable even in severely immunocompromised patients following its relief suggests that KS is not a true sarcoma. Clonality is often used to define a neoplasm, because a true malignancy originates from a single cell. X-linked inactivation assays have been attempted to establish clonality but provide conflicting findings (Rabkin et al., 1997; Gill et al., 1998) (Gill et al., 1998). However, HHV-8 clonality could be demonstrated in nodular lesions of KS (Judde et al., 2000), indicating that the establishment of latent HHV-8 infection precedes tumor growth. It would appear that KS in its early stages is a nonclonal proliferation of endothelial cells that then evolves into a true clonal disease.

HHV-8 DNA has been sought for and consistently detected by PCR from KS lesional tissues from various geographical regions, thereby linking the presence of HHV-8 DNA with all epidemiological forms of KS. However, the clinical disparities between the individual forms of KS suggest a role for cofactors that contribute to their pathogenesis. Coinfection by HIV-1 is clearly the major risk factor unique to AIDS-associated KS, contributing to its aggressive course.

HHV-8 DNA may also be amplified in PBMCs of HIV-positive individuals. Its detection serves to predict the subsequent development of KS. In paired PBMC samples taken before and after KS onset from AIDS-KS patients and high-risk HIV-positive MSM patients, and single PBMC samples from low-risk HIV-positive hemophiliacs, HHV-8 DNA was detected in 50% of AIDS-KS patients prior to the onset of KS and in 10% of members in the other groups (Moore et al., 1996c). Another study revealed that 55% of HIV+HHV-8+ patients without KS developed the disease within 30 months of follow-up compared with 9% of HHV-8–seronegative/HIV-seropositive patients (Whitby et al., 1995). Increase of antibody titers against ORF73 may be a predictor for KS development among HIV-seropositive MSM (Inoue et al., 2004).

Extensive epidemiologic studies in Italy have confirmed that high HHV-8 seropositivity rates are associated with areas where the incidence of classic KS is the highest (Calabro et al., 1998; Whitby et al., 1998; Ascoli et al., 2001; Santarelli et al., 2001). Similarly, despite the clinical heterogeneity of African KS, all cases are associated with HHV-8 seropositivity (Gao et al., 1996a; Lennette et al., 1996). However, African populations that show similar HHV-8 seroprevalences may have significant variations in KS incidences (Grossman et al., 2002). Such data intimate the close correlation between HHV-8 seroprevalence and the incidence of KS in Western countries, but not in Africa, where other cofactors may be involved (Ziegler, 1993).

HHV-8 seropositivity has also been associated with the development of iatrogenic KS. Indeed, the high frequency of iatrogenic KS in Saudi Arabia likely reflects the relatively high prevalence of HHV-8 in the general population (Qunibi et al., 1988). Transplant-associated KS is seen predominantly in kidney allograft recipients and not other solid-organ or bone marrow transplant recipients (Cattani et al., 2001). This selection may be associated with differences in immunosuppressive therapy; for example, the use of cyclosporine, which may favor HHV-8 reactivation in the kidney recipients (Penn, 1995), or sirolimus, which may suppress reactivation (Stallone et al., 2005). Moreover, the kidney may be a site of HHV-8 latency (Sarid et al., 2001). Studies have also confirmed that most iatrogenic KS patients are HHV-8 seropositive prior to transplantation, favoring the hypothesis that reactivation of latent viral infection leads to disease (Parravicini et al., 1997; Cattani et al., 2001; Jenkins et al., 2002).

6.2.3.3. Primary Effusion Lymphoma (PEL)

PEL (also known as body cavity–based lymphoma) is another neoplastic condition associated with HHV-8 (Malnati et al., 2003). It is seen primarily in homosexual men (Nador et al., 1996) and seldom in other groups not at risk for HIV infection (Boulanger et al., 2004a). First described among AIDS patients (Knowles et al., 1988), it is usually encountered during the advanced stages of the disease (Komanduri et al., 1996). Rare even in AIDS patients, it constitutes <0.2% of all AIDS-associated lymphomas in the United States, with previous KS diagnosis conferring an increased risk of PEL relative to all other AIDS-associated non-Hodgkin lymphomas (Mbulaiteye et al., 2002). In patients with AIDS, PEL is a fulminant lymphoproliferative disease, and the median survival time is less than 6 months (Komanduri et al., 1996; Nador et al., 1996). A more indolent course has been documented in immunocompetent patients (Boulanger et al., 2004a).

PEL is a distinct subtype of non-Hodgkin lymphoma that has morphological features shared by large-cell immunoblastic lymphomas and anaplastic large-cell lymphoma (Ansari et al., 1996; Cesarman et al., 1996), typically presenting as malignant effusions in the pleural, pericardial, or peritoneal cavities, usually without significant tumor mass or lymphadenopathy. Lymphomatous infiltration of serosal surfaces adjacent to the site of the primary malignant effusion is sometimes encountered (Komanduri et al., 1996). Morphologically, the cells bridge the features of large-cell immunoblastic and anaplastic large-cell lymphomas and are usually large and irregularly shaped, with abundant cytoplasm and variably chromatic and pleomorphic nuclei resembling a plasmacytoid morphology (Ansari et al., 1996). Its clonal nature has been established (Boulanger et al., 2005). The gene expression profile closely resembles that of malignant plasma cells (Jenner et al., 2003). Co-infection with EBV is common in PELs, and although EBV monoclonality is very common (Cesarman et al., 1995; Komanduri et al., 1996; Nador et al., 1996), HHV-8 monoclonality is less so (Boulanger et al., 2005).

6.2.3.4. Castleman's Disease

Castleman's disease, also referred to as angiofollicular or giant lymph node hyperplasia, is a rare, usually polyclonal, non-neoplastic disorder of unknown etiology. Two distinct histopathological variants with different clinical characteristics have been described: the hyaline vascular type and the plasma-cell type (Keller et al., 1972). The more common hyaline form presents as a solitary mass, is asymptomatic, and is usually curable surgically. The rarer plasma-cell type is typically characterized by generalized lymphadenopathy, defined by the presence of interfollicular plasmacytosis associated with lymphoid follicles that show either hyperplasia or regressive changes. The systemic form of the disease, also called multicentric Castleman's disease (MCD), is primarily of the plasma-cell type. The majority of MCD cases occur in patients with HIV infection (Oksenhendler et al., 1996), with a significant proportion of these associated with HHV-8 infection (Dupin et al., 2000). The HHV-8–associated lesions are characterized histologically by follicle dissolution resulting from infiltration of HHV-8–infected lymphocytes into the mantle zone boundary (Amin et al., 2003). The autocrine or paracrine production of v-IL6 from the infected cells is thought to play an important pathogenic role (Staskus et al., 1999). MCD adopts an aggressive clinical course with a poor prognosis, and patients are at increased risk of developing non-Hodgkin lymphoma and KS (Oksenhendler et al., 2002).

6.2.3.5. Other Lymphoproliferative Disorders

HHV-8 sequences have been found in non-HIV-infected patients with angioimmunoblastic lymphadenopathies. One of these is a distinct benign, non-HIV-related, lymphadenopathy histologically characterized by a predominantly follicular lesion with giant germinal center hyperplasia and increased vascularity (Luppi et al., 1996). Other lymphoproliferative disorders have been associated with HHV-8 DNA carriage and include non-Hodgkin lymphomas, Hodgkin disease, and reactive lymphadenopathies (Malnati et al., 2003). Other entities are AIDS-associated immunoblastic lymphoma (Engels et al., 2003), post-transplantation lymphoproliferative disorders (Kapelushnik et al., 2001), and pulmonary inflammatory myofibroblastic tumor (Gomez-Roman et al., 2001). In germinotropic lymphoproliferative disorder, HHV-8- and EBV-coinfected B-cell plasmablasts can be observed to invade lymphoid follicle germinal centers (Du et al., 2002). Detection of HHV-8 in mature T-cell lymphoproliferative disorders has also been reported (Sander et al., 1996), but that observation has not been confirmed (Henghold et al., 1997).

6.2.3.6. Other Neoplastic Disorders

HHV-8 DNA was reported to be detectable in cultured bone-marrow DCs of patients with multiple myeloma but not in their plasmablasts (Rettig et al., 1997; Said et al., 1997). The relationship between HHV-8 infection and the disease is controversial (Berenson and Vescio, 1999; Tarte et al., 1999; Cannon et al., 2000).

HHV-8 sequences have also been detected in some angiosarcomas (McDonagh et al., 1996) and tissue affected by angiolymphoid hyperplasia with eosinophilia (Gyulai et al., 1996); such findings could not be confirmed (Dictor et al., 1996). HHV-8 DNA has also been found in lesional tissue of patients with squamous cell or basal cell carcinomas (Rady et al., 1995), but, again, confirmatory studies have not been forthcoming (Dictor et al., 1996). The etiological connection between HHV-8 infection and most of these disorders is suspect.

6.2.3.7. Other Diseases

Primary but not secondary pulmonary hypertension has been found to be associated with HHV-8 infection (Bull et al., 2003; Cool et al., 2003). The cells in the plexiform lesions of the disorder showed histological similarities to the endothelial abnormalities of cutaneous KS and expressed HHV-8 LANA-1 and v-cyclin. There is as yet no definitive serological evidence that the patients with this disease have been infected by the virus (Henke-Gendo et al., 2004). The presence of HHV-8 has been found in lung tissue and bronchoalveolar lavage samples of predominantly (but not exclusively) HIV-infected patients with interstitial pneumonitis (Trovato et al., 1999; Tarp et al., 2001).

Association of HHV-8 with heart disease has been proposed. Individuals with PEL have been noted to have a high incidence of congestive heart failure, a condition also common to classic KS patients (Ascoli et al., 2002). Moreover, Italian patients with cardiovascular disease show a higher HHV-8 seroprevalence than the general population (Carletti et al., 2002). Furthermore, HIV-1–infected patients with KS are more likely to develop atheromas and aortic endothelial damage than those without KS (Grahame-Clarke et al., 2001). It is postulated that HHV-8–encoded chemokine vCCL-1 may mediate the chemotactic response of endothelial cells in response to the atherogenic apolipoprotein(a) through CCR8 (Haque et al., 2001).

The high prevalence of both HHV-8 DNA in lesional skin and in PBMCs and of HHV-8–specific IgG antibodies in patients with pemphigus suggest that HHV-8 infection might be a contributing factor in the development of this autoimmune disease (Wang et al., 2005a). More confirmatory studies are required. HHV-8 DNA was reported to be detectable in sarcoid tissues (Di Alberti et al., 1997b). Subsequent studies have failed to confirm this finding (di Gennaro et al., 2001).

6.2.4. Management

6.2.4.1. Antivirals

Many of the currently available antiherpesvirus drugs are DNA polymerase inhibitors, which are active against lytic but not latent herpesvirus infection. *In vitro* studies have revealed HHV-8 to be resistant to acyclovir and penciclovir but sensitive to ganciclovir, cidofovir, adefovir, and foscarnet (Kedes and Ganem, 1997; Medveczky et al., 1997; Neyts and De Clercq, 1997; Long et al., 2003; Friedrichs et al., 2004). However, as such antivirals do not inhibit episomal viral DNA synthesis (Medveczky et al., 1997), little benefit may be expected from their use in the treatment of neoplastic diseases associated with HHV-8 latency, for example, lymphomas (Staudt et al., 2004). In diseases associated with HHV-8 replication, like KS and MCD, treatment incorporating these agents might prove beneficial. Nonetheless, a pilot study of cidofovir for the treatment of KS indicates that it is not efficacious (Little et al., 2003). Some improvement in clinical course was observed with the use of ganciclovir in patients with MCD, but the study sample was small (Casper et al., 2004).

6.2.4.2. Anti-retroviral Protease Inhibitors

HAART regimes that incorporate the protease inhibitors used for the treatment of HIV infection have been found to lead to positive clinical outcomes in KS patients and to a reduction in HHV-8 viremia (Leao et al., 2000; Gill et al., 2002). Moreover, both protease inhibitor–based and non-nucleoside reverse transcriptase inhibitor–based anti-retroviral treatment combinations have been observed to result in KS regression (Gill et al., 2002). The efficacy of protease inhibitors may relate not only to restoration of the immune status but also to specific anti-angiogenic and anti-tumorigenic effects exerted by this class of drugs (Sgadari et al., 2002).

6.2.4.3. Other Approaches

The potency by which thalidomide exerts its anti-angiogenic and anti-inflammatory effects has been exploited in attempts to determine if this drug can lead to the regression of KS. A phase II trial showed a high frequency of toxicity, but significant decreases in the circulating HHV-8 were observed in patients who could tolerate the therapy (Fife et al., 1998). In a minority of patients, thalidomide therapy has led to disease regression (Krown, 2003). The experimental basis for cytokine-based therapeutic approaches is being investigated. IFN-α exerts potent effects *in vitro* and *in vivo* (see Section 6.2.1.3.1) and may be therapeutically explored. Treatment of a PEL cell line with the antiseizure drug valproate leads to HHV-8 lytic replication and induces apoptosis. As the production of virus was greatly decreased by concomitant treatment with foscarnet, therapeutic applications for HHV-8–associated malignancies using the two drugs in combination become a possibility (Klass et al., 2005).

References

Ablashi, D., Agut, H., Berneman, Z., Campadelli-Fiume, G., Carrigan, D., Ceccherini-Nelli, L., Chandran, B., Chou, S., Collandre, H., Cone, R., Dambaugh, T., Dewhurst, S., DiLuca, D., Foa-Tomasi, L., Fleckenstein, B., Frenkel, N., Gallo, R., Gompels, U., Hall, C., Jones, M., Lawrence, G., Martin, M., Montagnier, L., Neipel, F., Nicholas, J., Pellett, P., Razzaque, A., Torrelli, G., Thomson, B., Salahuddin, S., Wyatt, L., and Yamanishi, K. (1993). Human herpesvirus-6 strain groups: a nomenclature. *Arch. Virol. 129*, 363–366.

Ablashi, D.V., Schirm, S., Fleckenstein, B., Faggioni, A., Dahlberg, J., Rabin, H., Loeb, W., Armstrong, G., Peng, J.W., Aulahk, G., and Torrisi, M.R. (1985). Herpesvirus saimiri-induced lymphoblastoid rabbit cell line: growth characteristics, virus persistence, and oncogenic properties. *J. Virol. 55*, 623–633.

Adler, H., Messerle, M., and Koszinowski, U.H. (2003). Cloning of herpesviral genomes as bacterial artificial chromosomes. *Rev. Med. Virol. 13*, 111–121.

Akkapaiboon, P., Mori, Y., Sadaoka, T., Yonemoto, S., and Yamanishi, K. (2004). Intracellular processing of human herpesvirus 6 glycoproteins Q1 and Q2 into tetrameric complexes expressed on the viral envelope. *J. Virol. 78*, 7969–7983.

Akula, S.M., Ford, P.W., Whitman, A.G., Hamden, K.E., Shelton, J.G., and McCubrey, J.A. (2004). Raf promotes human herpesvirus-8 (HHV-8/KSHV) infection. *Oncogene 23*, 5227–5241.

Akula, S.M., Naranatt, P.P., Walia, N.S., Wang, F.Z., Fegley, B., and Chandran, B. (2003). Kaposi's sarcoma-associated herpesvirus (human herpesvirus 8) infection of human fibroblast cells occurs through endocytosis. *J. Virol. 77*, 7978–7990.

Akula, S.M., Pramod, N.P., Wang, F.Z., and Chandran, B. (2001). Human herpesvirus 8 envelope-associated glycoprotein B interacts with heparan sulfate-like moieties. *Virology 284*, 235–249.

Akula, S.M., Pramod, N.P., Wang, F.Z., and Chandran, B. (2002). Integrin alpha3beta1 (CD 49c/29) is a cellular receptor for Kaposi's sarcoma-associated herpesvirus (KSHV/HHV-8) entry into the target cells. *Cell 108*, 407–419.

Albright, A.V., Lavi, E., Black, J.B., Goldberg, S., O'Connor, M.J., and Gonzalez-Scarano, F. (1998). The effect of human herpesvirus-6 (HHV-6) on cultured human neural cells: oligodendrocytes and microglia. *J. Neurovirol. 4*, 486–494.

Amin, H.M., Medeiros, L.J., Manning, J.T., and Jones, D. (2003). Dissolution of the lymphoid follicle is a feature of the HHV8+ variant of plasma cell Castleman's disease. *Am. J. Surg. Pathol. 27*, 91–100.

An, F.Q., Compitello, N., Horwitz, E., Sramkoski, M., Knudsen, E.S., and Renne, R. (2005). The latency-associated nuclear antigen of Kaposi's sarcoma-associated herpesvirus modulates cellular gene expression and protects lymphoid cells from p16 INK4A-induced cell cycle arrest. *J. Biol. Chem. 280*, 3862–3874.

Andre-Garnier, E., Milpied, N., Boutolleau, D., Saiagh, S., Billaudel, S., and Imbert-Marcille, B.M. (2004). Reactivation of human herpesvirus 6 during ex vivo expansion of circulating CD34+ haematopoietic stem cells. *J. Gen. Virol. 85*, 3333–3336.

Andreoni, M., El Sawaf, G., Rezza, G., Ensoli, B., Nicastri, E., Ventura, L., Ercoli, L., Sarmati, L., and Rocchi, G. (1999). High seroprevalence of antibodies to human herpesvirus-8 in Egyptian children: evidence of nonsexual transmission. *J. Natl. Cancer Inst. 91*, 465–469.

Andreoni, M., Sarmati, L., Nicastri, E., El Sawaf, G., El Zalabani, M., Uccella, I., Bugarini, R., Parisi, S.G., and Rezza, G. (2002). Primary human herpesvirus 8 infection in immunocompetent children. *JAMA 287*, 1295–1300.

Angeloni, A., Heston, L., Uccini, S., Sirianni, M.C., Cottoni, F., Masala, M.V., Cerimele, D., Lin, S.F., Sun, R., Rigsby, M., Faggioni, A., and Miller, G. (1998). High prevalence of antibodies to human herpesvirus 8 in relatives of patients with classic Kaposi's sarcoma from Sardinia. *J. Infect. Dis. 177*, 1715–1718.

Ansari, M.Q., Dawson, D.B., Nador, R., Rutherford, C., Schneider, N.R., Latimer, M.J., Picker, L., Knowles, D.M., and McKenna, R.W. (1996). Primary body cavity-based AIDS-related lymphomas. *Am. J. Clin. Pathol. 105*, 221–229.

Aoki, Y. and Tosato, G. (2004). HIV-1 Tat enhances Kaposi sarcoma–associated herpesvirus (KSHV) infectivity. *Blood 104*, 810–814.

Arvanitakis, L., Geras-Raaka, E., Varma, A., Gershengorn, M.C., and Cesarman, E. (1997). Human herpesvirus KSHV encodes a constitutively active G-protein-coupled receptor linked to cell proliferation. *Nature 385*, 347–350.

Arvanitakis, L., Mesri, E.A., Nador, R.G., Said, J.W., Asch, A.S., Knowles, D.M., and Cesarman, E. (1996). Establishment and characterization of a primary effusion (body cavity-based) lymphoma cell line (BC–3) harboring kaposi's sarcoma-associated herpesvirus (KSHV/HHV-8) in the absence of Epstein-Barr virus. *Blood 88*, 2648–2654.

Ascoli, V., Belli, S., Benedetti, M., Trinca, S., Ricci, P., and Comba, P. (2001). High incidence of classic Kaposi's sarcoma in Mantua, Po Valley, Northern Italy (1989-1998). *Br. J. Cancer 85*, 379–382.

Ascoli, V., Lo, C.F., Torelli, G., Vallisa, D., Cavanna, L., Bergonzi, C., and Luppi, M. (2002). Human herpesvirus 8–associated primary effusion lymphoma in HIV-patients: a clinicpidemiologic variant resembling classic Kaposi's sarcoma. *Haematologica 87*, 339–343.

AuCoin, D.P., Colletti, K.S., Cei, S.A., Papouskova, I., Tarrant, M., and Pari, G.S. (2004). Amplification of the Kaposi's sarcoma-associated herpesvirus/human herpesvirus 8 lytic origin of DNA replication is dependent upon a cis-acting AT-rich region and an ORF50 response element and the trans–acting factors ORF50 (K-Rta) and K8 (K-bZIP). *Virology 318*, 542–555.

Babcock, G.J., Decker, L.L., Volk, M., and Thorley-Lawson, D.A. (1998). EBV persistence in memory B cells in vivo. *Immunity 9*, 395–404.

Baillargeon, J., Deng, J.H., Hettler, E., Harrison, C., Grady, J.J., Korte, L.G., Alexander, J., Montalvo, E., Jenson, H.B., and Gao, S.J. (2001). Seroprevalence of Kaposi's sarcoma-associated herpesvirus infection among blood donors from Texas. *Ann. Epidemiol. 11*, 512–518.

Bais, C., Santomasso, B., Coso, O., Arvanitakis, L., Raaka, E.G., Gutkind, J.S., Asch, A.S., Cesarman, E., Gershengorn, M.C., and Mesri, E.A. (1998). G-protein-coupled receptor of Kaposi's sarcoma-associated herpesvirus is a viral oncogene and angiogenesis activator. *Nature 391*, 86–89.

Ballestas, M.E., Chatis, P.A., and Kaye, K.M. (1999). Efficient persistence of extrachromosomal KSHV DNA mediated by latency-associated nuclear antigen. *Science 284*, 641–644.

Barclay, A.N., Wright, G.J., Brooke, G., and Brown, M.H. (2002). CD200 and membrane protein interactions in the control of myeloid cells. *Trends Immunol. 23*, 285–290.

Barillari, G. and Ensoli, B. (2002). Angiogenic effects of extracellular human immunodeficiency virus type 1 Tat protein and its role in the pathogenesis of AIDS-associated Kaposi's sarcoma. *Clin. Microbiol. Rev. 15*, 310–326.

Bayley, A.C. (1991). Occurrence, clinical behaviour and management of Kaposi's sarcoma in Zambia. *Cancer Surv. 10*, 53–71.

Belec, L., Cancre, N., Hallouin, M.C., Morvan, J., Si, M.A., and Gresenguet, G. (1998). High prevalence in Central Africa of blood donors who are potentially infectious for human herpesvirus 8. *Transfusion 38*, 771–775.

Bellows, D.S., Chau, B.N., Lee, P., Lazebnik, Y., Burns, W.H., and Hardwick, J.M. (2000). Antiapoptotic herpesvirus Bcl-2 homologs escape caspase-mediated conversion to proapoptotic proteins. *J. Virol. 74*, 5024–5031.

Beral, V., Peterman, T.A., Berkelman, R.L., and Jaffe, H.W. (1990). Kaposi's sarcoma among persons with AIDS: a sexually transmitted infection? *Lancet 335*, 123–128.

Berenson, J.R. and Vescio, R.A. (1999). HHV–8 is present in multiple myeloma patients. *Blood 93*, 3157–3159.

Bestetti, G., Renon, G., Mauclere, P., Ruffie, A., Mbopi Keou, F.X., Eme, D., Parravicini, C., Corbellino, M., de The, G., and Gessain, A. (1998). High seroprevalence of human herpesvirus-8 in pregnant women and prostitutes from Cameroon. *AIDS 12*, 541–543.

Bethge, W., Beck, R., Jahn, G., Mundinger, P., Kanz, L., and Einsele, H. (1999). Successful treatment of human herpesvirus-6 encephalitis after bone marrow transplantation. *Bone Marrow Transplant. 24*, 1245–1248.

Beyari, M.M., Hodgson, T.A., Cook, R.D., Kondowe, W., Molyneux, E.M., Scully, C.M., Teo, C.G., and Porter, S.R. (2003). Multiple human herpesvirus-8 infection. *J. Infect. Dis. 188*, 678–689.

Beyari, M.M., Hodgson, T.A., Kondowe, W., Molyneux, E.M., Scully, C.M., Porter, S.R., and Teo, C.G. (2004). Genotypic profile of human herpesvirus 8 (Kaposi's sarcoma-associated herpesvirus) in urine. *J. Clin. Microbiol. 42*, 3313–3316.

Biesinger, B., Muller-Fleckenstein, I., Simmer, B., Lang, G., Wittmann, S., Platzer, E., Desrosiers, R.C., and Fleckenstein, B. (1992). Stable growth transformation of human T lymphocytes by herpesvirus saimiri. *Proc. Natl. Acad. Sci. U. S. A. 89*, 3116–3119.

Biggar, R.J., Whitby, D., Marshall, V., Linhares, A.C., and Black, F. (2000). Human herpesvirus 8 in Brazilian Amerindians: a hyperendemic population with a new subtype. *J. Infect. Dis. 181*, 1562–1568.

Birkmann, A., Mahr, K., Ensser, A., Yaguboglu, S., Titgemeyer, F., Fleckenstein, B., and Neipel, F. (2001). Cell surface heparan sulfate is a receptor for human herpesvirus 8 and interacts with envelope glycoprotein K8.1. *J. Virol. 75*, 11583–11593.

Black, J.B., Inoue, N., Kite-Powell, K., Zaki, S., and Pellett, P.E. (1993). Frequent isolation of human herpesvirus 7 from saliva. *Virus Res. 29*, 91–98.

Black, J.B., Schwarz, T.F., Patton, J.L., Kite-Powell, K., Pellett, P.E., Wiersbitzky, S., Bruns, R., Muller, C., Jager, G., and Stewart, J.A. (1996). Evaluation of immunoassays for detection of antibodies to human herpesvirus 7. *Clin. Diagn. Lab Immunol. 3*, 79–83.

Blackbourn, D.J., Ambroziak, J., Lennette, E., Adams, M., Ramachandran, B., and Levy, J.A. (1997). Infectious human herpesvirus 8 in a healthy North American blood donor. *Lancet 349*, 609–611.

Blackbourn, D.J., Lennette, E.T., Ambroziak, J., Mourich, D.V., and Levy, J.A. (1998). Human herpesvirus 8 detection in nasal secretions and saliva. *J. Infect. Dis. 177*, 213–216.

Blackbourn, D.J., Osmond, D., Levy, J.A., and Lennette, E.T. (1999). Increased human herpesvirus 8 seroprevalence in young homosexual men who have multiple sex contacts with different partners. *J. Infect. Dis. 179*, 237–239.

Blauvelt, A., Sei, S., Cook, P.M., Schulz, T.F., and Jeang, K.T. (1997). Human herpesvirus 8 infection occurs following adolescence in the United States. *J. Infect. Dis. 176*, 771–774.

Boname, J.M., de Lima, B.D., Lehner, P.J., and Stevenson, P.G. (2004). Viral degradation of the MHC class I peptide loading complex. *Immunity 20*, 305–317.

Boname, J.M., May, J.S., and Stevenson, P.G. (2005). The murine gamma-herpesvirus-68 MK3 protein causes TAP degradation independent of MHC class I heavy chain degradation. *Eur. J. Immunol. 35*, 171–179.

Boname, J.M. and Stevenson, P.G. (2001). MHC class I ubiquitination by a viral PHD/LAP finger protein. *Immunity 15*, 627–636.

Boshoff, C. and Chang, Y. (2001). Kaposi's sarcoma-associated herpesvirus: a new DNA tumor virus. *Annu. Rev. Med 52*, 453–470.

Boshoff, C., Endo, Y., Collins, P.D., Takeuchi, Y., Reeves, J.D., Schweickart, V.L., Siani, M.A., Sasaki, T., Williams, T.J., Gray, P.W., Moore, P.S., Chang, Y., and Weiss, R.A. (1997). Angiogenic and HIV-inhibitory functions of KSHV–encoded chemokines. *Science 278*, 290–294.

Boshoff, C. and Weiss, R.A. (2001). Epidemiology and pathogenesis of Kaposi's sarcoma–associated herpesvirus. *Philos. Trans. R. Soc. Lond. B Biol. Sci. 356*, 517–534.

Boulanger, E., Duprez, R., Delabesse, E., Gabarre, J., Macintyre, E., and Gessain, A. (2005). Mono/oligoclonal pattern of Kaposi Sarcoma-associated herpesvirus (KSHV/HHV-8) episomes in primary effusion lymphoma cells. *Int. J. Cancer.* 115:511–518.

Boulanger, E., Hermine, O., Fermand, J.P., Radford-Weiss, I., Brousse, N., Meignin, V., and Gessain, A. (2004a). Human herpesvirus 8 (HHV-8)-associated peritoneal primary effusion lymphoma (PEL) in two HIV-negative elderly patients. *Am. J. Hematol. 76*, 88–91.

Boulanger, M.J., Chow, D.C., Brevnova, E., Martick, M., Sandford, G., Nicholas, J., and Garcia, K.C. (2004b). Molecular mechanisms for viral mimicry of a human cytokine: activation of gp130 by HHV–8 interleukin–6. *J. Mol. Biol. 335*, 641–654.

Bourboulia, D., Whitby, D., Boshoff, C., Newton, R., Beral, V., Carrara, H., Lane, A., and Sitas, F. (1998). Serologic evidence for mother-to-child transmission of Kaposi sarcoma-associated herpesvirus infection. *JAMA 280*, 31–32.

Braaten, D.C., Sparks-Thissen, R.L., Kreher, S., Speck, S.H., and Virgin, H.W.t. (2005). An optimized CD8+ T-cell response controls productive and latent gammaherpesvirus infection. *J. Virol. 79*, 2573–2583.

Brayfield, B.P., Kankasa, C., West, J.T., Muyanga, J., Bhat, G., Klaskala, W., Mitchell, C.D., and Wood, C. (2004). Distribution of Kaposi sarcoma-associated herpesvirus/human herpesvirus 8 in maternal saliva and breast milk in Zambia: implications for transmission. *J. Infect. Dis. 189*, 2260–2270.

Brinkmann, M.M., Glenn, M., Rainbow, L., Kieser, A., Henke-Gendo, C., and Schulz, T.F. (2003). Activation of mitogen-activated protein kinase and NF-kappaB pathways by a Kaposi's sarcoma–associated herpesvirus K15 membrane protein. *J. Virol. 77*, 9346–9358.

Brousset, P., Cesarman, E., Meggetto, F., Lamant, L., and Delsol, G. (2001). Colocalization of the viral interleukin-6 with latent nuclear antigen-1 of human herpesvirus-8 in endothelial spindle cells of Kaposi's sarcoma and lymphoid cells of multicentric Castleman's disease. *Hum. Pathol. 32*, 95–100.

Bull, T.M., Cool, C.D., Serls, A.E., Rai, P.R., Parr, J., Neid, J.M., Geraci, M.W., Campbell, T.B., Voelkel, N.F., and Badesch, D.B. (2003). Primary pulmonary hypertension, Castleman's disease and human herpesvirus–8. *Eur. Respir. J. 22*, 403–407.

Burd, E.M., Knox, K.K., and Carrigan, D.R. (1993). Human herpesvirus 6 associated suppression of growth factor-induced macrophage maturation in human bone marrow cultures. *Blood 81*, 1645–1650.

Burger, R., Neipel, F., Fleckenstein, B., Savino, R., Ciliberto, G., Kalden, J.R., and Gramatzki, M. (1998). Human herpesvirus type 8 interleukin-6 homologue is functionally active on human myeloma cells. *Blood 91*, 1858–1863.

Burysek, L. and Pitha, P.M. (2001). Latently expressed human herpesvirus 8-encoded interferon regulatory factor 2 inhibits double-stranded RNA-activated protein kinase. *J. Virol. 75*, 2345–2352.

Burysek, L., Yeow, W.S., Lubyova, B., Kellum, M., Schafer, S.L., Huang, Y.Q., and Pitha, P.M. (1999a). Functional analysis of human herpesvirus 8-encoded viral interferon regulatory factor 1 and its association with cellular interferon regulatory factors and p300. *J. Virol. 73*, 7334–7342.

Burysek, L., Yeow, W.S., and Pitha, P.M. (1999b). Unique properties of a second human herpesvirus 8-encoded interferon regulatory factor (vIRF-2). *J. Hum. Virol. 2*, 19–32.

Calabro, M.L., Gasperini, P., Barbierato, M., Ometto, L., Zanchetta, M., De Rossi, A., and Chieco-Bianchi, L. (2000). A search for human herpesvirus 8 (HHV-8) in HIV-1 infected mothers and their infants does not suggest vertical transmission of HHV–8. *Int. J. Cancer 85*, 296–297.

Calabro, M.L., Sheldon, J., Favero, A., Simpson, G.R., Fiore, J.R., Gomes, E., Angarano, G., Chieco-Bianchi, L., and Schulz, T.F. (1998). Seroprevalence of Kaposi's sarcoma-associated herpesvirus/human herpesvirus 8 in several regions of Italy. *J. Hum. Virol. 1*, 207–213.

Cannon, J.S., Nicholas, J., Orenstein, J.M., Mann, R.B., Murray, P.G., Browning, P.J., DiGiuseppe, J.A., Cesarman, E., Hayward, G.S., and Ambinder, R.F. (1999). Heterogeneity of viral IL–6 expression in HHV–8–associated diseases. *J. Infect. Dis. 180*, 824–828.

Cannon, M.J., Dollard, S.C., Black, J.B., Edlin, B.R., Hannah, C., Hogan, S.E., Patel, M.M., Jaffe, H.W., Offermann, M.K., Spira, T.J., Pellett, P.E., and Gunthel, C.J. (2003). Risk factors for Kaposi's sarcoma in men seropositive for both human herpesvirus 8 and human immunodeficiency virus. *AIDS 17*, 215–222.

Cannon, M.J., Dollard, S.C., Smith, D.K., Klein, R.S., Schuman, P., Rich, J.D., Vlahov, D., and Pellett, P.E. (2001). Blood-borne and sexual transmission of human herpesvirus 8 in women with or at risk for human immunodeficiency virus infection. *N. Engl. J. Med. 344*, 637–643.

Cannon, M.J., Flanders, W.D., and Pellett, P.E. (2000). Occurrence of primary cancers in association with multiple myeloma and Kaposi's sarcoma in the United States, 1973-1995. *Int. J Cancer 85*, 453–456.

Carletti, F., Mandolini, C., Rossi, A., Capobianchi, M.R., and Borgia, M.C. (2002). Prevalence of human herpesvirus (HHV)-8 infection among carriers of cardiovascular disease. *J. Biol. Regul. Homeost. Agents 16*, 110–113.

Carrigan, D.R. and Knox, K.K. (1994). Human herpesvirus 6 (HHV-6) isolation from bone marrow: HHV-6-associated bone marrow suppression in bone marrow transplant patients. *Blood 84*, 3307–3310.

Carroll, P.A., Brazeau, E., and Lagunoff, M. (2004). Kaposi's sarcoma-associated herpesvirus infection of blood endothelial cells induces lymphatic differentiation. *Virology 328*, 7–18.

Caruso, A., Favilli, F., Rotola, A., Comar, M., Horejsh, D., Alessandri, G., Grassi, M., Di Luca, D., and Fiorentini, S. (2003). Human herpesvirus-6 modulates RANTES production in primary human endothelial cell cultures. *J. Med. Virol. 70*, 451–458.

Caruso, A., Rotola, A., Comar, M., Favilli, F., Galvan, M., Tosetti, M., Campello, C., Caselli, E., Alessandri, G., Grassi, M., Garrafa, E., Cassai, E., and Di Luca, D. (2002). HHV-6 infects human aortic and heart microvascular endothelial cells, increasing their ability to secrete proinflammatory chemokines. *J. Med. Virol. 67*, 528–533.

Caserta, M.T., Hall, C.B., Schnabel, K., Long, C.E., and D'Heron, N. (1998). Primary human herpesvirus 7 infection: a comparison of human herpesvirus 7 and human herpesvirus 6 infections in children. *J. Pediatr. 133*, 386–389.

Casper, C., Krantz, E., Taylor, H., Dalessio, J., Carrell, D., Wald, A., Corey, L., and Ashley, R. (2002). Assessment of a combined testing strategy for detection of antibodies to human herpesvirus 8 (HHV-8) in persons with Kaposi's sarcoma, persons with asymptomatic HHV-8 infection, and persons at low risk for HHV-8 infection. *J. Clin. Microbiol. 40*, 3822–3825.

Casper, C., Nichols, W.G., Huang, M.L., Corey, L., and Wald, A. (2004). Remission of HHV-8 and HIV-associated multicentric Castleman disease with ganciclovir treatment. *Blood 103*, 1632–1634.

Cattani, P., Capuano, M., Cerimele, F., La Parola, I.L., Santangelo, R., Masini, C., Cerimele, D., and Fadda, G. (1999). Human herpesvirus 8 seroprevalence and evaluation of nonsexual transmission routes by detection of DNA in clinical specimens from human immunodeficiency virus–seronegative patients from central and southern Italy, with and without Kaposi's sarcoma. *J. Clin. Microbiol. 37*, 1150–1153.

Cattani, P., Capuano, M., Graffeo, R., Ricci, R., Cerimele, F., Cerimele, D., Nanni, G., and Fadda, G. (2001). Kaposi's sarcoma associated with previous human herpesvirus 8 infection in kidney transplant recipients. *J. Clin. Microbiol. 39*, 506–508.

Cattani, P., Capuano, M., Lesnoni, L.P., I, Guido, R., Santangelo, R., Cerimele, F., Masini, C., Nanni, G., Fadda, G., and Cerimele, D. (1998). Human herpesvirus 8 in Italian HIV-seronegative patients with Kaposi sarcoma. *Arch. Dermatol. 134*, 695–699.

Cerimele, F., Curreli, F., Ely, S., Friedman-Kien, A.E., Cesarman, E., and Flore, O. (2001). Kaposi's sarcoma-associated herpesvirus can productively infect primary human keratinocytes and alter their growth properties. *J. Virol. 75*, 2435–2443.

Cesarman, E., Moore, P.S., Rao, P.H., Inghirami, G., Knowles, D.M., and Chang, Y. (1995). In vitro establishment and characterization of two acquired immunodeficiency syndrome-related lymphoma cell lines (BC-1 and BC-2) containing Kaposi's sarcoma–associated herpesvirus-like (KSHV) DNA sequences. *Blood 86*, 2708–2714.

Cesarman, E., Nador, R.G., Aozasa, K., Delsol, G., Said, J.W., and Knowles, D.M. (1996). Kaposi's sarcoma-associated herpesvirus in non-AIDS related lymphomas occurring in body cavities. *Am. J. Pathol. 149*, 53–57.

Challoner, P.B., Smith, K.T., Parker, J.D., MacLeod, D.L., Coulter, S.N., Rose, T.M., Schultz, E.R., Bennett, J.L., Garber, R.L., Chang, M., Schad, P.A. , Stewart, P.M., Nowinski, R.C., Brown, J.P., and Burmer, G.C. (1995). Plaque-associated expression of human herpesvirus 6 in multiple sclerosis. *Proc. Natl. Acad. Sci. U. S. A. 92*, 7440–7444.

Chan, P.K., Li, C.K., Chik, K.W., Lee, V., Shing, M.M., Ng, K.C., Cheung, J.L., Fok, T.F., and Cheng, A.F. (2004). Risk factors and clinical consequences of human herpesvirus 7 infection in paediatric haematopoietic stem cell transplant recipients. *J. Med. Virol. 72*, 668–674.

Chang, P.J., Shedd, D., Gradoville, L., Cho, M.S., Chen, L.W., Chang, J., and Miller, G. (2002). Open reading frame 50 protein of Kaposi's sarcoma-associated herpesvirus directly activates the viral PAN and K12 genes by binding to related response elements. *J. Virol. 76*, 3168–3178.

Chatterjee, M., Osborne, J., Bestetti, G., Chang, Y., and Moore, P.S. (2002). Viral IL-6-induced cell proliferation and immune evasion of interferon activity. *Science 298*, 1432–1435.

Chen, N., Nelson, K.E., Jenkins, F.J., Suriyanon, V., Duerr, A., Costello, C., Robison, V., and Jacobson, L.P. (2004). Seroprevalence of human herpesvirus 8 infection in Northern Thailand. *Clin. Infect. Dis. 39*, 1052–1058.

Chen, S., Bacon, K.B., Li, L., Garcia, G.E., Xia, Y., Lo, D., Thompson, D.A., Siani, M.A., Yamamoto, T., Harrison, J.K., and Feng, L. (1998). In vivo inhibition of CC and CX3C chemokine-induced leukocyte infiltration and attenuation of glomerulonephritis in Wistar-Kyoto (WKY) rats by vMIP–II. *J. Exp. Med. 188*, 193–198.

Cheng, E.H., Nicholas, J., Bellows, D.S., Hayward, G.S., Guo, H.G., Reitz, M.S., and Hardwick, J.M. (1997). A Bcl-2 homolog encoded by Kaposi sarcoma-associated virus, human herpesvirus 8, inhibits apoptosis but does not heterodimerize with Bax or Bak. *Proc. Natl. Acad. Sci. U. S. A. 94*, 690–694.

Chintu, C., Athale, U.H., and Patil, P.S. (1995). Childhood cancers in Zambia before and after the HIV epidemic. *Arch. Dis. Child 73*, 100–104.

Choi, J.K., Ishido, S., and Jung, J.U. (2000a). The collagen repeat sequence is a determinant of the degree of herpesvirus saimiri STP transforming activity. *J. Virol. 74*, 8102–8110.

Choi, J.K., Lee, B.S., Shim, S.N., Li, M., and Jung, J.U. (2000b). Identification of the novel K15 gene at the rightmost end of the Kaposi's sarcoma-associated herpesvirus genome. *J. Virol. 74*, 436–446.

Chokunonga, E., Levy, L.M., Bassett, M.T., Mauchaza, B.G., Thomas, D.B., and Parkin, D.M. (2000). Cancer incidence in the African population of Harare, Zimbabwe: second results from the cancer registry 1993-1995. *Int. J. Cancer 85*, 54–59.

Chuh, A., Chan, H., and Zawar, V. (2004). Pityriasis rosea—evidence for and against an infectious aetiology. *Epidemiol. Infect. 132*, 381–390.

Chung, Y.H., Cho, N.H., Garcia, M.I., Lee, S.H., Feng, P., and Jung, J.U. (2004). Activation of Stat3 transcription factor by Herpesvirus saimiri STP-A oncoprotein. *J. Virol. 78*, 6489–6497.

Chung, Y.H., Means, R.E., Choi, J.K., Lee, B.S., and Jung, J.U. (2002). Kaposi's sarcoma-associated herpesvirus OX2 glycoprotein activates myeloid-lineage cells to induce inflammatory cytokine production. *J. Virol. 76*, 4688–4698.

Cirone, M., Campadelli-Fiume, G., Foa-Tomasi, L., Torrisi, M.R., and Faggioni, A. (1994). Human herpesvirus 6 envelope glycoproteins B and H-L complex are undetectable on the plasma membrane of infected lymphocytes. *AIDS Res. Hum. Retroviruses 10*, 175–179.

Ciufo, D.M., Cannon, J.S., Poole, L.J., Wu, F.Y., Murray, P., Ambinder, R.F., and Hayward, G.S. (2001). Spindle cell conversion by Kaposi's sarcoma-associated herpesvirus: Formation of colonies and plaques with mixed lytic and latent gene expression in infected primary dermal microvascular endothelial cell cultures. *J. Virol. 75*, 5614–5626.

Clark, D. (2004). Human herpesvirus type 6 and multiple sclerosis. *Herpes 11 (Suppl 2)*, 112A–119A.

Clark, D.A. (2002). Human herpesvirus 6 and human herpesvirus 7: emerging pathogens in transplant patients. *Int. J. Hematol. 76 (Suppl 2)*, 246–252.

Cockerell, C.J. (1991). Histopathological features of Kaposi's sarcoma in HIV infected individuals. *Cancer Surv. 10*, 73–89.

Cole, P.D., Stiles, J., Boulad, F., Small, T.N., O'Reilly, R.J., George, D., Szabolcs, P., Kiehn, T.E., and Kernan, N.A. (1998). Successful treatment of human herpesvirus 6 encephalitis in a bone marrow transplant recipient. *Clin. Infect. Dis. 27*, 653–654.

Cone, R.W., Huang, M.L., Corey, L., Zeh, J., Ashley, R., and Bowden, R. (1999). Human herpesvirus 6 infections after bone marrow transplantation: clinical and virologic manifestations. *J. Infect. Dis. 179*, 311–318.

Conti, C., Cirone, M., Sgro, R., Altieri, F., Zompetta, C., and Faggioni, A. (2000). Early interactions of human herpesvirus 6 with lymphoid cells: role of membrane protein components and glycosaminoglycans in virus binding. *J. Med. Virol. 62*, 487–497.

Cook, R.D., Hodgson, T.A., Waugh, A.C., Molyneux, E.M., Borgstein, E., Sherry, A., Teo, C.G., and Porter, S.R. (2002). Mixed patterns of transmission of human herpesvirus-8 (Kaposi's sarcoma–associated herpesvirus) in Malawian families. *J. Gen. Virol. 83*, 1613–1619.

Cook–Mozaffari, P., Newton, R., Beral, V., and Burkitt, D.P. (1998). The geographical distribution of Kaposi's sarcoma and of lymphomas in Africa before the AIDS epidemic. *Br. J. Cancer 78*, 1521–1528.

Cool, C.D., Rai, P.R., Yeager, M.E., Hernandez-Saavedra, D., Serls, A.E., Bull, T.M., Geraci, M.W., Brown, K.K., Routes, J.M., Tuder, R.M., and Voelkel, N.F. (2003). Expression of human herpesvirus 8 in primary pulmonary hypertension. *N. Engl. J. Med. 349*, 1113–1122.

Corchero, J.L., Mar, E.C., Spira, T.J., Pellett, P.E., and Inoue, N. (2001). Comparison of serologic assays for detection of antibodies against human herpesvirus 8. Clin. Diagn. *Lab Immunol. 8*, 913–921.

Coscoy, L. and Ganem, D. (2000). Kaposi's sarcoma-associated herpesvirus encodes two proteins that block cell surface display of MHC class I chains by enhancing their endocytosis. *Proc. Natl. Acad. Sci. U. S. A. 97*, 8051–8056.

Cotter, I.I. and Robertson, E.S. (1999). The latency-associated nuclear antigen tethers the Kaposi's sarcoma-associated herpesvirus genome to host chromosomes in body cavity-based lymphoma cells. *Virology 264*, 254–264.

Cunningham, C., Barnard, S., Blackbourn, D.J., and Davison, A.J. (2003). Transcription mapping of human herpesvirus 8 genes encoding viral interferon regulatory factors. *J. Gen. Virol. 84*, 1471–1483.

Daibata, M., Taguchi, T., Nemoto, Y., Taguchi, H., and Miyoshi, I. (1999). Inheritance of chromosomally integrated human herpesvirus 6 DNA. *Blood 94*, 1545–1549.

Daibata, M., Taguchi, T., Taguchi, H., and Miyoshi, I. (1998). Integration of human herpesvirus 6 in a Burkitt's lymphoma cell line. *Br. J. Haematol. 102*, 1307–1313.

Dairaghi, D.J., Fan, R.A., McMaster, B.E., Hanley, M.R., and Schall, T.J. (1999). HHV8-encoded vMIP-I selectively engages chemokine receptor CCR8. Agonist and antagonist profiles of viral chemokines. *J. Biol. Chem. 274*, 21569–21574.

Dal Canto, A.J., Virgin, H.W.t., and Speck, S.H. (2000). Ongoing viral replication is required for gammaherpesvirus 68-induced vascular damage. *J. Virol. 74*, 11304–11310.

De Bolle, L., Van Loon, J., De Clercq, E., and Naesens, L. (2005). Quantitative analysis of human herpesvirus 6 cell tropism. *J. Med. Virol. 75*, 76–85.

De Clercq, E., Naesens, L., De Bolle, L., Schols, D., Zhang, Y., and Neyts, J. (2001). Antiviral agents active against human herpesviruses HHV-6, HHV-7 and HHV-8. *Rev. Med. Virol. 11*, 381–395.

de Sanjose, S., Marshall, V., Sola, J., Palacio, V., Almirall, R., Goedert, J.J., Bosch, F.X., and Whitby, D. (2002). Prevalence of Kaposi's sarcoma-associated herpesvirus infection in sex workers and women from the general population in Spain. *Int. J. Cancer 98*, 155–158.

de The, G., Bestetti, G., van Beveren, M., and Gessain, A. (1999). Prevalence of human herpesvirus 8 infection before the acquired immunodeficiency disease syndrome-related epidemic of Kaposi's sarcoma in East Africa. *J. Natl. Cancer Inst. 91*, 1888–1889.

Deborska, D., Durlik, M., Sadowska, A., Nowacka-Cieciura, E., Pazik, J., Lewandowski, Z., Chmura, A., Galazka, Z., Paczek, L., and Lao, M. (2003). Human herpesvirus-6 in renal transplant recipients: potential risk factors for the development of human herpesvirus–6 seroconversion. *Transplant. Proc. 35*, 2199–2201.

Dedicoat, M., Newton, R., Alkharsah, K.R., Sheldon, J., Szabados, I., Ndlovu, B., Page, T., Casabonne, D., Gilks, C.F., Cassol, S.A., Whitby, D., and Schulz, T.F. (2004). Mother-to-child transmission of human herpesvirus-8 in South Africa. *J. Infect. Dis. 190*, 1068–1075.

Denes, E., Magy, L., Pradeau, K., Alain, S., Weinbreck, P., and Ranger–Rogez, S. (2004). Successful treatment of human herpesvirus 6 encephalomyelitis in immunocompetent patient. *Emerg. Infect. Dis. 10*, 729–731.

DesJardin, J.A., Cho, E., Supran, S., Gibbons, L., Werner, B.G., and Snydman, D.R. (2001). Association of human herpesvirus 6 reactivation with severe cytomegalovirus-associated disease in orthotopic liver transplant recipients. *Clin. Infect. Dis. 33*, 1358–1362.

DesJardin, J.A., Gibbons, L., Cho, E., Supran, S.E., Falagas, M.E., Werner, B.G., and Snydman, D.R. (1998). Human herpesvirus 6 reactivation is associated with cytomegalovirus infection and syndromes in kidney transplant recipients at risk for primary cytomegalovirus infection. *J. Infect. Dis. 178*, 1783–1786.

Desrosiers, R.C., Bakker, A., Kamine, J., Falk, L.A., Hunt, R.D., and King, N.W. (1985). A region of the Herpesvirus saimiri genome required for oncogenicity. *Science 228*, 184–187.

Desrosiers, R.C., Silva, D.P., Waldron, L.M., and Letvin, N.L. (1986). Nononcogenic deletion mutants of herpesvirus saimiri are defective for in vitro immortalization. *J. Virol. 57*, 701–705.

Dewhurst, S., Dollard, S.C., Pellett, P.E., and Dambaugh, T.R. (1993). Identification of a lytic-phase origin of DNA replication in human herpesvirus 6B strain Z29. *J. Virol. 67*, 7680–7683.

Dhepakson, P., Mori, Y., Jiang, Y.B., Huang, H.L., Akkapaiboon, P., Okuno, T., and Yamanishi, K. (2002). Human herpesvirus-6 rep/U94 gene product has single-stranded DNA-binding activity. *J. Gen. Virol. 83*, 847–854.

Di Alberti, L., Ngui, S.L., Porter, S.R., Speight, P.M., Scully, C.M., Zakrewska, J.M., Williams, I.G., Artese, L., Piattelli, A., and Teo, C.G. (1997a). Presence of human herpesvirus 8 variants in the oral tissues of human immunodeficiency virus-infected persons. *J. Infect. Dis. 175*, 703–707.

Di Alberti, L., Piatelli, A., Artese, L., Favia, G., Patel, S., Saunders, N., Porter, S.R., Scully, C.M., Ngui, S.L., Teo, C.G. (1997b). Human herpesvirus 8 variants in sarcoid tissues. *Lancet 350*, 1655–1661.

di Gennaro, G., Canzonieri, V., Schioppa, O., Nasti, G., Carbone, A., and Tirelli, U. (2001). Discordant HHV8 detection in a young HIV-negative patient with Kaposi's sarcoma and sarcoidosis. *Clin. Infect. Dis. 32*, 1100–1102.

Diamond, C., Brodie, S.J., Krieger, J.N., Huang, M.L., Koelle, D.M., Diem, K., Muthui, D., and Corey, L. (1998). Human herpesvirus 8 in the prostate glands of men with Kaposi's sarcoma. *J. Virol. 72*, 6223–6227.

Dictor, M., Rambech, E., Way, D., Witte, M., and Bendsoe, N. (1996). Human herpesvirus 8 (Kaposi's sarcoma-associated herpesvirus) DNA in Kaposi's sarcoma lesions, AIDS Kaposi's sarcoma cell lines, endothelial Kaposi's sarcoma simulators, and the skin of immunosuppressed patients. *Am. J. Pathol. 148*, 2009–2016.

Dietrich, J., Blumberg, B.M., Roshal, M., Baker, J.V., Hurley, S.D., Mayer-Proschel, M., and Mock, D.J. (2004). Infection with an endemic human herpesvirus disrupts critical glial precursor cell properties. *J. Neurosci. 24*, 4875–4883.

Dilnur, P., Katano, H., Wang, Z.H., Osakabe, Y., Kudo, M., Sata, T., and Ebihara, Y. (2001). Classic type of Kaposi's sarcoma and human herpesvirus 8 infection in Xinjiang, China. *Pathol. Int. 51*, 845–852.

Dittmer, D.P. (2003). Transcription profile of Kaposi's sarcoma-associated herpesvirus in primary Kaposi's sarcoma lesions as determined by real-time PCR arrays. *Cancer Res. 63*, 2010–2015.

Djerbi, M., Screpanti, V., Catrina, A.I., Bogen, B., Biberfeld, P., and Grandien, A. (1999). The inhibitor of death receptor signaling, FLICE-inhibitory protein defines a new class of tumor progression factors. *J. Exp. Med. 190*, 1025–1032.

Dockrell, D.H., Prada, J., Jones, M.F., Patel, R., Badley, A.D., Harmsen, W.S., Ilstrup, D.M., Wiesner, R.H., Krom, R.A., Smith, T.F., and Paya, C.V. (1997). Seroconversion to human herpesvirus 6 following liver transplantation is a marker of cytomegalovirus disease. *J. Infect. Dis. 176*, 1135–1140.

Doherty, P.C., Christensen, J.P., Belz, G.T., Stevenson, P.G., and Sangster, M.Y. (2001). Dissecting the host response to a gamma-herpesvirus. *Philos. Trans. R. Soc. Lond. B Biol. Sci. 356*, 581–593.

Dourmishev, L.A., Dourmishev, A.L., Palmeri, D., Schwartz, R.A., and Lukac, D.M. (2003). Molecular genetics of Kaposi's sarcoma-associated herpesvirus (human herpesvirus-8) epidemiology and pathogenesis. *Microbiol. Mol. Biol. Rev. 67*, 175–212.

Drago, F., Ranieri, E., Malaguti, F., Losi, E., and Rebora, A. (1997). Human herpesvirus 7 in pityriasis rosea. *Lancet 349*, 1367–1368.

Drobyski, W.R., Dunne, W.M., Burd, E.M., Knox, K.K., Ash, R.C., Horowitz, M.M., Flomenberg, N., and Carrigan, D.R. (1993). Human herpesvirus-6 (HHV-6) infection in allogeneic bone marrow transplant recipients: evidence of a marrow-suppressive role for HHV-6 in vivo. *J. Infect. Dis. 167*, 735–739.

Du, M.Q., Diss, T.C., Liu, H., Ye, H., Hamoudi, R.A., Cabecadas, J., Dong, H.Y., Harris, N.L., Chan, J.K., Rees, J.W., Dogan, A., and Isaacson, P.G. (2002). KSHV- and EBV-associated germinotropic lymphoproliferative disorder. *Blood 100*, 3415–3418.

Duboise, S.M., Guo, J., Czajak, S., Desrosiers, R.C., and Jung, J.U. (1998a). STP and Tip are essential for herpesvirus saimiri oncogenicity. *J. Virol. 72*, 1308–1313.

Duboise, S.M., Lee, H., Guo, J., Choi, J.K., Czajak, S., Simon, M., Desrosiers, R.C., and Jung, J.U. (1998b). Mutation of the Lck-binding motif of Tip enhances lymphoid cell activation by herpesvirus saimiri. *J. Virol. 72*, 2607–2614.

Dukers, N.H., Renwick, N., Prins, M., Geskus, R.B., Schulz, T.F., Weverling, G.J., Coutinho, R.A., and Goudsmit, J. (2000). Risk factors for human herpesvirus 8 seropositivity and seroconversion in a cohort of homosexual men. *Am. J. Epidemiol. 151*, 213–224.

Dupin, N., Diss, T.L., Kellam, P., Tulliez, M., Du, M.Q., Sicard, D., Weiss, R.A., Isaacson, P.G., and Boshoff, C. (2000). HHV-8 is associated with a plasmablastic variant of Castleman disease that is linked to HHV-8-positive plasmablastic lymphoma. *Blood 95*, 1406–1412.

Dutia, B.M., Stewart, J.P., Clayton, R.A., Dyson, H., and Nash, A.A. (1999). Kinetic and phenotypic changes in murine lymphocytes infected with murine gammaherpesvirus-68 in vitro. *J. Gen. Virol. 80*, 2729–2736.

Duus, K.M., Lentchitsky, V., Wagenaar, T., Grose, C., and Webster-Cyriaque, J. (2004). Wild-type Kaposi's sarcoma-associated herpesvirus isolated from the oropharynx of immune–competent individuals has tropism for cultured oral epithelial cells. *J. Virol. 78*, 4074–4084.

Dykstra, M.L., Longnecker, R., and Pierce, S.K. (2001). Epstein-Barr virus coopts lipid rafts to block the signaling and antigen transport functions of the BCR. *Immunity 14*, 57–67.

Edelman, D.C., Ketema, F., Saville, R.D., Herman, J., Sill, A.M., Gill, P.S., Blattner, W.A., and Constantine, N.T. (2000). Specifics on the refinement and application of two serological assays for the detection of antibodies to HHV-8. *J. Clin. Virol. 16*, 225–237.

Ellis, M., Chew, Y.P., Fallis, L., Freddersdorf, S., Boshoff, C., Weiss, R.A., Lu, X., and Mittnacht, S. (1999). Degradation of p27(Kip) cdk inhibitor triggered by Kaposi's sarcoma virus cyclin-cdk6 complex. *EMBO J. 18*, 644–653.

Emond, J.P., Marcelin, A.G., Dorent, R., Milliancourt, C., Dupin, N., Frances, C., Agut, H., Gandjbakhch, I., and Calvez, V. (2002). Kaposi's sarcoma associated with previous human herpesvirus 8 infection in heart transplant recipients. *J. Clin. Microbiol. 40*, 2217–2219.

Endres, M.J., Garlisi, C.G., Xiao, H., Shan, L., and Hedrick, J.A. (1999). The Kaposi's sarcoma-related herpesvirus (KSHV)-encoded chemokine vMIP-I is a specific agonist for the CC chemokine receptor (CCR)8. *J. Exp. Med. 189*, 1993–1998.

Engels, E.A., Eastman, H., Ablashi, D.V., Wilks, R.J., Braham, J., and Manns, A. (1999). Risk of transfusion-associated transmission of human herpesvirus 8. *J. Natl. Cancer Inst. 91*, 1773–1775.

Engels, E.A., Pittaluga, S., Whitby, D., Rabkin, C., Aoki, Y., Jaffe, E.S., and Goedert, J.J. (2003). Immunoblastic lymphoma in persons with AIDS-associated Kaposi's sarcoma: a role for Kaposi's sarcoma–associated herpesvirus. *Mod. Pathol. 16*, 424–429.

Engels, E.A., Sinclair, M.D., Biggar, R.J., Whitby, D., Ebbesen, P., Goedert, J.J., and Gastwirth, J.L. (2000). Latent class analysis of human herpesvirus 8 assay performance and infection prevalence in sub-Saharan Africa and Malta. *Int. J. Cancer 88*, 1003–1008.

Ensser, A., Glykofrydes, D., Niphuis, H., Kuhn, E.M., Rosenwirth, B., Heeney, J.L., Niedobitek, G.., Muller-Fleckenstein, I., and Fleckenstein, B. (2001). Independence of herpesvirus-induced T cell lymphoma from viral cyclin D homologue. *J. Exp. Med. 193*, 637–642.

Falk, L.A., Wolfe, L.G., and Deinhardt, F. (1972). Isolation of Herpesvirus saimiri from blood of squirrel monkeys (Saimiri sciureus). *J. Natl. Cancer Inst. 48*, 1499–1505.

Feldstein, A.E., Razonable, R.R., Boyce, T.G., Freese, D.K., El Youssef, M., Perrault, J., Paya, C.V., and Ishitani, M.B. (2003). Prevalence and clinical significance of human herpesviruses 6 and 7 active infection in pediatric liver transplant patients. *Pediatr. Transplant. 7*, 125–129.

Feng, P., Park, J., Lee, B.S., Lee, S.H., Bram, R.J., and Jung, J.U. (2002). Kaposi's sarcoma–associated herpesvirus mitochondrial K7 protein targets a cellular calcium–modulating cyclophilin ligand to modulate intracellular calcium concentration and inhibit apoptosis. *J. Virol. 76*, 11491–11504.

Feng, P., Scott, C.W., Cho, N.H., Nakamura, H., Chung, Y.H., Monteiro, M.J., and Jung, J.U. (2004). Kaposi's sarcoma-associated herpesvirus K7 protein targets a ubiquitin-like/ubiquitin-associated domain-containing protein to promote protein degradation. *Mol. Cell Biol. 24*, 3938–3948.

Fickenscher, H., Biesinger, B., Knappe, A., Wittmann, S., and Fleckenstein, B. (1996). Regulation of the herpesvirus saimiri oncogene stpC, similar to that of T-cell activation genes, in growth-transformed human T lymphocytes. *J. Virol. 70*, 6012–6019.

Fickenscher, H. and Fleckenstein, B. (2001). Herpesvirus saimiri. *Philos. Trans. R. Soc. Lond. B Biol. Sci. 356*, 545–567.

Field, N., Low, W., Daniels, M., Howell, S., Daviet, L., Boshoff, C., and Collins, M. (2003). KSHV vFLIP binds to IKK-gamma to activate IKK. *J Cell Sci 116*, 3721–3728.

Fife, K., Howard, M.R., Gracie, F., Phillips, R.H., and Bower, M. (1998). Activity of thalidomide in AIDS-related Kaposi's sarcoma and correlation with HHV8 titre. *Int. J. STD AIDS 9*, 751–755.

Fischl, M.A., Finkelstein, D.M., He, W., Powderly, W.G., Triozzi, P.L., and Steigbigel, R.T. (1996). A phase II study of recombinant human interferon-alpha 2a and zidovudine in patients with AIDS-related Kaposi's sarcoma. AIDS Clinical Trials Group. *J. Acquir. Immune Defic. Syndr. Hum. Retrovirol. 11*, 379–384.

Flamand, L., Stefanescu, I., and Menezes, J. (1996). Human herpesvirus-6 enhances natural killer cell cytotoxicity via IL-15. *J. Clin. Invest 97*, 1373–1381.

Flano, E., Kim, I.J., Woodland, D.L., and Blackman, M.A. (2002). Gamma–herpesvirus latency is preferentially maintained in splenic germinal center and memory B cells. *J. Exp. Med. 196*, 1363–1372.

Fleckenstein, B. and Desrosiers, R.C. (1982). Herpesvirus saimiri and Herpesvirus ateles. In: *The Herpesviruses*, B.Roizman, ed. (New York: Plenum), pp. 253–331.

Flore, O., Rafii, S., Ely, S., O'Leary, J.J., Hyjek, E.M., and Cesarman, E. (1998). Transformation of primary human endothelial cells by Kaposi's sarcoma-associated herpesvirus. *Nature 394*, 588–592.

Flowers, C.C., Flowers, S.P., and Nabel, G.J. (1998). Kaposi's sarcoma-associated herpesvirus viral interferon regulatory factor confers resistance to the antiproliferative effect of interferon-alpha. *Mol. Med. 4*, 402–412.

Foreman, K.E., Friborg, J., Jr., Kong, W.P., Woffendin, C., Polverini, P.J., Nickoloff, B.J., and Nabel, G.J. (1997). Propagation of a human herpesvirus from AIDS-associated Kaposi's sarcoma. *N. Engl. J. Med. 336*, 163–171.

Foster-Cuevas, M., Wright, G.J., Puklavec, M.J., Brown, M.H., and Barclay, A.N. (2004). Human herpesvirus 8 K14 protein mimics CD200 in down-regulating macrophage activation through CD200 receptor. *J. Virol. 78*, 7667–7676.

Fowler, P. and Efstathiou, S. (2004). Vaccine potential of a murine gammaherpesvirus-68 mutant deficient for ORF73. *J. Gen. Virol. 85*, 609–613.

Fowler, P., Marques, S., Simas, J.P., and Efstathiou, S. (2003). ORF73 of murine herpesvirus-68 is critical for the establishment and maintenance of latency. *J. Gen. Virol. 84*, 3405–3416.

Friborg, J., Jr., Kong, W., Hottiger, M.O., and Nabel, G.J. (1999). p53 inhibition by the LANA protein of KSHV protects against cell death. *Nature 402*, 889–894.

Friedman-Kien, A.E. (1981). Disseminated Kaposi's sarcoma syndrome in young homosexual men. *J. Am. Acad. Dermatol. 5*, 468–471.

Friedrichs, C., Neyts, J., Gaspar, G., De Clercq, E., and Wutzler, P. (2004). Evaluation of antiviral activity against human herpesvirus 8 (HHV-8) and Epstein-Barr virus (EBV) by a quantitative real-time PCR assay. *Antiviral Res. 62*, 121–123.

Fujimuro, M. and Hayward, S.D. (2003). The latency-associated nuclear antigen of Kaposi's sarcoma-associated herpesvirus manipulates the activity of glycogen synthase kinase-3beta. *J. Virol. 77*, 8019–8030.

Fujisaki, H., Tanaka–Taya, K., Tanabe, H., Hara, T., Miyoshi, H., Okada, S., and Yamanishi, K. (1998). Detection of human herpesvirus 7 (HHV-7) DNA in breast milk by polymerase chain reaction and prevalence of HHV-7 antibody in breast-fed and bottle-fed children. *J Med. Virol. 56*, 275–279.

Fukuda, K., Straus, S.E., Hickie, I., Sharpe, M.C., Dobbins, J.G., and Komaroff, A. (1994). The chronic fatigue syndrome: a comprehensive approach to its definition and study. International Chronic Fatigue Syndrome Study Group. *Ann. Intern. Med. 121*, 953–959.

Gandhi, M., Koelle, D.M., Ameli, N., Bacchetti, P., Greenspan, J.S., Navazesh, M., Anastos, K., and Greenblatt, R.M. (2004). Prevalence of human herpesvirus–8 salivary shedding in HIV increases with CD4 count. *J. Dent. Res. 83*, 639–643.

Gangappa, S., Kapadia, S.B., Speck, S.H., and Virgin, H.W.t. (2002a). Antibody to a lytic cycle viral protein decreases gammaherpesvirus latency in B-cell-deficient mice. *J. Virol. 76*, 11460–11468.

Gangappa, S., van Dyk, L.F., Jewett, T.J., Speck, S.H., and Virgin, H.W.t. (2002b). Identification of the in vivo role of a viral bcl-2. *J. Exp. Med. 195*, 931–940.

Gao, S.J., Boshoff, C., Jayachandra, S., Weiss, R.A., Chang, Y., and Moore, P.S. (1997). KSHV ORF K9 (vIRF) is an oncogene which inhibits the interferon signaling pathway. *Oncogene 15*, 1979–19785.

Gao, S.J., Kingsley, L., Hoover, D.R., Spira, T.J., Rinaldo, C.R., Saah, A., Phair, J., Detels, R., Parry, P., Chang, Y., and Moore, P.S. (1996a). Seroconversion to antibodies against Kaposi's sarcoma–associated herpesvirus-related latent nuclear antigens before the development of Kaposi's sarcoma. *N. Engl. J. Med. 335*, 233–241.

Gao, S.J., Kingsley, L., Li, M., Zheng, W., Parravicini, C., Ziegler, J., Newton, R., Rinaldo, C.R., Saah, A., Phair, J., Detels, R., Chang, Y., and Moore, P.S. (1996b). KSHV antibodies among Americans, Italians and Ugandans with and without Kaposi's sarcoma. *Nat. Med. 2*, 925–928.

Geras-Raaka, E., Varma, A., Clark-Lewis, I., and Gershengorn, M.C. (1998a). Kaposi's sarcoma-associated herpesvirus (KSHV) chemokine vMIP-II and human SDF-1alpha inhibit signaling by KSHV G protein-coupled receptor. *Biochem. Biophys. Res. Commun. 253*, 725–727.

Geras-Raaka, E., Varma, A., Ho, H., Clark-Lewis, I., and Gershengorn, M.C. (1998b). Human interferon-gamma-inducible protein 10 (IP-10) inhibits constitutive signaling of Kaposi's sarcoma–associated herpesvirus G protein-coupled receptor. *J. Exp. Med. 188*, 405–408.

Gershengorn, M.C., Geras-Raaka, E., Varma, A., and Clark-Lewis, I. (1998). Chemokines activate Kaposi's sarcoma-associated herpesvirus G protein-coupled receptor in mammalian cells in culture. *J. Clin. Invest. 102*, 1469–1472.

Gessain, A., Mauclere, P., van Beveren, M., Plancoulaine, S., Ayouba, A., Essame-Oyono, J.L., Martin, P.M., and de The, G. (1999). Human herpesvirus 8 primary infection occurs during childhood in Cameroon, Central Africa. *Int. J. Cancer 81*, 189–192.

Gill, J., Bourboulia, D., Wilkinson, J., Hayes, P., Cope, A., Marcelin, A.G., Calvez, V., Gotch, F., Boshoff, C., and Gazzard, B. (2002). Prospective study of the effects of antiretroviral therapy on Kaposi sarcoma-associated herpesvirus infection in patients with and without Kaposi sarcoma. *J. Acquir. Immune. Defic. Syndr. 31*, 384–390.

Gill, P.S., Tsai, Y.C., Rao, A.P., Spruck, C.H., III, Zheng, T., Harrington, W.A., Jr., Cheung, T., Nathwani, B., and Jones, P.A. (1998). Evidence for multiclonality in multicentric Kaposi's sarcoma. *Proc. Natl. Acad. Sci. U. S. A. 95*, 8257–8261.

Glaunsinger, B. and Ganem, D. (2004). Highly selective escape from KSHV-mediated host mRNA shutoff and its implications for viral pathogenesis. *J. Exp. Med 200*, 391–398.

Glenn, M., Rainbow, L., Aurade, F., Davison, A., and Schulz, T.F. (1999). Identification of a spliced gene from Kaposi's sarcoma-associated herpesvirus encoding a protein with similarities to latent membrane proteins 1 and 2A of Epstein-Barr virus. *J. Virol. 73*, 6953–6963.

Glykofrydes, D., Niphuis, H., Kuhn, E.M., Rosenwirth, B., Heeney, J.L., Bruder, J., Niedobitek, G., Muller-Fleckenstein, I., Fleckenstein, B., and Ensser, A. (2000). Herpesvirus saimiri vFLIP provides an antiapoptotic function but is not essential for viral replication, transformation, or pathogenicity. *J. Virol. 74*, 11919–11927.

Gobbi, A., Stoddart, C.A., Malnati, M.S., Locatelli, G., Santoro, F., Abbey, N.W., Bare, C., Linquist-Stepps, V., Moreno, M.B., Herndier, B.G., Lusso, P., and McCune, J.M. (1999). Human herpesvirus 6 (HHV-6) causes severe thymocyte depletion in SCID-hu Thy/Liv mice. *J. Exp. Med. 189*, 1953–1960.

Godden-Kent, D., Talbot, S.J., Boshoff, C., Chang, Y., Moore, P., Weiss, R.A., and Mittnacht, S. (1997). The cyclin encoded by Kaposi's sarcoma-associated herpesvirus stimulates cdk6 to phosphorylate the retinoblastoma protein and histone H1. *J. Virol. 71*, 4193–4198.

Goedert, J.J. (2000). The epidemiology of acquired immunodeficiency syndrome malignancies. *Semin. Oncol. 27*, 390–401.

Gomez-Roman, J.J., Sanchez-Velasco, P., Ocejo-Vinyals, G., Hernandez-Nieto, E., Leyva-Cobian, F., and Val-Bernal, J.F. (2001). Human herpesvirus-8 genes are expressed in pulmonary inflammatory myofibroblastic tumor (inflammatory pseudotumor). *Am. J. Surg. Pathol. 25*, 624–629.

Goodwin, D.J., Walters, M.S., Smith, P.G., Thurau, M., Fickenscher, H., and Whitehouse, A. (2001). Herpesvirus saimiri open reading frame 50 (Rta) protein reactivates the lytic replication cycle in a persistently infected A549 cell line. *J. Virol. 75*, 4008–4013.

Goudsmit, J., Renwick, N., Dukers, N.H., Coutinho, R.A., Heisterkamp, S., Bakker, M., Schulz, T.F., Cornelissen, M., and Weverling, G.J. (2000). Human herpesvirus 8 infections in the Amsterdam Cohort Studies (1984-1997): analysis of seroconversions to ORF65 and ORF73. *Proc. Natl. Acad. Sci. U. S. A. 97*, 4838–4843.

Grahame-Clarke, C., Alber, D.G., Lucas, S.B., Miller, R., and Vallance, P. (2001). Association between Kaposi's sarcoma and atherosclerosis: implications for gammaherpesviruses and vascular disease. *AIDS 15*, 1902–1904.

Greenstone, H.L., Santoro, F., Lusso, P., and Berger, E.A. (2002). Human herpesvirus 6 and measles virus employ distinct CD46 domains for receptor function. *J. Biol. Chem. 277*, 39112–39118.

Griffiths, P.D., Ait-Khaled, M., Bearcroft, C.P., Clark, D.A., Quaglia, A., Davies, S.E., Burroughs, A.K., Rolles, K., Kidd, I.M., Knight, S.N., Noibi, S.M., Cope, A.V., Phillips, A.N., and Emery, V.C. (1999). Human herpesviruses 6 and 7 as potential pathogens after liver transplant: prospective comparison with the effect of cytomegalovirus. *J. Med. Virol. 59*, 496–501.

Grivel, J.C., Santoro, F., Chen, S., Faga, G., Malnati, M.S., Ito, Y., Margolis, L., and Lusso, P. (2003). Pathogenic effects of human herpesvirus 6 in human lymphoid tissue ex vivo. *J. Virol. 77*, 8280–8289.

Grossman, Z., Iscovich, J., Schwartz, F., Azizi, E., Klepfish, A., Schattner, A., and Sarid, R. (2002). Absence of Kaposi sarcoma among Ethiopian immigrants to Israel despite high seroprevalence of human herpesvirus 8. *Mayo Clin. Proc. 77*, 905–909.

Grulich, A.E., Olsen, S.J., Luo, K., Hendry, O., Cunningham, P., Cooper, D.A., Gao, S.J., Chang, Y., Moore, P.S., and Kaldor, J.M. (1999). Kaposi's sarcoma-associated herpesvirus: a sexually transmissible infection? *J. Acquir. Immune. Defic. Syndr. Hum. Retrovirol. 20*, 387–393.

Guasparri, I., Keller, S.A., and Cesarman, E. (2004). KSHV vFLIP is essential for the survival of infected lymphoma cells. *J. Exp. Med. 199*, 993–1003.

Guo, H.G., Sadowska, M., Reid, W., Tschachler, E., Hayward, G., and Reitz, M. (2003). Kaposi's sarcoma-like tumors in a human herpesvirus 8 ORF74 transgenic mouse. *J. Virol. 77*, 2631–2639.

Guo, J., Williams, K., Duboise, S.M., Alexander, L., Veazey, R., and Jung, J.U. (1998). Substitution of ras for the herpesvirus saimiri STP oncogene in lymphocyte transformation. *J. Virol. 72*, 3698–3704.

Gwack, Y., Baek, H.J., Nakamura, H., Lee, S.H., Meisterernst, M., Roeder, R.G., and Jung, J.U. (2003a). Principal role of TRAP/mediator and SWI/SNF complexes in Kaposi's sarcoma–associated herpesvirus RTA-mediated lytic reactivation. *Mol. Cell Biol. 23*, 2055–2067.

Gwack, Y., Nakamura, H., Lee, S.H., Souvlis, J., Yustein, J.T., Gygi, S., Kung, H.J., and Jung, J.U. (2003b). Poly(ADP-ribose) polymerase 1 and Ste20-like kinase hKFC act as transcriptional repressors for gamma-2 herpesvirus lytic replication. *Mol. Cell. Biol. 23*, 8282–8294.

Gwack, Y., Byun, H., Hwang, S., Lim, C., and Choe, J. (2001). CREB-binding protein and histone deacetylase regulate the transcriptional activity of Kaposi's sarcoma-associated herpesvirus open reading frame 50. *J. Virol. 75*, 1909–1917.

Gyulai, R., Kemeny, L., Adam, E., Nagy, F., and Dobozy, A. (1996). HHV8 DNA in angiolymphoid hyperplasia of the skin. *Lancet 347*, 1837.

Hall, C.B., Caserta, M.T., Schnabel, K.C., Boettrich, C., McDermott, M.P., Lofthus, G.K., Carnahan, J.A., and Dewhurst, S. (2004). Congenital infections with human herpesvirus 6 (HHV6) and human herpesvirus 7 (HHV7). *J. Pediatr. 145*, 472–477.

Hall, C.B., Caserta, M.T., Schnabel, K.C., Long, C., Epstein, L.G., Insel, R.A., and Dewhurst, S. (1998). Persistence of human herpesvirus 6 according to site and variant: possible greater neurotropism of variant A. *Clin. Infect. Dis. 26*, 132–137.

Hall, C.B., Long, C.E., Schnabel, K.C., Caserta, M.T., McIntyre, K.M., Costanzo, M.A., Knott, A., Dewhurst, S., Insel, R.A., and Epstein, L.G. (1994). Human herpesvirus-6 infection in children. A prospective study of complications and reactivation. *N. Engl. J. Med. 331*, 432–438.

Haque, N.S., Fallon, J.T., Taubman, M.B., and Harpel, P.C. (2001). The chemokine receptor CCR8 mediates human endothelial cell chemotaxis induced by I-309 and Kaposi sarcoma herpesvirus-encoded vMIP-I and by lipoprotein(a)-stimulated endothelial cell conditioned medium. *Blood 97*, 39–45.

Harnett, G.B., Farr, T.J., Pietroboni, G.R., and Bucens, M.R. (1990). Frequent shedding of human herpesvirus 6 in saliva. *J. Med. Virol. 30*, 128–130.

Hartley, D.A., Amdjadi, K., Hurley, T.R., Lund, T.C., Medveczky, P.G., and Sefton, B.M. (2000). Activation of the Lck tyrosine protein kinase by the Herpesvirus saimiri tip protein involves two binding interactions. *Virology 276*, 339–348.

Hasegawa, H., Utsunomiya, Y., Yasukawa, M., Yanagisawa, K., and Fujita, S. (1994). Induction of G protein-coupled peptide receptor EBI 1 by human herpesvirus 6 and 7 infection in CD4+ T cells. *J. Virol. 68*, 5326–5329.

He, J., Bhat, G., Kankasa, C., Chintu, C., Mitchell, C., Duan, W., and Wood, C. (1998). Seroprevalence of human herpesvirus 8 among Zambian women of childbearing age without Kaposi's sarcoma (KS) and mother-child pairs with KS. *J. Infect. Dis. 178*, 1787–1790.

He, J., McCarthy, M., Zhou, Y., Chandran, B., and Wood, C. (1996). Infection of primary human fetal astrocytes by human herpesvirus 6. *J. Virol. 70*, 1296–1300.

Hengge, U.R., Ruzicka, T., Tyring, S.K., Stuschke, M., Roggendorf, M., Schwartz, R.A., and Seeber, S. (2002). Update on Kaposi's sarcoma and other HHV8 associated diseases. Part 1: epidemiology, environmental predispositions, clinical manifestations, and therapy. *Lancet Infect. Dis. 2*, 281–292.

Henghold, W.B., Purvis, S.F., Schaffer, J., Giam, C.Z., and Wood, G.S. (1997). No evidence of KSHV/HHV-8 in mycosis fungoides or associated disorders. *J. Invest Dermatol. 108*, 920–922.

Henke-Gendo, C., Schulz, T.F., and Hoeper, M.M. (2004). HHV-8 in pulmonary hypertension. *N. Engl. J. Med. 350*, 194–195.

Hewitt, E.W. (2003). The MHC class I antigen presentation pathway: strategies for viral immune evasion. *Immunology 110*, 163–169.

Hideshima, T., Chauhan, D., Teoh, G., Raje, N., Treon, S.P., Tai, Y.T., Shima, Y., and Anderson, K.C. (2000). Characterization of signaling cascades triggered by human interleukin-6 versus Kaposi's sarcoma-associated herpes virus-encoded viral interleukin 6. *Clin Cancer Res 6*, 1180–1189.

Hirata, Y., Kondo, K., and Yamanishi, K. (2001). Human herpesvirus 6 downregulates major histocompatibility complex class I in dendritic cells. *J. Med. Virol. 65*, 576–583.

Hochberg, D., Souza, T., Catalina, M., Sullivan, J.L., Luzuriaga, K., and Thorley-Lawson, D.A. (2004). Acute infection with Epstein-Barr virus targets and overwhelms the peripheral memory B-cell compartment with resting, latently infected cells. *J. Virol. 78*, 5194–5204.

Hoge, A.T., Hendrickson, S.B., and Burns, W.H. (2000). Murine gammaherpesvirus 68 cyclin D homologue is required for efficient reactivation from latency. *J. Virol. 74*, 7016–7023.

Hong, Y.K., Foreman, K., Shin, J.W., Hirakawa, S., Curry, C.L., Sage, D.R., Libermann, T., Dezube, B.J., Fingeroth, J.D., and Detmar, M. (2004). Lymphatic reprogramming of blood vascular endothelium by Kaposi sarcoma-associated herpesvirus. *Nat. Genet. 36*, 683–685.

Hor, S., Ensser, A., Reiss, C., Ballmer-Hofer, K., and Biesinger, B. (2001). Herpesvirus saimiri protein StpB associates with cellular Src. *J. Gen. Virol. 82*, 339–344.

Hoshino, K., Nishi, T., Adachi, H., Ito, H., Fukuda, Y., Dohi, K., and Kurata, T. (1995). Human herpesvirus-6 infection in renal allografts: retrospective immunohistochemical study in Japanese recipients. *Transpl. Int. 8*, 169–173.

Huang, L.M., Chao, M.F., Chen, M.Y., Shih, H., Chiang, Y.P., Chuang, C.Y., and Lee, C.Y. (2001). Reciprocal regulatory interaction between human herpesvirus 8 and human immunodeficiency virus type 1. *J. Biol. Chem. 276*, 13427–13432.

Huang, L.M., Huang, S.Y., Chen, M.Y., Chao, M.F., Lu, C.Y., Tien, H.F., Lee, C.Y., and Jeang, K.T. (2000). Geographical differences in human herpesvirus 8 seroepidemiology: a survey of 1, 201 individuals in Asia. *J. Med. Virol. 60*, 290–293.

Huang, L.M., Lee, C.Y., Chen, J.Y., Yang, C.S., Wang, J.D., Chang, M.H., Hsu, C.Y., and Kuo, P.F. (1992). Primary human herpesvirus 6 infections in children: a prospective serologic study. *J. Infect. Dis. 165*, 1163–1164.

Huang, Q., Petros, A.M., Virgin, H.W., Fesik, S.W., and Olejniczak, E.T. (2002). Solution structure of a Bcl-2 homolog from Kaposi sarcoma virus. *Proc. Natl. Acad. Sci. U. S. A. 99*, 3428–3433.

Hudnall, S.D., Chen, T., Rady, P., Tyring, S., and Allison, P. (2003). Human herpesvirus 8 seroprevalence and viral load in healthy adult blood donors. *Transfusion 43*, 85–90.

Hudson, A.W., Howley, P.M., and Ploegh, H.L. (2001). A human herpesvirus 7 glycoprotein, U21, diverts major histocompatibility complex class I molecules to lysosomes. *J. Virol. 75*, 12347–12358.

Humar, A., Kumar, D., Caliendo, A.M., Moussa, G., Ashi-Sulaiman, A., Levy, G., and Mazzulli, T. (2002). Clinical impact of human herpesvirus 6 infection after liver transplantation. *Transplantation 73*, 599–604.

Hymes, K.B., Cheung, T., Greene, J.B., Prose, N.S., Marcus, A., Ballard, H., William, D.C., and Laubenstein, L.J. (1981). Kaposi's sarcoma in homosexual men—a report of eight cases. *Lancet 2*, 598–600.

Imbert–Marcille, B.M., Tang, X.W., Lepelletier, D., Besse, B., Moreau, P., Billaudel, S., and Milpied, N. (2000). Human herpesvirus 6 infection after autologous or allogeneic stem cell transplantation: a single-center prospective longitudinal study of 92 patients. *Clin. Infect. Dis. 31*, 881–886.

Inoue, N., Dambaugh, T.R., Rapp, J.C., and Pellett, P.E. (1994). Alphaherpesvirus origin-binding protein homolog encoded by human herpesvirus 6B, a betaherpesvirus, binds to nucleotide sequences that are similar to ori regions of alphaherpesviruses. *J. Virol. 68*, 4126–4136.

Inoue, N., Mar, E.C., Dollard, S.C., Pau, C.P., Zheng, Q., and Pellett, P.E. (2000). New immunofluorescence assays for detection of Human herpesvirus 8-specific antibodies. *Clin. Diagn. Lab Immunol. 7*, 427–435.

Inoue, N. and Pellett, P.E. (1995). Human herpesvirus 6B origin-binding protein: DNA-binding domain and consensus binding sequence. *J. Virol. 69*, 4619–4627.

Inoue, N., Spira, T., Lam, L., Corchero, J.L., and Luo, W. (2004). Comparison of serologic responses between Kaposi's sarcoma-positive and -negative men who were seropositive for both human herpesvirus 8 and human immunodeficiency virus. *J. Med. Virol. 74*, 202–206.

Inoue, N., Winter, J., Lal, R.B., Offermann, M.K., and Koyano, S. (2003). Characterization of entry mechanisms of human herpesvirus 8 by using an Rta-dependent reporter cell line. *J. Virol.* 77, 8147–8152.

Iscovich, J., Boffetta, P., Franceschi, S., Azizi, E., and Sarid, R. (2000). Classic kaposi sarcoma: epidemiology and risk factors. *Cancer 88*, 500–517.

Isegawa, Y., Ping, Z., Nakano, K., Sugimoto, N., and Yamanishi, K. (1998). Human herpesvirus 6 open reading frame U12 encodes a functional beta-chemokine receptor. *J. Virol.* 72, 6104–6112.

Ishido, S., Choi, J.K., Lee, B.S., Wang, C., DeMaria, M., Johnson, R.P., Cohen, G.B., and Jung, J.U. (2000a). Inhibition of natural killer cell-mediated cytotoxicity by Kaposi's sarcoma-associated herpesvirus K5 protein. *Immunity 13*, 365–374.

Ishido, S., Wang, C., Lee, B.S., Cohen, G.B., and Jung, J.U. (2000b). Downregulation of major histocompatibility complex class I molecules by Kaposi's sarcoma-associated herpesvirus K3 and K5 proteins. *J. Virol.* 74, 5300–5309.

Isomura, H., Yamada, M., Yoshida, M., Tanaka, H., Kitamura, T., Oda, M., Nii, S., and Seino, Y. (1997). Suppressive effects of human herpesvirus 6 on in vitro colony formation of hematopoietic progenitor cells. *J. Med. Virol.* 52, 406–412.

Isomura, H., Yoshida, M., Namba, H., Fujiwara, N., Ohuchi, R., Uno, F., Oda, M., Seino, Y., and Yamada, M. (2000). Suppressive effects of human herpesvirus-6 on thrombopoietin-inducible megakaryocytic colony formation in vitro. *J. Gen. Virol.* 81, 663–673.

Isomura, H., Yoshida, M., Namba, H., and Yamada, M. (2003). Interaction of human herpesvirus 6 with human CD34 positive cells. *J. Med. Virol.* 70, 444–450.

Jacobs, U., Ferber, J., and Klehr, H.U. (1994). Severe allograft dysfunction after OKT3-induced human herpes virus–6 reactivation. *Transplant. Proc. 26*, 3121.

Janelle, M.E., Gravel, A., Gosselin, J., Tremblay, M.J., and Flamand, L. (2002). Activation of monocyte cyclooxygenase-2 gene expression by human herpesvirus 6. Role for cyclic AMP-responsive element-binding protein and activator protein-1. *J. Biol. Chem. 277*, 30665–30674.

Jenkins, F.J., Hoffman, L.J., and Liegey-Dougall, A. (2002). Reactivation of and primary infection with human herpesvirus 8 among solid-organ transplant recipients. *J. Infect. Dis. 185*, 1238–1243.

Jenner, R.G., Maillard, K., Cattini, N., Weiss, R.A., Boshoff, C., Wooster, R., and Kellam, P. (2003). Kaposi's sarcoma-associated herpesvirus-infected primary effusion lymphoma has a plasma cell gene expression profile. *Proc. Natl. Acad. Sci. U. S. A. 100*, 10399–10404.

Jones, J.L., Hanson, D.L., Dworkin, M.S., and Jaffe, H.W. (2000). Incidence and trends in Kaposi's sarcoma in the era of effective antiretroviral therapy. *J. Acquir. Immune. Defic. Syndr. 24*, 270–274.

Judde, J.G., Lacoste, V., Briere, J., Kassa–Kelembho, E., Clyti, E., Couppie, P., Buchrieser, C., Tulliez, M., Morvan, J., and Gessain, A. (2000). Monoclonality or oligoclonality of human herpesvirus 8 terminal repeat sequences in Kaposi's sarcoma and other diseases. *J. Natl. Cancer Inst. 92*, 729–736.

Jung, J.U. and Desrosiers, R.C. (1991). Identification and characterization of the herpesvirus saimiri oncoprotein STP-C488. *J. Virol. 65*, 6953–6960.

Jung, J.U. and Desrosiers, R.C. (1995). Association of the viral oncoprotein STP-C488 with cellular ras. *Mol. Cell. Biol. 15*, 6506–6512.

Jung, J.U., Lang, S.M., Friedrich, U., Jun, T., Roberts, T.M., Desrosiers, R.C., and Biesinger, B. (1995). Identification of Lck–binding elements in tip of herpesvirus saimiri. *J. Biol. Chem. 270*, 20660–20667.

Jung, J.U., Stager, M., and Desrosiers, R.C. (1994). Virus-encoded cyclin. *Mol. Cell. Biol. 14*, 7235–7244.

Jung, J.U., Trimble, J.J., King, N.W., Biesinger, B., Fleckenstein, B.W., and Desrosiers, R.C. (1991). Identification of transforming genes of subgroup A and C strains of Herpesvirus saimiri. *Proc. Natl. Acad. Sci. U. S. A. 88*, 7051–7055.

Kakimoto, M., Hasegawa, A., Fujita, S., and Yasukawa, M. (2002). Phenotypic and functional alterations of dendritic cells induced by human herpesvirus 6 infection. *J. Virol. 76*, 10338–10345.

Kapadia, S.B., Levine, B., Speck, S.H., and Virgin, H.W.t. (2002). Critical role of complement and viral evasion of complement in acute, persistent, and latent gamma-herpesvirus infection. *Immunity 17*, 143–155.

Kapelushnik, J., Ariad, S., Benharroch, D., Landau, D., Moser, A., Delsol, G., and Brousset, P. (2001). Post renal transplantation human herpesvirus 8-associated lymphoproliferative disorder and Kaposi's sarcoma. *Br. J. Haematol. 113*, 425–428.

Kasolo, F.C., Mpabalwani, E., and Gompels, U.A. (1997). Infection with AIDS–related herpesviruses in human immunodeficiency virus-negative infants and endemic childhood Kaposi's sarcoma in Africa. *J. Gen. Virol. 78*, 847–855.

Katsafanas, G.C., Schirmer, E.C., Wyatt, L.S., and Frenkel, N. (1996). In vitro activation of human herpesviruses 6 and 7 from latency. *Proc. Natl. Acad. Sci. U. S. A. 93*, 9788–9792.

Kedes, D.H. and Ganem, D. (1997). Sensitivity of Kaposi's sarcoma-associated herpesvirus replication to antiviral drugs. Implications for potential therapy. *J. Clin. Invest 99*, 2082–2086.

Kedes, D.H., Operskalski, E., Busch, M., Kohn, R., Flood, J., and Ganem, D. (1996). The seroepidemiology of human herpesvirus 8 (Kaposi's sarcoma-associated herpesvirus): distribution of infection in KS risk groups and evidence for sexual transmission. *Nat. Med. 2*, 918–924.

Keller, A.R., Hochholzer, L., and Castleman, B. (1972). Hyaline-vascular and plasma-cell types of giant lymph node hyperplasia of the mediastinum and other locations. *Cancer 29*, 670–683.

Keller, S.A., Schattner, E.J., and Cesarman, E. (2000). Inhibition of NF-kappaB induces apoptosis of KSHV-infected primary effusion lymphoma cells. *Blood 96*, 2537–42.

Kempf, W., Adams, V., Mirandola, P., Menotti, L., Di Luca, D., Wey, N., Muller, B., and Campadelli–Fiume, G. (1998). Persistence of human herpesvirus 7 in normal tissues detected by expression of a structural antigen. *J. Infect. Dis. 178*, 841–845.

Kempf, W., Adams, V., Wey, N., Moos, R., Schmid, M., Avitabile, E., and Campadelli-Fiume, G. (1997). CD68+ cells of monocyte/macrophage lineage in the environment of AIDS-associated and classic-sporadic Kaposi sarcoma are singly or doubly infected with human herpesviruses 7 and 6B. *Proc. Natl. Acad. Sci. U. S. A. 94*, 7600–7605.

Kempf, W., Muller, B., Maurer, R., Adams, V., and Campadelli, F.G. (2000). Increased expression of human herpesvirus 7 in lymphoid organs of AIDS patients. *J. Clin. Virol. 16*, 193–201.

Kidd, I.M., Clark, D.A., Sabin, C.A., Andrew, D., Hassan-Walker, A.F., Sweny, P., Griffiths, P.D., and Emery, V.C. (2000). Prospective study of human betaherpesviruses after renal transplantation: association of human herpesvirus 7 and cytomegalovirus co–infection with cytomegalovirus disease and increased rejection. *Transplantation 69*, 2400–2404.

Kim, I.J., Flano, E., Woodland, D.L., Lund, F.E., Randall, T.D., and Blackman, M.A. (2003). Maintenance of long term gamma-herpesvirus B cell latency is dependent on CD40-mediated development of memory B cells. *J. Immunol. 171*, 886–892.

Kirchhoff, S., Sebens, T., Baumann, S., Krueger, A., Zawatzky, R., Li-Weber, M., Meinl, E., Neipel, F., Fleckenstein, B., and Krammer, P.H. (2002). Viral IFN-regulatory factors inhibit activation-induced cell death via two positive regulatory IFN-regulatory factor 1-dependent domains in the CD95 ligand promoter. *J. Immunol. 168*, 1226–1234.

Kjellen, P., Amdjadi, K., Lund, T.C., Medveczky, P.G., and Sefton, B.M. (2002). The herpesvirus saimiri tip484 and tip488 proteins both stimulate lck tyrosine protein kinase activity in vivo and in vitro. *Virology 297*, 281–288.

Klass, C.M., Krug, L.T., Pozharskaya, V.P., and Offermann, M.K. (2005). The targeting of primary effusion lymphoma cells for apoptosis by inducing lytic replication of human herpesvirus 8 while blocking virus production. *Blood 105*, 4028–4034.

Kledal, T.N., Rosenkilde, M.M., Coulin, F., Simmons, G., Johnsen, A.H., Alouani, S., Power, C.A., Luttichau, H.R., Gerstoft, J., Clapham, P.R., Clark-Lewis, I., Wells, T.N., and Schwartz, T.W. (1997). A broad-spectrum chemokine antagonist encoded by Kaposi's sarcoma-associated herpesvirus. *Science 277*, 1656–9.

Kliche, S., Nagel, W., Kremmer, E., Atzler, C., Ege, A., Knorr, T., Koszinowski, U., Kolanus, W., and Haas, J. (2001). Signaling by human herpesvirus 8 kaposin A through direct membrane recruitment of cytohesin-1. *Mol. Cell 7*, 833–843.

Kliche, S., Kremmer, E., Hammerschmidt, W., Koszinowski, U., and Haas, J. (1998). Persistent infection of Epstein-Barr virus-positive B lymphocytes by human herpesvirus 8. *J. Virol. 72*, 8143–8149.

Knight, J.S., Cotter, M.A., II, and Robertson, E.S. (2001). The latency-associated nuclear antigen of Kaposi's sarcoma-associated herpesvirus transactivates the telomerase reverse transcriptase promoter. *J. Biol. Chem. 276*, 22971–22978.

Knowles, D.M., Chamulak, G.A., Subar, M., Burke, J.S., Dugan, M., Wernz, J., Slywotzky, C., Pelicci, G., Dalla-Favera, R., and Raphael, B. (1988). Lymphoid neoplasia associated with the acquired immunodeficiency syndrome (AIDS). The New York University Medical Center experience with 105 patients (1981-1986). *Ann. Intern. Med. 108*, 744–753.

Knox, K.K. and Carrigan, D.R. (1992). In vitro suppression of bone marrow progenitor cell differentiation by human herpesvirus 6 infection. *J. Infect. Dis. 165*, 925–929.

Koelle, D.M., Huang, M.L., Chandran, B., Vieira, J., Piepkorn, M., and Corey, L. (1997). Frequent detection of Kaposi's sarcoma-associated herpesvirus (human herpesvirus 8) DNA in saliva of human immunodeficiency virus-infected men: clinical and immunologic correlates. *J. Infect. Dis. 176*, 94–102.

Komanduri, K.V., Luce, J.A., McGrath, M.S., Herndier, B.G., and Ng, V.L. (1996). The natural history and molecular heterogeneity of HIV-associated primary malignant lymphomatous effusions. *J. Acquir. Immune. Defic. Syndr. Hum. Retrovirol. 13*, 215–226.

Komaroff, A.L. (1988). Chronic fatigue syndromes: relationship to chronic viral infections. *J. Virol. Methods 21*, 3–10.

Kondo, K., Kondo, T., Okuno, T., Takahashi, M., and Yamanishi, K. (1991). Latent human herpesvirus 6 infection of human monocytes/macrophages. *J. Gen. Virol. 72*, 1401–1408.

Kondo, K., Kondo, T., Shimada, K., Amo, K., Miyagawa, H., and Yamanishi, K. (2002a). Strong interaction between human herpesvirus 6 and peripheral blood monocytes/macrophages during acute infection. *J. Med. Virol. 67*, 364–369.

Kondo, K., Nagafuji, H., Hata, A., Tomomori, C., and Yamanishi, K. (1993). Association of human herpesvirus 6 infection of the central nervous system with recurrence of febrile convulsions. *J. Infect. Dis. 167*, 1197–1200.

Kondo, K., Sashihara, J., Shimada, K., Takemoto, M., Amo, K., Miyagawa, H., and Yamanishi, K. (2003). Recognition of a novel stage of betaherpesvirus latency in human herpesvirus 6. *J. Virol. 77*, 2258–2264.

Kondo, K., Shimada, K., Sashihara, J., Tanaka-Taya, K., and Yamanishi, K. (2002b). Identification of human herpesvirus 6 latency-associated transcripts. *J. Virol. 76*, 4145–4151.

Kretschmer, C., Murphy, C., Biesinger, B., Beckers, J., Fickenscher, H., Kirchner, T., Fleckenstein, B., and Ruther, U. (1996). A Herpes saimiri oncogene causing peripheral T-cell lymphoma in transgenic mice. *Oncogene 12*, 1609–16.

Krishnan, H.H., Naranatt, P.P., Smith, M.S., Zeng, L., Bloomer, C., and Chandran, B. (2004). Concurrent expression of latent and a limited number of lytic genes with immune modulation and antiapoptotic function by Kaposi's sarcoma-associated herpesvirus early during infection of primary endothelial and fibroblast cells and subsequent decline of lytic gene expression. *J. Virol. 78*, 3601–3620.

Krithivas, A., Young, D.B., Liao, G., Greene, D., and Hayward, S.D. (2000). Human herpesvirus 8 LANA interacts with proteins of the mSin3 corepressor complex and negatively regulates Epstein–Barr virus gene expression in dually infected PEL cells. *J. Virol. 74*, 9637–9645.

Krown, S.E. (2003). Therapy of AIDS-associated Kaposi's sarcoma: targeting pathogenetic mechanisms. *Hematol. Oncol. Clin. North Am. 17*, 763–783.

Krown, S.E., Paredes, J., Bundow, D., Polsky, B., Gold, J.W., and Flomenberg, N. (1992). Interferon-alpha, zidovudine, and granulocyte-macrophage colony-stimulating factor: a phase I AIDS Clinical Trials Group study in patients with Kaposi's sarcoma associated with AIDS. *J. Clin. Oncol. 10*, 1344–51.

Krug, L.T., Inoue, N., and Pellett, P.E. (2001a). Differences in DNA binding specificity among Roseolovirus origin binding proteins. *Virology 288*, 145–153.

Krug, L.T., Inoue, N., and Pellett, P.E. (2001b). Sequence requirements for interaction of human herpesvirus 7 origin binding protein with the origin of lytic replication. *J. Virol. 75*, 3925–3936.

Krug, L.T., Pozharskaya, V.P., Yu, Y., Inoue, N., and Offermann, M.K. (2004). Inhibition of infection and replication of human herpesvirus 8 in microvascular endothelial cells by alpha interferon and phosphonoformic acid. *J. Virol. 78*, 8359–8371.

Kusuhara, K., Takabayashi, A., Ueda, K., Hidaka, Y., Minamishima, I., Take, H., Fujioka, K., Imai, S., and Osato, T. (1997). Breast milk is not a significant source for early Epstein-Barr virus or human herpesvirus 6 infection in infants: a seroepidemiologic study in 2 endemic areas of human T-cell lymphotropic virus type I in Japan. Microbiol. *Immunol. 41*, 309–312.

Lacoste, V., Mauclere, P., Dubreuil, G., Lewis, J., Georges-Courbot, M.C., Rigoulet, J., Petit, T., and Gessain, A. (2000). Simian homologues of human gamma-2 and betaherpesviruses in mandrill and drill monkeys. *J. Virol. 74*, 11993–11999.

LaDuca, J.R., Love, J.L., Abbott, L.Z., Dube, S., Freidman-Kien, A.E., and Poiesz, B.J. (1998). Detection of human herpesvirus 8 DNA sequences in tissues and bodily fluids. *J. Infect. Dis. 178*, 1610–1615.

Lagunoff, M., Majeti, R., Weiss, A., and Ganem, D. (1999). Deregulated signal transduction by the K1 gene product of Kaposi's sarcoma-associated herpesvirus. *Proc. Natl. Acad. Sci. U. S. A. 96*, 5704–5709.

Lagunoff, M., Lukac, D.M., and Ganem, D. (2001). Immunoreceptor tyrosine-based activation motif-dependent signaling by Kaposi's sarcoma-associated herpesvirus K1 protein: effects on lytic viral replication. *J. Virol. 75*, 5891–5898.

Lam, L.L., Pau, C.P., Dollard, S.C., Pellett, P.E., and Spira, T.J. (2002). Highly sensitive assay for human herpesvirus 8 antibodies that uses a multiple antigenic peptide derived from open reading frame K8.1. *J. Clin. Microbiol. 40*, 325–329.

Laman, H., Coverley, D., Krude, T., Laskey, R., and Jones, N. (2001). Viral cyclin-cyclin-dependent kinase 6 complexes initiate nuclear DNA replication. *Mol. Cell. Biol. 21*, 624–635.

Lan, K., Kuppers, D.A., Verma, S.C., and Robertson, E.S. (2004). Kaposi's sarcoma-associated herpesvirus-encoded latency-associated nuclear antigen inhibits lytic replication by targeting Rta: a potential mechanism for virus-mediated control of latency. *J. Virol. 78*, 6585–6594.

Lautenschlager, I., Harma, M., Hockerstedt, K., Linnavuori, K., Loginov, R., and Taskinen, E. (2002). Human herpesvirus-6 infection is associated with adhesion molecule induction and lymphocyte infiltration in liver allografts. *J. Hepatol. 37*, 648–654.

Lautenschlager, I., Linnavuori, K., and Hockerstedt, K. (2000). Human herpesvirus-6 antigenemia after liver transplantation. *Transplantation 69*, 2561–2566.

Leach, C.T., Newton, E.R., McParlin, S., and Jenson, H.B. (1994). Human herpesvirus 6 infection of the female genital tract. *J. Infect. Dis. 169*, 1281–1283.

Leao, J.C., Kumar, N., McLean, K.A., Porter, S.R., Scully, C.M., Swan, A.V., and Teo, C.G. (2000). Effect of human immunodeficiency virus-1 protease inhibitors on the clearance of human herpesvirus 8 from blood of human immunodeficiency virus-1-infected patients. *J. Med. Virol. 62*, 416–420.

Lee, B.J., Koszinowski, U.H., Sarawar, S.R., and Adler, H. (2003). A gammaherpesvirus G protein–coupled receptor homologue is required for increased viral replication in response to chemokines and efficient reactivation from latency. *J. Immunol. 170*, 243–251.

Lee, B.S., Alvarez, X., Ishido, S., Lackner, A.A., and Jung, J.U. (2000). Inhibition of intracellular transport of B cell antigen receptor complexes by Kaposi's sarcoma-associated herpesvirus K1. *J. Exp. Med. 192*, 11–22.

Lee, H., Choi, J.K., Li, M., Kaye, K., Kieff, E., and Jung, J.U. (1999). Role of cellular tumor necrosis factor receptor-associated factors in NF-kappaB activation and lymphocyte transformation by herpesvirus Saimiri STP. *J. Virol. 73*, 3913–3919.

Lee, H., Guo, J., Li, M., Choi, J.K., DeMaria, M., Rosenzweig, M., and Jung, J.U. (1998a). Identification of an immunoreceptor tyrosine-based activation motif of K1 transforming protein of Kaposi's sarcoma-associated herpesvirus. *Mol. Cell Biol. 18*, 5219–5228.

Lee, H., Trimble, J.J., Yoon, D.W., Regier, D., Desrosiers, R.C., and Jung, J.U. (1997). Genetic variation of herpesvirus saimiri subgroup A transforming protein and its association with cellular src. *J. Virol. 71*, 3817–3825.

Lee, H., Veazey, R., Williams, K., Li, M., Guo, J., Neipel, F., Fleckenstein, B., Lackner, A., Desrosiers, R.C., and Jung, J.U. (1998b). Deregulation of cell growth by the K1 gene of Kaposi's sarcoma–associated herpesvirus. *Nat. Med. 4*, 435–440.

Lennette, E.T., Blackbourn, D.J., and Levy, J.A. (1996). Antibodies to human herpesvirus type 8 in the general population and in Kaposi's sarcoma patients. *Lancet 348*, 858–861.

Li, H., Wang, H., and Nicholas, J. (2001). Detection of direct binding of human herpesvirus 8-encoded interleukin-6 (vIL-6) to both gp130 and IL-6 receptor (IL-6R) and identification of amino acid residues of vIL-6 important for IL-6R-dependent and -independent signaling. *J. Virol. 75*, 3325–3334.

Li, M., Damania, B., Alvarez, X., Ogryzko, V., Ozato, K., and Jung, J.U. (2000). Inhibition of p300 histone acetyltransferase by viral interferon regulatory factor. *Mol. Cell. Biol. 20*, 8254–8263.

Li, M., Lee, H., Guo, J., Neipel, F., Fleckenstein, B., Ozato, K., and Jung, J.U. (1998). Kaposi's sarcoma-associated herpesvirus viral interferon regulatory factor. *J. Virol. 72*, 5433–5440.

Li, M., Lee, H., Yoon, D.W., Albrecht, J.C., Fleckenstein, B., Neipel, F., and Jung, J.U. (1997). Kaposi's sarcoma-associated herpesvirus encodes a functional cyclin. *J. Virol. 71*, 1984–1991.

Liang, Y., Chang, J., Lynch, S.J., Lukac, D.M., and Ganem, D. (2002). The lytic switch protein of KSHV activates gene expression via functional interaction with RBP-Jkappa (CSL), the target of the Notch signaling pathway. *Genes Dev. 16*, 1977–1989.

Lim, C., Sohn, H., Gwack, Y., and Choe, J. (2000). Latency-associated nuclear antigen of Kaposi's sarcoma–associated herpesvirus (human herpesvirus-8) binds ATF4/CREB2 and inhibits its transcriptional activation activity. *J. Gen. Virol. 81*, 2645–2652.

Lin, R., Genin, P., Mamane, Y., Sgarbanti, M., Battistini, A., Harrington, W.J., Jr., Barber, G.N., and Hiscott, J. (2001). HHV–8 encoded vIRF-1 represses the interferon antiviral response by blocking IRF–3 recruitment of the CBP/p300 coactivators. *Oncogene 20*, 800–811.

Little, R.F., Merced-Galindez, F., Staskus, K., Whitby, D., Aoki, Y., Humphrey, R., Pluda, J.M., Marshall, V., Walters, M., Welles, L., Rodriguez-Chavez, I.R., Pittaluga, S., Tosato, G., and Yarchoan, R. (2003). A pilot study of cidofovir in patients with kaposi sarcoma. *J. Infect. Dis. 187*, 149–153.

Liu, C., Okruzhnov, Y., Li, H., and Nicholas, J. (2001). Human herpesvirus 8 (HHV-8)-encoded cytokines induce expression of and autocrine signaling by vascular endothelial growth factor (VEGF) in HHV-8-infected primary-effusion lymphoma cell lines and mediate VEGF-independent antiapoptotic effects. *J. Virol. 75*, 10933–10940.

Liu, L., Eby, M.T., Rathore, N., Sinha, S.K., Kumar, A., and Chaudhary, P.M. (2002). The human herpes virus 8–encoded viral FLICE inhibitory protein physically associates with and persistently activates the Ikappa B kinase complex. *J. Biol. Chem. 277*, 13745–13751.

Ljungman, P., Wang, F.Z., Clark, D.A., Emery, V.C., Remberger, M., Ringden, O., and Linde, A. (2000). High levels of human herpesvirus 6 DNA in peripheral blood leucocytes are correlated to platelet engraftment and disease in allogeneic stem cell transplant patients. *Br. J. Haematol. 111*, 774–781.

Long, M.C., Bidanset, D.J., Williams, S.L., Kushner, N.L., and Kern, E.R. (2003). Determination of antiviral efficacy against lymphotropic herpesviruses utilizing flow cytometry. *Antiviral Res. 58*, 149–157.

Lorenzo, M.E., Jung, J.U., and Ploegh, H.L. (2002). Kaposi's sarcoma-associated herpesvirus K3 utilizes the ubiquitin-proteasome system in routing class major histocompatibility complexes to late endocytic compartments. *J. Virol. 76*, 5522–5531.

Lu, C., Zeng, Y., Huang, Z., Huang, L., Qian, C., Tang, G., and Qin, D. (2005). Human herpesvirus 6 activates lytic cycle replication of Kaposi's sarcoma-associated herpesvirus. *Am. J. Pathol. 166*, 173–183.

Lukac, D.M., Renne, R., Kirshner, J.R., and Ganem, D. (1998). Reactivation of Kaposi's sarcoma–associated herpesvirus infection from latency by expression of the ORF 50 transactivator, a homolog of the EBV R protein. *Virology 252*, 304–312.

Lukac, D.M., Garibyan, L., Kirshner, J.R., Palmeri, D., and Ganem, D. (2001). DNA binding by Kaposi's sarcoma–associated herpesvirus lytic switch protein is necessary for transcriptional activation of two viral delayed early promoters. *J. Virol. 75*, 6786–6799.

Luna, R.E., Zhou, F., Baghian, A., Chouljenko, V., Forghani, B., Gao, S.J., and Kousoulas, K.G. (2004). Kaposi's sarcoma-associated herpesvirus glycoprotein K8.1 is dispensable for virus entry. *J. Virol. 78*, 6389–6398.

Lund, T.C., Garcia, R., Medveczky, M.M., Jove, R., and Medveczky, P.G. (1997). Activation of STAT transcription factors by herpesvirus Saimiri Tip-484 requires p56lck. *J. Virol. 71*, 6677–6682.

Lund, T.C., Prator, P.C., Medveczky, M.M., and Medveczky, P.G. (1999). The Lck binding domain of herpesvirus saimiri tip-484 constitutively activates Lck and STAT3 in T cells. *J. Virol. 73*, 1689–1694.

Lundquist, A., Barre, B., Bienvenu, F., Hermann, J., Avril, S., and Coqueret, O. (2003). Kaposi sarcoma-associated viral cyclin K overrides cell growth inhibition mediated by oncostatin M through STAT3 inhibition. *Blood 101*, 4070–4077.

Luppi, M., Barozzi, P., Maiorana, A., Artusi, T., Trovato, R., Marasca, R., Savarino, M., Ceccherini-Nelli, L., and Torelli, G. (1996). Human herpesvirus-8 DNA sequences in human immunodeficiency virus-negative angioimmunoblastic lymphadenopathy and benign lymphadenopathy with giant germinal center hyperplasia and increased vascularity. *Blood 87*, 3903–3909.

Luppi, M., Barozzi, P., Marasca, R., and Torelli, G. (1994). Integration of human herpesvirus–6 (HHV–6) genome in chromosome 17 in two lymphoma patients. *Leukemia 8 (Suppl 1)*, S41–S45.

Luppi, M., Barozzi, P., Morris, C., Maiorana, A., Garber, R., Bonacorsi, G., Donelli, A., Marasca, R., Tabilio, A., and Torelli, G. (1999). Human herpesvirus 6 latently infects early bone marrow progenitors in vivo. *J. Virol. 73*, 754–759.

Luppi, M., Barozzi, P., Rasini, V., Riva, G., Re, A., Rossi, G., Setti, G., Sandrini, S., Facchetti, F., and Torelli, G. (2002). Severe pancytopenia and hemophagocytosis after HHV-8 primary infection in a renal transplant patient successfully treated with foscarnet. *Transplantation 74*, 131–132.

Luppi, M., Barozzi, P., Schulz, T.F., Setti, G., Staskus, K., Trovato, R., Narni, F., Donelli, A., Maiorana, A., Marasca, R., Sandrini, S., and Torelli, G. (2000). Bone marrow failure associated with human herpesvirus 8 infection after transplantation. *N. Engl. J. Med. 343*, 1378–1385.

Lusso, P., Malnati, M.S., Garzino-Demo, A., Crowley, R.W., Long, E.O., and Gallo, R.C. (1993). Infection of natural killer cells by human herpesvirus 6. *Nature 362*, 458–462.

Lusso, P., Secchiero, P., Crowley, R.W., Garzino-Demo, A., Berneman, Z.N., and Gallo, R.C. (1994). CD4 is a critical component of the receptor for human herpesvirus 7: interference with human immunodeficiency virus. *Proc. Natl Acad. Sci. U. S. A. 91*, 3872–3876.

Luttichau, H.R., Clark-Lewis, I., Jensen, P.O., Moser, C., Gerstoft, J., and Schwartz, T.W. (2003). A highly selective CCR2 chemokine agonist encoded by human herpesvirus 6. *J. Biol. Chem. 278*, 10928–10933.

Luttichau, H.R., Lewis, I.C., Gerstoft, J., and Schwartz, T.W. (2001). The herpesvirus 8-encoded chemokine vMIP-II, but not the poxvirus-encoded chemokine MC148, inhibits the CCR10 receptor. *Eur. J. Immunol. 31*, 1217–20.

Lybarger, L., Wang, X., Harris, M.R., Virgin, H.W., and Hansen, T.H. (2003). Virus subversion of the MHC class I Peptide-loading complex. *Immunity 18*, 121–130.

Maclean, C.M. (1963). Kaposi's sarcoma in Nigeria. *Br. J. Cancer 17*, 195–205.

Maeda, Y., Teshima, T., Yamada, M., Shinagawa, K., Nakao, S., Ohno, Y., Kojima, K., Hara, M., Nagafuji, K., Hayashi, S., Fukuda, S., Sawada, H., Matsue, K., Takenaka, K., Ishimaru, F., Ikeda, K., Niiya, K., and Harada, M. (1999). Monitoring of human herpesviruses after allogeneic peripheral blood stem cell transplantation and bone marrow transplantation. *Br. J. Haematol. 105*, 295–302.

Malmgaard, L. (2004). Induction and regulation of IFNs during viral infections. *J. Interferon Cytokine Res. 24*, 439–454.

Malnati, M.S., Dagna, L., Ponzoni, M., and Lusso, P. (2003). Human herpesvirus 8 (HHV-8/KSHV) and hematologic malignancies. *Rev. Clin. Exp. Hematol. 7*, 375–405.

Manichanh, C., Grenot, P., Gautheret-Dejean, A., Debre, P., Huraux, J.M., and Agut, H. (2000). Susceptibility of human herpesvirus 6 to antiviral compounds by flow cytometry analysis. *Cytometry 40*, 135–140.

Mann, D.J., Child, E.S., Swanton, C., Laman, H., and Jones, N. (1999). Modulation of p27(Kip1) levels by the cyclin encoded by Kaposi's sarcoma-associated herpesvirus. *EMBO J. 18*, 654–663.

Marcelin, A.G., Gorin, I., Morand, P., Ait-Arkoub, Z., Deleuze, J., Morini, J.P., Calvez, V., and Dupin, N. (2004). Quantification of Kaposi's sarcoma–associated herpesvirus in blood, oral mucosa, and saliva in patients with Kaposi's sarcoma. *AIDS Res. Hum. Retroviruses 20*, 704–708.

Marques, S., Efstathiou, S., Smith, K.G., Haury, M., and Simas, J.P. (2003). Selective gene expression of latent murine gammaherpesvirus 68 in B lymphocytes. *J. Virol. 77*, 7308–7318.

Martin, J.N. (2003). Diagnosis and epidemiology of human herpesvirus 8 infection. *Semin. Hematol. 40*, 133–142.

Martin, J.N., Amad, Z., Cossen, C., Lam, P.K., Kedes, D.H., Page-Shafer, K.A., Osmond, D.H., and Forghani, B. (2000). Use of epidemiologically well-defined subjects and existing immunofluorescence assays to calibrate a new enzyme immunoassay for human herpesvirus 8 antibodies. *J. Clin. Microbiol. 38*, 696–701.

Martin, J.N., Ganem, D.E., Osmond, D.H., Page-Shafer, K.A., Macrae, D., and Kedes, D.H. (1998). Sexual transmission and the natural history of human herpesvirus 8 infection. *N. Engl. J. Med. 338*, 948–954.

Martinez-Guzman, D., Rickabaugh, T., Wu, T.T., Brown, H., Cole, S., Song, M.J., Tong, L., and Sun, R. (2003). Transcription program of murine gammaherpesvirus 68. *J. Virol. 77*, 10488–10503.

Matta, H. and Chaudhary, P.M. (2004). Activation of alternative NF-kappa B pathway by human herpes virus 8-encoded Fas-associated death domain-like IL-1 beta-converting enzyme inhibitory protein (vFLIP). *Proc. Natl. Acad. Sci. U. S. A. 101*, 9399–9404.

Matta, H., Sun, Q., Moses, G., and Chaudhary, P.M. (2003). Molecular genetic analysis of human herpes virus 8-encoded viral FLICE inhibitory protein-induced NF-kappaB activation. *J. Biol. Chem. 278*, 52406–52411.

May, J.S., Coleman, H.M., Smillie, B., Efstathiou, S., and Stevenson, P.G. (2004). Forced lytic replication impairs host colonization by a latency-deficient mutant of murine gammaherpesvirus-68. *J. Gen. Virol. 85*, 137–146.

Mayama, S., Cuevas, L.E., Sheldon, J., Omar, O.H., Smith, D.H., Okong, P., Silvel, B., Hart, C.A., and Schulz, T.F. (1998). Prevalence and transmission of Kaposi's sarcoma-associated herpesvirus (human herpesvirus 8) in Ugandan children and adolescents. *Int. J. Cancer 77*, 817–820.

Mayne, M., Cheadle, C., Soldan, S.S., Cermelli, C., Yamano, Y., Akhyani, N., Nagel, J.E., Taub, D.D., Becker, K.G., and Jacobson, S. (2001). Gene expression profile of herpesvirus-infected T cells obtained using immunomicroarrays: induction of proinflammatory mechanisms. *J. Virol. 75*, 11641–11650.

Mbopi-Keou, F.X., Legoff, J., Piketty, C., Hocini, H., Malkin, J.E., Inoue, N., Scully, C.M., Porter, S.R., Teo, C.G., and Belec, L. (2004). Salivary production of IgA and IgG to human herpes virus 8 latent and lytic antigens by patients in whom Kaposi's sarcoma has regressed. *AIDS 18*, 338–340.

Mbulaiteye, S.M., Biggar, R.J., Goedert, J.J., and Engels, E.A. (2002). Pleural and peritoneal lymphoma among people with AIDS in the United States. *J. Acquir. Immune. Defic. Syndr. 29*, 418–421.

Mbulaiteye, S.M., Pfeiffer, R.M., Engels, E.A., Marshall, V., Bakaki, P.M., Owor, A.M., Ndugwa, C.M., Katongole-Mbidde, E., Goedert, J.J., Biggar, R.J., and Whitby, D. (2004). Detection of kaposi sarcoma-associated herpesvirus DNA in saliva and buffy-coat samples from children with sickle cell disease in Uganda. *J. Infect. Dis. 190*, 1382–1386.

Mbulaiteye, S.M., Pfeiffer, R.M., Whitby, D., Brubaker, G.R., Shao, J., and Biggar, R.J. (2003). Human herpesvirus 8 infection within families in rural Tanzania. *J. Infect. Dis. 187*, 1780–1785.

McClellan, J.S., Tibbetts, S.A., Gangappa, S., Brett, K.A., and Virgin, H.W.t. (2004). Critical role of CD4 T cells in an antibody-independent mechanism of vaccination against gammaherpesvirus latency. *J. Virol. 78*, 6836–45.

McDonagh, D.P., Liu, J., Gaffey, M.J., Layfield, L.J., Azumi, N., and Traweek, S.T. (1996). Detection of Kaposi's sarcoma-associated herpesvirus-like DNA sequence in angiosarcoma. *Am. J. Pathol. 149*, 1363–1368.

McGeoch, D.J., Dolan, A., and Ralph, A.C. (2000). Toward a comprehensive phylogeny for mammalian and avian herpesviruses. *J. Virol. 74*, 10401–10406.

Means, R.E., Ishido, S., Alvarez, X., and Jung, J.U. (2002). Multiple endocytic trafficking pathways of MHC class I molecules induced by a Herpesvirus protein. *EMBO J 21*, 1638–1649.

Medveczky, M.M., Horvath, E., Lund, T., and Medveczky, P.G. (1997). In vitro antiviral drug sensitivity of the Kaposi's sarcoma-associated herpesvirus. *AIDS 11*, 1327–1332.

Melbye, M., Cook, P.M., Hjalgrim, H., Begtrup, K., Simpson, G.R., Biggar, R.J., Ebbesen, P., and Schulz, T.F. (1998). Risk factors for Kaposi's-sarcoma-associated herpesvirus (KSHV/HHV-8) seropositivity in a cohort of homosexual men, 1981-1996. *Int. J. Cancer 77*, 543–548.

Melendez, L.V., Daniel, M.D., Hunt, R.D., and Garcia, F.G. (1968). An apparently new herpesvirus from primary kidney cultures of the squirrel monkey (Saimiri sciureus). *Lab Anim Care 18*, 374–381.

Meng, Y.X., Spira, T.J., Bhat, G.J., Birch, C.J., Druce, J.D., Edlin, B.R., Edwards, R., Gunthel, C., Newton, R., Stamey, F.R., Wood, C., and Pellett, P.E. (1999). Individuals from North America, Australasia, and Africa are infected with four different genotypes of human herpesvirus 8. *Virology 261*, 106–119.

Menotti, L., Mirandola, P., Locati, M., and Campadelli-Fiume, G. (1999). Trafficking to the plasma membrane of the seven-transmembrane protein encoded by human herpesvirus 6 U51 gene involves a cell-specific function present in T lymphocytes. *J. Virol. 73*, 325–333.

Mercader, M., Taddeo, B., Panella, J.R., Chandran, B., Nickoloff, B.J., and Foreman, K.E. (2000). Induction of HHV-8 lytic cycle replication by inflammatory cytokines produced by HIV-1-infected T cells. *Am. J. Pathol. 156*, 1961–1971.

Merlo, J.J. and Tsygankov, A.Y. (2001). Herpesvirus saimiri oncoproteins Tip and StpC synergistically stimulate NF-kappaB activity and interleukin-2 gene expression. *Virology 279*, 325–338.

Mesri, E.A., Cesarman, E., Arvanitakis, L., Rafii, S., Moore, M.A., Posnett, D.N., Knowles, D.M., and Asch, A.S. (1996). Human herpesvirus-8/Kaposi's sarcoma-associated herpesvirus is a new transmissible virus that infects B cells. *J. Exp. Med. 183*, 2385–2390.

Milligan, S., Robinson, M., O'Donnell, E., and Blackbourn, D.J. (2004). Inflammatory cytokines inhibit Kaposi's sarcoma-associated herpesvirus lytic gene transcription in in vitro-infected endothelial cells. *J. Virol. 78*, 2591–2596.

Milne, R.S., Mattick, C., Nicholson, L., Devaraj, P., Alcami, A., and Gompels, U.A. (2000). RANTES binding and down-regulation by a novel human herpesvirus-6 beta chemokine receptor. *J. Immunol. 164*, 2396–2404.

Mirandola, P., Secchiero, P., Pierpaoli, S., Visani, G., Zamai, L., Vitale, M., Capitani, S., and Zauli, G. (2000). Infection of CD34(+) hematopoietic progenitor cells by human herpesvirus 7 (HHV-7). *Blood 96*, 126–131.

Miyoshi, H., Tanaka–Taya, K., Hara, J., Fujisaki, H., Matsuda, Y., Ohta, H., Osugi, Y., Okada, S., and Yamanishi, K. (2001). Inverse relationship between human herpesvirus-6 and -7 detection after allogeneic and autologous stem cell transplantation. *Bone Marrow Transplant. 27*, 1065–1070.

Molden, J., Chang, Y., You, Y., Moore, P.S., and Goldsmith, M.A. (1997). A Kaposi's sarcoma-associated herpesvirus-encoded cytokine homolog (vIL-6) activates signaling through the shared gp130 receptor subunit. *J. Biol. Chem. 272*, 19625–19631.

Montaner, S., Sodhi, A., Molinolo, A., Bugge, T.H., Sawai, E.T., He, Y., Li, Y., Ray, P.E., and Gutkind, J.S. (2003). Endothelial infection with KSHV genes in vivo reveals that vGPCR initiates Kaposi's sarcomagenesis and can promote the tumorigenic potential of viral latent genes. *Cancer Cell 3*, 23–36.

Montaner, S., Sodhi, A., Pece, S., Mesri, E.A., and Gutkind, J.S. (2001). The Kaposi's sarcoma-associated herpesvirus G protein-coupled receptor promotes endothelial cell survival through the activation of Akt/protein kinase B. *Cancer Res. 61*, 2641–2648.

Montaner, S., Sodhi, A., Servitja, J.M., Ramsdell, A.K., Barac, A., Sawai, E.T., and Gutkind, J.S. (2004). The small GTPase Rac1 links the Kaposi sarcoma-associated herpesvirus vGPCR to cytokine secretion and paracrine neoplasia. *Blood 104*, 2903–2911.

Montejo, M., Ramon, F.J., Testillano, M., Valdivieso, A., Aguirrebengoa, K., Varas, C., Olaizola, A., and De Urbina, J.O. (2002). Encephalitis caused by human herpesvirus-6 in a liver transplant recipient. *Eur. Neurol. 48*, 234–235.

Mookerjee, B.P. and Vogelsang, G. (1997). Human herpes virus-6 encephalitis after bone marrow transplantation: successful treatment with ganciclovir. *Bone Marrow Transplant. 20*, 905–906.

Moore, P.S., Boshoff, C., Weiss, R.A., and Chang, Y. (1996a). Molecular mimicry of human cytokine and cytokine response pathway genes by KSHV. *Science 274*, 1739–1744.

Moore, P.S., Gao, S.J., Dominguez, G., Cesarman, E., Lungu, O., Knowles, D.M., Garber, R., Pellett, P.E., McGeoch, D.J., and Chang, Y. (1996b). Primary characterization of a herpesvirus agent associated with Kaposi's sarcomae [published erratum appears in *J. Virol.* 1996;70(12):9083]. *J. Virol. 70*, 549–558.

Moore, P.S., Kingsley, L.A., Holmberg, S.D., Spira, T., Gupta, P., Hoover, D.R., Parry, J.P., Conley, L.J., Jaffe, H.W., and Chang, Y. (1996c). Kaposi's sarcoma-associated herpesvirus infection prior to onset of Kaposi's sarcoma. *AIDS 10*, 175–180.

Moorman, N.J., Virgin, H.W.t., and Speck, S.H. (2003a). Disruption of the gene encoding the gammaHV68 v-GPCR leads to decreased efficiency of reactivation from latency. *Virology 307*, 179–190.

Moorman, N.J., Willer, D.O., and Speck, S.H. (2003b). The gammaherpesvirus 68 latency-associated nuclear antigen homolog is critical for the establishment of splenic latency. *J. Virol. 77*, 10295–10303.

Mori, Y., Akkapaiboon, P., Yang, X., and Yamanishi, K. (2003). The human herpesvirus 6 U100 gene product is the third component of the gH-gL glycoprotein complex on the viral envelope. *J. Virol. 77*, 2452–2458.

Mori, Y., Akkapaiboon, P., Yonemoto, S., Koike, M., Takemoto, M., Sadaoka, T., Sasamoto, Y., Konishi, S., Uchiyama, Y., and Yamanishi, K. (2004). Discovery of a second form of tripartite complex containing gH-gL of human herpesvirus 6 and observations on CD46. *J. Virol. 78*, 4609–4616.

Mori, Y., Dhepakson, P., Shimamoto, T., Ueda, K., Gomi, Y., Tani, H., Matsuura, Y., and Yamanishi, K. (2000). Expression of human herpesvirus 6B rep within infected cells and binding of its gene product to the TATA-binding protein in vitro and in vivo. *J. Virol. 74*, 6096–6104.

Moses, A.V., Jarvis, M.A., Raggo, C., Bell, Y.C., Ruhl, R., Luukkonen, B.G., Griffith, D.J., Wait, C.L., Druker, B.J., Heinrich, M.C., Nelson, J.A., and Fruh, K. (2002). Kaposi's sarcoma-associated herpesvirus-induced upregulation of the c-kit proto-oncogene, as identified by gene expression profiling, is essential for the transformation of endothelial cells. *J. Virol. 76*, 8383–8399.

Moses, A.V., Fish, K.N., Ruhl, R., Smith, P.P., Strussenberg, J.G., Zhu, L., Chandran, B., and Nelson, J.A. (1999). Long-term infection and transformation of dermal microvascular endothelial cells by human herpesvirus 8. *J. Virol. 73*, 6892–6902.

Mullick, J., Bernet, J., Singh, A.K., Lambris, J.D., and Sahu, A. (2003). Kaposi's sarcoma-associated herpesvirus (human herpesvirus 8) open reading frame 4 protein (kaposica) is a functional homolog of complement control proteins. *J. Virol. 77*, 3878–3881.

Muralidhar, S., Pumfery, A.M., Hassani, M., Sadaie, M.R., Kishishita, M., Brady, J.N., Doniger, J., Medveczky, P., and Rosenthal, L.J. (1998). Identification of kaposin (open reading frame K12) as a human herpesvirus 8 (Kaposi's sarcoma-associated herpesvirus) transforming gene. *J. Virol. 72*, 4980–4988.

Murphy, C., Kretschmer, C., Biesinger, B., Beckers, J., Jung, J., Desrosiers, R.C., Muller-Hermelink, H.K., Fleckenstein, B.W., and Ruther, U. (1994). Epithelial tumours induced by a herpesvirus oncogene in transgenic mice. *Oncogene 9*, 221–226.

Murthy, S.C., Trimble, J.J., and Desrosiers, R.C. (1989). Deletion mutants of herpesvirus saimiri define an open reading frame necessary for transformation. *J. Virol. 63*, 3307–3314.

Nador, R.G., Cesarman, E., Chadburn, A., Dawson, D.B., Ansari, M.Q., Sald, J., and Knowles, D.M. (1996). Primary effusion lymphoma: a distinct clinicopathologic entity associated with the Kaposi's sarcoma-associated herpes virus. *Blood 88*, 645–656.

Nakamura, H., Li, M., Zarycki, J., and Jung, J.U. (2001). Inhibition of p53 tumor suppressor by viral interferon regulatory factor. *J. Virol. 75*, 7572–7582.

Nakano, K., Isegawa, Y., Zou, P., Tadagaki, K., Inagi, R., and Yamanishi, K. (2003). Kaposi's sarcoma–associated herpesvirus (KSHV)-encoded vMIP-I and vMIP-II induce signal transduction and chemotaxis in monocytic cells. *Arch. Virol. 148*, 871–890.

Nash, A.A., Dutia, B.M., Stewart, J.P., and Davison, A.J. (2001). Natural history of murine gamma-herpesvirus infection. *Philos. Trans. R. Soc. Lond. B Biol. Sci. 356*, 569–579.

Nash, P.J., Avery, R.K., Tang, W.H., Starling, R.C., Taege, A.J., and Yamani, M.H. (2004). Encephalitis owing to human herpesvirus-6 after cardiac transplant. *Am. J. Transplant. 4*, 1200–1203.

Neyts, J. and De Clercq, E. (1997). Antiviral drug susceptibility of human herpesvirus 8. *Antimicrob. Agents Chemother. 41*, 2754–2756.

Nicholas, J., Cameron, K.R., and Honess, R.W. (1992). Herpesvirus saimiri encodes homologues of G protein-coupled receptors and cyclins. *Nature 355*, 362–365.

Nicholas, J., Ruvolo, V.R., Burns, W.H., Sandford, G., Wan, X., Ciufo, D., Hendrickson, S.B., Guo, H.G., Hayward, G.S., and Reitz, M.S. (1997). Kaposi's sarcoma-associated human herpesvirus-8 encodes homologues of macrophage inflammatory protein-1 and interleukin-6. *Nat Med 3*, 287–292.

Nielsen, L. and Vestergaard, B.F. (1996). Competitive ELISA for detection of HHV-6 antibody: sero-prevalence in a danish population. *J. Virol. Methods 56*, 221–230.

Nuvor, S.V., Katano, H., Ampofo, W.K., Barnor, J.S., and Sata, T. (2001). Higher prevalence of anti-bodies to human herpesvirus 8 in HIV-infected individuals than in the general population in Ghana, West Africa. *Eur. J. Clin. Microbiol. Infect. Dis. 20*, 362–364.

Oettle, A.G. (1962). Geographical and racial differences in the frequency of Kaposi's sarcoma as evidence of environmental or genetic causes. *Acta Unio. Int. Contra. Cancrum. 18*, 330–363.

Oksenhendler, E., Boulanger, E., Galicier, L., Du, M.Q., Dupin, N., Diss, T.C., Hamoudi, R., Daniel, M.T., Agbalika, F., Boshoff, C., Clauvel, J.P., Isaacson, P.G., and Meignin, V. (2002). High inci-dence of Kaposi sarcoma-associated herpesvirus-related non-Hodgkin lymphoma in patients with HIV infection and multicentric Castleman disease. *Blood 99*, 2331–2336.

Oksenhendler, E., Duarte, M., Soulier, J., Cacoub, P., Welker, Y., Cadranel, J., Cazals–Hatem, D., Autran, B., Clauvel, J.P., and Raphael, M. (1996). Multicentric Castleman's disease in HIV infection: a clinical and pathological study of 20 patients. *AIDS 10*, 61–67.

Okuno, T., Higashi, K., Shiraki, K., Yamanishi, K., Takahashi, M., Kokado, Y., Ishibashi, M., Takahara, S., Sonoda, T., Tanaka, K., Baba, K., and Kurata, T. (1990). Human herpesvirus 6 infection in renal transplantation. *Transplantation 49*, 519–522.

Okuno, T., Mukai, T., Baba, K., Ohsumi, Y., Takahashi, M., and Yamanishi, K. (1991). Outbreak of exanthem subitum in an orphanage. *J. Pediatr. 119*, 759–761.

Okuno, T., Oishi, H., Hayashi, K., Nonogaki, M., Tanaka, K., and Yamanishi, K. (1995). Human her-pesviruses 6 and 7 in cervixes of pregnant women. *J. Clin. Microbiol. 33*, 1968–1970.

Okuno, T., Takahashi, K., Balachandra, K., Shiraki, K., Yamanishi, K., Takahashi, M., and Baba, K. (1989). Seroepidemiology of human herpesvirus 6 infection in normal children and adults. *J. Clin. Microbiol. 27*, 651–653.

Olsen, S.J., Chang, Y., Moore, P.S., Biggar, R.J., and Melbye, M. (1998). Increasing Kaposi's sar-coma–associated herpesvirus seroprevalence with age in a highly Kaposi's sarcoma endemic region, Zambia in 1985. *AIDS 12*, 1921–1925.

Operskalski, E.A., Busch, M.P., Mosley, J.W., and Kedes, D.H. (1997). Blood donations and viruses. *Lancet 349*, 1327.

Osborne, J., Moore, P.S., and Chang, Y. (1999). KSHV-encoded viral IL-6 activates multiple human IL-6 signaling pathways. *Hum. Immunol. 60*, 921–927.

Osman, H.K., Peiris, J.S., Taylor, C.E., Warwicker, P., Jarrett, R.F., and Madeley, C.R. (1996). "Cytomegalovirus disease" in renal allograft recipients: is human herpesvirus 7 a co-factor for disease progression? *J. Med. Virol. 48*, 295–301.

Oster, B. and Hollsberg, P. (2002). Viral gene expression patterns in human herpesvirus 6B-infected T cells. *J. Virol. 76*, 7578–7586.

Parisi, S.G., Sarmati, L., Pappagallo, M., Mazzi, R., Carolo, G., Farchi, F., Nicastri, E., Concia, E., Rezza, G., and Andreoni, M. (2002). Prevalence trend and correlates of HHV-8 infection in HIV-infected patients. *J. Acquir. Immune. Defic. Syndr. 29*, 295–299.

Park, J., Cho, N.H., Choi, J.K., Feng, P., Choe, J., and Jung, J.U. (2003). Distinct roles of cellular Lck and p80 proteins in herpesvirus saimiri Tip function on lipid rafts. *J. Virol. 77*, 9041–9051.

Park, J., Seo, T., Jung, J., and Choe, J. (2004). Herpesvirus saimiri STP A11 protein interacts with STAT3 and stimulates its transcriptional activity. *Biochem. Biophys. Res. Commun. 320*, 279–285.

Parkin, D.M., Wabinga, H., Nambooze, S., and Wabwire-Mangen, F. (1999). AIDS-related cancers in Africa: maturation of the epidemic in Uganda. *AIDS 13*, 2563–2570.

Parravicini, C., Olsen, S.J., Capra, M., Poli, F., Sirchia, G., Gao, S.J., Berti, E., Nocera, A., Rossi, E., Bestetti, G., Pizzuto, M., Galli, M., Moroni, M., Moore, P.S., and Corbellino, M. (1997). Risk of Kaposi's sarcoma-associated herpes virus transmission from donor allografts among Italian posttransplant Kaposi's sarcoma patients. *Blood 90*, 2826–2829.

Paterson, D.L., Singh, N., Gayowski, T., Carrigan, D.R., and Marino, I.R. (1999). Encephalopathy associated with human herpesvirus 6 in a liver transplant recipient. *Liver Transpl. Surg. 5*, 454–455.

Pauk, J., Buchwald, D., and Corey, L. (2001). Letter to the editor: human herpesvirus 6 serologic responses. *J. Clin. Virol. 21*, 103–104.

Pauk, J., Huang, M.L., Brodie, S.J., Wald, A., Koelle, D.M., Schacker, T., Celum, C., Selke, S., and Corey, L. (2000). Mucosal shedding of human herpesvirus 8 in men. *N. Engl. J. Med. 343*, 1369–1377.

Pavlova, I.V., Virgin, H.W.t., and Speck, S.H. (2003). Disruption of gammaherpesvirus 68 gene 50 demonstrates that Rta is essential for virus replication. *J. Virol. 77*, 5731–5739.

Pellett, P.E., Wright, D.J., Engels, E.A., Ablashi, D.V., Dollard, S.C., Forghani, B., Glynn, S.A., Goedert, J.J., Jenkins, F.J., Lee, T.H., Neipel, F., Todd, D.S., Whitby, D., Nemo, G.J., and Busch, M.P. (2003). Multicenter comparison of serologic assays and estimation of human herpesvirus 8 seroprevalence among US blood donors. *Transfusion 43*, 1260–1268.

Penn, I. (1995). Sarcomas in organ allograft recipients. *Transplantation 60*, 1485–1491.

Perez, C., Tous, M., Gallego, S., Zala, N., Rabinovich, O., Garbiero, S., Martinez, M.J., Cunha, A.M., Camino, S., Camara, A., Costa, S.C., Larrondo, M., Francalancia, V., Landreau, F., and Bartomioli, M.A. (2004). Seroprevalence of human herpesvirus-8 in blood donors from different geographical regions of Argentina, Brazil, and Chile. *J. Med. Virol. 72*, 661–667.

Pertel, P.E. (2002). Human herpesvirus 8 glycoprotein B (gB), gH, and gL can mediate cell fusion. *J. Virol. 76*, 4390–4400.

Pfeiffer, B., Thomson, B., and Chandran, B. (1995). Identification and characterization of a cDNA derived from multiple splicing that encodes envelope glycoprotein gp105 of human herpesvirus 6. *J. Virol. 69*, 3490–3500.

Plancoulaine, S., Abel, L., van Beveren, M., Tregouet, D.A., Joubert, M., Tortevoye, P., de The, G., and Gessain, A. (2000). Human herpesvirus 8 transmission from mother to child and between siblings in an endemic population. *Lancet 356*, 1062–1065.

Pohl-Koppe, A., Blay, M., Jager, G., and Weiss, M. (2001). Human herpes virus type 7 DNA in the cerebrospinal fluid of children with central nervous system diseases. *Eur. J Pediatr. 160*, 351–358.

Poole, L.J., Zong, J.C., Ciufo, D.M., Alcendor, D.J., Cannon, J.S., Ambinder, R., Orenstein, J.M., Reitz, M.S., and Hayward, G.S. (1999). Comparison of genetic variability at multiple loci across the genomes of the major subtypes of Kaposi's sarcoma-associated herpesvirus reveals evidence for recombination and for two distinct types of open reading frame K15 alleles at the right-hand end. *J. Virol. 73*, 6646–6660.

Pozharskaya, V.P., Weakland, L.L., and Offermann, M.K. (2004a). Inhibition of infectious human herpesvirus 8 production by gamma interferon and alpha interferon in BCBL-1 cells. *J. Gen. Virol. 85*, 2779–2787.

Pozharskaya, V.P., Weakland, L.L., Zimring, J.C., Krug, L.T., Unger, E.R., Neisch, A., Joshi, H., Inoue, N., and Offermann, M.K. (2004b). Short duration of elevated vIRF-1 expression during lytic replication of human herpesvirus 8 limits its ability to block antiviral responses induced by alpha interferon in BCBL-1 cells. *J. Virol. 78*, 6621–6635.

Prakash, O., Tang, Z.Y., Peng, X., Coleman, R., Gill, J., Farr, G., and Samaniego, F. (2002). Tumorigenesis and aberrant signaling in transgenic mice expressing the human herpesvirus-8 K1 gene. *J. Natl. Cancer Inst. 94*, 926–935.

Pruksananonda, P., Hall, C.B., Insel, R.A., McIntyre, K., Pellett, P.E., Long, C.E., Schnabel, K.C., Pincus, P.H., Stamey, F.R., and Dambaugh, T.R. (1992). Primary human herpesvirus 6 infection in young children. *N. Engl. J. Med. 326*, 1445–1450.

Qunibi, W., Akhtar, M., Sheth, K., Ginn, H.E., Al Furayh, O., DeVol, E.B., and Taher, S. (1988). Kaposi's sarcoma: the most common tumor after renal transplantation in Saudi Arabia. *Am. J. Med. 84*, 225–232.

Rabkin, C.S., Janz, S., Lash, A., Coleman, A.E., Musaba, E., Liotta, L., Biggar, R.J., and Zhuang, Z. (1997). Monoclonal origin of multicentric Kaposi's sarcoma lesions. *N. Engl. J. Med. 336*, 988–993.

Rabkin, C.S., Schulz, T.F., Whitby, D., Lennette, E.T., Magpantay, L.I., Chatlynne, L., and Biggar, R.J. (1998). Interassay correlation of human herpesvirus 8 serologic tests. HHV–8 Interlaboratory Collaborative Group. *J. Infect. Dis. 178*, 304–309.

Radkov, S.A., Kellam, P., and Boshoff, C. (2000). The latent nuclear antigen of Kaposi sarcoma-associated herpesvirus targets the retinoblastoma-E2F pathway and with the oncogene Hras transforms primary rat cells. *Nat. Med 6*, 1121–1127.

Rady, P.L., Yen, A., Rollefson, J.L., Orengo, I., Bruce, S., Hughes, T.K., and Tyring, S.K. (1995). Herpesvirus-like DNA sequences in non-Kaposi's sarcoma skin lesions of transplant patients. *Lancet 345*, 1339–1340.

Rapaport, D., Engelhard, D., Tagger, G., Or, R., and Frenkel, N. (2002). Antiviral prophylaxis may prevent human herpesvirus-6 reactivation in bone marrow transplant recipients. *Transpl. Infect. Dis. 4*, 10–16.

Rapp, J.C., Krug, L.T., Inoue, N., Dambaugh, T.R., and Pellett, P.E. (2000). U94, the human herpesvirus 6 homolog of the parvovirus nonstructural gene, is highly conserved among isolates and is expressed at low mRNA levels as a spliced transcript. *Virology 268*, 504–516.

Ratnamohan, V.M., Chapman, J., Howse, H., Bovington, K., Robertson, P., Byth, K., Allen, R., and Cunningham, A.L. (1998). Cytomegalovirus and human herpesvirus 6 both cause viral disease after renal transplantation. *Transplantation 66*, 877–882.

Reeves, W.C., Stamey, F.R., Black, J.B., Mawle, A.C., Stewart, J.A., and Pellett, P.E. (2000). Human herpesviruses 6 and 7 in chronic fatigue syndrome: a case-control study. *Clin. Infect. Dis. 31*, 48–52.

Reiss, C., Niedobitek, G., Hor, S., Lisner, R., Friedrich, U., Bodemer, W., and Biesinger, B. (2002). Peripheral T-cell lymphoma in herpesvirus saimiri-infected tamarins: tumor cell lines reveal subgroup-specific differences. *Virology 294*, 31–46.

Renne, R., Zhong, W., Herndier, B., McGrath, M., Abbey, N., Kedes, D., and Ganem, D. (1996). Lytic growth of Kaposi's sarcoma-associated herpesvirus (human herpesvirus 8) in culture. *Nat. Med. 2*, 342–346.

Renne, R., Blackbourn, D., Whitby, D., Levy, J., and Ganem, D. (1998). Limited transmission of Kaposi's sarcoma-associated herpesvirus in cultured cells. *J. Virol. 72*, 5182–5188.

Renwick, N., Dukers, N.H., Weverling, G.J., Sheldon, J.A., Schulz, T.F., Prins, M., Coutinho, R.A., and Goudsmit, J. (2002). Risk factors for human herpesvirus 8 infection in a cohort of drug users in the Netherlands, 1985-1996. *J. Infect. Dis. 185*, 1808–1812.

Rettig, M.B., Ma, H.J., Vescio, R.A., Pold, M., Schiller, G., Belson, D., Savage, A., Nishikubo, C., Wu, C., Fraser, J., Said, J.W., and Berenson, J.R. (1997). Kaposi's sarcoma-associated herpesvirus infection of bone marrow dendritic cells from multiple myeloma patients. *Science 276*, 1851–1854.

Rickabaugh, T.M., Brown, H.J., Martinez-Guzman, D., Wu, T.T., Tong, L., Yu, F., Cole, S., and Sun, R. (2004). Generation of a latency-deficient gammaherpesvirus that is protective against secondary infection. *J. Virol. 78*, 9215–9223.

Roan, F., Zimring, J.C., Goodbourn, S., and Offermann, M.K. (1999). Transcriptional activation by the human herpesvirus-8-encoded interferon regulatory factor. *J. Gen. Virol. 80*, 2205–2209.

Rosenkilde, M.M., McLean, K.A., Holst, P.J., and Schwartz, T.W. (2004). The CXC chemokine receptor encoded by herpesvirus saimiri, ECRF3, shows ligand regulated signaling through Gi, Gq, and G12/13 proteins but constitutive signaling only through Gi and G12/13 proteins. *J. Biol. Chem. 279*, 32524–32533.

Rossi, C., Delforge, M.L., Jacobs, F., Wissing, M., Pradier, O., Remmelink, M., Byl, B., Thys, J.P., and Liesnard, C. (2001). Fatal primary infection due to human herpesvirus 6 variant A in a renal transplant recipient. *Transplantation 71*, 288–292.

Rotola, A., Ravaioli, T., Gonelli, A., Dewhurst, S., Cassai, E., and Di Luca, D. (1998). U94 of human herpesvirus 6 is expressed in latently infected peripheral blood mononuclear cells and blocks viral gene expression in transformed lymphocytes in culture. *Proc. Natl. Acad. Sci. U. S. A. 95*, 13911–13916.

Roy, D.J., Ebrahimi, B.C., Dutia, B.M., Nash, A.A., and Stewart, J.P. (2000). Murine gammaherpesvirus M11 gene product inhibits apoptosis and is expressed during virus persistence. *Arch. Virol. 145*, 2411–2420.

Russo, J.J., Bohenzky, R.A., Chien, M.C., Chen, J., Yan, M., Maddalena, D., Parry, J.P., Peruzzi, D., Edelman, I.S., Chang, Y., and Moore, P.S. (1996). Nucleotide sequence of the Kaposi sarcoma–associated herpesvirus (HHV8). *Proc. Natl. Acad. Sci. U. S. A. 93*, 14862–14867.

Said, J.W., Hoyer, K.K., French, S.W., Rosenfelt, L., Garcia-Lloret, M., Koh, P.J., Cheng, T.C., Sulur, G.G., Pinkus, G.S., Kuehl, W.M., Rawlings, D.J., Wall, R., and Teitell, M.A. (2001). TCL1 oncogene expression in B cell subsets from lymphoid hyperplasia and distinct classes of B cell lymphoma. *Lab. Invest. 81*, 555–564.

Said, J.W., Rettig, M.R., Heppner, K., Vescio, R.A., Schiller, G., Ma, H.J., Belson, D., Savage, A., Shintaku, I.P., Koeffler, H.P., Asou, H., Pinkus, G., Pinkus, J., Schrage, M., Green, E., and Berenson, J.R. (1997). Localization of Kaposi's sarcoma-associated herpesvirus in bone marrow biopsy samples from patients with multiple myeloma. *Blood 90*, 4278–4282.

Sander, C.A., Simon, M., Puchta, U., Raffeld, M., and Kind, P. (1996). HHV–8 in lymphoproliferative lesions in skin. *Lancet 348*, 475–476.

Santarelli, R., De Marco, R., Masala, M.V., Angeloni, A., Uccini, S., Pacchiarotti, R., Montesu, M.A., Satta, R., Cerimele, D., Faggioni, A., and Cottoni, F. (2001). Direct correlation between human herpesvirus-8 seroprevalence and classic Kaposi's sarcoma incidence in Northern Sardinia. *J. Med. Virol. 65*, 368–372.

Santoro, F., Greenstone, H.L., Insinga, A., Liszewski, M.K., Atkinson, J.P., Lusso, P., and Berger, E.A. (2003). Interaction of glycoprotein H of human herpesvirus 6 with the cellular receptor CD46. *J. Biol. Chem. 278*, 25964–25969.

Santoro, F., Kennedy, P.E., Locatelli, G., Malnati, M.S., Berger, E.A., and Lusso, P. (1999). CD46 is a cellular receptor for human herpesvirus 6. *Cell 99*, 817–827.

Sarid, R., Flore, O., Bohenzky, R.A., Chang, Y., and Moore, P.S. (1998). Transcription mapping of the Kaposi's sarcoma-associated herpesvirus (human herpesvirus 8) genome in a body cavity-based lymphoma cell line (BC-1). *J. Virol. 72*, 1005–1012.

Sarid, R., Pizov, G., Rubinger, D., Backenroth, R., Friedlaender, M.M., Schwartz, F., and Wolf, D.G. (2001). Detection of human herpesvirus-8 DNA in kidney allografts prior to the development of Kaposi's sarcoma. *Clin. Infect. Dis. 32*, 1502–1505.

Sarmati, L., Carlo, T., Rossella, S., Montano, M., Adalgisa, P., Rezza, G., and Andreoni, M. (2004). Human herpesvirus-8 infection in pregnancy and labor: lack of evidence of vertical transmission. *J. Med. Virol. 72*, 462–466.

Sashihara, J., Tanaka–Taya, K., Tanaka, S., Amo, K., Miyagawa, H., Hosoi, G., Taniguchi, T., Fukui, T., Kasuga, N., Aono, T., Sako, M., Hara, J., Yamanishi, K., and Okada, S. (2002). High incidence of human herpesvirus 6 infection with a high viral load in cord blood stem cell transplant recipients. *Blood 100*, 2005–2011.

Satoh, M., Toma, H., Sato, Y., Futenma, C., Kiyuna, S., Shiroma, Y., Kokaze, A., Sakurada, S., Sata, T., and Katano, H. (2001). Seroprevalence of human herpesvirus 8 in Okinawa, Japan. *Jpn. J. Infect. Dis. 54*, 125–126.

Saxinger, C., Polesky, H., Eby, N., Grufferman, S., Murphy, R., Tegtmeir, G., Parekh, V., Memon, S., and Hung, C. (1988). Antibody reactivity with HBLV (HHV-6) in U.S. populations. *J. Virol. Methods 21*, 199–208.

Schatz, O., Monini, P., Bugarini, R., Neipel, F., Schulz, T.F., Andreoni, M., Erb, P., Eggers, M., Haas, J., Butto, S., Lukwiya, M., Bogner, J.R., Yaguboglu, S., Sheldon, J., Sarmati, L., Goebel, F.D., Hintermaier, R., Enders, G., Regamey, N., Wernli, M., Sturzl, M., Rezza, G., and Ensoli, B.

(2001). Kaposi's sarcoma-associated herpesvirus serology in Europe and Uganda: multicentre study with multiple and novel assays. *J. Med. Virol. 65*, 123–132.

Schulze-Gahmen, U. and Kim, S.H. (2002). Structural basis for CDK6 activation by a virus-encoded cyclin. *Nat Struct Biol 9*, 177–181.

Secchiero, P., Sun, D., De Vico, A.L., Crowley, R.W., Reitz, M.S., Jr., Zauli, G., Lusso, P., and Gallo, R.C. (1997). Role of the extracellular domain of human herpesvirus 7 glycoprotein B in virus binding to cell surface heparan sulfate proteoglycans. *J. Virol. 71*, 4571–4580.

Seo, T., Lee, D., Lee, B., Chung, J.H., and Choe, J. (2000). Viral interferon regulatory factor 1 of Kaposi's sarcoma-associated herpesvirus (human herpesvirus 8) binds to, and inhibits transactivation of, CREB-binding protein. *Biochem. Biophys. Res. Commun. 270*, 23–27.

Seo, T., Park, J., Lee, D., Hwang, S.G., and Choe, J. (2001). Viral interferon regulatory factor 1 of Kaposi's sarcoma-associated herpesvirus binds to p53 and represses p53-dependent transcription and apoptosis. *J. Virol. 75*, 6193–6198.

Serraino, D., Franceschi, S., Dal Maso, L., and La Vecchia, C. (1995). HIV transmission and Kaposi's sarcoma among European women. *AIDS 9*, 971–973.

Severini, A., Sevenhuysen, C., Garbutt, M., and Tipples, G.A. (2003). Structure of replicating intermediates of human herpesvirus type 6. *Virology 314*, 443–450.

Sgadari, C., Barillari, G., Toschi, E., Carlei, D., Bacigalupo, I., Baccarini, S., Palladino, C., Leone, P., Bugarini, R., Malavasi, L., Cafaro, A., Falchi, M., Valdembri, D., Rezza, G., Bussolino, F., Monini, P., and Ensoli, B. (2002). HIV protease inhibitors are potent anti–angiogenic molecules and promote regression of Kaposi sarcoma. *Nat. Med. 8*, 225–232.

Sharma–Walia, N., Naranatt, P.P., Krishnan, H.H., Zeng, L., and Chandran, B. (2004). Kaposi's sarcoma–associated herpesvirus/human herpesvirus 8 envelope glycoprotein gB induces the integrin–dependent focal adhesion kinase-Src-phosphatidylinositol 3-kinase-Rho GTPase signal pathways and cytoskeletal rearrangements. *J. Virol. 78*, 4207–4223.

Sharp, T.V., Wang, H.W., Koumi, A., Hollyman, D., Endo, Y., Ye, H., Du, M.Q., and Boshoff, C. (2002). K15 protein of Kaposi's sarcoma-associated herpesvirus is latently expressed and binds to HAX–1, a protein with antiapoptotic function. *J. Virol. 76*, 802–816.

Simpson, G.R., Schulz, T.F., Whitby, D., Cook, P.M., Boshoff, C., Rainbow, L., Howard, M.R., Gao, S.J., Bohenzky, R.A., Simmonds, P., Lee, C., de Ruiter, A., Hatzakis, A., Tedder, R.S., Weller, I.V., Weiss, R.A., and Moore, P.S. (1996). Prevalence of Kaposi's sarcoma associated herpesvirus infection measured by antibodies to recombinant capsid protein and latent immunofluorescence antigen. *Lancet 348*, 1133–1138.

Singh, N., Carrigan, D.R., Gayowski, T., and Marino, I.R. (1997). Human herpesvirus-6 infection in liver transplant recipients: documentation of pathogenicity. *Transplantation 64*, 674–678.

Sitas, F., Carrara, H., Beral, V., Newton, R., Reeves, G., Bull, D., Jentsch, U., Pacella–Norman, R., Bourboulia, D., Whitby, D., Boshoff, C., and Weiss, R. (1999a). Antibodies against human herpesvirus 8 in black South African patients with cancer. *N. Engl. J. Med. 340*, 1863–1871.

Sitas, F., Newton, R., and Boshoff, C. (1999b). Increasing probability of mother-to-child transmission of HHV-8 with increasing maternal antibody titer for HHV-8. *N. Engl. J. Med. 340*, 1923.

Skrincosky, D., Hocknell, P., Whetter, L., Secchiero, P., Chandran, B., and Dewhurst, S. (2000). Identification and analysis of a novel heparin-binding glycoprotein encoded by human herpesvirus 7. *J. Virol. 74*, 4530–4540.

Smith, A., Santoro, F., Di Lullo, G., Dagna, L., Verani, A., and Lusso, P. (2003). Selective suppression of IL-12 production by human herpesvirus 6. *Blood 102*, 2877–2884.

Smith, N.A., Sabin, C.A., Gopal, R., Bourboulia, D., Labbet, W., Boshoff, C., Barlow, D., Band, B., Peters, B.S., de Ruiter, A., Brown, D.W., Weiss, R.A., Best, J.M., and Whitby, D. (1999). Serologic evidence of human herpesvirus 8 transmission by homosexual but not heterosexual sex. *J. Infect. Dis. 180*, 600–606.

Sodhi, A., Montaner, S., Patel, V., Gomez-Roman, J.J., Li, Y., Sausville, E.A., Sawai, E.T., and Gutkind, J.S. (2004). Akt plays a central role in sarcomagenesis induced by Kaposi's sarcoma herpesvirus-encoded G protein-coupled receptor. *Proc. Natl. Acad. Sci. U. S. A. 101*, 4821 4826.

Sodhi, A., Montaner, S., Patel, V., Zohar, M., Bais, C., Mesri, E.A., and Gutkind, J.S. (2000). The Kaposi's sarcoma-associated herpes virus G protein-coupled receptor up-regulates vascular endothelial growth factor expression and secretion through mitogen-activated protein kinase and p38 pathways acting on hypoxia-inducible factor 1alpha. *Cancer Res. 60*, 4873–4880.

Song, M.J., Brown, H.J., Wu, T.T., and Sun, R. (2001). Transcription activation of polyadenylated nuclear RNA by Rta in human herpesvirus 8/Kaposi's sarcoma-associated herpesvirus. *J. Virol. 75*, 3129–3140.

Sorokina, E.M., Merlo, J.J., Jr., and Tsygankov, A.Y. (2004). Molecular mechanisms of the effect of herpesvirus saimiri protein StpC on the signaling pathway leading to NF-kappaB activation. *J. Biol. Chem. 279*, 13469–13477.

Sosa, C., Benetucci, J., Hanna, C., Sieczkowski, L., Deluchi, G., Canizal, A.M., Mantina, H., Klaskala, W., Baum, M., and Wood, C. (2001). Human herpesvirus 8 can be transmitted through blood in drug addicts. *Medicina (B Aires) 61*, 291–294.

Sparks-Thissen, R.L., Braaten, D.C., Kreher, S., Speck, S.H., and Virgin, H.W.t. (2004). An optimized CD4 T-cell response can control productive and latent gammaherpesvirus infection. *J. Virol. 78*, 6827–6835.

Speck, S.H. and Virgin, H.W. (1999). Host and viral genetics of chronic infection: a mouse model of gamma-herpesvirus pathogenesis. *Curr. Opin. Microbiol. 2*, 403–409.

Spiller, O.B., Blackbourn, D.J., Mark, L., Proctor, D.G., and Blom, A.M. (2003). Functional activity of the complement regulator encoded by Kaposi's sarcoma-associated herpesvirus. *J. Biol. Chem. 278*, 9283–9289.

Spira, T.J., Lam, L., Dollard, S.C., Meng, Y.X., Pau, C.P., Black, J.B., Burns, D., Cooper, B., Hamid, M., Huong, J., Kite-Powell, K., and Pellett, P.E. (2000). Comparison of serologic assays and PCR for diagnosis of human herpesvirus 8 infection. *J. Clin. Microbiol. 38*, 2174–2180.

Stallone, G., Schena, A., Infante, B., Di Paolo, S., Loverre, A., Maggio, G., Ranieri, E., Gesualdo, L., Schena, F.P., Grandaliano, G. (2005). Sirolimus for Kaposi's sarcoma in renal-transplant recipients. *N. Engl. J. Med. 352*, 1317–23.

Staskus, K.A., Sun, R., Miller, G., Racz, P., Jaslowski, A., Metroka, C., Brett-Smith, H., and Haase, A.T. (1999). Cellular tropism and viral interleukin-6 expression distinguish human herpesvirus 8 involvement in Kaposi's sarcoma, primary effusion lymphoma, and multicentric Castleman's disease. *J. Virol. 73*, 4181–4187.

Staskus, K.A., Zhong, W., Gebhard, K., Herndier, B., Wang, H., Renne, R., Beneke, J., Pudney, J., Anderson, D.J., Ganem, D., and Haase, A.T. (1997). Kaposi's sarcoma-associated herpesvirus gene expression in endothelial (spindle) tumor cells. *J. Virol. 71*, 715–719.

Staudt, M.R., Kanan, Y., Jeong, J.H., Papin, J.F., Hines-Boykin, R., and Dittmer, D.P. (2004). The tumor microenvironment controls primary effusion lymphoma growth in vivo. *Cancer Res. 64*, 4790–4799.

Stevenson, P.G., Efstathiou, S., Doherty, P.C., and Lehner, P.J. (2000). Inhibition of MHC class I-restricted antigen presentation by gamma 2-herpesviruses. *Proc. Natl. Acad. Sci. U. S. A. 97*, 8455–8460.

Stevenson, P.G., May, J.S., Smith, X.G., Marques, S., Adler, H., Koszinowski, U.H., Simas, J.P., and Efstathiou, S. (2002). K3-mediated evasion of CD8(+) T cells aids amplification of a latent gamma-herpesvirus. *Nat. Immunol. 3*, 733–740.

Stine, J.T., Wood, C., Hill, M., Epp, A., Raport, C.J., Schweickart, V.L., Endo, Y., Sasaki, T., Simmons, G., Boshoff, C., Clapham, P., Chang, Y., Moore, P., Gray, P.W., and Chantry, D. (2000). KSHV-encoded CC chemokine vMIP–III is a CCR4 agonist, stimulates angiogenesis, and selectively chemoattracts TH2 cells. *Blood 95*, 1151–1157.

Suga, S., Suzuki, K., Ihira, M., Yoshikawa, T., Kajita, Y., Ozaki, T., Iida, K., Saito, Y., and Asano, Y. (2000). Clinical characteristics of febrile convulsions during primary HHV-6 infection. *Arch. Dis. Child 82*, 62–66.

Sun, Q., Matta, H., and Chaudhary, P.M. (2003). The human herpes virus 8-encoded viral FLICE inhibitory protein protects against growth factor withdrawal-induced apoptosis via NF-kappa B activation. *Blood 101*, 1956–1961.

Sun, R., Lin, S.F., Gradoville, L., Yuan, Y., Zhu, F., and Miller, G. (1998). A viral gene that activates lytic cycle expression of Kaposi's sarcoma-associated herpesvirus. *Proc. Natl. Acad. Sci. U. S. A. 95*, 10866–10871.

Sunil-Chandra, N.P., Arno, J., Fazakerley, J., and Nash, A.A. (1994). Lymphoproliferative disease in mice infected with murine gammaherpesvirus 68. *Am. J. Pathol. 145*, 818–826.

Sunil-Chandra, N.P., Efstathiou, S., Arno, J., and Nash, A.A. (1992a). Virological and pathological features of mice infected with murine gamma-herpesvirus 68. *J. Gen. Virol. 73*, 2347–2356.

Sunil-Chandra, N.P., Efstathiou, S., and Nash, A.A. (1992b). Murine gammaherpesvirus 68 establishes a latent infection in mouse B lymphocytes in vivo. *J. Gen. Virol. 73*, 3275–3279.

Swanton, C., Mann, D.J., Fleckenstein, B., Neipel, F., Peters, G., and Jones, N. (1997). Herpes viral cyclin/Cdk6 complexes evade inhibition by CDK inhibitor proteins. *Nature 390*, 184–187.

Szomolanyi, E., Medveczky, P., and Mulder, C. (1987). In vitro immortalization of marmoset cells with three subgroups of herpesvirus saimiri. *J. Virol. 61*, 3485–3490.

Takahashi, K., Segal, E., Kondo, T., Mukai, T., Moriyama, M., Takahashi, M., and Yamanishi, K. (1992). Interferon and natural killer cell activity in patients with exanthem subitum. *Pediatr. Infect. Dis. J. 11*, 369–373.

Takahashi, K., Sonoda, S., Higashi, K., Kondo, T., Takahashi, H., Takahashi, M., and Yamanishi, K. (1989). Predominant CD4 T-lymphocyte tropism of human herpesvirus 6–related virus. *J. Virol. 63*, 3161–3163.

Talbot, S.J., Weiss, R.A., Kellam, P., and Boshoff, C. (1999). Transcriptional analysis of human herpesvirus-8 open reading frames 71, 72, 73, K14, and 74 in a primary effusion lymphoma cell line. *Virology 257*, 84–94.

Tanaka, K., Kondo, T., Torigoe, S., Okada, S., Mukai, T., and Yamanishi, K. (1994). Human herpesvirus 7: another causal agent for roseola (exanthem subitum). *J Pediatr. 125*, 1–5.

Tanaka–Taya, K., Kondo, T., Mukai, T., Miyoshi, H., Yamamoto, Y., Okada, S., and Yamanishi, K. (1996). Seroepidemiological study of human herpesvirus-6 and -7 in children of different ages and detection of these two viruses in throat swabs by polymerase chain reaction. *J. Med. Virol. 48*, 88–94.

Tanaka-Taya, K., Kondo, T., Nakagawa, N., Inagi, R., Miyoshi, H., Sunagawa, T., Okada, S., and Yamanishi, K. (2000). Reactivation of human herpesvirus 6 by infection of human herpesvirus 7. *J. Med. Virol. 60*, 284–289.

Tanaka-Taya, K., Sashihara, J., Kurahashi, H., Amo, K., Miyagawa, H., Kondo, K., Okada, S., and Yamanishi, K. (2004). Human herpesvirus 6 (HHV-6) is transmitted from parent to child in an integrated form and characterization of cases with chromosomally integrated HHV-6 DNA. *J. Med. Virol. 73*, 465–473.

Tarp, B., Jensen-Fangel, S., Dahl, R., and Obel, N. (2001). Herpesvirus type 1-8 in BAL fluid from HIV-1-infected patients with suspected pneumonia and from healthy individuals. *Eur. Respir. J. 18*, 146–150.

Tarte, K., Chang, Y., and Klein, B. (1999). Kaposi's sarcoma-associated herpesvirus and multiple myeloma: lack of criteria for causality. *Blood 93*, 3159–3163.

Taylor, M.M., Chohan, B., Lavreys, L., Hassan, W., Huang, M.L., Corey, L., Ashley, M.R., Richardson, B.A., Mandaliya, K., Ndinya-Achola, J., Bwayo, J., and Kreiss, J. (2004). Shedding of human herpesvirus 8 in oral and genital secretions from HIV-1-seropositive and –seronegative Kenyan women. *J. Infect. Dis. 190*, 484–488.

Tedeschi, R., Caggiari, L., Silins, I., Kallings, I., Andersson-Ellstrom, A., De Paoli, P., and Dillner, J. (2000). Seropositivity to human herpesvirus 8 in relation to sexual history and risk of sexually transmitted infections among women. *Int. J. Cancer 87*, 232–235.

Thomas, J.A., Brookes, L.A., McGowan, I., Weller, I., and Crawford, D.H. (1996). HHV8 DNA in normal gastrointestinal mucosa from HIV seropositive people. *Lancet 347*, 1337–1338.

Thome, M., Schneider, P., Hofmann, K., Fickenscher, H., Meinl, E., Neipel, F., Mattmann, C., Burns, K., Bodmer, J.L., Schroter, M., Scaffidi, C., Krammer, P.H., Peter, M.E., and Tschopp, J. (1997). Viral FLICE-inhibitory proteins (FLIPs) prevent apoptosis induced by death receptors. *Nature 386*, 517–521.

Thompson, M.P. and Kurzrock, R. (2004). Epstein-Barr virus and cancer. *Clin Cancer Res 10*, 803–821.

Tibbetts, S.A., McClellan, J.S., Gangappa, S., Speck, S.H., and Virgin, H.W.t. (2003). Effective vaccination against long-term gammaherpesvirus latency. *J. Virol. 77*, 2522–2529.

Tibbetts, S.A., van Dyk, L.F., Speck, S.H., and Virgin, H.W.t. (2002). Immune control of the number and reactivation phenotype of cells latently infected with a gammaherpesvirus. *J. Virol. 76*, 7125–7132.

Tokimasa, S., Hara, J., Osugi, Y., Ohta, H., Matsuda, Y., Fujisaki, H., Sawada, A., Kim, J.Y., Sashihara, J., Amou, K., Miyagawa, H., Tanaka-Taya, K., Yamanishi, K., and Okada, S. (2002). Ganciclovir is effective for prophylaxis and treatment of human herpesvirus-6 in allogeneic stem cell transplantation. *Bone Marrow Transplant. 29*, 595–598.

Tong, C.Y., Bakran, A., Williams, H., Cheung, C.Y., and Peiris, J.S. (2000). Association of human herpesvirus 7 with cytomegalovirus disease in renal transplant recipients. *Transplantation 70*, 213–216.

Toomey, N.L., Deyev, V.V., Wood, C., Boise, L.H., Scott, D., Liu, L.H., Cabral, L., Podack, E.R., Barber, G.N., and Harrington, W.J., Jr. (2001). Induction of a TRAIL-mediated suicide program by interferon alpha in primary effusion lymphoma. *Oncogene 20*, 7029–7040.

Torelli, G., Barozzi, P., Marasca, R., Cocconcelli, P., Merelli, E., Ceccherini-Nelli, L., Ferrari, S., and Luppi, M. (1995). Targeted integration of human herpesvirus 6 in the p arm of chromosome 17 of human peripheral blood mononuclear cells in vivo. *J. Med. Virol. 46*, 178–188.

Torigoe, S., Kumamoto, T., Koide, W., Taya, K., and Yamanishi, K. (1995). Clinical manifestations associated with human herpesvirus 7 infection. *Arch. Dis. Child 72*, 518–519.

Torrisi, M.R., Gentile, M., Cardinali, G., Cirone, M., Zompetta, C., Lotti, L.V., Frati, L., and Faggioni, A. (1999). Intracellular transport and maturation pathway of human herpesvirus 6. *Virology 257*, 460–471.

Trovato, R., Luppi, M., Barozzi, P., Da Prato, L., Maiorana, A., Lico, S., Marasca, R., Torricelli, P., Torelli, G., and Ceccherini-Nelli, L. (1999). Cellular localization of human herpesvirus 8 in non-neoplastic lymphadenopathies and chronic interstitial pneumonitis by in situ polymerase chain reaction studies. *J. Hum. Virol. 2*, 38–44.

Tsygankov, A.Y. (2004). Cell transformation by Herpesvirus saimiri. *J. Cell. Physiol. 203*, 305–318.

Usherwood, E.J., Stewart, J.P., Robertson, K., Allen, D.J., and Nash, A.A. (1996). Absence of splenic latency in murine gammaherpesvirus 68-infected B cell-deficient mice. *J. Gen. Virol. 77*, 2819–2825.

van Dyk, L.F., Hess, J.L., Katz, J.D., Jacoby, M., Speck, S.H., and Virgin, H.I. (1999). The murine gammaherpesvirus 68 v-cyclin gene is an oncogene that promotes cell cycle progression in primary lymphocytes. *J. Virol. 73*, 5110–5122.

van Dyk, L.F., Virgin, H.W.t., and Speck, S.H. (2000). The murine gammaherpesvirus 68 v-cyclin is a critical regulator of reactivation from latency. *J. Virol. 74*, 7451–7461.

van Dyk, L.F., Virgin, H.W.t., and Speck, S.H. (2003). Maintenance of gammaherpesvirus latency requires viral cyclin in the absence of B lymphocytes. *J. Virol. 77*, 5118–5126.

Varnell, E.D., Kaufman, H.E., Hill, J.M., and Thompson, H.W. (1995). Cold stress–induced recurrences of herpetic keratitis in the squirrel monkey. *Invest. Ophthalmol. Vis. Sci. 36*, 1181–1183.

Verschuren, E.W., Hodgson, J.G., Gray, J.W., Kogan, S., Jones, N., and Evan, G.I. (2004). The role of p53 in suppression of KSHV cyclin-induced lymphomagenesis. *Cancer Res. 64*, 581–589.

Verzijl, D., Fitzsimons, C.P., Van Dijk, M., Stewart, J.P., Timmerman, H., Smit, M.J., and Leurs, R. (2004). Differential activation of murine herpesvirus 68- and Kaposi's sarcoma-associated herpesvirus-encoded ORF74 G protein-coupled receptors by human and murine chemokines. *J. Virol. 78*, 3343–3351.

Vieira, J., Huang, M.L., Koelle, D.M., and Corey, L. (1997). Transmissible Kaposi's sarcoma–associated herpesvirus (human herpesvirus 8) in saliva of men with a history of Kaposi's sarcoma. *J. Virol. 71*, 7083–7087.

Vieira, J., O'Hearn, P., Kimball, L., Chandran, B., and Corey, L. (2001). Activation of Kaposi's sarcoma–associated herpesvirus (human herpesvirus 8) lytic replication by human cytomegalovirus. *J. Virol. 75*, 1378–1386.

Vieira, J. and O'Hearn, P.M. (2004). Use of the red fluorescent protein as a marker of Kaposi's sarcoma-associated herpesvirus lytic gene expression. *Virology 325*, 225–240.

Virgin, H.W.t., Presti, R.M., Li, X.Y., Liu, C., and Speck, S.H. (1999). Three distinct regions of the murine gammaherpesvirus 68 genome are transcriptionally active in latently infected mice. *J. Virol. 73*, 2321–2332.

Vitale, F., Viviano, E., Perna, A.M., Bonura, F., Mazzola, G., Ajello, F., and Romano, N. (2000). Serological and virological evidence of non-sexual transmission of human herpesvirus type 8 (HHV8). *Epidemiol. Infect. 125*, 671–675.

Wakeling, M.N., Roy, D.J., Nash, A.A., and Stewart, J.P. (2001). Characterization of the murine gammaherpesvirus 68 ORF74 product: a novel oncogenic G protein-coupled receptor. *J. Gen. Virol. 82*, 1187–1197.

Wang, F.Z., Dahl, H., Linde, A., Brytting, M., Ehrnst, A., and Ljungman, P. (1996). Lymphotropic herpesviruses in allogeneic bone marrow transplantation. *Blood 88*, 3615–3620.

Wang, F.Z., Dahl, H., Ljungman, P., and Linde, A. (1999a). Lymphoproliferative responses to human herpesvirus–6 variant A and variant B in healthy adults. *J. Med. Virol. 57*, 134–139.

Wang, F.Z., Akula, S.M., Pramod, N.P., Zeng, L., and Chandran, B. (2001a). Human herpesvirus 8 envelope glycoprotein K8.1A interaction with the target cells involves heparan sulfate. *J. Virol. 75*, 7517–7527.

Wang, G.H., Garvey, T.L., and Cohen, J.I. (1999b). The murine gammaherpesvirus-68 M11 protein inhibits Fas- and TNF-induced apoptosis. *J. Gen. Virol. 80*, 2737–2740.

Wang, G.Q., Xu, H., Wang, Y.K., Gao, X.H., Zhao, Y., He, C., Inoue, N., and Chen, H.D. (2005a). Higher prevalence of human herpesvirus 8 DNA sequence and specific IgG antibodies in patients with pemphigus in China. *J. Am. Acad. Dermatol. 52*, 460–467.

Wang, H.W., Sharp, T.V., Koumi, A., Koentges, G., and Boshoff, C. (2002). Characterization of an anti-apoptotic glycoprotein encoded by Kaposi's sarcoma-associated herpesvirus which resembles a spliced variant of human survivin. *EMBO J. 21*, 2602–2615.

Wang, S., Liu, S., Wu, M.H., Geng, Y., and Wood, C. (2001b). Identification of a cellular protein that interacts and synergizes with the RTA (ORF50) protein of Kaposi's sarcoma–associated herpesvirus in transcriptional activation. *J. Virol. 75*, 11961–11973.

Wang, X., Connors, R., Harris, M.R., Hansen, T.H., and Lybarger, L. (2005b). Requirements for the selective degradation of endoplasmic reticulum-resident major histocompatibility complex class I proteins by the viral immune evasion molecule mK3. *J. Virol. 79*, 4099–4108.

Wang, X., Lybarger, L., Connors, R., Harris, M.R., and Hansen, T.H. (2004). Model for the interaction of gammaherpesvirus 68 RING-CH finger protein mK3 with major histocompatibility complex class I and the peptide-loading complex. *J. Virol. 78*, 8673–8686.

Wang, X.P., Zhang, Y.J., Deng, J.H., Pan, H.Y., Zhou, F.C., Montalvo, E.A., and Gao, S.J. (2001c). Characterization of the promoter region of the viral interferon regulatory factor encoded by Kaposi's sarcoma-associated herpesvirus. *Oncogene 20*, 523–530.

Watanabe, T., Kawamura, T., Jacob, S.E., Aquilino, E.A., Orenstein, J.M., Black, J.B., and Blauvelt, A. (2002). Pityriasis rosea is associated with systemic active infection with both human herpesvirus-7 and human herpesvirus-6. *J. Invest. Dermatol. 119*, 793–797.

Watanabe, T., Sugaya, M., Atkins, A.M., Aquilino, E.A., Yang, A., Borris, D.L., Brady, J., and Blauvelt, A. (2003). Kaposi's sarcoma-associated herpesvirus latency-associated nuclear antigen prolongs the life span of primary human umbilical vein endothelial cells. *J. Virol. 77*, 6188–6196.

Wawer, M.J., Eng, S.M., Serwadda, D., Sewankambo, N.K., Kiwanuka, N., Li, C., and Gray, R.H. (2001). Prevalence of Kaposi sarcoma-associated herpesvirus compared with selected sexually transmitted diseases in adolescents and young adults in rural Rakai District, Uganda. *Sex Transm. Dis. 28*, 77–81.

Weber, F., Kochs, G., and Haller, O. (2004). Inverse interference: how viruses fight the interferon system. *Viral Immunol. 17*, 498–515.

Weck, K.E., Dal Canto, A.J., Gould, J.D., O'Guin, A.K., Roth, K.A., Saffitz, J.E., Speck, S.H., and Virgin, H.W. (1997). Murine gamma-herpesvirus 68 causes severe large-vessel arteritis in mice lacking interferon-gamma responsiveness: a new model for virus-induced vascular disease. *Nat Med 3*, 1346–1353.

Wehner, L.E., Schroder, N., Kamino, K., Friedrich, U., Biesinger, B., and Ruther, U. (2001). Herpesvirus saimiri Tip gene causes T-cell lymphomas in transgenic mice. *DNA Cell Biol 20*, 81–88.

Whitby, D., Howard, M.R., Tenant-Flowers, M., Brink, N.S., Copas, A., Boshoff, C., Hatzioannou, T., Suggett, F.E., Aldam, D.M., and Denton, A.S. (1995). Detection of Kaposi sarcoma associated herpesvirus in peripheral blood of HIV-infected individuals and progression to Kaposi's sarcoma. *Lancet 346*, 799–802.

Whitby, D., Luppi, M., Barozzi, P., Boshoff, C., Weiss, R.A., and Torelli, G. (1998). Human herpesvirus 8 seroprevalence in blood donors and lymphoma patients from different regions of Italy. *J. Natl. Cancer Inst. 90*, 395–397.

Whitby, D., Luppi, M., Sabin, C., Barozzi, P., Di Biase, A.R., Balli, F., Cucci, F., Weiss, R.A., Boshoff, C., and Torelli, G. (2000). Detection of antibodies to human herpesvirus 8 in Italian children: evidence for horizontal transmission. *Br. J. Cancer 82*, 702–704.

Willer, D.O. and Speck, S.H. (2003). Long-term latent murine Gammaherpesvirus 68 infection is preferentially found within the surface immunoglobulin D-negative subset of splenic B cells in vivo. *J. Virol. 77*, 8310–8321.

Wu, T.T., Tong, L., Rickabaugh, T., Speck, S., and Sun, R. (2001). Function of Rta is essential for lytic replication of murine gammaherpesvirus 68. *J. Virol. 75*, 9262–9273.

Wu, T.T., Usherwood, E.J., Stewart, J.P., Nash, A.A., and Sun, R. (2000). Rta of murine gammaherpesvirus 68 reactivates the complete lytic cycle from latency. *J. Virol. 74*, 3659–3667.

Wu, W., Rochford, R., Toomey, L., Harrington, W., Jr., and Feuer, G. (2005). Inhibition of HHV–8/KSHV infected primary effusion lymphomas in NOD/SCID mice by azidothymidine and interferon-alpha. *Leuk Res 29*, 545–55.

Wyatt, L.S., Rodriguez, W.J., Balachandran, N., and Frenkel, N. (1991). Human herpesvirus 7: antigenic properties and prevalence in children and adults. *J. Virol. 65*, 6260–6265.

Xu, Y., AuCoin, D.P., Huete, A.R., Cei, S.A., Hanson, L.J., and Pari, G.S. (2005). A Kaposi's sarcoma-associated herpesvirus/human herpesvirus 8 ORF50 deletion mutant is defective for reactivation of latent virus and DNA replication. *J. Virol. 79*, 3479–3487.

Yalcin, S., Karpuzoglu, T., Suleymanlar, G., Mutlu, G., Mukai, T., Yamamoto, T., Isegawa, Y., and Yamanishi, K. (1994). Human herpesvirus 6 and human herpesvirus 7 infections in renal transplant recipients and healthy adults in Turkey. *Arch. Virol. 136*, 183–190.

Yalcin, S., Mukai, T., Kondo, K., Ami, Y., Okawa, T., Kojima, A., Kurata, T., and Yamanishi, K. (1992). Experimental infection of cynomolgus and African green monkeys with human herpesvirus 6. *J. Gen. Virol. 73*, 1673–1677.

Yamanishi, K., Okuno, T., Shiraki, K., Takahashi, M., Kondo, T., Asano, Y., and Kurata, T. (1988). Identification of human herpesvirus-6 as a causal agent for exanthem subitum. *Lancet 1*, 1065–1067.

Yang, T.Y., Chen, S.C., Leach, M.W., Manfra, D., Homey, B., Wiekowski, M., Sullivan, L., Jenh, C.H., Narula, S.K., Chensue, S.W., and Lira, S.A. (2000). Transgenic expression of the chemokine receptor encoded by human herpesvirus 8 induces an angioproliferative disease resembling Kaposi's sarcoma. *J. Exp. Med 191*, 445–454.

Yasukawa, M., Hasegawa, A., Sakai, I., Ohminami, H., Arai, J., Kaneko, S., Yakushijin, Y., Maeyama, K., Nakashima, H., Arakaki, R., and Fujita, S. (1999a). Down-regulation of CXCR4 by human herpesvirus 6 (HHV-6) and HHV-7. *J. Immunol. 162*, 5417–5422.

Yasukawa, M., Inoue, Y., Ohminami, H., Sada, E., Miyake, K., Tohyama, T., Shimada, T., and Fujita, S. (1997). Human herpesvirus 7 infection of lymphoid and myeloid cell lines transduced with an adenovirus vector containing the CD4 gene. *J. Virol. 71*, 1708–1712.

Yasukawa, M., Ohminami, H., Sada, E., Yakushijin, Y., Kaneko, M., Yanagisawa, K., Kohno, H., Bando, S., and Fujita, S. (1999b). Latent infection and reactivation of human herpesvirus 6 in two novel myeloid cell lines. *Blood 93*, 991–999.

Yasukawa, M., Yakushijin, Y., Furukawa, M., and Fujita, S. (1993). Specificity analysis of human CD4+ T-cell clones directed against human herpesvirus 6 (HHV-6), HHV-7, and human cytomegalovirus. *J. Virol. 67*, 6259–6264.

Ye, F.C., Zhou, F.C., Yoo, S.M., Xie, J.P., Browning, P.J., and Gao, S.J. (2004). Disruption of Kaposi's sarcoma-associated herpesvirus latent nuclear antigen leads to abortive episome persistence. *J. Virol. 78*, 11121–11129.

Yen-Moore, A., Hudnall, S.D., Rady, P.L., Wagner, R.F., Jr., Moore, T.O., Memar, O., Hughes, T.K., and Tyring, S.K. (2000). Differential expression of the HHV-8 vGCR cellular homolog gene in AIDS-associated and classic Kaposi's sarcoma: potential role of HIV-1 Tat. *Virology 267*, 247–51.

Yoshida, H., Matsunaga, K., Ueda, T., Yasumi, M., Ishikawa, J., Tomiyama, Y., and Matsuzawa, Y. (2002). Human herpesvirus 6 meningoencephalitis successfully treated with ganciclovir in a patient who underwent allogeneic bone marrow transplantation from an HLA-identical sibling. *Int. J. Hematol. 75*, 421–425.

Yoshida, M., Yamada, M., Tsukazaki, T., Chatterjee, S., Lakeman, F.D., Nii, S., and Whitley, R.J. (1998). Comparison of antiviral compounds against human herpesvirus 6 and 7. *Antiviral Res. 40*, 73–84.

Yoshikawa, T., Asano, Y., Ihira, M., Suzuki, K., Ohashi, M., Suga, S., Kudo, K., Horibe, K., Kojima, S., Kato, K., Matsuyama, T., and Nishiyama, Y. (2002). Human herpesvirus 6 viremia in bone marrow transplant recipients: clinical features and risk factors. *J. Infect. Dis. 185*, 847–853.

Yoshikawa, T., Ihira, M., Suzuki, K., Suga, S., Asano, Y., Asonuma, K., Tanaka, K., and Nishiyama, Y. (2001). Primary human herpesvirus 6 infection in liver transplant recipients. *J. Pediatr. 138*, 921–925.

Yoshikawa, T., Ihira, M., Suzuki, K., Suga, S., Iida, K., Saito, Y., Asonuma, K., Tanaka, K., and Asano, Y. (2000). Human herpesvirus 6 infection after living related liver transplantation. *J. Med. Virol. 62*, 52–59.

Yoshikawa, T., Suga, S., Asano, Y., Nakashima, T., Yazaki, T., Ono, Y., Fujita, T., Tsuzuki, K., Sugiyama, S., and Oshima, S. (1992). A prospective study of human herpesvirus-6 infection in renal transplantation. *Transplantation 54*, 879–883.

Yoshikawa, T., Suga, S., Asano, Y., Yazaki, T., Kodama, H., and Ozaki, T. (1989). Distribution of antibodies to a causative agent of exanthem subitum (human herpesvirus-6) in healthy individuals. *Pediatrics 84*, 675–677.

Yoshikawa, T., Yoshida, J., Hamaguchi, M., Kubota, T., Akimoto, S., Ihira, M., Nishiyama, Y., and Asano, Y. (2003). Human herpesvirus 7-associated meningitis and optic neuritis in a patient after allogeneic stem cell transplantation. *J. Med. Virol. 70*, 440–443.

Yu, Y., Wang, S.E., and Hayward, G.S. (2005). The KSHV immediate-early transcription factor RTA encodes ubiquitin E3 ligase activity that targets IRF7 for proteosome-mediated degradation. *Immunity 22*, 59–70.

Zerr, D.M., Corey, L., Kim, H.W., Huang, M.L., Nguy, L., and Boeckh, M. (2005a). Clinical outcomes of human herpesvirus 6 reactivation after hematopoietic stem cell transplantation. *Clin. Infect. Dis. 40*, 932–940.

Zerr, D.M., Gooley, T.A., Yeung, L., Huang, M.L., Carpenter, P., Wade, J.C., Corey, L., and Anasetti, C. (2001). Human herpesvirus 6 reactivation and encephalitis in allogeneic bone marrow transplant recipients. *Clin. Infect. Dis. 33*, 763–771.

Zerr, D.M., Gupta, D., Huang, M.L., Carter, R., and Corey, L. (2002). Effect of antivirals on human herpesvirus 6 replication in hematopoietic stem cell transplant recipients. *Clin. Infect. Dis. 34*, 309–317.

Zerr, D.M., Meier, A.S., Selke, S.S., Frenkel, L.M., Huang, M.L., Wald, A., Rhoads, M.P., Nguy, L., Bornemann, R., Morrow, R.A., and Corey, L. (2005b). A population-based study of primary human herpesvirus 6 infection. *N. Engl. J Med. 352*, 768–776.

Zhang, Y., Hatse, S., De Clercq, E., and Schols, D. (2000). CXC-chemokine receptor 4 is not a coreceptor for human herpesvirus 7 entry into CD4(+) T cells. *J. Virol. 74*, 2011–2016.

Zhu, F.X., King, S.M., Smith, E.J., Levy, D.E., and Yuan, Y. (2002). A Kaposi's sarcoma-associated herpesviral protein inhibits virus-mediated induction of type I interferon by blocking IRF-7 phosphorylation and nuclear accumulation. *Proc. Natl. Acad. Sci. U. S. A. 99*, 5573–5578.

Ziegler, J.L. (1993). Endemic Kaposi's sarcoma in Africa and local volcanic soils. *Lancet 342*, 1348–1351.

Ziegler, J.L. and Katongole-Mbidde, E. (1996). Kaposi's sarcoma in childhood: an analysis of 100 cases from Uganda and relationship to HIV infection. *Int. J. Cancer 65*, 200–203.

Zimring, J.C., Goodbourn, S., and Offermann, M.K. (1998). Human herpesvirus 8 encodes an interferon regulatory factor (IRF) homolog that represses IRF-1-mediated transcription. *J. Virol. 72*, 701–707.

Zong, J., Ciufo, D.M., Viscidi, R., Alagiozoglou, L., Tyring, S., Rady, P., Orenstein, J., Boto, W., Kalumbuja, H., Romano, N., Melbye, M., Kang, G.H., Boshoff, C., and Hayward, G.S. (2002).

Genotypic analysis at multiple loci across Kaposi's sarcoma herpesvirus (KSHV) DNA molecules: clustering patterns, novel variants and chimerism. *J. Clin. Virol.* *23*, 119–148.

Zong, J.C., Ciufo, D.M., Alcendor, D.J., Wan, X., Nicholas, J., Browning, P.J., Rady, P.L., Tyring, S.K., Orenstein, J.M., Rabkin, C.S., Su, I.J., Powell, K.F., Croxson, M., Foreman, K.E., Nickoloff, B.J., Alkan, S., and Hayward, G.S. (1999). High-level variability in the ORF-K1 membrane protein gene at the left end of the Kaposi's sarcoma-associated herpesvirus genome defines four major virus subtypes and multiple variants or clades in different human populations. *J. Virol.* *73*, 4156–4170.

Zong, J.C., Metroka, C., Reitz, M.S., Nicholas, J., and Hayward, G.S. (1997). Strain variability among Kaposi sarcoma-associated herpesvirus (human herpesvirus 8) genomes: evidence that a large cohort of United States AIDS patients may have been infected by a single common isolate. *J. Virol.* *71*, 2505–2511.

Zou, P., Isegawa, Y., Nakano, K., Haque, M., Horiguchi, Y., and Yamanishi, K. (1999). Human herpesvirus 6 open reading frame U83 encodes a functional chemokine. *J. Virol.* *73*, 5926–5933.

Section III: Emerging Viruses in Asia

7. Nipah and Hendra Viruses Encephalitis

KHEAN JIN GOH, KUM THONG WONG, AND CHONG TIN TAN

7.1. Introduction

Nipah and Hendra viruses are two new zoonotic viruses that have emerged during the past decade (Murray et al., 1995b; Chua et al., 2000a). Both are members of the Paramyxoviridae family, and they share similar antigenic, serologic, as well as ultrastructural characteristics. Molecular studies have also shown that they are closely related in terms of their nucleotide and amino acid sequences (Harcourt et al., 2000). Because of their homology and the fact that these two viruses differ much more from other members of the Paramyxoviridae family, a new genus called *Henipavirus* (*He*ndra + *Nipa*h) was created for these two viruses (Wang et al., 2000, 2001; Bossart et al., 2002).

Hendra virus first appeared in 1994 when it caused a disease affecting horses, which subsequently involved three human cases in Queensland, Australia. Between 1998 and 1999, Nipah virus resulted in widespread infection of pigs and humans in Malaysia and, to a lesser extent, Singapore (Murray et al., 1995a; Selvey et al., 1995; Chua et al., 1999). Between 2001 and 2004, several further outbreaks of Nipah virus have also occurred in Bangladesh (Hsu et al., 2004; ICCDR, B, 2004; Quddus et al., 2004; WHO, 2004).

7.2. Hendra Virus Infection

In August–September 1994, an outbreak of an acute respiratory illness among horses occurred in Australia, in which 13 of 20 affected horses died (Murray et al., 1995a, 1995b). The infection affected two humans, a horse trainer and a stablehand, who suffered from acute respiratory disease, from which the horse trainer died despite hospitalization (Selvey et al., 1995). The stablehand recovered subsequently. A new virus was isolated from tissues of infected horses and was named Hendra virus after the Brisbane, Queensland, suburb where the original outbreak occurred. A second human death occurred in October 1995, when a farmer from Mackay, about 1000 km north of Brisbane, died from a neurological illness (O'Sullivan et al., 1997). He had had close contact with two ill horses about a year earlier and had become ill with mild meningoencephalitis but recovered. After being asymptomatic for more than a year, he developed seizures, coma, and died. He tested seropositive for Hendra virus, and retrospective tests on tissues from the Mackay horses revealed the presence of Hendra virus. In January 1999, an isolated equine death occurred in Cairns, north Queensland, with no evidence of further infection (Barclay and Paton, 2000).

7.2.1. Epidemiology

The outbreak of Hendra virus infection primarily occurred among horses. Human infection occurred in individuals who had had close personal contact with infected horses, for example, nursed ill horses (Murray et al., 1995a, 1995b; Selvey et al., 1995; O'Sullivan et al., 1997). Noninfected individuals associated with the outbreak premises were serologically negative, and no human-to-human transmission has been reported (Selvey et al., 1995). Hendra virus was isolated from the oral cavity and urine of infected horses as well as in the urine of experimentally infected cats and guinea pigs (Williamson et al., 1998). Horses could be infected experimentally through infected urine contaminating their feed.

The natural reservoir for the Hendra virus is likely to be fruit bats of the *Pteropus* species, also known as flying foxes, although the bats remain asymptomatic. Neutralizing antibodies for Hendra virus have been demonstrated in all four species of *Pteropus* in Australia, and the virus has been isolated from fetal tissue and uterine fluid of these bats (Young et al., 1996; Halpin et al., 2000). However, there was no serological evidence of infection in persons with close and prolonged contact with bats (Selvey et al., 1996). The mechanism by which the virus could have spread to horses is unknown, although it has been noted that the outbreaks occurred during the breeding season of the fruit bats. The isolation of the virus from fetal tissues and fluid suggests that contact with aborted fetuses and products of the birthing process could be a possible mechanism of transmission (Halpin et al., 2000).

7.2.2. Clinical Features

Infected horses developed an acute febrile respiratory illness. Human infection resulted in an acute influenza-like illness with marked respiratory symptoms, fever, and myalgia in the Hendra cases (Selvey et al., 1995). One of the two patients (the horse trainer) died despite intensive care treatment after a week of illness, whereas the other patient (the stablehand) recovered over a 6-week period.

On the other hand, the patient from Mackay presented primarily with neurological symptoms with an unusual temporal pattern (O'Sullivan et al., 1997). A history of exposure was followed by a mild meningoencephalitic illness from which he recovered. He then remained asymptomatic for about 13 months before developing a severe encephalitic illness and died. The patient presented with irritability followed by focal seizures. He then developed a right hemiplegia and became comatose. He died after 25 days without recovering consciousness.

7.2.3. Diagnosis

Serological diagnosis of Hendra virus infection has been carried out by demonstrating antibodies using enzyme-linked immunosorbent assay (ELISA) or serum neutralization tests. Viral isolation was initially carried out from postmortem tissues, but as the virus has been classified as a biohazard level 4 pathogen, this cannot be readily done except in appropriate facilities.

MRI brain imaging of the patient with neurological illness revealed distinctive focal high signal cortical changes on T2-weighted sequences, and the electroencephalogram (EEG) showed persistent periodic epileptiform discharges (O'Sullivan et al., 1997). His cerebrospinal fluid examination showed increased leukocytes with a predominance of lymphocytes, raised protein, but normal glucose levels.

7.2.4. Pathology

Postmortem studies showed severe interstitial pneumonia in the first patient with respiratory illness (Selvey, et al., 1995). On the other hand, in the second fatal human case, the main abnormalities were in the brain, and findings were focal necrosis in the cortex, basal ganglia, brain stem, and cerebellum. Multinucleated endothelial cells were seen in several organs (O'Sullivan et al., 1997). Immunohistochemistry indicated the presence of viral antigens in the neuronal cytoplasm as well as the neuropil (felt work of interwoven cytoplasmic process of nerve cells in gray matter).

7.3. Nipah Virus Infection

Between September 1998 and June 1999, there was an outbreak of acute viral encephalitis in several pig-farming villages in Peninsular

Malaysia. (CDC, 1999a, 1999b; Chua et al., 1999; Goh et al., 2000). The outbreak started near Ipoh, in the northern state of Perak, but subsequently spread to involve villages 300 km to the south in Negeri Sembilan in the Sikamat and Bukit Pelanduk districts, including Sungai Nipah village, where patients, whose specimens yielded the first viral isolates, lived (Chua et al., 2000a). Overall, more than 265 patients were affected in Malaysia with more than 105 deaths (Parashar et al., 2000). Several abattoir workers in Singapore, which imports pigs from Malaysia, were also affected (Chew et al., 2000; Lee et al., 1999; Paton et al., 1999). The outbreak ended with the mass culling of pigs in the affected areas.

More recently, several outbreaks of acute Nipah encephalitis occurred in Bangladesh: in the Meherpur and the Naogaon districts in 2001 and 2003 (Hsu et al., 2004) and in the Rajbari, Faridpur, Golpagonj, Manikgonj, Joypurat, and Naogoan districts in January 2004 and the Faridpur district in April 2004 (ICCDR, B, 2004; Quddus et al., 2004; WHO, 2004). Unlike the earlier Malaysian outbreak of Nipah virus infection, no significant diseases among animals were noted, and exactly how the infection was transmitted to humans is uncertain.

7.3.1. Epidemiology

In the Nipah outbreak in Malaysia, direct contact with infected pigs, their secretions, or fresh pig products was responsible for viral transmission to humans. Patients were originally thought to have Japanese encephalitis (JE) because it occurred in pig-farming villages, but distinguishing features included infection predominantly in adults rather than children, clustering of cases in members of the same home with an attack rate much higher than JE, a high proportion of patients in direct contact with pigs as opposed to unaffected individuals living in the same neighbourhood, a history of illness in the pigs belonging to the affected farmers, and the fact that many patients had prior immunization against JE (Chua et al., 1999; Goh et al., 2000). These observations were confirmed by case-control studies showing that patients had activities with more direct contact with pigs. Parashar et al. (2000) found that Nipah-infected patients were more likely than community farm controls (persons from farms without reported Nipah infection) to have ill/dying pigs (59% vs. 24%) and were more likely than case farm controls (persons from infected farms without illness) to have had activities requiring direct contact with pigs (86% vs. 50%). Other affected occupations included abattoir workers, pork sellers, as well as army personnel brought in to cull infected pigs (Tan et al., 1999; Chew et al., 2000; Premalatha et al., 2000; Ali et al., 2001). Exposure to ill animals other than pigs (e.g., dogs) were also reported in a few patients suggesting possible viral transmission from other animals (Tan et al., 1999; Parashar et al., 2000).

The risk of nosocomial transmission of Nipah virus during the Malaysian outbreak was thought to be low. In a study on 338 health care workers exposed to infected patients during the outbreak, three subjects were positive for IgG antibodies on enzyme-linked immunosorbent assay (ELISA) but as their serum anti-Nipah IgM and neutralizing antibodies were negative, they were felt to be false positives (Mounts et al., 2001). However, in an MRI study of asymptomatic seropositive cases, MRI findings in the brain typical of Nipah infection was demonstrated in a nurse who had cared for Nipah-infected patients. She had no exposure to infected animals and is likely a case of human-to-human transmission, probably from exposure to infected patients' secretions (Tan et al., 2000; Tan and Tan, 2001). This is not surprising as the Nipah virus could be isolated from patients' respiratory secretions and urine (Chua et al., 2001a).

On the other hand, in the outbreaks in Bangladesh, no clusters of ill animals were observed (Hsu et al., 2004; WHO, 2004). A variety of animals were tested for antibodies to Nipah antigens but were negative except for bats (*P. giganteus*) (Hsu et al., 2004). Nipah-infected patients were more likely than nonpatients to have close contact with other Nipah-infected patients. The likelihood therefore was that in Bangladesh, the transmission occurred due to close contact with other infected persons.

The primary reservoir for Nipah virus is likely to be the fruit bat, of the species *Pteropus*. In a study of 324 bats from 14 species, serum neutralizing antibodies to Nipah virus were demonstrated in five species, including *P. vampyrus* and *P. hypomelanus,* but attempts to isolate the virus or amplify viral sequences from these bats were negative (Yob et al., 2001). However, the Nipah virus was isolated from the urine of *P. hypomelanus* roosting in fruit trees in Tioman, an island off the east coast of Peninsular Malaysia (Chua et al., 2002). In the search for the natural host for Nipah virus, another new paramyxovirus was discovered in urine of *P. hypomelanus* as well: Tioman virus (Chua et al., 2001b). The latter virus is as yet not known to cause any human or animal disease. In a serological survey of the inhabitants of Tioman Island, no individual was found to be seropositive for Nipah or Tioman antibodies, suggesting that direct viral transmission from bats to humans does not occur (Chong et al., 2003).

If the fruit bat is the reservoir host, half-eaten fruits could have been ingested by pigs, in which the virus was then amplified and transmitted to human beings. In fact, the virus has been isolated from such fruits (Chua et al., 2002). In the case of the Bangladesh outbreaks, the exact mechanism of the spread of virus to humans is unknown, although direct contact with bat secretions is a possibility (Hsu et al., 2004; WHO et al., 2004).

Subsequent person-to-person spread may have occurred as evidenced by clustering of cases in certain households (ICCDR, B, 2004).

7.3.2. Clinical Features

Nipah virus primarily caused an encephalitic illness both in the Malaysia/Singapore and the Bangladesh outbreaks. The incubation period ranged from a few days to 2 weeks (Chong et al., 2000; Goh et al., 2000). Most persons who were exposed to the virus became symptomatic, with the ratio of symptomatic versus asymptomatic (subclinical) infection assessed to be 3:1 (Tan et al., 1999).

The main clinical features were fever, headache, dizziness, vomiting, seizures, and reduced level of consciousness (Chong et al., 2000; Goh et al., 2000). In fact, more than 50% of patients with acute Nipah encephalitis had a reduced level of consciousness during the acute infection. This together with the presence of abnormal pupillary reflexes, absent doll's-eye reflex, a profound tachycardia and hypertension (suggesting involvement of the medullary vasomotor center) in many seriously ill patients suggested involvement of the brain stem (Goh et al., 2000). Persistent segmental myoclonus characterized by focal rhythmic jerking of muscles, occurring in about one-third to one-half of patients, was a distinctive feature, and the involvement especially of the diaphragm as well as the head and neck muscles suggested brain stem and/or upper cervical involvement. Another distinctive feature was hypotonia and areflexia, seen in about one-half of the patients. This was believed to be due to spinal root involvement secondary to meningeal inflammation (Chew et al., 2000). Other clinical features included seizures, nystagmus, cerebellar ataxia, tremor, dysarthria, and dysphasia.

Pneumonia was reported in 3 of the 11 patients from Singapore with abnormal chest radiograph findings (Paton et al., 1999). However, in Malaysian patients, respiratory tract symptoms (such as cough) were minor and occurred in about 14% in the series from the University of Malaya Medical Centre, Kuala Lumpur (Goh et al., 2000). A small number of patients presented with systemic symptoms, but no evidence for encephalitis both clinically and on cerebrospinal fluid examination, and were considered to have nonencephalitic infection (Goh et al., 2000). Mortality during the acute infection was high and estimated overall to be about 40% (Parashar et al., 2000). Mortality was associated with severe brain stem involvement, the presence of the Nipah virus in the cerebrospinal fluid suggesting high virus replication in the central nervous system and concomitant diabetes mellitus, probably due to immunoparesis (Chua et al., 2000b; Chong et al., 2001b; Goh et al., 2000).

Clinical descriptions of cases from the Bangladesh outbreaks similarly describe an acute febrile illness associated with headache and diminishing consciousness in the majority of patients and seizures (Hsu et al., 2004; ICCDR, B, 2004; Quddus et al., 2004; WHO, 2004). Respiratory symptoms (e.g., cough and dyspnea) also occurred, and chest radiographs in some patients demonstrated bilateral infiltrates consistent with acute respiratory distress syndrome (ARDS) (Hsu et al., 2004; ICCDR, B, 2004; WHO, 2004).

7.3.3. Investigations

In the majority of patients, cerebrospinal fluid (CSF) examination showed features typical of viral encephalitis with raised mononuclear leukocytes, elevated protein, and normal glucose levels. Blood investigation revealed nonspecific thrombocytopenia and leukopenia with raised alanine and aspartate transaminases in up to two-thirds of patients (Chong et al., 2000; Goh et al., 2000).

Diagnosis is confirmed by the detection of IgM and IgG antibodies against Nipah viral antigens in serum and CSF, using an IgM-capture enzyme-linked immunosorbent assay (ELISA) test and an indirect IgG ELISA test. The ELISA tests for Nipah antibodies had a high specificity and are therefore useful screening tests (Daniels et al., 2001). In the Malaysian outbreak, the rate of positive IgM was 60% to 70% by the 4th day and 100% by the 12th day of illness. IgG antibody was 100% positive by the 25th day of illness (Ramasundrum et al., 2000). Prior to the complete characterization of the virus, Nipah virus was suspected to be "Hendra-like" because cells infected with Nipah virus reacted strongly to anti-Hendra antibodies. Nipah and Hendra viruses shared enough epitopes for Hendra viral antigens to be used in the prototype serologic test sensitive enough to detect Nipah virus antigens (CDC, 1999a).

Viral isolation is not routinely carried out as Nipah virus is classified as a biosafety level 4 agent and requires specialized facilities. However, the virus was isolated from CSF, urine, and respiratory secretions of patients during the Malaysian outbreak (Chua et al., 2000b, 2001a). Direct visualization by electron microscopy in negatively stained CSF specimens was found to be useful but unable to differentiate between Nipah and Hendra viruses (Chow et al., 2000). In cell cultures, it was possible to differentiate between the various paramyxoviruses using features such as the types and distribution of nucleocapsid aggregates and viral envelope differences. The presence of single-fringe viral envelope and peripherally distributed, type 1 nucleocapsid is characteristic of Nipah virus (Hyatt et al., 2001).

Brain MRI is a useful diagnostic investigation. Ahmad Sarji et al. (2000) carried out MRI brain scans in 23 patients with Nipah encephalitis, 14 during the acute illness (during the first week) and a further 10 during the later phase of illness (about 54 days after onset) and demonstrated small and discrete high-signal-intensity lesions, measuring 2 to 7 mm in diameter, in the subcortical and deep white matter of the brain. These were best seen in the T2-weighted fluid attenuated inversion recovery (FLAIR) sequences (Fig. 7.1). These lesions were multiple and disseminated without specific predilection to any site in the brain and probably corresponded with the necrotic plaques seen in postmortem tissues (see below). No correlation appeared to exist between MRI findings and clinical focal neurological signs. MRI investigations of asymptomatic seropositive subjects revealed similar changes in about 16%, suggesting that these lesions can occur without any clinical symptoms or signs (Tan et al., 2000).

Electroencephalography (EEG) showed diffuse slow waves with the degree of slowing correlating with the severity of illness. In deeply comatosed patients, bitemporal, independent periodic complexes were seen and were associated with 100% mortality (Chew et al., 1999).

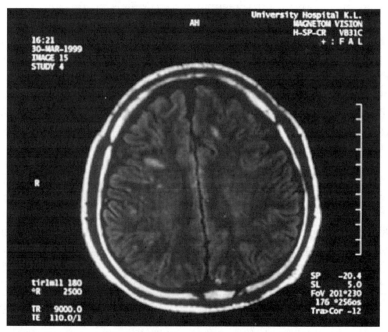

Figure 7.1. T2-weighted fluid attenuated inversion recovery (FLAIR) MRI showing multiple discrete subcortical lesions in a patient with acute Nipah virus encephalitis.

7.3.4. Treatment and Outcome

Treatment is mainly supportive with mechanical ventilatory support for seriously ill patients. Seizures were treated with anticonvulsants. Ribavirin, a broad-spectrum antiviral agent, was tried on an empirical basis in patients in the Malaysian outbreak. Ribavirin was administered orally initially and then intravenously, when available, to those who were unable to take it orally. In a comparison of 140 treated patients with 54 untreated patients serving as historical controls (i.e., those who developed the illness before ribavirin was made available), it was found that fewer treated patients died (32% vs. 54%, p = 0.011), suggesting that ribavirin reduced the mortality of patients (Chong et al., 2001a). However, it was possible that treated patients who were seen later in the outbreak were also given better general medical care than untreated patients seen earlier, as physicians became more experienced in the outbreak.

7.3.5. Relapsed and Late-Onset Encephalitis

Several patients who had recovered from the original encephalitis developed second and occasionally third episodes of neurological dysfunction. These patients constitute about 7.5% of the survivors and re-developed symptoms about 8.4 months after exposure (Tan et al., 2002). In addition, about 3.4% who were either asymptomatic or had mild nonencephalitic illness initially developed a late-onset neurological illness (late-onset encephalitis). Common clinical features in relapsed or late-onset disease were fever, headache, seizures, and focal neurological deficits. Mortality was 18%. MRI brain scan findings in these patients were markedly different from that of acute encephalitis and showed large, patchy, confluent lesions involving the cortex (Ahmad Sarji et al., 2000; Tan et al., 2002) (Fig. 7.2). These clinical and radiological features were strikingly similar to the fatal case of Hendra viral encephalitis (O'Sullivan et al., 1997).

7.3.6. Pathology

Several autopsy examinations were carried out during the Malaysian outbreak. Wong et al. (2002a) reported on the pathological findings. Macroscopically, features were nonspecific, although occasionally, small lesions suggestive of necrosis could be observed. One of the earliest histopathological findings was the formation of multinucleated syncytium in the vascular endothelium. More commonly, vasculitis with endothelial ulceration and varying degrees of inflammation and fibrinoid necrosis and associated with thrombosis were seen (Fig. 7.3).

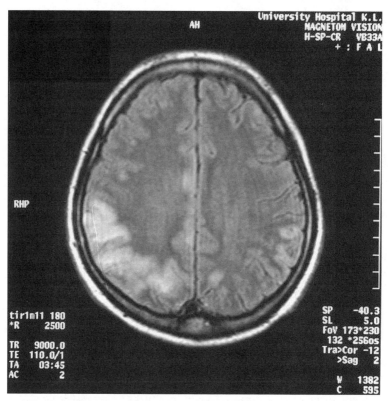

Figure 7.2. T2-weighted FLAIR MRI sequence in a patient with relapsed Nipah encephalitis showing large, patchy, confluent lesions involving the cortex.

Immunohistochemistry demonstrated the presence of viral antigen within
the vascular endothelium. These vascular lesions were most widespread
in the brain affecting the small but sparing the larger blood vessels.
Surrounding these vessels were necrotic plaques believed to be a combination of microinfarction (from thrombosis) and direct viral infection of
surrounding extravascular parenchyma. Some surviving neurons demonstrate cytoplasmic or nuclear inclusions, which were viral inclusions on
immunohistochemistry. Electron microscopy showed that these inclusions were viral nucleocapsids (Hyatt et al., 2001).

Other organs were also involved, and after the central nervous system,
the most severely affected organ was the lung in which there was focal fibrinoid necrosis of the lung parenchyma associated with vasculitis. In addition, there was inflammation associated with multinucleated giant cells in
the alveolar spaces. Again, the presence of viral antigens was confirmed on
immunohistochemistry in these giant cells, blood vessels, and, in one rare
case, in the bronchial epithelium (Wong et al., 2002a).

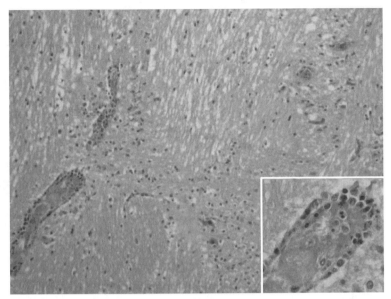

Figure 7.3. Vasculitis-induced thrombosis in two small blood vessels in the pons causing adjacent microinfarction (necrotic plaque) in the upper half of the figure (H&E; magnification, ×10 objective). The inset shows a close-up of the vasculitic vessel with thrombus within its lumen (magnification, ×40 objective).

Pathology of relapse encephalitis was different (Wong et al., 2002a). In the one autopsy case studied, vasculitis, perivascular cuffing, and necrotic plaques were not seen and instead viral inclusions were much more extensive and prominent, occupying the entire neuronal cytoplasm as well as being abundant in the neuropil. This suggested that relapse was due to viral reinfection rather than postinfectious demyelination (Wong et al., 2002a, 2002b).

7.3.7. Pathogenesis

After viral exposure, probably via the respiratory or alimentary tracts, and virus replication at site or sites presently unknown, viremia occurs with systemic spread of the virus, as evidenced by widespread vasculitis (Wong et al., 2002a, 2002b). The endothelium, being susceptible to viral infection, could be a secondary site for viral replication. In the brain, vasculitis would have resulted in a breach in the blood–brain barrier, allowing the spread of the virus into brain parenchyma. The predominatly central nervous system symptoms would have resulted from a combination of cerebral ischemia/microinfarction (from vasculitis and thrombosis) as well as from direct neuronal invasion.

7.4. Conclusion

Hendra and Nipah viruses are but two of the several recently discovered viruses isolated from bats. Others include other paramyxoviruses, viz. Menangle and Tioman viruses, and new members of the genus *Rubulavirus* (Chant et al., 1998; Philbey et al., 1998; Chua et al., 2001b). The former caused stillbirths among piglets and an influenza-like illness and rash in two human workers, whereas the latter has not yet been shown to cause human disease.

The implication of these new viral infections is that the virus can jump the species barrier, infect a naive animal host, and cross over to humans; occasionally at great cost, as can be seen in the Nipah and to a lesser extent the Hendra virus outbreaks. How the virus spreads from bats to the secondary animal hosts is not yet known for certain, and there is also the question of safety of human populations living near bats. Although the surveys in Australia and Malaysia showed no evidence of direct viral transmission from bats to humans (Selvey et al., 1996; Chong et al., 2003), the appearance of Nipah outbreaks in Bangladesh (Hsu et al., 2004; ICCDR, B, 2004; Quddus et al., 2004; WHO, 2004), with no apparent intermediate animal host and possible human-to-human transmission, makes it an all the more important question to answer. Factors that may influence viral transmission (both epidemiological and clinical) also remain to be elucidated.

Development of animal models for these infections will help further the understanding of their pathology and pathogenesis (Wong et al., 2003) as well as the development and testing of vaccines and antiviral therapy.

References

Ahmad Sarji, S., Abdullah, B. J. J., Goh, K. J., Tan, C. T., Wong, K. T. (2000). MR imaging features of Nipah encephalitis. *Am. J. Radiology* 175: 437–442.

Ali, R., Mounts, A. W., Parashar, U. D., Sahani, M., Lye, M. S., Isa, M. M., Balathevan, K., Arif, M. T., and Ksiazek, T. G. (2001). Nipah virus infection among military personnel involved in pig culling during an outbreak of encephalitis in Malaysia, 1998-1999. *Emerg. Infect. Dis.* 7(4): 759–761.

Barclay, A. J., Paton, D. J. (2000). Hendra (Equine Morbillivirus). *Vet. J.* 160: 169–176.

Bossart, K. N., Wang, L. F., Flora, M. N., Chua, K. B., Lam, S. K., Eaton, B. T., and Broder, C. C. (2002). Membrane fusion tropism and heterotypic functional activities of the Nipah virus and Hendra virus envelope glycoproteins. *J. Virol.* 76: 11186–11198.

CDC (1999a). Outbreak of Hendra-like virus—Malaysia and Singapore, 1998-1999. *MMWR Morb. Mortal. Wkly. Rep.* 48: 265.

CDC (1999b). Update: outbreak of Nipah virus—Malaysian and Singapore, 1998-1999. *MMWR Morb. Mortal. Wkly. Rep.* 48: 335.

Chant, K., Chan, R., Smith, M., Dwyer, D. E., Kirkland, P. D., and NSW Expert Group. (1998). Probable human infection with a newly described virus in the family paramyxoviridae. *Emerg. Infect. Dis.* 4: 273–275.

Chew, M. H., Arguin, P. M., Shay, D. K., Goh, K. T., Rollin, P. E., Shieh, W. J., Zaki, S. R., Rota, P. A., Ling, A. E., Ksiazek, T. G., Chew, S. K., and Anderson, L. J. (2000). Risk factors for Nipah virus infection among abattoir workers in Singapore. *J. Infect. Dis.* 181: 1760–1763.

Chew, N. K., Goh, K. J., Tan, C. T., Ahmad Sarji, S., and Wong, K. T. (1999). Electroencephalography in acute Nipah encephalitis. *Neurol. J. Southeast Asia* 4: 45–51.

Chew, N. K., Goh, K. J., and Tan, C. T. (2000). The mechanism of areflexia in patients with Nipah encephalitis. *Neurol. J. Southeast Asia* 5: 29–33.

Chong, H. T., Kunjapan, S. R., Thayaparan, T., Tong, J. M. G., Petharunam, V., Jusoh, M. R., and Tan, C. T. (2000). Nipah encephalitis outbreak in Malaysia: clinical features in patients from Seremban. *Neurol. J. Southeast Asia* 5: 61–67.

Chong, H. T., Kamarulzaman, A., Tan, C. T., Goh, K. J., Thayaparan, T., Kunjapan, S. R., Chew, N. K., Chua, K. B., and Lam, S. K. K. (2001a). Treatment of acute Nipah encephalitis with ribavirin. *Ann. Neurol.* 49: 810–813.

Chong, H. T., Tan, C. T., Goh, K. J., Chew, N. K., Kunjapan, S. R., Petharunam, V., and Thayaparan, T. (2001b). Occupational exposure, age, diabetes mellitus and outcome of acute Nipah encephalitis. *Neurol. J. Southeast Asia* 6: 7–11.

Chong, H. T., Tan, C. T., Goh, K. J., Lam S. K., Chua, K. B. (2003) The risk of human Nipah virus infection directly from bats (*Pteropus hypomelanus*) is low *Neurol. J. Southeast Asia* 8: 31–34.

Chow, V. T., Tambyah, P. A., Yeo, W. M., Phoon, M. C., and Howe, J. (2000). Diagnosis of Nipah virus encephalitis by electron microscopy of cerebrospinal fluid. *J. Clin. Virol.* 19: 143–147.

Chua, K. B., Goh, K. J., Wong, K. T., Kamarulzaman, A., Tan, P. S. K., Ksiazek, T. G., Zaki, S. R., Paul, G., Lam, S. K., Tan C. T. (1999). Fatal encephalitis due to Nipah virus among pig-farmers in Malaysia. *Lancet* 354: 1257–1259.

Chua, K. B., Bellini, W. J., Rota, P. A., Harcourt, B. H., Tamin, A., Lam, S. K. K., Ksiazek, T. G., Rollin, P. E., Zaki, S. R., Shieh, W. J., Goldsmith, C. S., Gubler, D. J., Roehrig, J. T., Eaton, B. T., Gould, A. R., Olson, J., Field, H. E., Daniels, P. W., Ling, A. E., Peters, C. J., Anderson, L. J., and Mahy, B. W. J. (2000a). Nipah virus: a recently emergent deadly paramyxovirus. *Science* 288: 1432–1435.

Chua, K. B., Lam, S. K. K., Tan, C. T., Hooi, P. S., Goh, K. J., Chew, N. K., Tan, K. S., Kamarulzaman, A., and Wong, K. T. (2000b). High mortality in Nipah encephalitis is associated with presence of virus in cerebrospinal fluid. *Ann. Neurol.* 48: 802–805.

Chua, K. B., Lam, S. K. K., Goh, K. J., Hooi, P. S., Ksiazek, T. G., Kamarulzaman, A., Olson, J., and Tan, C. T. (2001a). The presence of Nipah virus in respiratory secretions and urine of patients during an outbreak of Nipah virus encephalitis in Malaysia. *J. Infect.* 42: 40–43.

Chua, K. B., Wang, L. F., Lam, S. K. K., Crameri, G. C., Yu, M., Wise, T., Boyle, D. B., Hyatt, A. D., and Eaton, B. T. (2001b). Tioman virus, a novel paramyxovirus isolated from fruit bats in Malaysia. *Virology* 283: 215–229.

Chua, K. B., Koh, C. L., Hooi, P. S., Wee, K. F., Khong, J. H., Chua, B. H., Chan, Y. P., Lim, M. E., and Lam, S. K. K. (2002). Isolation of Nipah virus from Malaysian Island flying foxes. *Microbes Infect.* 4: 145–151.

Daniels, P. W., Ksiazek, T. G., and Eaton, B. T. (2001). Laboratory diagnosis of Nipah and Hendra virus infections. *Microbes Infect.* 3: 289–295.

Goh, K. J., Tan, C. T., Chew, N. K., Tan, P. S. K., Kamarulzaman, A., Ahmad Sarji, S., Wong, K. T., Abdullah, B. J. J., Chua, K. B., and Lam, S. K. K. (2000). Clinical features of Nipah virus encephalitis among pig farmers in Malaysia. *N. Engl. J. Med.* 342: 1229–1235.

Halpin, K., Young, P. L., Field, H. E., and MacKenzie, J. S. (2000). Isolation of Hendra virus from pteropid bats: a natural reservoir of Hendra virus. *J. Gen. Virol.* 81: 1927–1932.

Harcourt, B. H., Tamin, A., Ksiazek, T. G., Rollin, P. E., Anderson, L. J., Bellini, W. J., and Rota, P. A. (2000). Molecular characterization of Nipah virus, a newly emergent paramyxovirus. *Virology* 271: 334–349.

Hsu, V. P., Hossain, M. J., Parashar, U. D., Ali, M. M., Ksiazek, T. G., Kuzmin, I., Niezgoda, M., Upprecht, C., Bresee, J. and Breiman, R. F. (2004). Nipah virus encephalitis re-emergence, Bangladesh. *Emerg. Infect. Dis.* 10: 2082–2086.

Hyatt, A. D., Zaki, S. R., Goldsmith, C. S., Wise, T., and Hengstberger, S. G. (2001). Ultra structure of Hendra virus and Nipah virus within cultured cells and host animals. *Microbes Infect.* 3: 297–306.

ICCDR, B, Centre for Health and Population Research. (2004). Person-to-person transmission of Nipah virus during the outbreak in Faridpur District, 2004. *Health Sci. Bull.* 2: 5–9.

Lee, K. E., Umapathi, T., Tan, C. B., Tjia, H. T. L., Chua, T. S., Oh, H. M. L., Fock, K. M., Kurup, A., Das, A., Tan, A. K. Y., and Lee, W. L. (1999). The neurological manifestations of Nipah virus encephalitis, a novel paramyxovirus. *Ann. Neurol.* 46: 428–432.

Mounts, A.W., Kaur, H., Parashar, U.D., Ksiazek, T.G., Cannon, D., Arokiasamy, J.T., Anderson, L.J., and Lye, M.S. (2001). A cohort study of health care workers to assess nosocomial transmissibility of Nipah virus, Malaysia. (1999). *J. Infect. Dis.* 183: 810–813.

Murray, P. K., Rogers, R. J., Selvey, L. A., Selleck, P. W., Hyatt, A. D., Gould, A. R., Gleeson, L. J., Hooper, P. T., and Westbury, H. A. (1995a). A novel Morbillivirus pneumonia of horses and its transmission to humans. *Emerg. Infect. Dis.* 1: 31–33.

Murray, P. K., Selleck, P. W., Hooper, P. T., Hyatt, A. D., Gould, A. R., Gleeson, L. J., Westbury, H. A., Hiley, L., Selvey, L. A., Rodwell, B. J., and Ketterer, P. J. (1995b). A Morbillivirus that caused fatal disease in horses and humans. *Science* 268: 94–97.

O'Sullivan, J. D., Allworth, A. M., Paterson, D. L., Snow, T. M., Boots, R., Gleeson, L. J., Gould, A. R., Hyatt, A. D., Bradfield, J. (1997). Fatal encephalitis due to a novel paramyxovirus transmitted from horses. *Lancet* 349: 93–95.

Parashar, U. D., Sunn, L. M., Ong, F., Mounts, A. W., Arif, M. T., Ksiazek, T. G., Kamaluddin, M. A., Mustafa, A. N., Kaur, H., Ding, L. M., Othman, G., Radzi, H. M., Kitsutani, P. T., Stockton, P. C., Arokiasamy, J. T., Gary, H. E. Jr., Anderson, L. J. (2000). Case control study of risk factors for human infection with a new zoonotic paramyxovirus, Nipah virus, during a 1998-1999 outbreak of severe encephalitis in Malaysia. *J. Infect. Dis.* 181: 1755–1759.

Paton, N. I., Leo, Y. S., Zaki, S. R., Auchus, A. P., Lee, K. E., Ling, A. E., Chew, S. K., Ang, B. S. P., Rollin, P. E., Umapathi, T., Sng, I., Lee, C. C., Lim, E., and Ksiazek, T. G. (1999). Outbreak of Nipah-virus infection among abattoir workers in Singapore. *Lancet* 354: 1253–1256.

Philbey, A. W., Kirkland, P. D., Ross, A. D., Davis, R. J., Gleeson, A. B., Love, R. J., Daniels, P. W., Gould, A. R., and Hyatt, A. D. (1998). An apparently new virus (family paramyxoviridae) infectious for pigs, humans and fruit bats. *Emerg. Infect. Dis.* 4: 269–271.

Premalatha, G. D., Lye, M. S., Arokiasamy, J. T., Parashar, U. D., Rahmat, R., Lee, B. Y., and Ksiazek, T. G. (2000). Assessment of Nipah virus transmission among pork sellers in Seremban, Malaysia. *Southeast Asian J. Trop. Med. Public Health* 31: 307–309.

Quddus, R., Alam, S., Majumdar, M. A., Anwar, S., Khan, M. R., Zahid Mahmud Khan, A. K. S., Arif, S. M., Siddique, F. M., Tan, C. T., and Faiz, M. A.. (2004). A report of 4 patients with Nipah encephalitis from Rajbari district, Bangladesh in the January 2004 outbreak. *Neurol. Asia* 9: 33–37.

Ramasundrum, V., Tan, C. T., Chua, K. B., Chong, H. T., Goh, K. J., Chew, N. K., Tan, K. S., Thayaparan, T., Kunjapan, S. R., Petharunam, V., Loh, Y. L., Ksiazek, T. G., and Lam, S. K. K. (2000). Kinetics of IgM and IgG seroconversion of Nipah virus infection. *Neurol. J. Southeast Asia* 5: 23–28.

Selvey, L. A., Wells, R. M., McCormack, J. G., Ansford, A. J., Murray, K., Rogers, R. J., Lavercombe, P. S., Selleck, P., Sheridan, J. W. (1995). Infection of humans and horses by a newly described morbillivirus. *Med. J. Aust.* 162: 642–645.

Selvey, L. A., Taylor, R., Arklay, A., and Gerrard, J. (1996). Screening of bat carers for antibodies to Equine Morbillivirus. *Comm. Dis. Intell.* 20: 477–478.

Tan, C. T. and Tan, K. S. (2001). Nosocomial transmissibility of Nipah virus. *J. Infect. Dis.* 184: 1367.

Tan, C. T., Goh, K. J., Wong, K. T., Ahmad Sarji, S., Chua, K. B., Chew, N. K., Murugasu, P., Loh, Y. L., Chong, H. T., Tan, K. S., Thayaparan, T., Kumar, S., and Jusoh, M. R. (2002). Relapsed and late-onset Nipah encephalitis. *Ann. Neurol.* 51: 703–708.

Tan, C. T. and Wong, K. T. (2003). Nipah encephalitis outbreak in Malaysia. *Ann. Acad. Med. Singapore* 32: 112–117.

Tan, K. S., Tan, C. T., and Goh, K. J. (1999). Epidemiological aspects of Nipah virus infection. *Neurol. J. Southeast Asia* 4: 77–81.

Tan, K.S., Ahmad Sarji, S., Tan, C.T., Abdullah, B.J.J., Chong, H.T., Thayaparan, T., and Koh, C.N. (2000). Patients with asymptomatic Nipah virus infection may have abnormal cerebral MR imaging. *Neurol. J. Southeast Asia* 5: 69–73.

Wang, L. F., Yu, M., Hansson, E., Pritchard, L. I., Shiell, B. J., Michalski, W. P., and Eaton, B. T. (2000). The exceptionally large genome of Hendra virus: support for creation of a new genus within the family paramyxoviridae. *J. Virol.* 74: 9972–9979.

Wang, L. F., Harcourt, B. H., Yu, M., Tamin, A., Rota, P. A., Bellini, W. J., and Eaton, B. T. (2001). Molecular biology of Hendra and Nipah viruses. *Microbes Infect.* 3: 279–287.

Williamson, M. M., Hooper, P. T., Selleck, P. W., Gleeson, L. J., Daniels, P. W., Westbury, H. A., and Murray, P. K. (1998). Transmission studies of Hendra virus (Equine Morbillivirus) in fruit bats, horses and cats. *Aust. Vet. J.* 76: 813–818.

World Health Organization (2004) Nipah virus outbreak(s) in Bangladesh, January-April 2004. *Wkly Epidemiol Record* 79: 168–171.

Wong, K. T., Shieh, W. J., Kumar, S., Norain, K., Abdullah, W., Guarner, J., Goldsmith, C. S., Chua, K. B., Lam, S. K. K., Tan, C. T., Goh, K. J., Chong, H. T., Jusoh, M. R., Rollin, P. E., Ksiazek, T. G., and Zaki, S. R. (2002a). Nipah virus infection: pathology and pathogenesis of an emerging paramyxoviral zoonosis. *Am. J. Pathol.* 161: 2153–2167.

Wong, K. T., Shieh, W. J., Zaki, S. R., and Tan, C. T. (2002b). Nipah virus infection, an emerging paramyxoviral zoonosis. *Springer Semin Immunopathol* 24: 215–228.

Wong, K. T., Grosjean, I., Brisson, C., Blanquier, B., Fevre-Montagne, M., Bernard, A., Loth, P., Georges-Courbot, M. C., Chevallier, M., Akaoka, H., Marianneau, P., Lam, S. K., Wild, T. F., and Deubel, V. (2003). A golden hamster model for human acute Nipah virus infection. *Am. J. Pathol.* 163: 2127–2137.

Yob, J. M., Field, H. E., Azmin, M. R., Morrissy, C., White, J. R., Van der Heide, B., Daniels, P. W., Aziz, A. J., and Ksiazek, T. G. (2001). Serological evidence of infection with Nipah virus in bats (order Chiroptera) in peninsular Malaysia. *Emerg. Infect. Dis.* 7: 439–441.

Young, P. L., Halpin, K., Selleck, P. W., Field, H. E., Gravel, J. L., Kelly, M. A., and MacKenzie, J. S. (1996). Serologic evidence for the presence in Pteropus bats of a paramyxovirus related to Equine Morbillivirus. *Emerg. Infect. Dis.* 2: 239–240.

8. Enterovirus 71 Encephalitis

Luan-Yin Chang, Shin-Ru Shih, Li-Min Huang, and
Tzou-Yien Lin

8.1. Virology

Enterovirus 71 (EV71) was first described in 1974 after it was isolated from patients in California (Schmidt et al., 1974) and has been associated with sporadic cases or outbreaks of a wide spectrum of diseases, including hand, foot, and mouth disease (HFMD), herpangina, aseptic meningitis, encephalitis, cerebellar ataxia, poliomyelitis-like syndrome, and even fatal disease. Since the poliovirus has been eradicated, EV71 has become one of the most important enteroviruses known to cause fatalities and sequelae in children. Therefore, understanding its virology, epidemiology, clinical manifestations, treatment management, diagnosis, and prevention is important.

8.1.1. Virological Classification of Enterovirus 71

Enterovirus 71 is an enterovirus. Enteroviruses belong to Picornaviridae, a family of single-stranded, positive-sense RNA viruses. They can be classified into four groups: enteroviruses (e.g., poliovirus), rhinoviruses (e.g., human rhinovirus), cardioviruses (e.g., Mengo virus), and aphthovirus (e.g., foot-and-mouth virus). The rhinovirus and enterovirus genera are most closely related; the cardioviruses fall halfway between the two closely related ones and the foot-and-mouth virus, FMDV.

Serologic studies, using neutralization tests with antisera against enteroviruses, have identified more than 67 human enterovirus serotypes: poliovirus serotypes 1–3, 23 coxsackie A virus serotypes, 6 coxsackie B virus serotypes, 31 echovirus serotypes, and the numbered enterovirus serotypes (enteroviruses 68–71).

8.1.2. General Characteristics of Enterovirus

Most enteroviruses replicate in primate cells. The specific receptor on the surface of the host cell can be used to identify the host range and tissue tropism. The specific receptors of poliovirus and rhinovirus have been identified as belonging to the superimmunoglobulin family of proteins. About 90% of all rhinoviruses use intercellular adhesion molecule-1 (ICAM-1; an immunoglobulin-like molecule with five domains) as a receptor (Greve et al., 1989), whereas polioviruses use PVR (CD155, an immunoglobulin-like molecule with three domains) (Mendelsohn et al., 1989). Echoviruses use integrin very late antigen, VLA-2 (an integrin-like molecule) (Bergelson et al., 1992) or decay accelerating factor (DAF; CD55) as their receptors. Coxsackievirus B uses coxsackie-adenovirus receptor (CAR) and enterovirus 70 uses DAF as its receptor. The specific receptor for enterovirus 71 remains unidentified.

8.1.3. Virion Structure of Enterovirus

Structurally, enterovirus is a small, nonenveloped, icosahedrally symmetrical spherical particle ~30 nm in diameter. The virus has a single-stranded, positive-sense RNA and simple protein capsid. The protein capsid has 60 copies of each of the structural proteins VP1, VP2, VP3, and VP4 (Rossmann et al., 1985). The protein capsid protects viral RNA from nuclease cleavage, recognizes the receptors on the surfaces of the specific host cells, and displays antigenicity.

VP1-3, located on the virion surface, are the neutralization epitopes. Sequence comparisons and phylogenetic reconstructions suggest that VP1 contains serotype-specific information, which can be used to identify viruses and study evolution. Because enterovirus serotypic differentiation is based on neutralization and the VP1 sequence correlates with neutralization type, it is logical to assume that molecular diagnosis could be used to target the VP1 coding region and should be able to produce typing results that correlate with the serotype identified by neutralization with type-specific antisera (Rigonan et al., 1998).

VP4, which is located within the capsid and anchors the RNA genome to the capsid, interacts with the N termini of VP1 to enhance the genomic stability. Each of the proteins, VP 1–3, contains different amino acid sequences, but all share an eight-stranded, antiparallel β-barrel motif with a similar tertiary structure. Interestingly, a special structure, the hydrophobic pocket, is located beneath the canyon floor on the surface of VP1. According to the "canyon hypothesis" (Rossmann, 1989a, 1989b), cell attachment occurs at a depression on the surface, which is inaccessible to neutralizing antibody. This depression can be said to shield the invading virus from immune surveillance. Such depressions have been found on the surface of HRV14, poliovirus, and Mengo virus, and corroborative evidence supports their existence in the case of HRV.

8.1.4. Replication Cycle of Enterovirus

Enterovirus infection begins with the virus attaching itself to a single receptor unit on the host cells. This binding is reversible. After attachment, the virion undergoes an irreversible conversion to form the 135S, or A, particle. The 135S particle has a lower sedimentation coefficient than the native virion particle (135S vs. 160S for the poliovirus), and the antigenic and proteolytic properties of the 135S particle change and become different from those of the unattached virus. Upon conversion, cell attachment is mediated by externalized VP4 and the N termini of VP1. The externalized N termini of VP1 form an amphipathic helix and is inserted into the cell membrane to produce a pore through which the viral RNA can leave the capsid. This stage is called the uncoating stage. Later, the 135S particle releases its RNA during its conversion to the 80S (or H) particle, and the viral RNA can be used as the translation template to synthesize viral proteins and to amplify viral positive-sense RNA genome (Belnap et al., 2000; Huang et al., 2000). During advanced infection, viral capsid proteins VP 1–4 form the capsid, and the progeny viral RNAs are packaged into mature virion. The newly synthesized viruses can infect neighboring cells by disrupting the old cells and causing their release.

Picornavirus replication is rapid, and a cycle is completed in 5–10 h. After ~1–2 h of initial infection/attachment, the host cellular macromolecular synthesis sharply declines in a process called "shutoff," and chromatin marginates. From 2.5 to 3 h postinfection, viral proteins begin synthesis and cytoplasm vacuolates. At 6 h postinfection, newly synthesized viral RNA and proteins assemble in the cytoplasm. The infected cell lyses and releases the virus particle at 6–10 h after being infected.

8.1.5. Genotypes and Neurovirulence of EV71

In order to understand the virological basis of neurovirulence, Shih et al. (2000b) analyzed the nucleotide sequence of VP1, which is important for serotypic specificity, and the 5′-non-coding region (5′-NCR), which is important for efficient replication. Phylogenic analysis of both VP1 and 5′-NCR of nine EV71 isolates derived from specimens of fatal patients and seven isolates derived from uncomplicated HFMD patients of the 1998 epidemic showed that all but one isolate could be categorized as being of the genotype C. The one distinct isolate (TW/1743/98) from a case of uncomplicated HFMD belonged to genotype B and was clustered along with one strain (TW/253/86) that was isolated from the southern Taiwan in 1986 (Shih et al., 2000b).

Shih et al. (2000b) further analyzed complete sequences of two selected EV71 strains from the spinal cord of a fatal case and from vesicles of a patient with a mild case of HFMD, both from the 1998 epidemic. There was a high degree of identity (97–100%) in nucleotide sequence throughout the entire genome, except in the focal regions of 3C encoding viral protease and 3′-NCR, where the nucleotide homology was 90–91%.

Wang et al. (2002) also found that most EV71 isolates from the 1998 epidemic belonged to genotype C, whereas only one-tenth of the isolates were genotype B. However, most isolates from years 1999, 2000, and 2001 belonged to genotype B (Wang et al., 2002). Both B and C genotypes of EV71 can cause severe clinical illness.

Shimizu et al. (1999), analyzing EV71 from fatal and nonfatal cases of HFMD epidemics in Malaysia, Japan, and Taiwan, found the isoloates to be geographically and temporally heterogeneous. Cardosa et al. (2003) studied the molecular epidemiology of human enterovirus 71 strains and recent outbreaks in the Asia-Pacific region. Phylogenetic analysis of the VP4 and VP1 genes of recent EV71 strains indicates that several genotypes of the virus have been circulating in the Asia-Pacific region since 1997. The first of these recent outbreaks, described in Sarawak (Malaysian Borneo) in 1997, was caused by genotype B3. The large outbreak in Taiwan in 1998 was mainly caused by genotype C2, and in Perth (Western Australia) in 1999, the viruses belonging to genotypes B3 and C2 cocirculated. Singapore, Taiwan, and Sarawak had EV71 epidemics in 2000, caused predominantly by viruses belonging to genotype B4, though during that epidemic only Taiwan suffered a large number of fatalities. An epidemic of HFMD in Korea was found to be caused by EV71, which constituted a new genotype C3.

Two studies reported that 3C and 2A protease of EV71 can induce apoptotic cell death in neuronal or non-neuronal cells (Kuo et al., 2002; Li et al., 2002), and these two proteases may to some extent account for viral neurovirulence. However, the most important viral neurovirulence or virulence has not been clarified and needs further investigation.

8.2. Transmission and Incubation Period

8.2.1. Route of Transmission

Human beings are the only natural hosts of enteroviruses. Enterovirus can infect humans through gastrointestinal cells as well as the respiratory tract. Enterovirus is usually transmitted through fecal–oral contact and sometimes through droplet transmission. Furthermore, enterovirus can live for more than 24 h in stainless-steel containers, and such contaminated objects may be one way that it is transmitted. It can live in low-pH conditions (pH = 3) and is resistant to 70% ethanol and ether. The virus can remain active at room temperature for several days.

We found that the isolation rate of EV71 was significantly higher in throat swabs (93%) than rectal swabs or feces (30%) in EV71 cases with acute illnesses (Chang et al., 1999b), which suggests that oral–oral route or droplet transmission might be a more important route of transmission than the fecal–oral route during acute EV71 illness.

8.2.2. The Rate of Household Transmission

How high is the rate of enterovirus transmission? The secondary household transmission rates of enteroviruses vary, as has been found in those for poliovirus, enterovirus 70, and coxsackievirus A24 (Gelfand et al., 1957; Kogon et al., 1969; Morens et al., 1991).

EV71 seropositivity was found to be concordant among siblings in our previous seroepidemiological study, suggesting that household transmission plays an important role in the spread of EV71 (Chang et al., 2002). Therefore, we did a prospective family cohort study of EV71 household transmission. We studied 433 family members from 94 families in which EV71 positively isolated. The overall enterovirus 71 transmission rate of household contacts was 52% (176/339): 84% (70/83) siblings, 83% (19/23) cousins, 41% (72/175) parents, 28% (10/36) grandparents, and 26% (5/19) uncles/aunts. So, enterovirus 71 household transmission rates are high for children, medium for parents, and low for other adults. Being male and being less than 6 years old were associated with increased risk of EV71 infection (Chang et al., 2004a). EV71 isolation rate from children household contacts was 39% (41/106), significantly higher than the 4.3% (10/233) EV71 isolation rate from adult household contacts (p < 0.001). Adult household contacts have lower isolation rates possibly from partial protective antibodies from previous exposure or lower concentration of virus in secretions. From these figures, we can imply that infected children are more able to transmit the virus than adults.

Why is the household transmission rate for children so high? Long periods of viral shedding may account for widespread transmission of enteroviral diseases, which is certainly the case for polio and coxsackievirus infections (Gelfand et al., 1957). In a previous study, we found EV71 to be present in the stool of infected patients for up to 5 weeks (Chung et al., 2001). Therefore, close household contact, higher viral load, and long viral shedding periods may account for the high household transmission rate among children.

8.2.3. Incubation Period

Most secondary cases in the family develop diseases 3 to 4 days after the index cases. Case-to-case interval is shown in Figure 8.1. The incubation period is usually 3 to 4 days and can be as long as 10 or more days. The reason that some members of the same household develop the disease on the same day or one day later is more than likely because they contracted their infections from the same asymptomatic person.

8.3. Epidemiology

8.3.1. Worldwide Epidemiology

Enterovirus 71 was first isolated in 1969 in California, USA. Four epidemic outbreaks with high mortality rates occurred in Bulgaria in 1975 with 44 deaths (Shindarov et al., 1979), in Hungary in 1978 with 47 deaths (Nagy et al., 1982), in Malaysia in 1997 with at least 31 deaths (Chan et al., 2000), and in Taiwan in 1998 with 78 deaths (Ho et al., 1999).

In addition to these four well-known EV71 outbreaks, sporadic cases or small outbreaks with some mortality have occurred in the United States, Sweden, Japan, mainland China, Hong Kong, Australia, and Singapore (Blomberg et al., 1974; Deibel et al., 1975; Tagaya and Tachibana, 1975; Gilbert et al., 1988). A study in Singapore showed that the age-specific EV71 seroprevalence in children 5 years old and above leveled out at

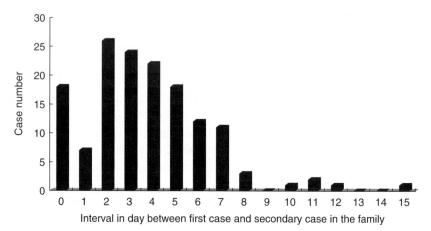

Figure 8.1. The interval in days between first case and secondary case in the same household. There were 18 households with at least 2 cases who became ill on the same day, and all 18 households did not have an identified extra-household source of EV71 infection. This indicated they might have had contact with the same asymptomatic EV71-infected person within the household or outside the household.

approximately 50% between 1996 and 1997 (Ooi et al., 2002). In Brazil, EV71 has been reported to cause polio-like syndrome even after the poliovirus had been eradicated there (Da Silva et al., 1996), and in that country the EV71 seropositive rate in children 12 to 15 years old has been reported to be as high as 69.2% (Gomes et al., 2002). A Taiwanese EV71 seroepidemiology study in 1999 also found about a 60% seropositive rate in people over 6 years of age (Chang et al., 2002). With EV71 sero-prevalence rates between 60% and 70% in the general population of these countries, EV71 infection cannot be considered uncommon, and what documented cases we have just reflect a small proportion of the actual number of infections.

8.3.2. Epidemiology in Taiwan

The EV71 outbreak in Taiwan in 1998 is very well-known and it certainly drew people's attention to the virus, but EV71 already existed in Taiwan before that outbreak. Our seropidemiological study before the 1998 outbreak showed preepidemic (1997) EV71 seroprevalence rates to be 57% and 67% in adults and children older than 6 years of age (Chang et al., 2002). Lu et al. (2002) examined serial serum antibody titers to EV71 in 81 children who were born in 1988 and who had yearly blood samples saved from 1989 to 1994 as well as in 1997 and 1999. They discovered that EV71 seroconversion occurred with a yearly incidence of 3% to 11% between 1989 and 1997 and that 68% of these children had serological evidence of EV71 infections by 1997 (Chang et al., 2002). In addition, EV71 had been isolated from patients with HFMD and poliomyelitis-like paralysis in Taiwan as early as 1980 and 1986 (Ho et al., 1999; Chu et al., 2001).

These findings indicate that EV71 had circulated in Taiwan for at least 17 years before 1998, though its clinical significance in Taiwan had not been investigated before 1998. It is likely that severe cases of EV71 had occurred but were not recognized. The pre-epidemic EV71 sero-prevalence rates were inversely correlated with mortality and morbidity (Chang et al., 2002). Among a cohort of 81 children, Lu et al. (2002) found that the annual EV71 seroconversion rates (3% to 4%) between 1994 and 1997 were significantly lower than the rate (7% to 11%) before 1994. It is likely that there was lower incidence of EV71 infection between 1994 and 1997, and accumulation of susceptible hosts over the threshold density might have triggered the 1998 outbreak. However, changes in EV71 neurovirulence and host genetic factors are also thought to affect clinical outcomes.

A physician-based sentinel surveillance system for infectious diseases was established in Taiwan in 1989 and has been operated by the

Ministry of Health since that time (Wu et al., 1999). This system included 850 physicians, 8.7% of the primary physicians in Taiwan. Hand, foot, and mouth disease and herpangina were included in the system after an outbreak of EV71-related HFMD in Malaysia in 1997. Compared with the case numbers of HFMD in 1997, HFMD was found to have increased noticeably by March 1998 (Wu et al., 1999). Because of a rapid increase in severe and fatal cases of HFMD, a hospital-based reporting system for monitoring severe and fatal cases was started in May 1998. From June 1998, both physician-based and hospital-based surveillance systems were maintained simultaneously (Wu et al., 1999). With the availability of EV71-specific monoclonal antibody, pediatricians in Taiwan linked EV71 with the deaths of young children by unexplained acute illnesses, usually preceding HFMD followed by sudden onset of pulmonary edema. Both the physician-based and hospital-based surveillance systems provided the critical information leading to the recognition of the EV71 outbreaks and provided the opportunity for the study of EV71 infections.

There were two peaks of HFMD epidemic in 1998. The first and bigger one peaked during the week of June 7 and encompassed all four regions of Taiwan. The second and smaller one occurred during the week of October 4, mainly in the southern part of Taiwan. The total number of HFMD/herpangina cases reported by the physician-based sentinel surveillance system were 129,106 (Ho et al., 1999), which probably represents less than 10% of the estimated total number of cases. The severe cases peaked in early June around the same time as the peak of HFMD. There were 405 severe cases with 78 deaths (Ho et al., 1999). Complications included encephalitis, aseptic meningitis, pulmonary edema or hemorrhage, acute flaccid paralysis, and myocarditis. Ninety-one percent of the fatalities were 5 years of age or younger. Of the patients who died, 65 (83%) had pulmonary edema or pulmonary hemorrhage. Among patients from whom a virus was isolated, 48.7% of the outpatients with uncomplicated HFMD or herpangina, 75% of the hospitalized patients, and 92% of patients who died had EV71. Therefore, during the 1998 epidemic, EV71 infection was associated with most of the serious clinical manifestations and with nearly all the deaths. Most of those who died were young and they died predominantly from pulmonary edema and pulmonary hemorrhage.

In an EV71 seroepidemiology study in 1999, we found that the postepidemic EV71-seropositive rates among children below 3 years old ranged from 0% to 36% (Fig. 8.2). An increased incidence of EV71 infection in young children occurred more often in geographic areas with increased mortality rates (Chang et al., 2002). For 3- to 6-year-old children, the seropositive rates ranged between 26% and 51%.

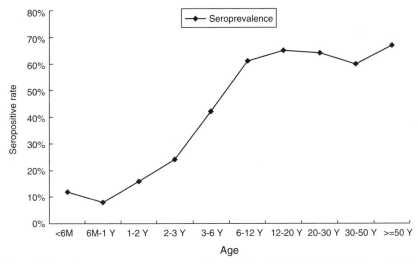

Figure 8.2. Age-specific seropositive rates against EV71 strain TW/2272/98 in Taiwan after the 1998 Taiwan EV71 epidemic, in January–July, 1999.

One year after the large outbreaks in 1998, the number of cases of EV71 infection decreased dramatically with only one fatal EV71 case occurring in 1999. However, there were recurrences of severe and fatal EV71, causing the death of 25 children in 2000 and 26 children in 2001 (Lin et al., 2003b). Outbreaks of EV71 will probably continue to occur for the next several years in Taiwan.

8.4. Clinical Spectrum

Although EV71 can infect both adults and children, their clinical outcomes diverge a lot. From our household EV71 study (Chang et al., 2004a), we found that only 6% of 183 infected children, were asymptomatic, 73% (133/183) had uncomplicated illnesses of HFMD, herpangina, or nonspecific febrile illness, and 21% (39/183) suffered from complications of central nervous system involvement and/or cardiopulmonary failure. During the 6-month follow-up, 10 died and 13 had sequelae, which included problems swallowing, cranial nerve palsy, central hypoventilation, or limb weakness/atrophy. On the contrary, 53% (46/87) of 87 infected adults were asymptomatic, 39% (34/87) had nonspecific illnesses with fever, sore throat, or gastrointestinal discomfort, and only 8% (7/87) had HFMD. All symptomatic adults recovered completely from uncomplicated illnesses (Chang et al., 2004a).

Overall serious complications, sequelae, and death are associated with young children, although two adult fatalities have been reported in Bulgaria and Singapore.

8.4.1. Asymptomatic Infection

The EV71 household study showed that only 6% of infected children were asymptomatic, whereas 53% of infected adults were asymptomatic (Chang et al., 2004a). Interestingly, in the seroepidemiologic study (Chang et al., 2002), only 29% of the preschool children infected with EV71 developed HFMD/HA, indicating about 70% of community-acquired infected children might be asymptomatic. Therefore, household transmission produced a higher rate of clinical symptoms (94%) than extra-household transmission (29%). Viral load or host genetic factors may account for this difference, but this hypothesis will need further confirmation. However, we cannot exclude that recall bias from retrospective nature of the seroepidemiologic study (Chang et al., 2002) may underestimate the true rate of clinical symptoms for extra-household transmission.

According to our clinical studies (Chang et al., 1999a, 2004b), symptomatic enterovirus 71 (EV71) infection can progress through four stages: HFMD/herpangina (stage 1), CNS involvement (stage 2), cardiopulmonary failure (stage 3), and convalescence (stage 4). Most EV71 cases in those studies stayed at stage 1, some progressed to stage 2, and a few would advance to the most severe condition, stage 3.

8.4.2. Stage 1: Uncomplicated EV71 Illness

The uncomplicated EV71 illnesses include HFMD, herpangina, pharyngitis, nonspecific febrile illness, generalized viral exanthema, and enteritis. The cases may have fever for 1 to 3 days, reaching sometimes higher than 39°C. HFMD patients have oral ulcers on the tongue and buccal mucosa, plus vesicular rash or small erythematous maculopapular rash on the hands, the feet, the knees, or the buttocks (Figs. 8.3A and 8.3B). The EV71-induced vesicular or maculopapular rash over the extremities is sometimes so tiny that it may be overlooked by parents and even doctors (Fig. 8.3C). Herpangina includes oral ulceration on anterior tonsillar pillars, the soft palate, buccal mucosa, or the uvula. Oral ulceration causes pain while eating or drinking, and patients may need intravenous fluid supplement if dehydration occurs. About 10% to 20% of the EV71 cases have febrile illness or pharyngitis without the usual HFMD/herpangina.

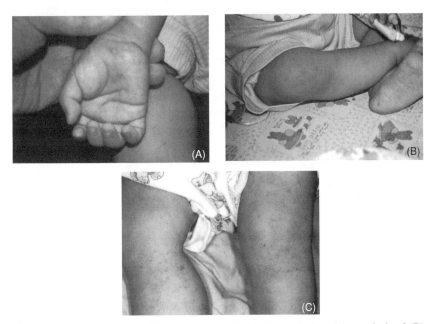

Figure 8.3. Vesicular rash of EV71 hand, foot, and mouth disease. Lesions (A) over the hand, (B) over the lower leg and foot, and (C) tiny, easily overlooked vesicular rash over the knees.

8.4.3. Stage 2: Complicated EV71 Illness with CNS Involvement

Human EV71 diseases may develop complicated conditions 1 to 5 days after the onset of the illness. After suffering the initial HFMD, herpangina, or febrile illness and an intermittent fever that usually lasts from 3 to 7 days, some patients may begin to suffer CNS involvement including meningitis, encephalitis, polio-like syndrome, or encephalomyelitis with or without pulmonary edema. Although the clinical manifestations, CSF pleocytosis, and image studies all show evidence of CNS involvement, seldom is EV71 ever isolated from a patient's cerebrospinal fluid. Huang et al. (1999) described three EV71 neurologic syndromes in the Taiwan outbreak: aseptic meningitis, acute flaccid paralysis, and rhombencephalitis (brain stem encephalitis).

8.4.3.1. EV71 Aseptic Meningitis

EV71 cases with aseptic meningitis usually have myoclonic jerk during sleep, vomiting, headache, or irritable crying. They have mild if any neck stiffness. They usually recover 3 to 7 days after hospitalization.

8.4.3.2. EV71 Encephalitis

The most common initial symptoms of EV71 encephalitis are myoclonic jerks during sleep, which is followed by other symptoms or signs of encephalitis. Patients may also show signs of changes in consciousness such as lethargy, sleepiness or coma, seizure attacks, ataxia, and cranial nerve palsy, such as abducens palsy, facial palsy, dysphagia, upward gaze, and nystagmus. Patients have also shown subtle symptoms of increased sympathetic tone, such as insomnia, profuse sweating, paralytic ileus, neurogenic bladder, and panic or increased startle reflex. If cases of encephalitis do not advance to stage 3, they usually recover without sequelae 5 to 10 days later.

8.4.3.3. Polio-like Syndrome

EV71 cases with poliomyelitis-like syndrome have asymmetric acute limb weakness plus decreased reflex without disturbance of limb sensation. Children suddenly cannot walk or raise their arms or they easily fall down 3 to 7 days after HFMD or herpangina. About one-half to two-thirds of EV71 polio-like cases have had long-term sequelae of limb weakness and atrophy.

8.4.3.4. Encephalomyelitis

Patients have symptoms of both encephalitis and poliomyelitis-like syndrome.

8.4.3.5. Image Studies for CNS Involvement

Brain or spinal CTs usually give negative findings in cases with EV71 CNS infection and are not the image study of choice. MRI is a better choice. MRI studies usually show hyperintensity in the CNS lesions on T2-weighted images. The major CNS lesions of brain-stem encephalitis and cerebellitis have been in the medulla oblongata, pons, midbrain, and the dentate nuclei of the cerebellum. For polio-like syndrome, the lesions have involved the anterior horn of the spinal cord (Fig. 8.4). Some might have normal MRI results. Cases of encephalomyelitis might have both lesions of the brain stem and spinal cord (Figs. 8.5A and 8.5B). In the follow-up MRI examinations of patients with sequelae, the lesions may persist 1 to 3 years after their acute illness.

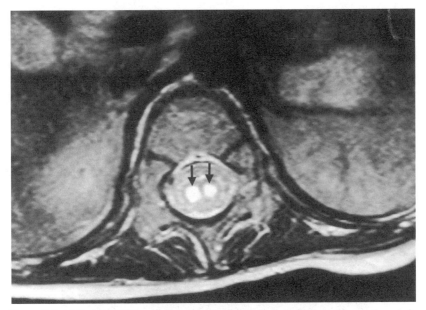

Figure 8.4. MRI of the EV71 polio-like case. Hyperintensity lesions (arrows) are in the anterior horn of the spinal cord on T2-weighted image.

8.4.4. Stage 3: Cardiopulmonary Failure or Pulmonary Edema

Several hours to 2 days after the onset of CNS involvement, some patients may advance into stage 3 at which time they have sudden signs of tachypnea, tachycardia (range 135–250 beats per minute) and cyanosis. Patients are usually alert except for mild lethargy and have sometimes been found to have transient hypertension. Laboratory findings include hyperglycemia and leukocytosis. Chest x-ray films show alveolar density and no cardiomegaly. Most became completely white within 12 h during the 1998 epidemic. Electrocardiographic examination shows sinus tachycardia and no arrhythmia. Ejection fractions on cardiac echography have been about 40% to 80%. Once intubated, children produce a white frothy secretion, followed by a pink frothy fluid and then fresh blood from endotracheal tube. Patients have frequently had persistent fever and profuse sweating at critical points during pulmonary edema/hemorrhage.

Progressive hypotension or shock, oliguria or anuria, tachycardia, and decreased levels of consciousness have been found if their disease progresses into stage 3B. Nearly 80% of these children died within 12 h of intubation during the 1998 epidemic, but the fatality rate had decreased to 30 40% in 2000 to 2002. The significantly lower mortality rate may be due to earlier and better intensive care.

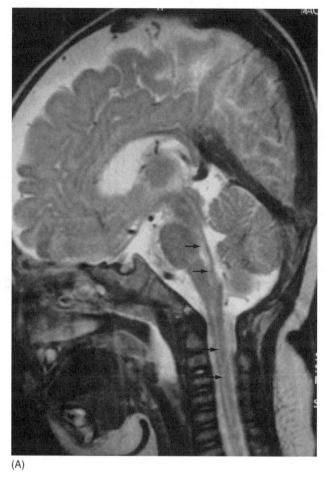

(A)

Figure 8.5. MRI of the EV71 encephalomyelitis plus pulmonary edema. (A) Saggital view of T2-weighted image shows hyperintensity lesions in the posterior portion of the pons and the medulla and also in the anterior portion of the C-spinal cord.

8.4.4.1. Pathogenesis of EV71-related Cardiopulmonary Failure

Pathological studies of cases with pulmonary edema have revealed extensive inflammation in the central nervous system (CNS), with predominant lesions in the brain stem and spinal cord (Hsueh et al., 2000). Also reported has been marked pulmonary edema with focal hemorrhage without evidence of myocarditis. EV71 has been isolated from CNS tissues but not from other tissues. Autopsy findings in Taiwan have been similar to those reported in Malaysia (Lum et al., 1998). EV71 was isolated usually from the brain; medulla; cervical, thoracic, and lumbar spinal cords; as well as from throat and rectal swabs, sometimes from the

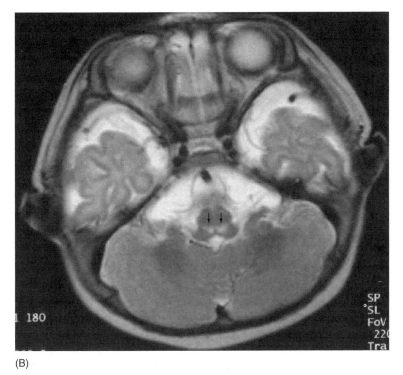

(B)

Figure 8.5. (*Continued*) (B) Coronal view shows hyperintensity lesions in the posterior portion of the pons–medulla junction.

blood. The MR imaging study of cases with pulmonary edema have usually showed hyperintensity of the posterior aspect of the medulla (Fig. 8.5B) with or without involvement of the cervical spinal cord on T2-weighted image.

Immunopathogenesis studies have found EV71 cases with both encephalitis and pulmonary edema to have much higher levels of white blood cell count, blood glucose, systemic proinflammatory cytokines such as interleukin-6, tumor necrosis factor-α, interleukin 1β, γ-interferon, IL-10, and IL-13 than those patients who have had EV71 encephalitis alone (Lin et al., 2002; Wang et al., 2003). Levels of CSF IL-6 in EV71 study patients have been found to be consistently higher during the initial 2 days of central nervous system (CNS) involvement regardless of pulmonary edema. Patients with pulmonary edema had lower circulating CD4(+) T cells, CD8(+) T cells, and natural killer (NK) cells (Wang et al., 2003). The CD40-ligand expression on T cells has been found to be significantly decreased in children with meningoencephalitis (Yang et al., 2001). However, EV71 neutralizing antibody titers are detectable in children with pulmonary edema, with meningoencephalitis alone, and with uncomplicated illness, but they have not differed in EV71 neutralizing titers.

Therefore, based on the above evidence, the combination of severe brain-stem encephalitis, especially the medullary vasomotor center, and severe systemic inflammatory response may trigger EV71-related cardiopulmonary collapse.

8.4.5. Stage 4: Convalescence and Long-term Sequelae

In a follow-up study (1 to 6 years after their EV71 CNS infection) of patients with EV71 CNS infection, we found some still needing tracheostomy with ventilator support and nasogastric tube feeding, and some with limb weakness, psychomotor developmental delay, lower IQs, or attention deficiency hyperactive disorder. Their sequelae are compatible with MRI findings, which usually reveal high signal intensity from the pons to cervical spinal cord (Fig. 8.5A).

8.4.6. Factors Associated with Complications

Univariate analysis of clinical data found fever, fever for more than 3 days, peak body temperatures over 39°C, headaches, lethargy, vomiting, seizures, and hyperglycemia to be significant risk factors of CNS involvement. Fever for more than 3 days, peak body temperatures over 39°C, headache, lethargy, vomiting, and seizure were included in the multivariate analysis. After multiple logistic analysis, lethargy and fever for more than 3 days were found to be the most significant factors (OR = 6.8, 95% CI 2.5–18.5, p = 0.0002; OR = 3.8, 95% CI 1.0–16, p = 0.05, respectively).

Once there is CNS involvement, there is a risk of pulmonary edema. The risk factors for developing pulmonary edema after CNS involvement are hyperglycemia, leukocytosis, and limb weakness. Hyperglycemia is the most significant prognostic factor for pulmonary edema (OR = 21.5, 95% CI 3–159, p = 0.003; Chang et al., 1999a).

These above risk factors may alert clinicians of the need to hospitalize high-risk patients as early as possible and put the most severe cases into the intensive care unit. These measures may help decrease mortality or sequelae.

8.4.7. EV71 Versus Coxsackievirus A16

Coxsackievirus A16 also causes HFMD, but it seldom causes severe disease. In a study comparing the clinical manifestations of EV71 and coxsackievirus A16 (Chang et al., 1999b), we found that 120 (68%) of EV71 cases were uncomplicated cases of HFMD, but 57 (32%) of the cases had complications, including 13 (7.3%) cases of aseptic meningitis, 18 (10%) cases of encephalitis, 4 (2.3%) cases of polio-like syndrome, 8 (4.5%) cases of encephalomyelitis, and 12 (6.8%) cases of fatal pulmonary edema. Fourteen (7.9%) patients died, including 12 cases of fatal pulmonary edema and 2 cases of encephalitis; 7 (4%) patients had sequelae. In contrast, 60 (94%) of the 64 cases of HFMD caused by Cox A16 infection were uncomplicated cases of HFMD and only 4 (6.3%) cases were complicated by aseptic meningitis; no fatalities nor sequelae were observed. Multivariate analysis showed significantly more frequent vomiting (p = 0.01) and fevers higher than 39°C lasting for longer than 3 days (p = 0.02) among the EV71 group. In other words, EV71-induced illnesses are more severe with significantly greater frequency of serious complications and fatalities than illnesses caused by coxsackievirus A16.

8.5. Diagnosis

8.5.1. Virus Isolation and Identification

Like other enteroviruses, isolation of enterovirus 71 can be performed in clinical virology laboratories with the use of RD, Vero, or MRC-5 cells. Neutralization test (NT) is considered the gold standard for identifying EV71. The EV71-specific antibody is used to neutralize the cytopathic effect (CPE) induced by EV71. Immunofluorescence assay (IFA) has also been a popular method for diagnosing EV71 in the clinical laboratory. A good method of confirming an EV71 diagnosis is molecular diagnosis by RT-PCR with the use of EV71-specific primers followed by sequence analysis (Tsao et al., 2002b).

8.5.2. Gene Chips

DNA microarray is a highly effective technology for investigating gene expression patterns in diverse organisms (Bowtell, 1999; Duggan et al., 1999) and can be used in such applications as drug discovery, genome mapping, and mutation detection. DNA microarray technology is also highly promising for diagnosing viral infection. Li et al. (2001) have reported using DNA microchip arrays for typing and subtyping influenza virus, and Lapa et al. (2002) have described a method for the species-specific detection of orthopoxviruses with the use of oligonucleotide microchips. A microchip to be used in the detection of EV71 was developed as an alternative diagnostic method. This novel approach is based on hybridization of amplified DNA specimens with oligonucleotide DNA probes immobilized on a microchip. Two oligonucletides were used as detection probes, the pan-enterovirus sequence located in the 5'-noncoding region (5'-NCR) and the EV71-specific sequence located in the VP2 region. The diagnostic procedure took 6 h. One hundred specimens identified as enteroviruses by viral cultures were tested using this microchip, including 67 EV71 specimens. The sensitivity of the novel method was 89.6% and its specificity was 90.9%. The EV71 microchip can detect the amplicon derived from viral RNA corresponding with 1 to 10 virions in a clinical specimen (Shih et al., 2003).

8.5.3. Serology Test

8.5.3.1. Neutralizing Antibody

Laboratory methods for measuring EV71 neutralizing antibody follow standard protocol for performing the neutralization test on microtiter plates. Serum was heat treated at 56° for 30 min. Then, serum and 50 μl of EV71, containing one hundred 50% tissue culture infective doses ($TCID_{50}$) of EV71 strain, were mixed and incubated onto the microtiter plates with RD cells at 35°C in a 5% CO_2 incubator. Each tested sample was run simultaneously with cell control, serum control, and virus back titration. Cytopathic effect (CPE) was observed under an inverted microscope after an incubation period of 2 to 7 days, and the neutralizing antibody titer was determined at the time when CPE was observed in one $TCID_{50}$ of the virus back titration. The neutralizing antibody titer was defined as the highest dilution of serum that would prevent the occurrence of CPE. Seropositivity was defined as a neutralizing antibody titer ≥8.

We found that the EV71 serotiter had already risen to 1:64 to 1:1024 from the third or fourth day of disease onset and that titer did not differ from convalescence. We seldom detected fourfold change in titer in cases with acute EV71 infection unless we happened to have their sera on the first 2 days of patient illness. EV71 cases of varying severities were not found to have different neutralizing antibody titers, either.

8.5.3.2. EV71 IgM

A rapid serology assay has been developed for the detection of the IgM to EV71 (Shih et al., 2000a; Tsao et al., 2002a). EV71 isolate was amplified and purified as an antigen for IgM-capture ELISA. The sensitivity and specificity of this in-house IgM-capture enzyme linked-immunosorbent assay (ELISA) was assessed by analyzing 213 serum samples. Among 82 sera from 70 EV71-infected patients, 75 were found positive with this newly developed ELISA. With the conventional virus culture as a standard method, this newly developed immunoassay had a sensitivity and specificity of 91.5% and 93.1%, respectively (Shih et al., 2000a; Tsao et al., 2002a). This method allows for the detection of the IgM responses from the patients either infected by genotype B or genotype C of enterovirus 71. With it, IgM can be detected as early as the second day from the onset of disease. IgM responses exhibit 100% positive rate from EV71-infected patients with CNS complications and fatal cases.

8.6. Management

Nearly 90% of the patients with cardiopulmonary failure died in 1998 in Taiwan (Chang et al., 1999a). In 2000, to improve the survival, we developed a disease management program that varied according to the different stages of EV71 infection with the approval of Taiwan's Enterovirus Ad Hoc Committee and the Center for Disease Control in Taiwan (Chang et al., 2004b; Table 8.1).

Table 8.1.   Clinical staging and management

Stages	Clinical Manifestations	Management
1	HFMD/herpangina	Symptomatic treatment only
2	CNS involvement	Fluid restriction, osmotic diuretics for increased intracranial pressure (IICP), and furosemide for fluid overloaded (CVP>8 cmH2O), intravenous immunoglobulin (IVIG) for encephalitis and/or polio-like syndrome and close monitoring of heart rate, blood pressure, oxygenation, coma scale and blood glucose
3	Cardiopulmonary failure	
3A	Hypertension/pulmonary Edema	Phosphodiesterase inhibitor, milrinone, to increase cardiac output, early intubation with positive pressure mechanical ventilation with increased positive end expiratory pressure for pulmonary edema, and high frequency oscillatory ventilator if pulmonary edema/hemorrhage persists or severe hypoxemia develops
3B	Hypotension	Adding inotropic agents such as dopamine and epinephrine
4	Convalescence	Rehabilitation for limb weakness, dysphagia, apnea/ or central hypoventilation, and sufficient chest care to avoid recurrent pneumonia

HFMD denotes hand, foot, and mouth disease; CVP, central venous pressure; CNS, central nervous system.

8.6.1. Stage-based Management

The clinical stages have been described above. Patients with stage 1 (uncomplicated illness) required treatment of symptoms only. Patients identified as havingstage 2 (complicated illness with CNS involvement) were hospitalized, and their treatment included fluid restriction and administration of osmotic diuretics for those with signs of increased intracranial pressure (IICP) and furosemide for those suspected of having fluid overload. Intravenous immunoglobulin (IVIG) was administered, and blood pressure, oximeter, coma scale, and blood sugar were closely monitored. Patients were managed in the ICU if they were found to have tachypnea/apnea, hypertension/hypotension, signs of IICP, or hyperglycemia.

Patients identified as having stage 3 (cardiopulmonary failure or pulmonary edema) were put on ventilator support and inotropic agents. We subdivided these patients into stage 3A (having hypertension and pulmonary edema) and stage 3B (having hypotension). Treatment of stage 3A included intensive care management with continuous fluid restriction, administration of milrinone to control severe hypertension and to increase cardiac output, and early intubation with positive-pressure mechanical ventilation with increased positive end expiratory pressure for pulmonary edema. High-frequency oscillatory ventilator was considered if pulmonary edema or hemorrhage persisted or if patients developed severe hypoxemia. When a patient's blood pressure drops below the normal range for his or her age, the disease is considered to have moved into stage 3B. In some cases, blood pressure is very unstable, requiring fine adjustments of inotropic agents such as dopamine and epinephrine.

For stage 4 (convalescence) patients, rehabilitation is provided for limb weakness/atrophy, dysphagia, diaphragm dysfunction, apnea or central hypoventilation. Sufficient chest care is necessary to avoid recurrent pneumonia, and some cases may need long-term tracheostomies and may need to be transferred to respiratory care centers.

The above stage-based management reduced the case-fatality rate of EV71-related cardiopulmonary failure compared with the cases in 1998, but two-thirds of the survivors had severe sequelae. Therefore, better preventive and treatment strategies for EV71 are sorely needed.

8.6.2. Antiviral Agents

Since EV71 can cause severe diseases resulting in death and sequelae, EV71-specific antiviral therapy may improve the clinical outcome. Until the 1980s, amantadine (Rubessa et al., 1997) was the only approved antiviral drug, but since then antiviral chemotherapy has come of age.

Enteroviruses and rhinoviruses are responsible for most human viral diseases, and currently no specific treatment exists for them. The replication cycle of enteroviruses involves several steps, some potential targets for the development of antiviral drugs. Some potential steps to be targeted by such drugs could be viral attachment, uncoating, viral RNA replication, and viral protein synthesis and processing. Among the most promising antiviral drugs are capsid-binding agents, which prevent viral attachment and receptor-mediated uncoating (Shih et al., 2004a).

The VP1 hydrophobic pocket generally contains unidentified natural molecules (pocket factor), which may stabilize the integrity of the virus and modulate the uncoating of its receptors.

8.6.2.1. Inhibitors of Virion Attachment for Enteroviruses

8.6.2.1.1. Receptor Blockade. Ninety percent of all rhinoviruses use ICAM-1 as a receptor to gain entry to the host cell, and viral receptor antagonists can effectively inhibit a broad spectrum of rhinoviruses. Colonno (1986) and co-workers were the first to verify the practicality of this idea when they did so by using a murine monoclonal antibody directed at the major cellular receptor to rhinovirus 14. The high-affinity monoclonal antibody is effective in competing against bound virus and is not cytotoxic to host cells. However, whether high doses of antibody or prolonged dosing would achieve a lasting effect is unclear.

8.6.2.1.2. Soluble Receptor. Marlin et al. (1987) demonstrated that the soluble form of ICAM-1 (extracellular domain) produced in CHO cells can effectively prevent rhinovirus replication in cell culture. One potential advantage of the soluble-form ICAM-1 approach to inhibiting rhinovirus infection is that the virus should not easily develop resistance to the inhibitors. However, using this treatment for a cold would be extremely expensive.

8.6.2.1.3. Capsid-binding Agents. A 25 Å deep depression, or canyon, encircled each fivefold axis of symmetry on the virion surface. Pevear et al. (1989) demonstrated that antiviral WIN compounds that raise the canyon floor did so as a result of conformational changes arising from binding in a hydrophobic pocket beneath the canyon and also inhibited attachment. These capsid-binding agents influenced the attachment of all the major receptor group rhinoviruses such as rhinovirus 14, while having no influence on minor receptor group viruses similar to the behavior of rhinovirus 1A. The key difference between the two groups of rhinoviruses is thought to be that the minor receptor group rhinoviruses do no display conformational changes in the canyon upon compound binding (Mallamo et al., 1992).

8.6.2.2. Inhibitors of Uncoating for Enteroviruses

After attachment to the cellular receptor, enteroviruses are thought to enter cells through a process of endocytosis (Zeichhardt et al., 1985). After penetrating the cell membrane, the eclipsed viruses become acidified within the endocytic vesicle. The uncoating process requires that the virion increase its stability in the extracellular environment, but not so much as to withstand the receptor and pH-induced conformational changes that are required for efficient RNA release. Increasing the stability of the virion is expected to make the virion resistant to low pH and receptor-induced uncoating pressure (Madshus et al., 1984). Another possible uncoating mechanism that can be blocked by drug binding is based on the dependence of the extensive conformational changes required for virion disassembly on the empty pocket of rhinovirus 14. The presence of capsid-binding agents makes the unoccupied pocket unnecessary, thus maintaining the integrity of the virion. Hydrophobicity is a common physical property of this uncoating inhibitor, and consequently the binding site within the virus may be mainly hydrophobic. Included in this capsid-binding agents group are VP 63843 or plecornail (Rogers et al., 1999; Rotbart, 1999; Billich, 2000; Romero, 2001; Sawyer, 2001), WIN 54954 (Woods et al., 1989; See and Tilles, 1992, 1993), WIN 51711 or disoxaril (Diana, 1985; McKinlay, 1985; Otto et al., 1985; Mosser et al. 1994; Dove and Racaniello, 2000; Nikolaeva and Galabov, 2000), R77975 (Andries, et al., 1992, 1994; Rombaut et al., 1996), R61387 (Andries et al., 1988; Chapman et al., 1991; Moeremans et al., 1992; Dewindt et al, 1994; Dove and Racaniello, 2000), BW683C or dichloroflavan (Dearden et al., 1989; Almela et al., 1991; Dewindt et al., 1994), Ro 09-0410, Ro 09-0696, RMI 15,731,44,081 R.P, BW4294, MDL 20,610, and SCH-38057 (Rozhon et al., 1993; Zhang et al., 1993). Some of the above failed in clinical trials, and currently pleconaril seems to have the most potential because it is easily absorbed and is excellent at inhibiting the activity of most enteroviruses.

8.6.2.3. Pleconaril (VP 63843) and Novel Anti-EV71 Agents

Pleconaril is a novel agent for treating picornaviral infections, including enteroviruses and rhinoviruses. Absorption of the drug through the gastrointestinal tract is good, and concentrations in serum and cerebrospinal fluid exceeding 0.1 mg/ml are easily attained after oral administration of a standard dose of the liquid formulation. Pleconaril has excellent antiviral activity against most enteroviruses *in vitro*. Furthermore, Groarke and Pevear (Groarke and Pevear, 1999) reported activity of pleconaril when given orally in three animal models of lethal enterovirus infection: coxsackievirus serotype A9 infection in suckling mice, coxsackievirus serotype A21 strain Kenny infection in weanling mice, and coxsackievirus serotype B3 strain M infection in adult mice. Treatment with pleconaril increased the survival rate in all three models for both prophylactic and therapeutic dosing regimens. This drug is undergoing late-stage clinical trials for the treatment of viral meningitis and viral respiratory infections (VRIs). The pleconaril-resistant strain of coxsackievirus B3 was selected and tested with the murine model. The variants exhibited reduced thermal stability and reduced capacity to replicate and could cause lethal infection in mice.

Pleconaril has not been found to neutralize the cytopathic effect (CPE) of cultured cells induced by enterovirus 71 isolates from the 1998 outbreak in Taiwan (Shia et al., 2002). However, using the skeleton of pleconaril and its related molecules, so-called WIN compounds, as a template, the rational design, synthesis, and structure–activity relationship (SAR) studies have led to the development of a novel class of imidazolidinones with significant antiviral activity (Shia et al., 2002). These synthetic compounds were evaluated for anti-EV71 activity. Some analogues were found, in addition to inhibiting all of the genotypes of EV71, to possess antiviral activity against coxsackieviruses A9, A24, B1, B3, and B5, echovirus 9, and enterovirus 68.

Pyridyl imidazolidinone was identified using computer-assisted drug design. A virological investigation has demonstrated that BPR0Z-194, one of the pyridyl imidazolidinones, targets enterovirus 71 capsid protein VP1. Time-course experiments revealed that BPR0Z-194 effectively inhibited virus replication in the early stages, implying that the compound might be able to inhibit viral adsorption and/or viral RNA uncoating. BPR0Z-194 was used to select and characterize the drug-resistant viruses. Sequence analysis of the VP1 region showed that the resistant variants differed consistently by seven amino acids in VP1 region from their parental drug-sensitive strains. Side-directed mutagenesis of enterovirus 71 infectious cDNA revealed that a single amino acid alteration at the position 192 of VP1 can confer resistance to the inhibitory effects of BPR0Z-194 (Shih et al., 2004b).

In addition to pyridyl imidazolidinone, a series of pyrazolo[3,4-d]pyrimidines were synthesized and their antiviral activities evaluated in plaque reduction assays. There has been remarkable evidence showing this class of compounds to be very specific for human enteroviruses, including EV71. Some derivatives have proved to be highly effective in inhibiting enterovirus replication at nanomolar concentrations. SAR studies revealed that the phenyl group at the N-1 position and the hydrophobic diarylmethyl group at the piperazine largely influenced the *in vitro* anti-enteroviral activity of this new class of potent antiviral agents. It was found that the pyrazolo[3,4-d]pyrimidines with a thiophene substituent, for example compounds 20–24, in general exhibited high activity against coxsackievirus B3 ($IC_{50} = 0.063$ to 0.089 μM) and moderate activity against enterovirus 71 ($IC_{50} = 0.32$ to 0.65 μM) with no apparent cytotoxic effect toward RD (rhabdomyosarcoma) cell lines ($CC_{50} > 25$ μM) (Chern et al., 2004).

These promising anti-EV71 drugs are being tested in animal studies in Taiwan and may go into clinical trials if the animal studies show positive results.

8.7. Prevention

8.7.1. Hand Washing and Isolation

Hand-washing precautions have been in practice since the 1998 epidemic in Taiwan. Hand washing is the standard preventive measure targeting the fecal–oral transmission route but has limited effect on preventing droplet transmission. Furthermore, younger infected children have higher virus isolation rates as well as higher transmission ability, and these young children are usually not able to consistently follow adequate hand-washing routines.

Previous research has demonstrated a higher rate of EV71 isolation from throat swabs than from rectal swabs or stool (90% vs. 32%, respectively) (Chang et al., 1999b) and very high household transmission among children (Chang et al., 2004a). We speculate that respiratory transmission by large droplets from the oral cavity may explain the high secondary infection rate within households and in kindergartens in Taiwan, despite hand-washing precautions. Therefore, isolation of infected patients within single rooms and masks for the patients and their close contacts may be recommended for the prevention of respiratory droplet transmission of EV71. In Taiwan, home isolation was suggested for 1 or 2 weeks to prevent droplet transmission within kindergartens or schools if the infected children were kindergarteners or elementary school students. It was suggested that younger children (<3 years old) refrain from going to kindergartens during the EV71 epidemic to decrease the risk of exposure to EV71.

Enterovirus excretion through stool can persist for up to 11 weeks. Therefore, hand washing or general hygiene precaution should be advocated at convalescence. We found that subclinical EV infection could occur, and that live vaccine poliovirus did not interfere with the invasion of other non-polio EV (Chung et al., 2001).

8.7.2. EV71-related Disease and Laboratory Surveillance

The 1998 EV71 epidemic was detected by the sentinel surveillance system of infectious diseases. Taiwan CDC also established virological surveillance for the enterovirus and influenza, and there were 10 viral laboratories for surveillance in different areas of Taiwan in 2000. These systems, both clinical and laboratory, serve public health workers where EV71 exists and allow for possible earlier control and prevention measures so that the spread of EV71 can be contained or limited.

8.7.3. Vaccination

Although the above preventive measures have been in practice for 5 years in Taiwan, there were still fatal EV71 cases from 2000 to 2002. Therefore, development of a vaccine may be the only effective measure against it. Since poliovirus was eradicated by the polio vaccination, EV71 has become the most important enterovirus to affect children and is the candidate for future vaccine development.

Because EV71 receptor has not been found, no transgenic mouse model has been made available, so a newborn mouse model has been used instead (Yu et al., 2000). In that study, experimental infection with EV71 induced death in neonatal mice in an age- and dose-dependent manner. The mortality rate was 100% after intraperitoneal inoculation of 1-day-old ICR mice, and this gradually decreased as the age at the time of inoculation increased (60% in 3-day-old mice, and no deaths occurred in mice older than 6 days of age). Two studies in Taiwan have demonstrated that inactivated EV71 virus vaccine can protect against lethal enterovirus 71 infection in newborn mice by passive immunization from immunized mice mother or adult mice (Yu, 2000; Wu, 2001).

Yu et al. (2000) found that protection against EV71 challenge in neonatal mice could be seen after passive transfer of serum from actively immunized adult mice 1 day after inoculation with the virus. Pups from hyperimmune dams were resistant to EV71 challenge. Additionally, maternal immunization with a formalin-inactivated whole-virus vaccine prolonged the survival of pups after EV71 lethal challenge.

In a study by Wu et al. (2001), the inactivated virus vaccine (10 μg protein/mouse), subunit vaccines—VP1 DNA vaccine (100 μg/mouse) or recombinant VP1protein (10 μg/mouse)—was injected into the female dams to elicit maternal antibody and to provide protection against lethal infection of EV71 in suckling mice. With a challenge dose of 2300 LD_{50} virus/mouse, suckling mice born to dams immunized with inactivated virus showed 80% survival. The subunit vaccines provided protection only at a lower challenge dosage of 230 LD_{50} per mouse, with 40% survival for DNA vaccine and 80% survival for VP1 protein. In addition, the inactivated virus elicited a much greater immune response than the subunit vaccines, including total IgG, all four IgG subtypes, and T-helper-cell responses. The data has indicated that inactivated virus is the choice for vaccine preparation. The ideal virus strain for vaccine production has also been found by this group.

The newborn mice animal studies are still in progress, and monkey or chimpanzee studies may be done in the near future. Hopefully, EV71 vaccine can be developed to control future epidemics in the Asia-Pacific area.

8.8. Future Directions

For the future, it is important to continue EV71 disease and laboratory surveillance, to do molecular genetic studies, to find host factors for susceptibility and severe disease, viral neurovirulent factors, and EV71 receptor, and to develop antiviral therapy and vaccine. Anti-EV71 drugs and vaccine development may be the most promising in the control of epidemics, but better animal models are needed. Finding the EV71 receptor and developing a better animal model (possible EV71-receptor transgenic mice) may be necessary for further drug and vaccine development.

Currently in Taiwan, much research is being done on the development of effective control measures (i.e., antiviral drugs and EV71 vaccine). We hope for success in the near future.

References

Almela, M. J., Gonzalez, M. E., and L. Carrasco. (1991). Inhibitors of poliovirus uncoating efficiently block the early membrane permeabilization induced by virus particles. *J. Virol.* 65:2572–2577.

Andries, K., Dewindt, B., De Brabander, M., Stokbroekx, R., and Janssen, P.A. (1988). In vitro activity of R 61837, a new antirhinovirus compound. *Arch. Virol.* 101:155–167.

Andries, K., Dewindt, B., Snoeks, J., Willebrords, R., van Eemeren, K., Stokbroekx, R., and Janssen, P. A. (1992). In vitro activity of pirodavir (R 77975), a substituted phenoxy-pyridazinamine with broad-spectrum antipicornaviral activity. *Antimicrob. Agents Chemother.* 36:100–107.

Andries, K., Rombaut, B., Dewindt, B., and Boeye, A. (1994). Discrepancy between infectivity and antigenicity stabilization of oral poliovirus vaccine by a capsid-binding compound. *J. Virol.* 68:3397–3400.

Belnap, D. M., Filman, D. J., Trus, B. L., Cheng, N., Booy, F. P., Conway, J. F., Curry, S., Hiremath, C. N., Tsang, S. K., Steven, A. C., and Hogle, J. M. (2000). Molecular tectonic model of virus structural transitions: the putative cell entry states of poliovirus. *J. Virol.* 74:1342–1354.

Bergelson, J. M., Shepley, M. P., Chan, B. M., Hemler, M. E., and Finberg, R. W. (1992). Identification of the integrin VLA-2 as a receptor for echovirus 1. *Science.* 255:1718–1720.

Billich, A. (2000). Pleconaril Sanofi Synthelabo/ViroPharma. *Curr. Opin. Invest. Drugs.* 1:303–307.

Blomberg, J., Lycke, E., Ahlfors, K., Johnsson, T., Wolontiss, S., and Von Eeipel, G. (1974). New enterovirus type associated with epidemic of aseptic meningitis and/or hand, foot, and mouth disease. *Lancet* 7872:112.

Bowtell, D. D. (1999). Options available—from start to finish—for obtaining expression data by microarray. *Nat. Genet.* 21:25–32.

Cardosa, M. J., Perera, D., Brown, B. A., Cheon, D., Chan, H. M., Chan, K. P., Cho, H., McMinn, P. (2003). Molecular epidemiology of human enterovirus 71 strains and recent outbreaks in the Asia-Pacific region: comparative analysis of the VP1 and VP4 genes. *Emerg. Infect. Dis.* 9:461–468.

Chan, L. G., Parashar, U. D., Lye, M. S., Ong, F. G., Zaki, S. R., Alexander, J. P., Ho, K. K., Han, L. L., Pallansch, M. A., Suleiman, A. B., Jegathesan, M., Anderson, L. J. (2000). Deaths of children during an outbreak of hand, foot, and mouth disease in sarawak, malaysia: clinical and pathological characteristics of the disease. For the Outbreak Study Group. *Clin. Infect. Dis.* 31:678–683.

Chang, L. Y., Lin, T. Y., Hsu, K. H., Huang, Y. C., Lin, K. L., Hsueh, C., Shih, S. R., Ning, H. C., Hwang, H. S., Wang, H. S., and Lee, C. Y. (1999a). Clinical features and risk factors of pulmonary edema after enterovirus-71-related hand, foot, and mouth disease. *Lancet.* 354:1682–1686.

Chang, L. Y., Lin, T. Y., Huang, Y. C., Tsao, K. C., Shih, S. R., Kuo, M. L., Ning, H. C., Chung, P. W., Kang, C. M. (1999b). Comparison of enterovirus 71 and coxsackie-virus A16 clinical illnesses during the Taiwan enterovirus epidemic, 1998. *Pediatr. Infect. Dis. J.* 18:1092–1096.

Chang, L. Y., King, C. C., Hsu, K. H., Ning, H. C., Tsao, K. C., Li, C. C., Huang, Y. C., Shih, S. R., Chiou, S. T., Chen, P. Y., Chang, H. J. and Lin, T. Y. (2002). Risk factors of Enterovirus 71 infection and associated hand-foot-and-mouth-disease/herpangina in children during an epidemic in Taiwan. *Pediatrics* 109;e88.

Chang, L. Y., Tsao, K. C., Hsia, S. H., Shih, S. R., Huang, C. G., Chan, W. K., Hsu, K. H., Fang, T. Y., Huang, Y. C., and Lin, T. Y. (2004a). Transmission and clinical features of enterovirus 71 infections in household contacts in Taiwan. *JAMA.* 291:222–227.

Chang LY, Hsia SH, Wu CT, Huang, Y. C., Lin, K. L., Fang, T. Y., and Lin, T. Y. (2004b). Outcome of EV71 infections with or without stage-based management, 1998-2002. *Ped. Infect. Dis. J.* 23:327–331.

Chapman, M. S., Minor, I., Rossmann, M. G., Diana, G.. D., and Andries, K. (1991). Human rhinovirus 14 complexed with antiviral compound R 61837. *J. Mol. Biol.* 217:455–463.

Chern, J. H., Shia, K. S., Hsu, T. A., Tai, C. L., Lee, C. C., Lee, Y. C., Chang, C. S., Tseng, S. N., and Shih. S. R. (2004). Design, synthesis, and structure-activity relationships of pyrazolo[3,4-d]pyrimidines: a novel class of potent enterovirus inhibitors. *Bioorg. Med. Chem. Lett.* 14:2519–2525.

Chu, P. Y., Lin, K. H., Hwang, K. P., Chou, L. C., Wang, C. F., Shih, S. R., Wang, J. R., Shimada, Y., and Ishiko, H. (2001). Molecular epidemiology of enterovirus 71 in Taiwan. *Arch. Virol.* 146:589–600.

Chung, P. W., Huang, Y. C., Chang, L. Y., Lin, T. Y., and Ning, H. C. (2001). Duration of enterovirus shedding in stool. *J. Microl. Immunol. Infect.* 34:167–170.

Colonno, R. J., Callahan, P. L., and Long, W. J. (1986). Isolation of a monoclonal antibody that blocks attachment of the major group of human rhinoviruses. *J. Virol.* 57:7–12.

Da Silva EE, Winkler MT, and Pallansch MA. (1996). Role of enterovirus 71 in acute flaccid paralysis after the eradication of poliovirus in Brazil. *Emerg. Infect. Dis.* 2:231–233.

Dearden, C., al-Nakib, W., Andries, K., Woestenborghs, R., and Tyrrell, D. A. (1989). Drug resistant rhinoviruses from the nose of experimentally treated volunteers. *Arch. Virol.* 109:71–81.

Deibel, R., Gross, L. L., and Collins, D. N. (1975). Isolation of a new enterovirus. *Proc. Soc. Exp. Biol. Med.* 148: 203–207.

Dewindt, B., van Eemeren, K., and Andries, K. (1994). Antiviral capsid-binding compounds can inhibit the adsorption of minor receptor rhinoviruses. *Antiviral Res.* 25:67–72.

Diana, G.. D., McKinlay, M. A., Otto, M. J., Akullian, V., and Oglesby, C. (1985). [[(4,5-Dihydro-2-oxazolyl)phenoxy]alkyl]isoxazoles. Inhibitors of picornavirus uncoating. *J. Med. Chem.* 28:1906–1910.

Dove, A. W., and Racaniello, V. R. (2000). An antiviral compound that blocks structural transitions of poliovirus prevents receptor binding at low temperatures. *J. Virol.* 74:3929–3931.

Duggan, D. J., Bittner, M., Chen, Y., Meltzer, P., and Trent, J. M. (1999). Expression profiling using cDNA microarrays. *Nat. Genet.* 21:10–14.

Gelfand, H. M., LeBlanc, D. R., Fox, J. P., and Conwell, D. P. (1957). Studies on the development of natural immunity to poliomyelitis in Louisiana. II. Description and analysis of episodes of infection observed in study group households. *Am. J. Hyg.* 65:367–385.

Gilbert, G. L., Dickson, K.E., Waters, M. J., Kennett, M. L., and Land, S. A. Sneddon M. (1988). Outbreak of enterovirus 71 infection in Victoria, Australia, with a high incidence of neurologic involvement. *Pediatr. Infect. Dis. J.* 7: 484–488.

Gomes ML, de Castro CM, Oliveira MJ, da Silva EE. (2002). Neutralizing antibodies to enterovirus 71 in Belem, Brazil. *Memorias do Instituto Oswaldo Cruz.* 97:47–49.

Greve, J. M., Davis, G.., Meyer, A. M., Forte, C. P., Yost, S. C., Marlor, C. W., Kamarck, M. E., and McClelland, A. (1989). The major human rhinovirus receptor is ICAM-1. *Cell.* 56:839–847.

Groarke, J. M., and Pevear, D. C. (1999). Attenuated virulence of pleconaril-resistant coxsackievirus B3 variants. *J. Infect. Dis.* 179:1538–1541.

Ho, M., Chen, E. R., Hsu, K. H., Twu, S. J., Chen, K. T., Tsai, S. F., Wang, J. R., and Shih, S. R. (1999). The enterovirus type 71 epidemic of Taiwan, 1998. *N. Engl. J. Med.* 341: 929–935.

Hsueh, C., Jung, S. M., Shih, S. R., Lin, T. Y., Shieh, W. J., Chang, L. Y., Yen, D. C., Zaki, S., and Kuo, T. T. (2000). Acute encephalomyelitis during an outbreak of enterovirus type 71 infection in Taiwan. Report of an autopsy case with pathologic, immunofluorescence, and molecular studies. *Mod. Pathol.* 13: 1200–1205.

Huang, C. C., Liu, C. C., Chang, Y. C., Chen, C. Y., Wang, S.T., and Yeh, T. F. (1999). Neurologic complications in children with enterovirus 71 infection. *N. Engl. J. Med.* 341:936–942.

Huang, Y., Hogle, J. M., and Chow, M. (2000). Is the 135S poliovirus particle an intermediate during cell entry? *J. Virol.* 74:8757–8761.

Kogon, A., Spigland, I., Frothingham, T. E., Elveback, L., Williams, C., Hall, C. E., and Fox, J. P. (1969) The Virus Watch program: a continuing surveillance of viral infections in metropolitan New York families. VII. Observations on viral excretion, seroimmunity, intrafamilial spread and illness association in coxsackie and echovirus infections. *Am. J. Epidemiol.* 89:51–61.

Kuo, R. L., Kung, S. H., Hsu, Y. Y., and Liu, W. T. (2002). Infection with enterovirus 71 or expression of its 2A protease induces apoptotic cell death. *J. Gen. Virol.* 83:1367–1376.

Lapa, S., Mikheev, M., Shchelkunov, S., Mikhailovich, V., Sobolev, A., Blinov, V., Babkin, I., Guskov, A., Sokunova, E., Zasedatelev, A., Sandakhchiev, L., and Mirzabekov, A. (2002). Species-level identification of orthopoxviruses with an oligonucleotide microchip. *J. Clin. Microbiol.* 40:753–757.

Li, J., Chen, S., and Evans, D. H. (2001). Typing and subtyping influenza virus using DNA microarrays and multiplex reverse transcriptase PCR. *J. Clin. Microbiol.* 39:696–704.

Li, M. L., Hsu, T. A., Chen, T. C., Chang, S. C., Lee, J. C., Chen, C. C., Stollar, V., Shih, S. R. (2002). The 3C protease activity of enterovirus 71 induces human neural cell apoptosis. *Virology.* 15;293:386–395.

Lin, T. Y., Chang, L. Y., Huang, Y. C., Hsu, K. H., Chiu, C. H., and Yang, K. D. (2002). Different proinflammatory reactions in fatal and nonfatal enterovirus 71 infections: implications for early recognition and therapy. *Acta. Paediatrica.* 91:632–635.

Lin, T. Y., Hsia, S. H., Huang, Y. C., Wu, C. T., Chang, L. Y. (2003a). Proinflammatory cytokine reactions of cerebrospinal fluid in enterovirus 71 central nervous system infections. *Clin. Infect. Dis.* 36:269–274.

Lin, T. Y., Twu, S. J., Ho, M. S., Chang, L. Y., Lee, C. Y. (2003b). Enterovirus 71 outbreaks in Taiwan: occurrence and recognition. *Emerg. Infect. Dis.* 9:291–293.

Lu, C. Y., Lee, C. Y., Kao, C. L., Shao, W. Y., Lee, P. I., Twu, S. J., Yeh, C. C., Lin, S. C., Shih, W. Y., Wu, S. I., and Huang, L. M. (2002). Incidence and case-fatality rates resulting from the 1998 enterovirus 71 outbreak in Taiwan. *J. Med. Virol.* 67: 217–223.

Lum, L. C. S., Wong, K. T., Lam, S. K., Chua, K. B., Gob, A. Y. T., Lin, W. L., Ong, B. B., Paul, G., AbuBakar, S., and Lambert, M. (1998). Fatal enterovirus 71 encephalomyelitis. *J. Pediatr.* 133:795–798.

Madshus, I. H., Olsnes, S., and Sandvig, K. (1984). Different pH requirements for entry of the two picornaviruses, human rhinovirus 2 and murine encephalomyocarditis virus. *Virology.* 139:346–357.

Mallamo, J. P., Diana, G. D., Pevear, D. C., Dutko, F. J., Chapman, M. S., Kim, K. H., Minor, I., Oliveira, M., and Rossmann, M. G.. (1992). Conformationally restricted analogues of disoxaril: a comparison of the activity against human rhinovirus types 14 and 1A. *J. Med. Chem.* 35:4690–4695.

Marlin, S. D., and Springer, T. A. (1987). Purified intercellular adhesion molecule-1 (ICAM-1) is a ligand for lymphocyte function-associated antigen 1 (LFA-1). *Cell.* 51:813–819.

McKinlay, M. A. (1985). WIN 51711, a new systematically active broad-spectrum antipicornavirus agent. *J. Antimicrob. Chemother.* 16:284–286.

Mendelsohn, C. L., Wimmer, E., and Racaniello, V. R. (1989). Cellular receptor for poliovirus: molecular cloning, nucleotide sequence, and expression of a new member of the immunoglobulin superfamily. *Cell* 56:855–865.

Moeremans, M., De Raeymaeker, M., Daneels, G.., De Brabander, M., Aerts, F., Janssen, C., and Andries, K. (1992). Study of the parameters of binding of R 61837 to human rhinovirus 9 and immunobiochemical evidence of capsid-stabilizing activity of the compound. *Antimicrob. Agents Chemother.* 36:417–424.

Morens, D. M., Pallansch, M. A., and Moore, M. (1991). Polioviruses and other enteroviruses. In: Belshe RB, ed. *Textbook of Human Virology*, 2nd ed. St. Louis, MO: Mosby Yearbook; 427–497.

Mosser, A. G.., Sgro, J. Y., and Rueckert, R. R. (1994). Distribution of drug resistance mutations in type 3 poliovirus identifies three regions involved in uncoating functions. *J. Virol.* 68:8193–8201.

Nagy, G., Takatsy, S., Kukan, E., Mihaly, I., and Domok, I. (1982). Virological diagnosis of enterovirus type 71 infections: experiences gained during an epidemic of acute CNS disease in Hungary in 1978. *Arch. Virol.* 71: 217–227.

Nikolaeva, L., and Galabov, A. S. (2000). Antiviral effect of the combination of enviroxime and disoxaril on coxsackievirus B1 infection. *Acta. Virol.* 44:73–78.

Ooi, E. E., Phoon, M. C., Ishak, B., Chan, S. H. (2002). Seroepidemiology of human enterovirus 71, Singapore. *Emerg. Infect. Dis.* 8:995–997.

Otto, M. J., Fox, M. P., Fancher, M. J., Kuhrt, M. F., Diana, G. D., and McKinlay, M. A. (1985). In vitro activity of WIN 51711, a new broad-spectrum antipicornavirus drug. *Antimicrob. Agents Chemother.* 27:883–886.

Pevear, D. C., Fancher, M. J., Felock, P. J., Rossmann, M. G.., Miller, M. S., Diana, G., Treasurywala, A. M., McKinlay, M. A., and Dutko, F. J. (1989). Conformational change in the floor of the human rhinovirus canyon blocks adsorption to HeLa cell receptors. *J. Virol.* 63:2002–2007.

Rigonan, A. S., Mann, L., and Chonmaitree, T. (1998). Use of monoclonal antibodies to identify serotypes of enterovirus isolates. *J. Clin. Microbiol.* 36:1877–1881.

Rogers, J. M., Diana, G. D., and McKinlay, M. A. (1999). Pleconaril. A broad spectrum antipicornaviral agent. *Adv. Exp. Med. Biol.* 458:69–76.

Rombaut, B., Andries, K., and Boeye, A. (1996). Stabilisation of poliovirus with pirodavir. *Dev. Biol. Stand.* 87:173–180.

Romero, J. R. (2001). Pleconaril: a novel antipicornaviral drug. *Expert. Opin. Invest. Drugs.* 10:369–379.

Rossmann, M. G.. (1989a). The canyon hypothesis. *Viral. Immunol.* 2:143–161.

Rossmann, M. G.. (1989b). The canyon hypothesis. Hiding the host cell receptor attachment site on a viral surface from immune surveillance. *J. Biol. Chem.* 264:14587–14590.

Rossmann, M. G.., Arnold, E., Erickson, J. W., Frankenberger, E. A., Griffith, J. P., Hecht, H. J., Johnson, J. E., Kamer, G.., Luo, M., and Mosser, A. G.. (1985). Structure of a human common cold virus and functional relationship to other picornaviruses. *Nature* 317:145–153.

Rotbart, H. A. (1999). Antiviral therapy for enteroviral infections. *Pediatr. Infect. Dis. J.* 18:632–633.

Rozhon, E., Cox, S., Buontempo, P., O'Connell, J., Slater, W., De Martino, J., Schwartz, J., Miller, G.., Arnold, E., and Zhang, A. (1993). SCH 38057: a picornavirus capsid-binding molecule with antiviral activity after the initial stage of viral uncoating. *Antiviral. Res.* 21:15–35.

Rubessa, F., Runti, C., Ulian, F., Vio, L., and Zonta, F. (1977). [Antiviral agents. XIX. Amantadine derivatives and several others]. *Farmaco. [Sci].* 32:129–140.

Sawyer, M. H. (2001). Enterovirus infections: diagnosis and treatment. *Curr. Opin. Pediatr.* 13:65–69.

Schmidt, N. J., Lennett, E, H., and Ho, H. H. (1974). An apparently new enterovirus isolated from patients with disease of the central nervous system. *J. Infect. Dis.* 129: 304–309.

See, D. M., and J. G., Tilles. (1992). Treatment of Coxsackievirus A9 myocarditis in mice with WIN 54954. *Antimicrob. Agents Chemother.* 36:425–428.

See, D. M., and Tilles, J. G.. (1993). WIN 54954 treatment of mice infected with a diabetogenic strain of group B coxsackievirus. *Antimicrob. Agents Chemother.* 37:1593–1598.

Shia, K. S., Li, W. T., Chang, C. M., Hsu, M. C., J. Chern, H., Leong, M. K., Tseng, S. N., Lee, C. C., Lee, Y. C., Chen, S. J., Peng, K. C., Tseng, H. Y., Chang, Y. L., Tai, C. L., and Shih, S. R. (2002). Design, synthesis, and structure-activity relationship of pyridyl imidazolidinones: a novel class of potent and selective human enterovirus 71 inhibitors. *J. Med. Chem.* 45:1644–1655.

Shih, S. R., Li, Y. S., Chiou, C. C., Suen, P. C., Lin, T. Y., Chang, L. Y., Huang, Y. C., Tsao, K. C., Ning, H. C., Wu, T. Z., and Chan, E. C. (2000a). Expression of capsid protein VP1 for use as antigen for the diagnosis of enterovirus 71 infection. *J. Med. Virol.* 61:228–234.

Shih, S. R., Ho, M. S., Lin, K. H., Wu, S. L., Chen, Y. T., Wu, C. N., Lin, T. Y., Chang, L. Y., Tsao, K. C., Ning, H. C., Chang, P. Y., Jung, S. M., Hsueh, C., and Chang, K.S. (2000b). Genetic analysis of enterovirus 71 isolated from fatal and nonfatal cases of hand, foot, and mouth disease during an epidemic in Taiwan. *Virus. Res.* 68:127–136.

Shih, S. R., Wang, Y. W., Chen, G. W., Chang, L. Y., Lin, T. Y., Tseng, M. C., Chiang, C., Tsao, K. C., Huang, C. G., Shio, M. R., Tai, J. H., Wang, S. H., Kuo, R. L., and Liu, W. T. (2003). Serotype-specific detection of enterovirus 71 in clinical specimens by DNA microchip array. *J. Virol. Methods* 111:55–60.

Shih, S. R., Chen, S. J., Hakimelahi, G.. H., Liu, H. J., Tseng, C. T., and Shia, K. S. (2004a). Selective human enterovirus and rhinovirus inhibitors: An overview of capsid-binding and protease-inhibiting molecules. *Med. Res. Rev.* 24:449–474.

Shih, S. R., Tsai, M. C., Tseng, S. N., Won, K. F., Shia, K. S., Li, W. T., Chern, J. H., Chen, G. W., Lee, C. C., Lee, Y. C., Peng, K. C., and Chao, Y. S. (2004b). Mutation in enterovirus 71 capsid protein vp1 confers resistance to the inhibitory effects of pyridyl imidazolidinone. *Antimicrob. Agents Chemother.* 48:3523–3529.

Shimizu, H., Utama, A., Yoshii, K., Yoshida, H., Yoneyama, T., Sinniah, M., Yusof, M. A., Okuno, Y., Okabe, N., Shih, S. R., Chen, H. Y., Wang, G. R., Kao, C. L., Chang, K. S., Miyamura, T., and Hagiwara, A. (1999). Enterovirus 71 from fatal and nonfatal cases of hand, foot and mouth disease epidemics in Malaysia, Japan and Taiwan in 1997-1998. *Jpn. J. Infect. Dis.* 52:12–15.

Shindarov, L. M., Chumakov, M. P., Bojinov, S., Tasilenoko, S. M., Iordanov, I., Kirov, I.D., Kamenov, E., Leshchinskaya, E. V., Mitov, G., Robinson, I. A., Sivchev, S., and Staikov, S. (1979). Epidemiological, clinical, and pathomorphological characteristics of epidemic poliomyelitis-like disease caused by enterovirus 71. *J. Hyg. Epidemiol. Microbiol. Immunol.* 23:284–295.

Tagaya, I., and Tachibana, K. (1975). Epidemic of hand, foot, and mouth disease in Japan. 1972-1973: difference in epidemiologic and virologic features from the previous one. *Jpn. J. Med. Sci. Biol.* 28:231–234.

Tsao, K. C., Chan, E. C., Chang, L. Y., Chang, P. Y., Huang, C. G.., Chen, Y. P., Chang, S. C., Lin, T. Y., Sun, C. F., and Shih. S. R. (2002a). Responses of IgM for enterovirus 71 infection. *J. Med. Virol.* 68:574–580.

Tsao, K. C., Chang, P. Y., Ning, H. C., Sun, C. F., Lin, T. Y., Chang, L. Y., Huang, Y. C., and Shih, S. R. (2002b). Use of molecular assay in diagnosis of hand, foot and mouth disease caused by enterovirus 71 or coxsackievirus A 16. *J. Virol. Methods* 102:9–14.

Wang, J. R., Tuan, Y. C., Tsai, H. P., Yan, J. J., Liu, C. C., Su, I. J. (2002). Change of major genotype of enterovirus 71 in outbreaks of hand-foot-and-mouth disease in Taiwan between 1998 and 2000. *J. Clin. Microbiol.* 40:10–15.

Wang, S. M., Lei, H. Y., Huang, K. J., Wu, J. M., Wang, J. R., Yu, C. K., Su, I. J., Liu, C. C. (2003). Pathogenesis of enterovirus 71 brainstem encephalitis in pediatric patients: roles of cytokines and cellular immune activation in patients with pulmonary edema. *J. Infect. Dis.* 188:564–570.

Woods, M. G., Diana, G.. D., Rogge, M. C., Otto, M. J., Dutko, F. J., and McKinlay, M. A. (1989). In vitro and in vivo activities of WIN 54954, a new broad-spectrum antipicornavirus drug. *Antimicrob. Agents Chemother.* 33:2069–2074.

Wu, C. N., Lin, Y. C., Fann, C., Liao, N. S., Shih, S. R., Ho, M. S. (2001). Protection against lethal enterovirus 71 infection in newborn mice by passive immunization with subunit VP1 vaccines and inactivated virus. *Vaccine* 20:895–904.

Wu, T. N., Tsai, S. F., Li, S. F., Lee, T. F., Huang, T. M., Wang, M. L., Hsu, K. H., and Shen, C. Y. (1999). Sentinel surveillance for enterovirus 71, Taiwan, 1998. *Emerg. Infect. Dis.* 5:458–460.

Yang, K. D., Yang, M. Y., Li, C. C., Lin, S. F., Chong, M. C., Wang, C. L., Chen, R. F., and Lin, T. Y. (2001). Altered cellular but not humoral reactions in children with complicated enterovirus 71 infections in Taiwan. *J. Infect. Dis.* 183:850–856.

Yu, C. K., Chen, C. C., Chen, C. L., Wang, J. R., Liu, C. C., Yan JJ, and Su, I. J. (2000). Neutralizing antibody provided protection against enterovirus type 71 lethal challenge in neonatal mice. *J. Biomed. Sci.* 7:523–528.

Zeichhardt, H., Wetz, K., Willingmann, P., and Habermehl, K. O. (1985). Entry of poliovirus type 1 and Mouse Elberfeld (ME) virus into HEp-2 cells: receptor-mediated endocytosis and endosomal or lysosomal uncoating. *J. Gen. Virol.* 66:483–92.

Zhang, A., Nanni, R. G.., Li, T., Arnold, G. F., Oren, D. A., Jacobo-Molina, A., Williams, R. L., Kamer, G.., Rubenstein, D. A., and Li, Y. (1993). Structure determination of antiviral compound SCH 38057 complexed with human rhinovirus 14. *J. Mol. Biol.* 230:857–67.

9. Avian Influenza Viruses and Pandemic Influenza

MENNO DOUWE DE JONG

9.1. Introduction

Human influenza viruses can hardly be labeled as reemerging pathogens because they cause annual human epidemics of symptomatic disease, affecting approximately 20% of children and 5% of adults worldwide, and have probably done so since ancient times. Around the year 400 B.C., Hippocrates recorded "epidemic catarrhs associated with seasonal periods," which may well have been attributable to influenza viruses. Periodically, however, completely novel antigenic subtypes of influenza viruses were introduced in the human population, causing large-scale global outbreaks with high death tolls. These pandemic strains can certainly be regarded as (re)emerging pathogens. The "Athen's plague" described by Hippocrates' contemporary Thucydides is believed by some to constitute the first account of such a devastating influenza epidemic. Since the 16th century, many large-scale outbreaks of influenza-like illnesses have been described in Europe. In 1580, one of such outbreaks spread from Europe into Africa and Asia, possibly making it the first recorded influenza pandemic. The most devastating influenza pandemic in modern recorded history, known as the "Spanish flu," occurred in 1918–1919, killing up to 100 million people worldwide. Other less destructive pandemics during the past century occurred in 1957 and 1968. Avian influenza A viruses are key to the emergence of human influenza pandemics. The virus strains implicated in the 20th century's influenza pandemics originated directly from avian influenza viruses, either through genetic reassortment between human and avian influenza strains (1957, 1968) or possibly through adaptation of purely avian strains to humans (1918). It was long thought that the host range of avian influenza viruses precluded direct transmission to humans and that the emergence of pandemic strains required genetic reassortment between avian and human strains. However, occurrences of direct bird-to-human transmission of avian influenza viruses have increasingly been reported in recent years, culminating in the ongoing outbreaks of influenza A (H5N1) among poultry and wild birds in several Asian, European and African countries with continuing instances of human infections. These unprecedented developments have resulted in increasing global concerns about the (re)emergence of pandemic influenza A strains and the role of avian influenza viruses in this.

9.2. Virology

9.2.1. Biological Properties

Influenza viruses are pleomorphic, enveloped RNA viruses belonging to the family Orthomyxoviridae. Protruding from the lipid envelope are two distinct glycoproteins: the hemagglutinin (HA) and neuraminidase (NA). HA attaches to cell-surface sialic acid receptors, thereby facilitating entry of the virus into host cells. Because it is the most important antigenic determinant to which neutralizing antibodies are directed, HA represents a crucial component of current vaccines. NA is the second major antigenic determinant for neutralizing antibodies. By catalyzing the cleavage of glycosidic linkages to sialic acid on host cell and virion surfaces, this glycoprotein prevents aggregation of virions thus facilitating the release of progeny virus from infected cells. Inhibition of this important function represents the most effective antiviral treatment strategy to date. A third membrane protein, the M2 protein, is present in small quantities in influenza A viruses. By functioning as an ion channel, this protein regulates the internal pH of the virus, which is essential for uncoating of the virus during the early stages of viral replication. This function is blocked by the antiviral drugs amantadine and rimantadine.

The genome of influenza viruses is segmented, consisting of eight single-stranded, negative-sense RNA molecules that encode 10 proteins. The RNA segments are contained within the viral envelope in association with the nucleoprotein (NP) and three subunits of viral polymerase (PA, PB1, and PB2), which together form the ribonucleoprotein (RNP) complex responsible for RNA replication and transcription. Additional proteins contained within the virion include M2 and the viral nuclear export protein (NEP), which function in assembly and budding and in export of RNP from the nucleus, respectively. The only nonstructural protein of influenza A viruses is NS1, which has multiple functions in viral replication and is also thought to counteract interferon activity of the host thereby evading the immune response.

9.2.2. Classification

Based on antigenic differences in NP and M proteins, influenza viruses are classified as types A, B, and C. Influenza B and C viruses are not divided into subtypes. All avian influenza viruses are classified as type A. Further subtyping of influenza A viruses is based on antigenic differences between the two surface glycoproteins HA and NA. To date, 16 HA subtypes (H1–H16) and 9 NA subtypes (N1–N9) of influenza A viruses have been identified (Fouchier et al., 2005). The standard nomenclature for influenza viruses include the influenza type, the host of origin (excluding humans), the place of isolation, the strain number, the year of isolation, and finally the influenza A subtype in parentheses (e.g., A/Duck/Vietnam/11/04 [H5N1]).

9.2.3. Natural Hosts

The natural reservoir of influenza A viruses are aquatic birds, in which the viruses appear to have achieved an optimal level of host adaptation and do not cause disease (Webster et al., 1992). From this principal reservoir, viruses are occasionally transmitted to other animals, including mammals and domestic poultry, causing transitory infections and outbreaks. Through adaptation by mutation or genetic reassortment, some of these viruses may establish species-specific permanent lineages of influenza A viruses and cause epidemics or epizootics in the new host. In the human population, the establishment of these lineages in the 20th century was preceded by influenza pandemics. Transmission of viruses and transitory infections may also occur among the new hosts (e.g., between humans and pigs or chickens and humans).

Although all HA and NA subtypes are found in aquatic birds, the number of subtypes that have crossed the species barrier and established stable lineages in mammals is limited. Only three HA and two NA subtypes (i.e., H1N1, H1N2, H2N2, and H3N2) have circulated in humans since 1918. In horses, only two influenza A subtypes (H7N7 and H3N8) are found, while, despite susceptibility to all avian subtypes in experimental settings, the only subtypes recovered from pigs in nature are H1, H3, N1, and N2. The molecular, biological, or ecological factors determining the apparent subtype-specific ability of viruses to cross species barriers and spread among a range of hosts remain largely unresolved.

9.2.4. Determinants of Host Range

Although interspecies transmission does occur at times, there certainly are host-range restrictions. For example, avian influenza viruses usually do not replicate efficiently in humans and vice versa (Hinshaw et al., 1983; Beare and Webster 1991). Relatively little is known about the viral and host factors governing the host range of influenza viruses and the mechanisms by which species barriers are crossed. However, in view of their role in entry of the virus, the viral HA glycoproteins and their sialic acid receptors on host cells clearly are important determinants of host-range restrictions. Human influenza strains preferentially bind to sialic acid residues linked to galactose by the α2,6 linkage, and avian and equine influenza strains recognize sialic acid linked to galactose by α2,3 linkage (Rogers et al., 1983; Rogers and Paulson 1983; Rogers and D'Souza 1989; Connor et al., 1994; Gambaryan et al., 1997; Matrosovich et al., 1997, 2004). Correspondingly, human respiratory epithelial cells predominantly contain α2,6 sialic acid–galactose linkages, whereas the host cells in birds and horses mainly contain α2,3 linkages (Couceiro et al., 1993; Ito et al., 1998; Matrosovich et al., 2004). Interestingly, in contrast with the human respiratory tract, epithelial cells in the human eye predominantly contain α2,3-linked sialic acid receptors, which may explain why conjunctivitis is a common symptom of human infections with avian influenza viruses (Paulsen et al., 1998; Terraciano et al., 1999; Diebold et al., 2003). It has been hypothesized that, by serving as the main port of entry and site of initial replication, the eye may play a role in the adaptation of avian influenza viruses to humans (Olofsson et al., 2005). The presence of α2, 3-linked sialic acid receptors has also recently been demonstrated in the lower respiratory tract of humans, i.e. on bronchiolar and alveolar cells, which may explain the propensity of avian H5N1 viruses to cause pneumonia and not upper respiratory illnesses, in humans (Shinya et al., 2006; van Riel et al., 2006).

Respiratory epithelial cells in the pig contain both α2,3 and α2,6 linkages, which explains why this animal is susceptible to both human and avian influenza viruses (Ito et al., 1998). Because of this trait, the pig is widely regarded as a potential source of new pandemic strains, because it could serve as a nonselective host in which mixed infection of avian and human strains efficiently occurs, potentially resulting in new reassortant viruses, or in which purely avian strains can adapt to human receptor recognition (Figure 9.1).

The receptor specificity of HA for either of the two sialic acid–galactose linkages is determined by the structure of the receptor-binding site of HA. Although several residues have been implicated, the amino acids at positions 226 and 228 particularly seem to determine HA receptor specificity, that is, Glu-226 and Gly-228 are predicted to have affinity for avian and equine receptors, whereas Leu-226 and Ser-228 confer specificity for human receptors (Wilson et al., 1981; Rogers et al.,

1983; Naeve et al., 1984; Weis et al., 1988; Suzuki et al., 1989). Albeit less important, substrate specificity of NA for either α2,3- or α2,6-linked sialic acid also contributes to the efficiency of viral replication in different hosts (Hinshaw et al., 1983). This is illustrated by the fact that during its evolution in humans, the NA of H2N2 viruses, which were of avian origin and therefore highly specific for hydrolization of α2,3-linked sialic acids, acquired high affinity for the human α2,6-linked sialic acids (Baum and Paulson, 1991) In addition to the surface glycoproteins, laboratory experiments with reassortant viruses suggest that the genes encoding internal proteins, such as M, NP, PB1 and PB2, may also play a role in determining the host range (Almond 1977; Scholtissek et al., 1978a; Snyder et al., 1987; Subbarao et al., 1993). However, because most of these experiments evaluated reassortant viruses with different constellations of gene segments, it remains difficult to interpret whether the proteins themselves contribute to host-range restrictions or whether certain combinations of gene segments from different origins are incompatible. Manipulation of the genome using reverse genetics approaches will undoubtedly provide more definitive insight in the role of other host range determinants.

9.2.5. Antigenic Variation and the Emergence of Pandemic Influenza Strains

9.2.5.1. Antigenic Drift

Antigenic variation of influenza A viruses can occur gradually by accumulation of point mutations (antigenic drift) or drastically by genetic reassortment (antigenic shift). Antigenic drift, driven by immunological pressure on HA and NA, allows the virus to evade the immune response and is the reason that influenza viruses manage to cause yearly epidemics. It is also because of antigenic drift that periodic replacements of human vaccine strains are needed. In contrast with human and other non-avian influenza strains, antigenic drift in avian viruses is very limited despite similar mutation rates (Austin and Webster, 1986; Kida et al., 1987; Liu et al., 2004). Most likely, this reflects optimal adaptation of these viruses to the host resulting in limited immunological pressure and consequent evolutionary stasis of these viruses in their natural reservoir.

9.2.5.2. Antigenic Shift

Drastic changes in antigenicity can occur through the acquisition of completely new surface proteins by genetic reassortment (Webster et al., 1982). The segmented nature of the influenza virus genome facilitates the exchange of genes between two viruses (e.g., human and avian strains) that coinfect a host cell. Although such exchange can result in 256 possible combinations of the eight different genomic segments of the virus, antigenic shift only arises when the reassortment at least includes the HA gene. Provided that the reassortant virus is efficiently transmissible from infected to noninfected hosts, such an antigenically novel virus strain has pandemic potential when introduced in a population that completely lacks immunity against the new surface protein (Figure 9.1A). The pig is regarded as the ideal host for reassortment in view of its equal susceptibility for human and avian influenza strains (Ito et al., 1998). However, the increasing reports of bird-to-human transmissions of avian viruses indicate that coinfections, and consequently reassortments, could also take place in humans.

Beside genetic reassortment, antigenic shift is also caused by direct transmission of non-human influenza viruses to humans, as occurred or is still occurring on a relatively large scale in Hong Kong in 1997 (H5N1), in The Netherlands in 2003 (H7N7), and in Asia, the Middle East, Europe and Africa since 2004 (H5N1) (Yuen et al., 1998; Fouchier et al., 2004; Hien et al., 2004a). As is true for reassortant viruses, these viruses are of pandemic potential when acquiring the ability for efficient transmission between humans through adaptation in either humans or an intermediate host (Figure 9.1B).

Finally, antigenic shift can occur when a previously circulating human influenza virus reemerges after an extended period of time. This happened in 1977 when H1N1 virus, which circulated in the 1950s, reappeared in the human population ("Russian flu"), possibly after escaping a laboratory (Nakajima et al., 1978; Scholtissek et al., 1978b). The reemergence of this virus gave rise to a relatively mild pandemic affecting mainly young persons who were still immunologically naive to this subtype. The same could have happened in 2005, when H2N2 virus, which had disappeared from the human population after the emergence of H3N2 viruses in 1968, was inadvertently sent to more than 3000 laboratories worldwide as part of an external quality assurance scheme (Enserink, 2005).

9.3. Pathogenesis of Avian Influenza

9.3.1. Avian Influenza Virus Infections in Natural Hosts

Avian influenza viruses can infect a wide range of domestic and wild birds, including (but not restricted to) chickens, ducks, turkeys, geese, quail, pheasants, seabirds, shore birds, and migratory birds. In these natural hosts, influenza viruses replicate in the gastrointestinal tract and are secreted in large amounts into the feces (Webster et al., 1978).

Transmission between birds occurs directly or indirectly through fecally contaminated aerosols, water, feed, and other materials.

The spectrum of disease in birds ranges from asymptomatic infection, to mild respiratory illness, to severe and rapidly fatal systemic disease. Most avian influenza viruses isolated from birds are avirulent (i.e., result in asymptomatic infection or only mild disease). Avian influenza viruses capable of causing outbreaks of severe disease (fowl plague) in chickens or turkeys are classified as highly pathogenic and are currently restricted to H5 and H7 subtypes. Typically, these highly pathogenic strains do not cause disease in ducks or geese. Infection of poultry by highly pathogenic avian influenza viruses is characterized by disseminated infection and clinically manifested by decreased egg production, respiratory signs, excessive lacrimation, edema of the head, diarrhea, neurological symptoms, and death.

9.3.2. Viral Determinants of Pathogenicity

The knowledge concerning the viral factors that determine the pathogenicity of influenza viruses is limited and is primarily derived from studies of highly pathogenic avian influenza viruses. A broad tissue tropism and the ability to replicate systemically are the hallmarks of these viruses. The most important and well-studied molecular correlate of these properties resides in the cleavability of the HA precursor glycoprotein (Webster and Rott, 1987; Garten and Klenk, 1999; Steinhauer, 1999). In the viral life cycle, post-translational cleavage of the precursor HA molecule into two subunits (HA1 and HA2) by host proteases is essential for infection to proceed. This cleavage generates a fusogenic domain at the amino terminus of HA2 that mediates fusion between the viral envelope and the endosomal membrane. HAs of avirulent avian influenza strains are cleaved only in a limited number of cell types, resulting in localized respiratory or gastrointestinal infections and mild illness. In contrast, HAs of highly pathogenic H5 and H7 strains can be cleaved in several different host cells, resulting in a broad cell tropism and the ability of causing systemic infection (Klenk and Garten, 1994; Senne et al., 1996). This apparent promiscuity of HA for a broad range of cellular proteases is determined by the structure of the HA cleavage site: HAs with high cleavability (i.e., from highly pathogenic strains) have multiple basic amino acid residues immediately upstream of the cleavage site, whereas HAs from avirulent subtypes usually have only a single arginine residue at this site (Bosch et al., 1981; Walker and Kawaoka, 1993; Senne et al., 1996; Chen et al., 1998). Evidence for the correlation between a multibasic cleavage site, susceptibility for proteases and virulence has been provided by experiments in which viruses were generated with altered cleavage sites in otherwise unchanged genetic backgrounds (Ohuchi et al., 1991; Horimoto and Kawaoka, 1994). The reason why multibasic cleavage sites seem restricted to the HAs of H5 and H7 subtypes is unclear but may suggest that the number of basic residues is limited by structural features of HA. Analyses of nucleotide sequences of H5 and H7 HA genes has shown the occurrence of direct repeats of purine-rich sequences (AAGAAA) at the cleavage site in many cases (Hirst et al., 2004). Such repeats may arise because of pausing of the transcriptase-complex at a region of secondary structure, resulting in slippage of the complex and insertion of a short repeat sequence. Additionally, recombination events between two genes of the same virus (e.g., from M or NP to HA) may result in the insertion at the cleavage site of short sequences that code for multibasic amino acid residues (Orlich et al., 1994; Suarez et al., 2004). In addition to the presence of multiple basic amino acids, susceptibility to ubiquitous proteases is also determined by the loss of a glycosylation site in the vicinity of the cleavage site (Deshpande et al., 1987; Kawaoka and Webster, 1988, 1989).

Although HA clearly is an important determinant of viral pathogenicity, animal studies indicate that virulence in mammals is a polygenic trait involving a constellation of other genes that can vary with the specific virus strain and host (Lipatov et al., 2004). However, besides HA, two genes have specifically been implicated in viral pathogenicity in mammals; that is, PB2 and NS.

By reverse genetics experiments, it has been shown that a lysine residue at position 627 (Lys627) of PB2 seems essential for high virulence and systemic replication in mice of highly pathogenic influenza H5N1 viruses responsible for the outbreak among poultry and humans in Hong Kong in 1997 (H5N1/97) (Hatta et al., 2001). The presence of Lys627 in PB2 of H5N1/97 viruses appears to determine the viral replicative efficiency in mouse cells (and not avian cells) but does not increase the tissue tropism of the virus in mice (Shinya et al., 2004). Lys627 has also been found in PB2s of some, but not all highly pathogenic H7N7 and H5N1 viruses isolated from humans during the outbreaks of these viruses among poultry and humans in 2003 (The Netherlands) and 2004 (Viet Nam, Thailand), respectively (Fouchier et al., 2004; Li et al., 2004). Interestingly, a lysine residue at position 627 of PB2 is also present in all human influenza subtypes (H1, H2, H3) (Webster, 2001). Furthermore, single-gene reassortant viruses carrying a PB2 gene of avian origin and all other genes from a human virus showed efficient replication in avian but not mammalian cells (Subbarao et al., 1993). This host cell restriction could be traced to a glutamic acid residue at position 627 of the avian PB2 instead of a lysine residue at the same position in the human virus (Subbarao et al., 1993). These observations suggest that an amino acid change to Lys627 in PB2 may help avian viruses to adapt to efficient replication in mice and possibly other mammals, thereby increasing the virulence in these hosts. Reverse genetics experiments with highly pathogenic avian influenza H5N1 and H7N7 viruses have indicated that other members of the viral polymerase complex beside PB2, i.e. PA and PBI, likely also play a role in adaptation of avian viruses to the mammalian host, suggesting that host factors are important for viral polymerase activity (Gabriel et al., 2005; Salomon et al., 2006).

In addition to PB2, the NS gene seems to play a role in the pathogenesis of avian and human influenza virus infections. This gene encodes two proteins: the nuclear export protein (NEP) and the only non-structural protein of influenza viruses, NS1. The NS1 gene or its product contribute to viral pathogenesis by allowing the virus to evade the interferon response of the host (Garcia-Sastre, 2001, 2002; Krug et al., 2003). This evasion may occur through multiple mechanisms, including interference with the activation of cell-signaling pathways and protein kinases involved in interferon induction or interference with the maturation of cellular pre-mRNA at the post-transcriptional level. The NS gene has also been implicated in determining the high pathogenicity of influenza H5N1/97 viruses in mammals. Experiments in pigs using recombinant viruses showed that the presence of the NS gene of H5N1/97 viruses greatly increased the pathogenicity of an H1N1 virus, possibly by escaping the antiviral effects of interferons and tumor necrosis factor alpha (TNF-α) (Seo and Webster 2002; Seo et al., 2002, 2004). This enhanced virulence in pigs required the presence of glutamate instead of aspartate at position 92 (Glu-92) of the H5N1 NS gene, but this amino acid change has not been found in all highly pathogenic H5N1 viruses isolated from humans or animals (Seo et al., 2002).

Beside the apparent cytokine resistance of H5N1/97 viruses, *in vitro* studies in human macrophages and respiratory cells showed that these viruses also seem to induce the transcription of proinflammatory cytokines, in particular TNF-α and interferon-β, and that the NS gene contributes to this induction (Cheung et al., 2002; Chan et al., 2005). Similar results were obtained in mice, in which infection with a recombinant H1N1 virus containing the H5N1/97 NS gene caused a cytokine imbalance in mouse lungs, characterized by increased concentrations of proinflammatory cytokines and decreased levels of anti-inflammatory cytokincs (Lipatov et al., 2005a). Cytokine dysregulation by H5N1/97 viruses is also suggested by observations in human infections.

Pathological examination of patients who died of influenza H5N1 infection during the 1997 outbreak in Hong Kong showed reactive hemophagocytic syndrome, which is believed to be a cytokine-driven condition, as the most prominent feature (To et al., 2001). In addition, exceptionally high levels of certain chemokines were observed in the serum of human cases with avian influenza H5N1 (Peiris et al., 2004). Together, these observations may suggest that a combination of increased resistance against, and high induction of cytokines by the virus synergistically lead to a profound cytokine dysregulation that may play a role in explaining the severity of illness in mammals, including humans. Although the NS gene seems to play a crucial role in this, it is likely that other particular gene constellations involving different internal genes also contribute.

9.3.3. Host Factors

The virulence of highly pathogenic avian influenza viruses is clearly influenced by the specific host. Two variants of the H5N1/97 virus, one of which was isolated from a human patient with mild repiratory illness and the other from a fatal human case, displayed similar differential pathogenicity in mice (Zitzow et al., 2002). However, in ferrets, both variants caused indistinguishable severe systemic disease (Zitzow et al., 2002). Conversely, experimental infection with H5N1/97 viruses exhibiting high virulence in mice caused localized respiratory illness without systemic spread in primates and only viral replication in the respiratory tract without clinical illness in pigs (Shortridge et al., 1998; Rimmelzwaan et al., 2001). The host factors determining the clinical outcome in animals are unclear.

The clinical outcome of human influenza is influenced by factors such as the patient's age, the level of preexisting immunity, immunosuppression, comorbidities, pregnancy, and smoking habits, indicating that host-related factors certainly contribute to pathogenesis in humans. Most of the above factors may be explained by differences in local, innate, or specific immunity at different stages of life or under specific circumstances, but other factors likely also play a role. For example, the observation that influenza-related encephalopathy seems well-recognized in Japan but less so in other countries may suggest that there are differences in proneness for certain disease manifestations among populations, possibly related to genetic differences (Morishima et al., 2002; Sugaya, 2002). Although evidence is lacking at present, it is not unlikely that host factors also play a role in the the susceptibility and pathogenesis of human infections with avian influenza viruses.

9.4. Avian Influenza Viruses Infecting Humans

9.4.1. Pandemics of the 20th Century

Introduction of an influenza A virus with a novel HA gene in a population that lacks immunity to this HA has the potential to cause a pandemic when the virus posesses the ability to spread efficiently among humans (Figure 9.1). During the 20th century, this has happened three times, in 1918, 1957, and 1968, killing millions of people worldwide. In all three pandemics, the viruses originated from avian influenza viruses.

The virus strains responsible for the influenza pandemics of 1957 and 1968 both first emerged in southeastern Asia, and both arose through reassortment of genes between avian viruses and the prevailing human influenza strain (Scholtissek et al., 1978c). The "Asian influenza" pandemic of 1957 was caused by an H2N2 virus that had acquired three genes (H2, N2, and PB1) from avian viruses infecting wild ducks, in a backbone of the circulating H1N1 human influenza strain. As the Asian flu strain emerged and established a permanent lineage, the H1N1 strains soon disappeared from the human population for unclear reasons. Similarly, the H3N2 virus causing the "Hong Kong influenza" pandemic of 1968

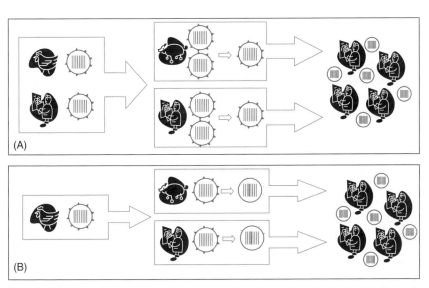

Figure 9.1. Mechanisms for generation of a pandemic influenza A strain. Pandemic influenza A strains could result from genetic reassortment involving the hemagglutinin gene between avian and human strains in coinfected pigs or humans, followed by adaptation to human receptors in either host and human-to-human transmission (A); or through adaptation to humans of a purely avian influenza strain, either in humans or in an intermediate host such as the pig (B). Mechanism A was implicated in the "Asian" (1957) and "Hong Kong" (1968) influenza pandemics. The H1N1 virus that caused the "Spanish flu" influenza pandemic of 1918 likely resulted from mechanism B.

consisted of two genes from a duck virus (H3 and PB1) in a background of the human H2N2 strain circulating at that time. The latter virus disappeared with the emergence of the H3N2 virus and since then has not been detected in humans. Sequence analysis of the hypothetical precursor strain that immediately preceded the pandemic H3N2 virus suggested that fewer than six amino acids in HA had changed during the avian-to-human transition (Bean et al., 1992). Interestingly, a number of these changes may reflect adaptation to the new host because they modified the area surrounding the receptor-binding pocket of HA, including a Glu to Leu change at position 226, which is particluarly implicated in determining specificity for human receptors (see Section 9.2.4). The fact that beside one or two novel surface glycoproteins, both pandemic strains also posessed a PB1 gene of avian origin is intriguing and may suggest a role of this gene in interspecies transmission (Kawaoka et al., 1989).

Although millions of people died during the 1957 and 1968 pandemics, the viruses involved did not appear particularly virulent, suggesting that lack of immunity was the main reason for the excess mortality. This was different during the "Spanish flu" pandemic of 1918, in which lack of immunity in the human population was combined with an apparent extremely high virulence of the virus, resulting in the demise of up to 100 million people worldwide. Because the 1918 pandemic occurred before viruses were identified as the causative agents, no intact virus has been available for analysis. This and the similar lack of available human and animal influenza strains circulating before 1918 has made it difficult to determine the exact origin of the pandemic H1N1 virus and the reason for its extreme virulence. However, valuable insight has been provided by the recovery of fragments of viral RNA isolated from archived autopsy specimens and tissue from Alaskan flu victims buried in the permafrost (Taubenberger et al., 1997). This enabled sequence analysis of all eight genes of the virus (Reid et al., 2004; Taubenberger et al., 2005). Phylogenetic analyses of these genes suggest that the 1918 H1N1 virus may not have arisen by the same mechanism as the 1957 and 1968 pandemic viruses (i.e., by reassortment of avian and human influenza viruses) but perhaps by direct transmission from an avian source after adaptation in humans or another permissive mammalian host, such as the pig (Reid et al., 2004; Taubenberger et al., 2005). This is supported by the observation that human H1N1 strains, including the 1918 pandemic strain, have retained the amino acid residues at positions 226 and 228 of HA predictive for binding to avian receptors (see Section 9.2.4) (Taubenberger et al., 1997). Recent crystallographic studies showed that structural changes in the H1 HA allowed the virus to recognize human receptors despite the presence of these avian-like residues, which may explain why the virus could nevertheless efficiently infect and spread among humans (Gamblin et al., 2004; Stevens et al., 2004). The possibility that the 1918 strain had retained the structure and biological properties of its avian ancestors while acquiring the ability to recognize and efficiently infect human cells may explain the high virulence of this virus. Mathematical modeling studies have suggested that the transmissability of the 1918 virus was not remarkably different than regular human influenza strains, indicating that extremely efficient spread did not account for the high morbidity and mortality (Mills et al., 2004). Although part of the high mortality of the 1918 pandemic could be explained by the lack of antibiotics to treat secondary bacterial pneumonia and poor living conditions, the extremely rapid and severe clinical course implies high pathogenicity of the virus as the major cause. The molecular basis for this high virulence remains unclear. The 1918 H1 HA lacks the multibasic cleavage site characteristic of highly pathogenic avian influenza viruses (see Section 9.3.2) (Taubenberger et al., 1997; Reid et al., 1999). There are conflicting observations concerning the role of the NS gene in the 1918 pandemic strain. In mice, the presence of the complete NS or only the NS1 segment seemed to confer decreased, rather than enhanced pathogenicity of reassortant H1N1 viruses (Basler et al., 2001). In contrast, *in vitro* experiments in human lung cells suggested more efficient inhibition of interferon-regulated genes by H1N1 virus in the presence of the 1918 NS gene (Geiss et al., 2002). The most convincing evidence implicates HA as an important determinant of the high virulence. The presence of HA of the 1918 virus conferred high pathogenicity in mice to human strains that were otherwise non-pathogenic in this host (Kobasa et al., 2004). Furthermore, these infections were associated with severe hemorrhagic pneumonia and the induction of high levels of macrophage-derived cytokines and chemokines, strikingly reminiscent of clinical observations in humans during the Spanish flu pandemic, as well as of recent *in vitro* and *in vivo* observations of infections with highly pathogenic avian influenza H5N1 viruses (Oxford 2000; To et al., 2001; Cheung et al., 2002; Peiris et al., 2004).

9.4.2. H7N7 Viruses

Before the year 2003, a few isolated cases of human infections with highly pathogenic H7N7 viruses were reported. These infections concerned laboratory accidents involving exposure to viral cultures or infected animals, and in one case presumed exposure to infected waterfowl in the absence of an overt outbreak (DeLay et al., 1967; Campbell et al., 1970; Taylor and Turner, 1977; Webster et al., 1981; Kurtz et al.,

1996). All reported cases, except one, were clinically characterized by self-limiting conjunctivitis. Influenza H7N7 virus was isolated from blood of one patient wih hepatitis, but the clinical relevance of this finding was unclear as was the source of this infection (DeLay et al., 1967; Campbell et al., 1970).

In 2003, a large-scale outbreak of H7N7 viruses decimated the poultry industry in The Netherlands and was associated with several human infections (Fouchier et al., 2004; Koopmans et al., 2004). After diagnosing the first case of human infection with H7N7 virus, active case finding among exposed persons and their close contacts identified a total of 89 laboratory-confirmed infections in humans (Koopmans et al., 2004). This amounted to approximately 2% of the estimated number of people potentially exposed to the virus. Highest infection rates were observed in veterinarians and chicken cullers.

Of the 89 H7N7 cases, 83 persons presented with conjunctivitis, of whom 5 also complained of influenza-like symptoms (Fouchier et al., 2004; Koopmans et al. 2004). It cannot be excluded that the remaining six patients also had conjunctivitis. Although two individuals reported an influenza-like illness only, one had suffered a previous eye injury that precluded evaluation of conjunctivitis, while the other had chronic blepharitis. Four individuals did not fit any case definition, either because of missing data or because they complained of red eyes only and therefore did not meet the criteria for a diagnosis of conjunctivitis. The prominence of conjunctivitis as the presenting syndrome in these and other reported human cases of influenza H7N7 is striking and may be explained by the presence of $\alpha2,3$-linked sialic acid receptors in the eye, which are preferentially recognized by HA of avian influenza viruses, including H7N7 subtypes (see Section 9.2.4) (Olofsson et al., 2005). The observation that, in contrast with human influenza strains, viral loads in conjunctival specimens of the Dutch H7N7-infected individuals seemed higher than in respiratory specimens, supports the notion that H7N7 virus may replicate efficiently in cells in or near the eye and not in the respiratory tract (Fouchier et al., 2004).

Six of the seven cases of influenza-like illnesses were mild. One patient, a previously healthy 57-year-old veterinarian, complained of fever and headache 2 days after visiting an infected farm (Fouchier et al., 2004). He subsequently developed pneumonia complicated by acute respiratory distress syndrome and multiorgan failure, of which he died 13 days after the onset of illness. Autopsy revealed pathologic changes in the lungs similar to those found in influenza H5N1–infected humans and no significant abnormalities in other organs. Direct human-to-human transmission of H7N7 virus during the Dutch outbreak is suggested by the fact that three individuals with confirmed infections had not been in direct contact with infected poultry but were family members of poultry workers with H7N7 conjunctivitis (Koopmans et al., 2004).

The H7N7 virus causing the outbreak in The Netherlands most likely evolved from a low pathogenic virus from wild ducks after the introduction of this virus into the poultry population (Fouchier et al., 2004). In agreement with its classification as a highly pathogenic avian influenza virus, the HA contained multiple basic amino acids at the cleavage site. Sequence comparison of virus isolates from chickens and humans, including those implicated in human-to-human transmission, revealed virtually no differences, indicating no significant accumulation of mutations on bird-to-human or human-to-human transmission. The only exception was the virus isolated from the fatal case, which showed a total of 14 amino acid substitutions not seen in the other isolates. Most of these substitutions involved the HA, NA, and PB2 genes, which have all been implicated as determinants of host range and pathogenicity. Intriguingly, the mutations in PB2 included a glutamine to lysine change at positions 627, associated with high virulence of H5N1 viruses in mice (see Section 9.3.2) (Fouchier et al., 2004).

The H7N7 outbreak in poultry was effectively contained by the culling of approximately 30 million chickens, which amounts to about 28% of the total chicken population in The Netherlands (Koopmans et al., 2004). After the first human infections were identified, individuals exposed to potentially infected chickens were vaccinated with the available human vaccine to prevent possible dual infection with human and avian strains and the resulting risk of reassortment. As the outbreak progressed, the recommendation for vaccination was extended to all poultry farmers in a 3-km radius of infected farms and to persons suspected of H7N7 infection. In addition, a prophylactic regimen of the neuraminidase-inhibitor oseltamivir was started for all people handling potentially infected poultry to prevent bird-to-human transmission and human-to-human transmission of avian viruses. Prophylactic treatment was to be continued for 2 days after the last exposure. These control measures may serve as a model for the control of emerging influenza viruses because they, at least theoretically, minimize the possibility that the virus spreads among the human population.

9.4.3. H7N3 Viruses

In early 2004, an outbreak of highly pathogenic H7N3 viruses occurred in poultry farms in British Columbia, Canada (Tweed et al., 2004). The causative virus probably had evolved by homologous recombination between the HA and M genes in a low pathogenic H7N3 virus (Hirst et al., 2004). This recombination event resulted in the introduction of a multi-basic sequence at the cleavage site of HA.

Surveillance among potentially exposed people identified two laboratory-confirmed cases of H7N3 infection. In these cases, conjunctivitis and mild influenza-like symptoms (coryza, headache) developed 1–3 days after exposure (Tweed et al., 2004). Both were treated with oseltamivir and recovered fully. No secondary cases were identified. The outbreak among poultry was contained by extensive culling. Control measures in potentially exposed people were similar to those during the Dutch H7N7 outbreak.

9.4.4. H9N2 Viruses

In 1999, human infections with H9N2 viruses were reported in two unrelated children from Hong Kong, aged 1 and 4 years (Peiris et al., 1999). Both children had a mild influenza-like syndrome, associated with mild lymphopenia in one, and slightly raised transaminase levels in the other child. Neither child developed pneumonia and both recovered uneventfully within 3–7 days. There was a history of probable contact with live chickens in one of the patients, but otherwise the source of transmission was unclear. No serological evidence of H9N2 infection was found in the children's family members or health care workers. Three serum samples from 150 volunteer blood donors in Hong Kong showed the presence of neutralizing antibodies against H9N2 virus, suggesting that additional infections had occurred in Hong Kong (Peiris et al., 1999). Around the same time as the infections in Hong Kong, five additional, similarly mild cases of human H9N2 in humans were reported from mainland China (Guo et al., 1999).

The human infections in Hong Kong and mainland China were caused by non-highly pathogenic H9N2 viruses of two disinct lineages. The Hong Kong virus was related to a quail H9N2 virus (A/quail/HK/G1/97 [H9N2]) and possessed internal genes similar to the H5N1 virus that caused the outbreak in poultry and humans in 1997 (Guan et al., 1999, 2000; Lin et al., 2000). This may suggest that the quail H9N2 virus has been the donor of all internal genes to the H5N1 outbreak strain (Guan et al., 1999). The strains isolated from humans in mainland China were related to a different lineage of H9N2 viruses found in ducks and chickens (A/duck/HK/Y280/97 [H9N2] and A/Chicken/HK/G9/97 [H9N2]) (Guo et al., 2000). Most H9N2 strains isolated since 1999 seem to be related antigenically to the latter virus but posess a variety of internal gene constellations, including those of H5N1/97-like origin (Choi et al., 2004; Lipatov et al., 2004).

Interestingly and perhaps concerning, H9N2 viruses isolated from poultry have acquired a preference for binding to the human-like $\alpha2,6$ sialic acid–galactose linkages, which may suggest that certain species of poultry could act as an intermediate host in the zoonotic transmission of influenza viruses from their natural reservoir in acquatic birds to mammals, including humans (Matrosovich et al., 2001). Indeed, H9N2 viruses have also been isolated from pigs in Southeastern China, indicating widening of the host range (Peiris et al., 2001). In addition, contemporary human H3N2 strains are cocirculating in southeastern Chinese pigs, providing ideal circumstances for potential genetic reassortment leading to the emergence of viruses with pandemic potential (Peiris et al., 2001).

9.4.5. H5N1 Viruses

9.4.5.1. Outbreaks of Influenza H5N1 in Poultry and Humans

In recent years it has become clear that, in contrast with the usually mild illnesses caused by H7 and H9N2 viruses, human infections with highly pathogenic influenza H5N1 viruses are associated with severe, often fatal disease. In May 1997, after outbreaks of influenza H5N1 among poultry on three farms in the New Territories of Hong Kong, an influenza H5N1 virus was isolated from a 3-year-old boy in Hong Kong, who died of severe pneumonia complicated by acute respiratory distress syndrome and Reye syndrome (Subbarao et al., 1998). In November and December of the same year, concomittant with outbreaks of influenza H5N1 among chickens in poultry markets and on farms in Hong Kong, 17 additional cases of human H5N1 infections were identified, five of which were fatal (Yuen et al., 1998; Chan 2002). The outbreak was contained after the slaughtering of all 1.5 million chickens in Hong Kong. In response to the outbreak, influenza surveillance in poultry was intensified permitting early recognition of other outbreaks of avian influenza in 2001 and 2002. No further human H5N1 infections were reported until February 2003, when two laboratory-confirmed cases and one probable case were identified in one family from Hong Kong (Peiris et al., 2004). The daughter died of an undiagnosed respiratory infection while visiting Fujian Province in mainland China. Upon their return to Hong Kong, the father and son developed severe respiratory illnesses of which the father died. H5N1 virus was isolated from both patients.

In December 2003, an outbreak of highly pathogenic H5N1 virus was identified among poultry in the Republic of Korea (Lee et al., 2005). Subsequently, outbreaks by antigenically related viruses were reported among poultry in Thailand, Viet Nam, Japan, China,

Cambodia, Laos, Malaysia, and Indonesia. The reason for this apparent simultaneous occurrence of H5N1 outbreaks in many Asian countries remains unclear. However, H5N1 viruses have also been found in dead migratory birds, which may suggest a role of wild birds in the spread of H5N1 viruses in the region (Li et al., 2004).Since 2005, migratory birds indeed have also been responsible of spreading the virus to regions outside Asia, including several countries in the Middle East, Europe and Africa.

Human infections during the Southeast Asian outbreaks were first reported in early 2004 from Viet Nam and Thailand, (Hien et al., 2004a; Chotpitayasunondh et al., 2005). Since then, concurrent with the spread of the virus by migrating birds and consequent poultry outbreaks elsewhere, human H5N1 infections have been reported in several other countries in Asia (China, Cambodia, Indonesia), Eurasia and Europe (Azerbaijan, Iraq, Turkey), and Africa (Egypt, Djibouti). At the time of this writing (May 2006) more than 200 human infections have been reported worldwide of which more than half were fatal (WHO, 2005). It cannot be excluded and may even be likely that additional cases have gone unnoticed in affected countries due to a lack of clinical awaress, active surveillance, or diagnostic facilities (Hien et al., 2004b).

Although many countries initially affected by poultry outbreaks in 2004 have been declared free of the virus, H5N1 virus seems to have reached endemic levels in poultry and aquatic birds in several Asian countries, despite attempts to contain the outbreak by extensive culling of poultry. This is also suggested by the establishment of multiple geographically distinct sublineages of H5N1 influenza viruses in Asia (Chen et al., 2006). Continuing occurrences of bird-to-human transmissions increase the opportunity of the virus to adapt to humans and acquire the ability to spread between humans. In addition, continuing cocirculation of avian and human viruses in countries, where humans live in close proximity with poultry and pigs, increases the risk of reassortment between both in coinfected humans or other mammalian hosts, such as the pig. The isolation of H5N1 viruses from pigs in China and Indonesia is concerning in this respect (Chen et al., 2004). For all these reasons, the current developments in Asia and other regions in the world seem to justify the global concern that, similar to 1957 and 1968, a new pandemic influenza strain may emerge in the near future.

9.4.5.2. The Clinical Spectrum of Human H5N1 Infections

At presentation, most cases of human H5N1 infections were characterized by a severe influenza syndrome, clinically indistinguishable from severe human influenza, with symptoms of fever, cough, and shortness of breath, and radiological evidence of pneumonia (Yuen et al., 1998; Hien et al., 2004a; Chotpitayasunondh et al., 2005). Abnormalities on chest radiographs at presentation included extensive, usually bilateral infiltration, lobar collapse, focal consolidation, and air bronchograms (Figure 9.2). Radiological evidence of pulmonary damage could still be observed in surviving patients several months after the illness (T.T. Hien, personal communication). Beside respiratory symptoms, a large proportion of patients also complained of gastrointestinal symptoms such as diarrhea, vomiting, and abdominal pain, which are common in children with human influenza, but not in adults. In some cases, diarrhea was the only presenting symptom, preceding other clinical manifestations (Apisarnthanarak et al., 2004; de Jong et al., 2005). Unlike human infections with H7 or H9 viruses, conjunctivitis was not prominent in H5N1-infected patients. The clinical course of the illness in severe cases was characterized by rapid development of severe bilateral pneumonia necessitating ventilatory support within days after onset. Complications included acute respiratory distress syndrome, renal failure, and multiorgan failure. Evidence that the clinical spectrum of human H5N1 infections is not restricted to pulmonary symptoms was provided by a reported case of possible central nervous system involvement in a Vietnamese boy who presented with diarrhea, followed by coma and death. Influenza H5N1 virus was isolated from throat, rectal, blood, and cerebrospinal fluid specimens, suggesting widely disseminated viral replication (de Jong et al., 2005). His sister had died of a similar illness 2 weeks earlier, but no diagnostic specimens were obtained. Although highly virulent H5N1 viruses have shown neurotropism in mammals such as mice and

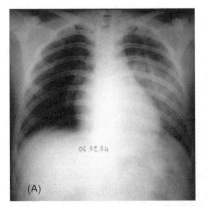 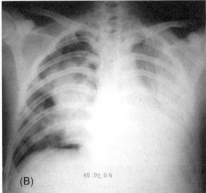

Figure 9.2. Influenza H5N1 pneumonia. Chest radiographs of an influenza H5N1 patient obtained at admission (A) and 4 days later (B).

cats (Lipatov et al., 2003; Tanaka et al., 2003; Keawcharoen et al., 2004), these cases may be similarly rare as central nervous system manifestations associated with human influenza (Morishima et al., 2002; Sugaya, 2002). Genetic predisposition of the host to such manifestations may play a role.

Striking routine laboratory results in H5N1-infected patients, especially in severe cases, were an early onset of lymphopenia, with a pronounced inversion of the CD4+/CD8+ ratio, thrombocytopenia, and increased levels of serum transaminases (Yuen et al., 1998; Hien et al., 2004a; Chotpitayasunondh et al., 2005). High levels of cytokines and chemokines have been observed in several H5N1-infected patients, suggesting a role of immune-mediated pathology in the pathogenesis of H5N1 infections (see Section 9.3.2) (To et al., 2001; Peiris et al., 2004). This was supported by pathological examination in two patients who died during the outbreak in Hong Kong, which showed reactive hemophagocytosis as the most prominent feature (To et al., 2001). Other findings included diffuse alveolar damage with interstitial fibrosis, hepatic central lobular necrosis, acute renal tubular necrosis, and lymphoid depletion. Although the gastrointestinal, hepatic, renal, and hematologic manifestations could suggest wider tissue tropism, there was no evidence of viral replication in organs outside the respiratory tract (To et al., 2001).

Although many laboratory-confirmed H5N1 infections were associated with severe, often fatal disease, milder cases have also been reported, especially during the outbreak in Hong Kong (Yuen et al., 1998; Chan 2002). An increasing number of milder cases also seemed to occur in Viet Nam, as the outbreak progressed in 2005 (WHO, 2005). Although increased clinical awareness and surveillance may account for such observations, progressive adaptation of the virus to humans is the dreaded alternative explanation. Detailed monitoring of virus evolution during outbreaks is obviously important and may help to distinguish between both possibilities. The occurrence of mildly symptomatic and asymptomatic infections have also been suggested during the outbreak in Hong Kong by seroepidemiological studies in household members of H5N1-infected patients and health care workers. In these studies, 8 of 217 exposed and 2 of 309 nonexposed health care workers were seropositive for H5N1-specific antibodies (Bridges et al., 2002). Seroconversion was documented in two exposed nurses, one of whom reported a respiratory illness 2 days after exposure to an H5N1-infected patient. More importantly than showing the occurrence of asymptomatic infections, these data indicated that nosocomial person-to-person transmission had occurred, albeit limited to a few cases. An additional case of possible human-to-human transmission during the Hong Kong outbreak was suggested by

H5N1-seropositivity in a household contact of a patient, who had no history of poultry exposure (Katz et al., 1999). Seroepidemiological studies in health care workers involved in the care of H5N1-infected patients in Thailand and Viet Nam in 2004 have not shown evidence of person-to-person transmission, despite the absence of adequate infection control measures in the Vietnamese cohort at the time of study (Apisarnthanarak et al., 2005; Liem and Lim, 2005; Schultsz et al., 2005). During the outbreak in Thailand in 2004, extensive epidemiological investigations have suggested person-to-person transmission from a child, who died of presumed H5N1 infection, to her mother who had no history of exposure to poultry and had provided prolonged unprotected nursing care to her daughter (Ungchusak et al., 2005). An aunt of the child may have been infected by the same route because her last exposure to poultry before infection had been 17 days, considerably longer than the estimated incubation period of 2–10 days. There have been several similar family clusters of H5N1 cases in other affected countries, which have all ignited concerns about the possibility of human-to-human transmission, but most of which could be explained by common exposure to poultry. Although there has been no evidence of efficient transmission of influenza H5N1 virus between humans to date, caution and detailed investigations obviously remain warranted in case of any cluster of infections, especially in view of the relatively rapid evolution H5N1 viruses have exhibited in recent years.

9.4.5.3. The Evolution of H5N1 Viruses, 1997–2004

In 1996, an H5N1 virus was isolated from geese during an outbreak in Guangdong Province in China (influenza A/Goose/Guangdong/1/96 [A/G/Gd/96]) (Xu et al., 1999). This virus proved to be the donor of the HA gene of the reassortant H5N1 viruses causing the outbreak among poultry and humans in Hong Kong in 1997. The internal genes of the Hong Kong H5N1 viruses were closely related to those of an H9N2 virus isolated from quail (see Section 9.4.3) (Guan et al., 1999). The origin of the NA gene remains unclear but was notable for a 19-amino-acid deletion in the stalk region (Subbarao et al., 1998). Such deletions may be associated with adaptation of influenza viruses to land-based poultry (Matrosovich et al., 1999). The HA gene contained multibasic sequences at the cleavage site, in accordance with its classification as a highly pathogenic strain (Claas et al., 1998; Matrosovich et al., 1999). The role of other genes potentially involved in its pathogenicity is reviewed in Section 9.3.2.

After the eradication of the 1997 Hong Kong strain, the goose precursor viruses continued to circulate in geese in southeastern China

(Cauthen et al., 2000; Webster et al., 2002). Through reassortment between this virus and other avian viruses, multiple antigenically similar genotypes, which were highly pathogenic in chickens but not in ducks, emerged and again were eradicated in Hong Kong in 2001 and 2002 (Guan et al., 2002). Then, in late 2002, H5N1 strains isolated from wild migratory birds and resident waterfowl in two Hong Kong parks showed marked antigenic drift and exhibited high pathogenicity in ducks (Guan et al., 2004; Sturm-Ramirez et al., 2004). The latter property is rarely found in nature and had not been observed in strains isolated during previous years. An antigenically and molecularly similar virus caused the two confirmed human infections in early 2003 in a family from Hong Kong (see Section 9.4.5.1) (Guan et al., 2004; Peiris et al., 2004).

H5N1 influenza viruses isolated from healthy ducks in southern China between 1999 and 2002 were all antigenically similar to the precursor influenza A/G/Gd/96 virus (Chen et al., 2004). It is thought that these ducks played a central role in the generation of the virus responsible for the outbreaks in Southeast Asia since 2003. Detailed genetic analyses of H5N1 strains isolated during the period 2000–2004 from poultry and humans in China, Hong Kong, Indonesia, Thailand, and Viet Nam demonstrated that a series of genetic reassortment events, all traceable to the A/G/Gd/96-precursor virus, ultimately gave rise to a dominant H5N1 genotype (genotype Z) in chickens and ducks (Li et al., 2004). This genotype is implicated in the human cases in Hong Kong in 2003 and the outbreaks among poultry and humans since 2004.

The evolution of H5N1 viruses in recent years has been associated with increasing virulence and an expanding host range, which beside terrestrial poultry and wild birds also includes mammals. Although all H5N1 viruses isolated from ducks in China between 1999 and 2002 were highly pathogenic in chickens, an increasing level of pathogenicity was observed in mice with the progression of time: virus isolated in 1999 and 2000 were less pathogenic than those isolated in 2001 and 2002 (Chen et al., 2004). It has been suggested that the increasing ability to replicate in mammals has resulted from transmission between ducks and pigs The expanding host range is also illustrated by successful experimental infection of domestic cats and natural infections of cats, tigers and leopards with recent H5N1 strains (Keawcharoen et al., 2004; Kuiken et al., 2004; Songserm et al., 2006).

In summary, continued evolution of H5N1 viruses since 1997, involving multiple genetic reassortment events between A/G/Gd/96-like viruses and other avian viruses and perhaps transmission between birds and pigs or other mammalian hosts, has resulted in a highly virulent genotype with an expanded host range that is causing widespread outbreaks among wild birds, poultry and humans affecting several regions in the world. Although transmission between birds and humans at present still seems inefficient, as does transmission between humans, this may change when the virus is allowed to continue its evolution through adaptation and reassortment.

9.5. Laboratory Diagnosis of Avian Influenza

In clinical trials, human influenza has been clinically diagnosed correctly in approximately two-thirds of adults with influenza-like symptoms, despite the lack of pathognomomic features (Monto et al., 2000). Although virus isolation remains the gold standard of diagnosis and indispensable for virus characterization, rapid laboratory confirmation of suspected human influenza in routine diagnostic laboratories is usually performed by immunochromatographic or immunofluorescent detection of influenza virus antigens or by reverse transcriptase (RT)-PCR detection of viral nucleic acids in respiratory specimens. In addition, serological evidence of human influenza A virus infection can be obtained by commercially available ELISA kits that detect antibodies to conserved viral antigens, such as the nucleoprotein. In the absence of cocirculating avian influenza strains in the human population, further subtyping of influenza viruses or detection of subtype-specific antibodies are usually not done by routine diagnostic laboratories but are restricted to reference laboratories involved in epidemiological analyses and planning of vaccine strains. However, in case of an outbreak of avian influenza, efforts to further subtype the virus (e.g., by subtype-specific RT-PCR methods) should be made by routine laboratories because immediate knowledge about the infecting influenza subtype is essential for infection control and timely epidemiological investigations. Dependence on reference laboratories, which in the case of many Southeast Asian countries affected by avian influenza outbreaks are situated abroad, potentially results in unacceptable delays and hampers timely recognition of outbreaks and institution of adequate control measures (Hien et al., 2004b). However, the reality is that diagnostic facilities in many affected countries are scarce and often not sufficiently equipped for virological diagnostics, let alone subtyping of influenza viruses. Global efforts to improve diagnostic capacity in resource-poor countries may prove an important step toward the prevention and control of pandemic influenza (Hien et al., 2004b).

9.5.1. Virus Isolation

Similar to human influenza viruses, avian viruses can be isolated in embryonated eggs or in cell culture, using permissive cells such as Madin

Darby canine kidney (MDCK) cells or rhesus monkey kidney (LLC-MK2) cells. Unlike human strains and avirulent avian strains and in accordance with their promiscuity for cellular proteases, highly pathogenic avian viruses do not require the addition of exogenous trypsine for efficient replication in cell culture. For safety purposes, the isolation of highly pathogenic avian influenza virus requires biosafety level 3 laboratory facilities or higher. Cytopathic effects in cell culture are nonspecific. Initial identification of influenza A virus can be performed by immunofluorescence staining with monoclonal antibodies against the nucleoprotein. Further HA and NA subtyping is performed by subtype-specific RT-PCRs of culture supernatant or hemagglutination inhibition and neuraminidase inhibition assays using a panel of reference antisera against various subtypes. In human infections, avian influenza viruses have mostly been isolated from conjunctival swabs and respiratory specimens such as throat or nasal secretions or washings (Yuen et al., 1998; Fouchier et al., 2004; Hien et al., 2004a). In one case of H5N1 infection, virus was also isolated from serum, cerebrospinal fluid, and a rectal swab (de Jong et al., 2005).

9.5.2. Antigen Detection

Detection of influenza A viral antigens in clinical specimens by direct immunofluorescence or by rapid immunochromatographic assays is widely used for diagnosis of human influenza because of their ability for rapid diagnosis. However, in patients with avian influenza, the usefulness of these assays seems limited due to low sensitivity, possibly because of lower viral loads than during human influenza (Yuen et al., 1998; Peiris et al., 2004). In addition, some rapid antigen detection kits do not distnguish between influenza types A and B, and none of the currently available immunofluoresence and immunochromatographic assays distnguishes between influenza A subtypes. However, developments of H5N1-specific rapid antigen detection tests are ongoing (Xu et al., 2005).

9.5.3. RT-PCR

RT-PCR methods allow for sensitive and specific detection of viral nucleic acids and have shown to increase the diagnostic sensitivity for many viral pathogens when compared with culture or antigen detection methods. During the H5N1 outbreaks in Hong Kong and Southeast Asia, RT-PCR methods for specific detection of H5N1 viral nucleic acids proved valuable and seem to be the diagnostic methods of choice in case of an outbreak of avian influenza (Yuen et al., 1998; Hien et al., 2004a; Chotpitayasunondh et al., 2005). Especially when using real-time PCR technology, a reliable subtype-specific diagnostic result can be generated within a few hours after specimen collection. A disadvantage of RT-PCR methods is its proneness for contamination and the consequent risk of false-positive results, which should be minimized by proper precautions, including physical separation of laboratories for PCR preparation and amplification. In addition, the inclusion of an internal control in RT-PCR assays is highly desirable to monitor for false-negative results due to inefficient nucleic acid extraction, cDNA synthesis, or amplification.

9.5.4. Serology

During outbreaks of avian influenza, the detection of subtype-specific antibodies is particularly important for epidemiological investigations. Hemagglutination inhibition (HI) assays are the gold standard for detection of antibodies against human influenza viruses. However, their usefulness for detection of antibodies against avian viruses in mammalian species, including humans, seems limited (Hinshaw et al., 1981; Beare and Webster, 1991; Kida et al., 1994). Several studies have shown a failure to detect HI antibodies against avian viruses in mammals, even in cases where infection was confirmed by virus isolation. Possible reasons for this failure include poor immunogenicity of some avian viruses and lack of sensitivity to detect low-titered or less avid antibodies induced by avian viruses (Hinshaw et al., 1981; Lu et al., 1982; Kida et al., 1994; Rowe et al., 1999). It has been demonstrated that HI testing with subunit HA, but not with intact virus, could detect antibodies against an avian H2N2 virus (Lu et al., 1982). However, neutralizing antibodies against this virus could readily be detected with intact virus. A direct comparison of HI testing with a microneutralization assay in H5N1-infected persons from the 1997 Hong Kong outbreak indeed showed the latter to be more sensitive (Rowe et al., 1999). Although an indirect ELISA assay using recombinant HA from H5N1/97 showed at least equal sensitivity as the microneutralization assay, the specificity in adult sera was inferior, most likely due to the presence of cross-reactive epitopes common to all HAs (Rowe et al., 1999). Based on these observations, neutralization assays are the methods of choice for detection of antibodies against avian viruses in humans.

Using these assays, it has been shown that the kinetics of the antibody response against H5N1 virus in patients infected during the Hong Kong outbreak are similar to the primary response to human influenza viruses (Katz et al., 1999). Neutralizing antibodies were generally detected 14 or more days after the onset of symptoms, and titers equal to or higher than 1:640 were observed 20 or more days after onset. Using neutralization assays, antibodies against H9N2 could be detected in a small number of blood donors from Hong Kong (Peiris et al., 1999). However, in two laboratory-confirmed H7N3-infected patients with conjunctivitis, no neutralizing antibodies could be detected in sera obtained more than 20 days after onset of the illness (Tweed et al., 2004). Similarly, no HI antibodies could be detected in an H7N7-infected patient with conjunctivitis (Webster et al., 1981). Although the reason for this apparent failure to mount an antibody response remains unclear, it has been suggested that this could be secondary to the highly localized nature of the infection in these cases (Tweed et al., 2004).

9.6. Treatment and Prevention

9.6.1. Antiviral Treatment

Currently, two classes of drugs are available with antiviral activity against influenza viruses: inhibitors of the ion channel activity of the M2 membrane protein, amantadine and rimantadine; and inhibitors of the neuraminidase, oseltamivir and zanamivir. The therapeutic efficacy of amantadine in human influenza is unclear due to a paucity of reliable clinical studies, but reductions of fever or illness by 1 day have been observed in adults and children (Nicholson et al., 2003). Major disadvantages of amantadine include neurotoxicity and a rapid development of drug resistance during treatment. Resistance is conferred by single nucleotide changes resulting in amino acid substitutions at positions 26, 27, 30, 31, or 34 of the M2 protein. Rates of resistance against amantadine in human influenza viruses has increased from less than 0.5% in 1994-1995 to more than 12% in 2003-2004. Particularly high resistance frequencies of up to 61% were observed in viruses isolated in Asia (Bright et al., 2005). Rimantadine causes less neurological side effects but is not available in most parts of the world. Although several H5N1-infected patients have been treated with amantadine during the 1997 H5N1 outbreak in Hong Kong, the numbers were too small to draw any meaningful conclusions concerning its activity against this virus (Yuen et al., 1998). *In vitro* sensitivity testing of virus isolated from the first patient during this outbreak showed normal susceptibility to amantadine (Subbarao et al., 1998). Strikingly, the sublineage of genotype Z H5N1 viruses prevalent in Thailand, Viet Nam, Cambodia and Malaysia in 2004 invariably showed an amantadine-resistance conferring amino acid substitution at position 31 of the M2 protein, while this mutation was mostly not present in sublineages of H5N1 viruses isolated in other geographic regions (Li et al., 2004; Puthavathana et al., 2005; Cheung et al., 2006).

Both oseltamivir and zanamivir have proven efficacy in the treatment of human influenza when started early during the course of illness and are particularly effective as seasonal or postexposure prohylaxis (Nicholson et al., 2003). Zanamivir has poor oral availability and is therefore administered by inhalation, which has limited its use in the elderly and may induce bronchospasm. Oseltamivir can be given orally. The development of drug resistance during treatment has been reported for both drugs and is associated with mutations in the active site of neuraminidase or in the hemagglutinin. The latter mutations decrease the affinity of HA for the cellular receptor, thereby obviating the need for neuraminidase to escape the cells.

Data on the efficacy of neuraminidase inhibitors in avian influenza virus infections are scarce. The H5N1 strains implicated in the 1997 Hong Kong outbreak were susceptible *in vitro* to oseltamivir and zanamivir (Leneva et al., 2000; Govorkova et al., 2001). Oral oseltamivir and topical zanamivir also showed therapeutic and protective activities against Hong Kong H5N1 isolates in murine animal models (Gubareva et al., 1998; Leneva et al., 2001). Recent murine studies suggest that, perhaps due to higher virulence, higher doses of oseltamivir and longer durations of treatment are necessary to achieve antiviral effects in mice against H5N1 strains causing the Southeast Asian outbreak since 2004, when compared with the 1997 Hong Kong H5N1 strain (Yen et al., 2005). *In vitro* sensitivity testing of H7N7 isolates during the 2003 outbreak of this virus in The Netherlands showed normal susceptibility to zanamivir and oseltamivir (Koopmans et al., 2004). H7N7 infection was detected in 1 of 90 persons who reportedly received prophylactic treatment with oseltamivir during that outbreak, compared with 5 of 52 persons who had not taken oseltamivir prophylaxis (Koopmans et al., 2004).

Oseltamivir treatment has been given to several patients infected with avian influenza viruses, including H7N7, H7N3, and H5N1 subtypes, but no conclusions can be made concerning its efficacy. However, the timing of antiviral treatment may not have been optimal in many human cases of avian influenza so far. Beneficial effects of antiviral treatment in human influenza are optimal when started within 48 h after onset of the illness. During the H5N1 outbreak in Viet Nam in 2004, H5N1-infected patients were admitted 5 days or later after onset of symptoms (Hien et al., 2004a). Earlier recognition of avian influenza in humans may improve the efficacy of antiviral treatment. Nevertheless, favourable virological responses associated with a beneficial clinical outcome have been reported in H5N1-injected patients despite late initiation of treatment (de Jong et al., 2005). The emergence of drug-resistant H5N1 variants during prophylaxis or treatment with oseltamivir has also been reported, and may be associated with clinical failure of treatment (de Jong et al., 2005; Le et al., 2005). Treatment strategies which minimize the risk of resistance development, such as antiviral combination treatment, deserve attention. In addition, parenteral formulations of antiviral drugs may be desirable to guarantee systemic drug levels in H5N1 patients with severe disease. A novel intravenously administered neuraminidase inhibitor, peramivir, is currently in clinical development.

Although several H5N1-infected patients have received steroids in addition to oseltamivir, the potential benefits of this need formal evaluation in clinical studies (Hien et al., 2004a). Considering the observed cytokine dysregulation in H5N1-infected animals and humans, a beneficial effect of immunomodulating agents could be hypothesized and perhaps requires further study. Finally, neutralizing monoclonal antibodies have been shown effective in treating established influenza A virus infection in mice with severe combined immunodeficiency (Palladino et al., 1995). Although mice are not men, this strategy deserves attention in the treatment of a severe illness such as influenza H5N1.

9.6.2. Infection Control and Prophylaxis

Birds infected with avian influenza excrete large amounts of virus in feces and other secretions, which contaminate the direct environment, such as dust, soil, water, cages, tools, and other fomites. Avian influenza virus may remain infectious in soil, water, or contaminated equipment for weeks to months, depending on the temperature and humidity (i.e., longer in colder climates). Illness in birds caused by highly pathogenic avian influenza viruses results in systemic replication and the presence of infectious virus in their eggs and many tissues and organs. Transmission of avian influenza viruses between birds occurs directly or indirectly through contact with fecally contaminated aerosols, water, feed, and other materials. Bird-to-human transmission likely occurs via the same route (i.e., direct contact with birds or contaminated fomites).

Most, but not all human infections with avian influenza viruses involved handling of affected poultry or direct exposure to live poultry in the week before onset of the illness (Mounts et al., 1999; Hien et al., 2004a; Koopmans et al., 2004). Case-control studies during the 1997 H5N1 outbreak in Hong Kong identified visiting a stall or market selling live poultry during the week before the illness as a risk factor, whereas eating or preparing poultry products were not risk factors (Mounts et al., 1999). In cases in which no apparent direct exposure to poultry could be identified, contact with contaminated environment, such as water, has been suggested (de Jong et al., 2005). Of note, it has been shown that ducks infected by the currently circulating H5N1 strain in Southeast Asia remain healthy but excrete large amounts of virus for prolonged periods of time (Hulse-Post et al., 2005). Because water in ponds and canals in which large flocks of ducks reside is widely used for bathing and drinking in rural areas of many Southeast Asian countries, it may not be unlikely that such water represents a source of transmission when contaminated by infected ducks. In fact, contact with contaminated water is regarded as the most important mode of transmission between aquatic birds.

A limited number of possible human-to-human transmissions have been reported, which involved prolonged, close, and unprotected contact with infected patients (Katz et al., 1999; Koopmans et al., 2004; Ungchusak et al., 2005). Similar to human influenza, droplet and contact transmission are probably the most effective means of transmission of avian influenza virus between humans, should the the virus acquire the ability for efficient spread, but airborne transmission remains a possibility. The occurrence of diarrhea in H5N1-infected patients, which may contain infectious virus, represents a potential nonrespiratory route of transmission that needs to be considered in infection control practices (Apisarnthanarak et al., 2004; Hien et al., 2004a; de Jong et al., 2005). Data concerning excretion patterns and periods of potential infectivity are lacking for human infections with avian influenza viruses. Based on exposure histories, the incubation time for human H5N1-infections has been estimated at 2–10 days, but it is not known whether excretion of virus occurs during this time (Yuen et al., 1998; Hien et al., 2004a). Based on the current (lack of) knowledge, infection control measures during contact with potentially infected birds or environment or with patients with suspected or confirmed infection should prevent contact, droplet, and airborne transmission. These measures include mask (preferably high-efficiency masks, with surgical masks as a second alternative), gown, face shield or goggles, and gloves.

The efficacy of neuraminidase inhibitors as seasonal or postexposure prohylaxis against human influenza is high (Nicholson et al., 2003). Offering prophylactic treatment to potentially exposed people in the setting of a poultry outbreak of avian influenza, as has been done during H7-outbreaks in The Netherlands and Canada (Koopmans et al., 2004; Tweed et al., 2004), is rational but hardly feasible during the ongoing outbreak in Asia and Africa for logistical and financial reasons. Postexposure prophylaxis to unprotected health care workers and close contacts of infected patients needs serious consideration. The potential use of specific monoclonal antibodies for prophylaxis warrants further investigation.

Eliminating the source of infection (i.e., infected birds) remains the most effective infection control measure. Culling of all infected poultry has proved succesful during avian influenza outbreaks in Hong Kong, The Netherlands, and Canada (Chan, 2002; Koopmans et al., 2004; Tweed et al., 2004). However, considering the geographic extensiveness of the outbreak, the different farming practices in affected regions, and the occurence of infection in migratory birds, it is doubtful whether culling of poultry will be able to contain the outbreaks in the various regions.

9.6.3. Vaccination

The bulk of human influenza vaccines are produced from inactivated viruses grown in embryonated eggs. Vaccine production against highly pathogenic avian influenza viruses is complicated because of the requirement for high biosafety containment facilities and the difficulty, in some cases, to obtain high virus yields in embryonated eggs because of the virus' pathogenicity (Stephenson et al., 2004; Wood and Robertson, 2004). Several other approaches have been used in an attempt to overcome these obstacles, including the use of reverse genetics techniques, generation of recombinant hemagglutinin, DNA vaccination, and the use of related apathogenic H5 viruses with and without different adjuvants (Nicholson et al., 2003; Stephenson et al., 2004; Webby et al., 2004; Wood and Robertson, 2004). Experimental H5N1 vaccines in which important virulence determinants were altered using plasmid-based reverse genetics have shown protective efficacy to homologous and heterologous H5 strains in animal models and may prove an attractive approach (Li et al., 1999; Takada et al., 1999; Lipatov et al., 2005b). Studies in humans using an H5N3 vaccine developed from a 1997 apathogenic avian virus showed high rates of seroconversions to the vaccine strain and heterologous H5N1 strains after 3 doses, but only when the vaccine was given with the adjuvant MF59 (Stephenson et al., 2005). In animal models, baculovirus-derived recombinant H5 vaccines were immunogenic and protective, but results in humans were disappointing even when using high doses (Crawford et al., 1999; Treanor et al., 2001). In a study using a subvirion influenza H5N1 vaccine, neutralizing antibody responses were observed in approximately half of the subjects receiving the highest dose of the vaccine (two intramuscular injections of 90 micrograms) (Treanor et al., 2006). H5 DNA vaccines protected mice from infection by homologous, but not by heterologous H5N1 viruses (Kodihalli et al., 1999; Epstein et al., 2002).

9.7. Pandemic Preparedness and Future Directives

The increasing frequency of outbreaks with highly pathogenic avian influenza viruses among poultry and wild birds, and direct transmission of these viruses to humans, has ignited grave concerns about an imminent influenza pandemic. Indeed, two of three prerequisites for a human pandemic have been met in the H5N1 outbreaks since 1997: the emergence of an antigenically novel strain to which the population has no immunity, and the transmission of this strain to humans in whom it can cause severe disease. To date, there fortunately is no evidence of efficient spread of H5N1 virus between humans, but continued circulation of this strain, which now has reached levels of endemicity among poultry in several Asian countries, increases the opportunity to adapt to humans through mutation or genetic reassortment in humans or intermediate mammalian hosts. As suggested by the "Spanish flu" pandemic of 1918, extremely high transmissibility is no prerequisite for a severe pandemic killing tens of millions of people, and as shown by the severe acute respiratory syndrome (SARS) virus epidemic in 2003, viruses can rapidly spread across the globe in the current age of intense global travel.

As a consequence of all this, pandemic preparedness has become an increasingly important issue, and pandemic plans are being developed by an increasing number of countries worldwide. Control measures based on case identification (e.g., contact tracing and quarantine) were essential for the control of SARS. However, during an influenza epidemic, such measures may not be as effective because of short incubation periods and the potential infectivity before the onset of case-defining symptoms. Much of the preparedness therefore will rely on clinical management and vaccination. Mathematical modelling studies have suggested the possibility of containing an influenza pandemic at the source by antiviral prophylaxis and other preventive measures (Ferguson et al., 205; Longini et al., 2005). Many developed countries are now stockpiling antiviral drugs for initial management of illness or prophylaxis during the first months of a pandemic, when vaccines are in development and not yet available. In case of an influenza pandemic, there will be limitations on the timeliness and availability of vaccines (Stohr and Esveld, 2004). It has been estimated that it could take at least 6 months for the first vaccine doses to be produced after identifying a pandemic strain. Currently, global production capacity for influenza vaccines is insufficient for worldwide coverage in case of a pandemic, especially because vaccination for the novel influenza strain likely requires two doses, and interruption of annual production of the human influenza vaccine is undesirable (Schwartz and Gellin, 2005). In response to the pandemic threat by the H5N1 outbreak in Southeast Asia, plans have been made to stockpile candidate H5N1 vaccines based on the currently circulating strain. However, there is no certainty whether the next pandemic will indeed be caused by H5N1 virus, and if so, whether antigenic drift will not have rendered the stockpiled vaccine less effective by the time pandemic spread occurs. In the latter event, such vaccines may still mitigate the illness, which is beneficial for vaccinated people but may also carry a risk of prolonged excretion and increased spread of the virus. Similar worries exist when poultry would be vaccinated with a suboptimal vaccines.

In case of an influenza pandemic, all possibilities for rapid production of vaccines, as well as potential methods to reduce doses without affecting immunogenicity should be considered. This would require the use of alternative, currently not officially approved methods for vaccine production, such as reverse genetics techniques and cell culture–based vaccine production, and the use of alternative adjuvants that may enable dose reduction (Webby and Webster, 2003; Stephenson et al., 2004; Wood and Robertson, 2004; Schwartz and Gellin, 2005). In addition, vaccine doses may be spared by alternative administration routes. It has been shown that intradermal, instead of intramuscular vaccination for human influenza may require less antigen by recruiting efficient antigen-presenting cells present in the dermis (Belshe et al., 2004; Kenney et al., 2004) .

Notwithstanding the importance of current efforts to prepare for a possible H5N1 pandemic, more structural and longer term global efforts are needed to allow for early recognition of emerging novel influenza viruses in the future. In 2002, a WHO Global Agenda for Influenza Surveillance and Control has been adopted, of which the main objectives are to strengthen surveillance, improve knowledge of the disease burden, increase vaccine use, and accelerate pandemic preparedness (Stohr, 2003). It is essential that these objectives are increasingly focused on the Southeast Asian region, which has been the source of previous pandemics and is the epicenter of the current pandemic threat. However, many Southeast Asian countries currently lack the expertise, financial means, and infrastructure for human and animal surveillance. Global investments to improve public health care infrastructures and laboratory facilities and to transfer clinical, epidemiological, and technical knowledge to these countries are much needed (Hien et al., 2004b). The window of opportunity in the era of global travel is narrow. Local capacity, and less dependence on foreign laboratories and expertise, will allow for earlier recognition and quicker responses to epidemics. In addition, local availability of clinical, scientific, and laboratory capacity facilitates and expedites clinical, virological, and epidemiological analyses needed to optimize outbreak control, infection control, and clinical managment and guarantees the timely availability of virus strains for monitoring virus evolution and planning of vaccines by reference laboratories.

In response to the 1997 H5N1 outbreak in Hong Kong, influenza surveillance in poultry was intensified, which permitted early recognition of outbreaks by other avian influenza strains and timely interventions and has helped to keep Hong Kong free of H5N1 influenza despite the outbreak of this virus in many other countries in the region. The Hong Kong response may serve as a model, but wider implementation of this approach will require global efforts.

References

Almond, J. W. (1977). A single gene determines the host range of influenza virus. *Nature* 270: 617–618.

Apisarnthanarak, A., Kitphati, R., Thongphubeth, K., Patoomanunt, P., Anthanont, P., Auwanit, W., Thawatsupha, P., Chittaganpitch, M., Saeng-Aroon, S., Waicharoen, S., Apisarnthanarak, P., Storch, G. A., Mundy, L. M. and Fraser, V. J. (2004). Atypical avian influenza (H5N1). *Emerg Infect Dis* 10: 1321–1324.

Apisarnthanarak, A., Erb, S., Stephenson, I., Katz, J. M., Chittaganpitch, M., Sangkitporn, S., Kitphati, R., Thawatsupha, P., Waicharoen, S., Pinitchai, U., Apisarnthanarak, P., Fraser, V. J. and Mundy, L. M. (2005). Seroprevalence of anti-H5 antibody among Thai health care workers after exposure to Avian influenza (H5N1) in a tertiary care center. *Clin Infect Dis* 40: e16–18.

Austin, F. J. and Webster, R. G. (1986). Antigenic mapping of an avian H1 influenza virus haemagglutinin and interrelationships of H1 viruses from humans, pigs and birds. *J Gen Virol* 67 (Pt 6): 983–992.

Basler, C. F., Reid, A. H., Dybing, J. K., Janczewski, T. A., Fanning, T. G., Zheng, H., Salvatore, M., Perdue, M. L., Swayne, D. E., Garcia-Sastre, A., Palese, P. and Taubenberger, J. K. (2001). Sequence of the 1918 pandemic influenza virus nonstructural gene (NS) segment and characterization of recombinant viruses bearing the 1918 NS genes. *Proc Natl Acad Sci U S A* 98: 2746–2751.

Baum, L. G. and Paulson, J. C. (1991). The N2 neuraminidase of human influenza virus has acquired a substrate specificity complementary to the hemagglutinin receptor specificity. *Virology* 180: 10–15.

Bean, W. J., Schell, M., Katz, J., Kawaoka, Y., Naeve, C., Gorman, O. and Webster, R. G. (1992). Evolution of the H3 influenza virus hemagglutinin from human and nonhuman hosts. *J Virol* 66: 1129–1138.

Beare, A. S. and Webster, R. G. (1991). Replication of avian influenza viruses in humans. *Arch Virol* 119: 37–42.

Belshe, R. B., Newman, F. K., Cannon, J., Duane, C., Treanor, J., Van Hoecke, C., Howe, B. J. and Dubin, G. (2004). Serum antibody responses after intradermal vaccination against influenza. *N Engl J Med* 351: 2286–2294.

Bosch, F. X., Garten, W., Klenk, H. D. and Rott, R. (1981). Proteolytic cleavage of influenza virus hemagglutinins: primary structure of the connecting peptide between HA1 and HA2 determines proteolytic cleavability and pathogenicity of Avian influenza viruses. *Virology* 113: 725–735.

Bridges, C. B., Lim, W., Hu–Primmer, J., Sims, L., Fukuda, K., Mak, K. H., Rowe, T., Thompson, W. W., Conn, L., Lu, X., Cox, N. J. and Katz, J. M. (2002). Risk of influenza A (H5N1) infection among poultry workers, Hong Kong, 1997-1998. *J Infect Dis* 185: 1005–1010.

Bright, R. A., Medina, M. J., Xu, X., Perez-Oronoz, G., Wallis, T. R., Davis, X. M., Porinelli, L., Cox, N. J. and Klimov (2005). Incidence of adamantane resistance among influenza A (H3N2) viruses isolated worldwide from 1994 to 2005: a cause for concern. *Lancet* 366: 1175–1181.

Campbell, C. H., Webster, R. G. and Breese, S. S., Jr. (1970). Fowl plague virus from man. *J Infect Dis* 122: 513 516.

Cauthen, A. N., Swayne, D. E., Schultz-Cherry, S., Perdue, M. L. and Suarez, D. L. (2000). Continued circulation in China of highly pathogenic avian influenza viruses encoding the hemagglutinin gene associated with the 1997 H5N1 outbreak in poultry and humans. *J Virol* 74: 6592–6599.

Chan M. C., Cheung, C. Y., Chui, W. H., Tsao, S. W., Nicholls, J. M., Chan, R. W., Long, H. T., Poon, L. L., Guan, Y. and Peiris, J. S. (2005). Proinflammatory cytokine responses induced by influenza A (H5N1) viruses to primaty human alveolar and bronchial epithelial cells. *Respir Res* 6: 135.

Chan, P. K. (2002). Outbreak of avian influenza A(H5N1) virus infection in Hong Kong in 1997. *Clin Infect Dis* 34 Suppl 2: S58–64.

Chen, H., Deng, G., Li, Z., Tian, G., Li, Y., Jiao, P., Zhang, L., Liu, Z., Webster, R. G. and Yu, K. (2004). The evolution of H5N1 influenza viruses in ducks in southern China. *Proc Natl Acad Sci U S A* 101: 10452–10457.

Chen, H., Smith, G. J., Li, K. S., Wang, J., Fan, X. H., Rayner, J. M., Vijaykrishna, D., Wu, J. X., Lu, H. R., Chen, Y., Xia, N. S., Naipospos, T. S., Yuen, K. Y., Hassan, S. S., Bahri, S., Nguyen, T. D., Webster, R. G., Peiris, J. S. and Guan, Y. (2006). Establishment of multiple sublineages of H5N1 influenza virus in Asia: Implications for pandemic control. *Proc Natl Acad Sci U S A*. The World health Organization Global Influenza Program Surveillance Network. Evolution of H5N1 avian influenza viruses in Asia. *Emerg Infect Dis* 11: 1515–1521.

Chen, J., Lee, K. H., Steinhauer, D. A., Stevens, D. J., Skehel, J. J. and Wiley, D. C. (1998). Structure of the hemagglutinin precursor cleavage site, a determinant of influenza pathogenicity and the origin of the labile conformation. *Cell* 95: 409–417.

Cheung, C. Y., Poon, L. L., Lau, A. S., Luk, W., Lau, Y. L., Shortridge, K. F., Gordon, S., Guan, Y. and Peiris, J. S. (2002). Induction of proinflammatory cytokines in human macrophages by influenza A (H5N1) viruses: a mechanism for the unusual severity of human disease? *Lancet* 360: 1831–1837.

Cheung, C. L., Rayner, J. M., Smith, G. J., Wang, P., Naispospos, T. S., Zhang, J., Yuen, K. Y., Webster, R. G., Peiris, J. S., Guan, Y. and Chen, H. (2006). Distribution of Amantadine-Resistant H5N1 Avian Influenza Variants in Asia. *J Infect Dis* 193: 1626–1629.

Choi, Y. K., Ozaki, H., Webby, R. J., Webster, R. G., Peiris, J. S., Poon, L., Butt, C., Leung, Y. H. and Guan, Y. (2004). Continuing evolution of H9N2 influenza viruses in Southeastern China. *J Virol* 78: 8609–8614.

Chotpitayasunondh, T., Ungchusak, K., Hanshaoworakul, W., Chunsuthiwat, S., Sawanpanyalert, P., Kijphati, R., Lochindarat, S., Srisan, P., Suwan, P., Osotthanakorn, Y., Anantasetagoon, T., Kanjanawasri, S., Tanupattarachai, S., Weerakul, J., Chaiwirattana, R., Maneerattanaporn, M., Poolsavathitikool, R., Chokephaibulkit, K., Apisarnthanarak, A. and Dowell, S. F. (2005). Human disease from influenza A (H5N1), Thailand, 2004. *Emerg Infect Dis* 11: 201–209.

Claas, E. C., Osterhaus, A. D., van Beek, R., De Jong, J. C., Rimmelzwaan, G. F., Senne, D. A., Krauss, S., Shortridge, K. F. and Webster, R. G. (1998). Human influenza A H5N1 virus related to a highly pathogenic avian influenza virus. *Lancet* 351: 472–477.

Connor, R. J., Kawaoka, Y., Webster, R. G. and Paulson, J. C. (1994). Receptor specificity in human, avian, and equine H2 and H3 influenza virus isolates. *Virology* 205: 17–23.

Couceiro, J. N., Paulson, J. C. and Baum, L. G. (1993). Influenza virus strains selectively recognize sialyloligosaccharides on human respiratory epithelium; the role of the host cell in selection of hemagglutinin receptor specificity. *Virus Res* 29: 155–165.

Crawford, J., Wilkinson, B., Vosnesensky, A., Smith, G., Garcia, M., Stone, H. and Perdue, M. L. (1999). Baculovirus-derived hemagglutinin vaccines protect against lethal influenza infections by avian H5 and H7 subtypes. *Vaccine* 17: 2265–2274.

de Jong, M. D., Bach, V. C., Phan, T. Q., Vo, M. H., Tran, T. T., Nguyen, B. H., Beld, M., Le, T. P., Truong, H. K., Nguyen, V. V., Tran, T. H., Do, Q. H. and Farrar, J. (2005). Fatal avian influenza A (H5N1) in a child presenting with diarrhea followed by coma. *N Engl J Med* 352: 686–691.

de Jong, M. D., Tran, T. T., Truong, H. K., Vo, M. H., Smith, G. J., Nguyen, V. C., Bach, V. C., Phan, T. Q., Do, Q. H., Guan, Y., Peiris, J. S., Tran, T. H. and Farrar, J. (2005). Oseltamivir resistance during treatment of influenza A (H5N1) infection. *N Engl J Med* 353: 2667–2672.

DeLay, P. D., Casey, H. L. and Tubiash, H. S. (1967). Comparative study of fowl plague virus and a virus isolated from man. *Public Health Rep* 82: 615–620.

Deshpande, K. L., Fried, V. A., Ando, M. and Webster, R. G. (1987). Glycosylation affects cleavage of an H5N2 influenza virus hemagglutinin and regulates virulence. *Proc Natl Acad Sci U S A* 84: 36–40.

Diebold, Y., Calonge, M., Enriquez de Salamanca, A., Callejo, S., Corrales, R. M., Saez, V., Siemasko, K. F. and Stern, M. E. (2003). Characterization of a spontaneously immortalized cell line (IOBA-NHC) from normal human conjunctiva. *Invest Ophthalmol Vis Sci* 44: 4263–4274.

Enserink, M. (2005). Influenza. Test kit error is wake-up call for 50-year-old foe. *Science* 308: 476.

Epstein, S. L., Tumpey, T. M., Misplon, J. A., Lo, C. Y., Cooper, L. A., Subbarao, K., Renshaw, M., Sambhara, S. and Katz, J. M. (2002). DNA vaccine expressing conserved influenza virus proteins protective against H5N1 challenge infection in mice. *Emerg Infect Dis* 8: 796–801.

Ferguson, N. M., Cummings, D. A., Cauchemez, S., Fraser, C., Riley, S., Meeyai, A., Iamsirithaworn, S. and Burke, D. S. (2005). Strategies for containing an emerging influenza pandemic in Southeast Asia. *Nature* 437: 209–214.

Fouchier, R. A., Schneeberger, P. M., Rozendaal, F. W., Broekman, J. M., Kemink, S. A., Munster, V., Kuiken, T., Rimmelzwaan, G. F., Schutten, M., Van Doornum, G. J., Koch, G., Bosman, A., Koopmans, M. and Osterhaus, A. D. (2004). Avian influenza A virus (H7N7) associated with human conjunctivitis and a fatal case of acute respiratory distress syndrome. *Proc Natl Acad Sci U S A* 101: 1356–1361.

Fouchier, R. A., Munster, V., Wallensten, A., Bestebroer, T. M., Herfst, S., Smith, D., Rimmelzwaan, G. F., Olsen, B. and Osterhaus, A. D. (2005). Characterization of a novel influenza A virus hemagglutinin subtype (H16) obtained from black-headed gulls. *J Virol* 79: 2814–2822.

Gabriel, G., Dauber, B., Wolff, T., Planz, O., Klenk, H. D. and Stech, J. (2005). The viral polymerase mediates adaptation of an avian influenza virus to a mammalian host. *Proc Natl Acad Sci U S A* 102: 18590–18595.

Gambaryan, A. S., Tuzikov, A. B., Piskarev, V. E., Yamnikova, S. S., Lvov, D. K., Robertson, J. S., Bovin, N. V. and Matrosovich, M. N. (1997). Specification of receptor–binding phenotypes of influenza virus isolates from different hosts using synthetic sialylglycopolymers: non-egg-adapted human H1 and H3 influenza A and influenza B viruses share a common high binding affinity for 6'-sialyl(N-acetyllactosamine). *Virology* 232: 345–350.

Gamblin, S. J., Haire, L. F., Russell, R. J., Stevens, D. J., Xiao, B., Ha, Y., Vasisht, N., Steinhauer, D. A., Daniels, R. S., Elliot, A., Wiley, D. C. and Skehel, J. J. (2004). The structure and receptor binding properties of the 1918 influenza hemagglutinin. *Science* 303: 1838–1842.

Garcia-Sastre, A. (2001). Inhibition of interferon-mediated antiviral responses by influenza A viruses and other negative-strand RNA viruses. *Virology* 279: 375–384.

Garcia-Sastre, A. (2002). Mechanisms of inhibition of the host interferon alpha/beta-mediated antiviral responses by viruses. *Microbes Infect* 4: 647–655.

Garten, W. and Klenk, H. D. (1999). Understanding influenza virus pathogenicity. *Trends Microbiol* 7: 99–100.

Geiss, G. K., Salvatore, M., Tumpey, T. M., Carter, V. S., Wang, X., Basler, C. F., Taubenberger, J. K., Bumgarner, R. E., Palese, P., Katze, M. G. and Garcia-Sastre, A. (2002). Cellular transcriptional profiling in influenza A virus-infected lung epithelial cells: the role of the nonstructural NS1 protein in the evasion of the host innate defense and its potential contribution to pandemic influenza. *Proc Natl Acad Sci U S A* 99: 10736–10741.

Govorkova, E. A., Leneva, I. A., Goloubeva, O. G., Bush, K. and Webster, R. G. (2001). Comparison of efficacies of RWJ-270201, zanamivir, and oseltamivir against H5N1, H9N2, and other avian influenza viruses. *Antimicrob Agents Chemother* 45: 2723–2732.

Guan, Y., Shortridge, K. F., Krauss, S. and Webster, R. G. (1999). Molecular characterization of H9N2 influenza viruses: were they the donors of the "internal" genes of H5N1 viruses in Hong Kong? *Proc Natl Acad Sci U S A* 96: 9363–9367.

Guan, Y., Shortridge, K. F., Krauss, S., Chin, P. S., Dyrting, K. C., Ellis, T. M., Webster, R. G. and Peiris, M. (2000). H9N2 influenza viruses possessing H5N1-like internal genomes continue to circulate in poultry in southeastern China. *J Virol* 74: 9372–9380.

Guan, Y., Peiris, J. S., Lipatov, A. S., Ellis, T. M., Dyrting, K. C., Krauss, S., Zhang, L. J., Webster, R. G. and Shortridge, K. F. (2002). Emergence of multiple genotypes of H5N1 avian influenza viruses in Hong Kong SAR. *Proc Natl Acad Sci U S A* 99: 8950–8955.

Guan, Y., Poon, L. L., Cheung, C. Y., Ellis, T. M., Lim, W., Lipatov, A. S., Chan, K. H., Sturm–Ramirez, K. M., Cheung, C. L., Leung, Y. H., Yuen, K. Y., Webster, R. G. and Peiris, J. S. (2004). H5N1 influenza: a protean pandemic threat. *Proc Natl Acad Sci U S A* 101: 8156–8161.

Gubareva, L. V., McCullers, J. A., Bethell, R. C. and Webster, R. G. (1998). Characterization of influenza A/HongKong/156/97 (H5N1) virus in a mouse model and protective effect of zanamivir on H5N1 infection in mice. *J Infect Dis* 178: 1592–1596.

Guo, Y., Li, J. and Cheng, X. (1999). [Discovery of men infected by avian influenza A (H9N2) virus]. *Zhonghua Shi Yan He Lin Chuang Bing Du Xue Za Zhi* 13: 105–108.

Guo, Y. J., Krauss, S., Senne, D. A., Mo, I. P., Lo, K. S., Xiong, X. P., Norwood, M., Shortridge, K. F., Webster, R. G. and Guan, Y. (2000). Characterization of the pathogenicity of members of the newly established H9N2 influenza virus lineages in Asia. *Virology* 267: 279–288.

Hatta, M., Gao, P., Halfmann, P. and Kawaoka, Y. (2001). Molecular basis for high virulence of Hong Kong H5N1 influenza A viruses. *Science* 293: 1840–1842.

Hien T.T.. H., Nguyen, T. L., Nguyen, T. D., Luong, T. S., Pham, P. M., Nguyen, V. C., Pham, T. S., Vo, C. D., Le, T. Q., Ngo, T. T., Dao, B. K., Le, P. P., Nguyen, T. T., Hoang, T. L., Cao, V. T., Le, T. G., Nguyen, D. T., Le, H. N., Nguyen, K. T., Le, H. S., Le, V. T., Christiane, D., Tran, T. T., de Jong, M.D.., Schultsz, C., Cheng, P., Lim, W., Horby, P. and Farrar, J. (2004a). Avian influenza A (H5N1) in 10 patients in Vietnam. *N Engl J Med* 350: 1179–1188.

Hien, T. T., de Jong, M. and Farrar, J. (2004b). Avian influenza—challenge to global health care structures. *N Engl J Med* 351: 2363–2365.

Hinshaw, V. S., Webster, R. G., Easterday, B. C. and Bean, W. J., Jr. (1981). Replication of avian influenza A viruses in mammals. *Infect Immun* 34: 354–361.

Hinshaw, V. S., Webster, R. G., Naeve, C. W. and Murphy, B. R. (1983). Altered tissue tropism of human-avian reassortant influenza viruses. *Virology* 128: 260–263.

Hirst, M., Astell, C. R., Griffith, M., Coughlin, S. M., Moksa, M., Zeng, T., Smailus, D. E., Holt, R. A., Jones, S., Marra, M. A., Petric, M., Krajden, M., Lawrence, D., Mak, A., Chow, R., Skowronski, D. M., Tweed, S. A., Goh, S., Brunham, R. C., Robinson, J., Bowes, V., Sojonky, K., Byrne, S. K., Li, Y., Kobasa, D., Booth, T. and Paetzel, M. (2004). Novel avian influenza H7N3 strain outbreak, British Columbia. *Emerg Infect Dis* 10: 2192–2195.

Horimoto, T. and Kawaoka, Y. (1994). Reverse genetics provides direct evidence for a correlation of hemagglutinin cleavability and virulence of an avian influenza A virus. *J Virol* 68: 3120–3128.

Hulse-Post, D. J., Sturm-Ramirez, K. M., Humbred, J., Seiler, P., Govorkova, E. A., Krauss, S., Scholtissek, C., Puthavathana, P., Buranathai, C., Nguyen, T. D., Long, H. T., Naipospos, T. S., Chen, H., Ellis, T. M., Guan, Y., Peiris, J. S., and Webster, R. G. (2005). Role of domestic ducks in the propagation and biological evolution of highly pathogenic H5N1 influenza viruses in Asia. *Proc Natl Acad Sci U S A* 102: 10682–10687.

Ito, T., Couceiro, J. N., Kelm, S., Baum, L. G., Krauss, S., Castrucci, M. R., Donatelli, I., Kida, H., Paulson, J. C., Webster, R. G. and Kawaoka, Y. (1998). Molecular basis for the generation in pigs of influenza A viruses with pandemic potential. *J Virol* 72: 7367–7373.

Katz, J. M., Lim, W., Bridges, C. B., Rowe, T., Hu–Primmer, J., Lu, X., Abernathy, R. A., Clarke, M., Conn, L., Kwong, H., Lee, M., Au, G., Ho, Y. Y., Mak, K. H., Cox, N. J. and Fukuda, K. (1999). Antibody response in individuals infected with avian influenza A (H5N1) viruses and detection of anti-H5 antibody among household and social contacts. *J Infect Dis* 180: 1763–1770.

Kawaoka, Y. and Webster, R. G. (1988). Molecular mechanism of acquisition of virulence in influenza virus in nature. *Microb Pathog* 5: 311–318.

Kawaoka, Y. and Webster, R. G. (1989). Interplay between carbohydrate in the stalk and the length of the connecting peptide determines the cleavability of influenza virus hemagglutinin. *J Virol* 63: 3296–3300.

Kawaoka, Y., Krauss, S. and Webster, R. G. (1989). Avian-to-human transmission of the PB1 gene of influenza A viruses in the 1957 and 1968 pandemics. *J Virol* 63: 4603–4608.

Keawcharoen, J., Oraveerakul, K., Kuiken, T., Fouchier, R. A., Amonsin, A., Payungporn, S., Noppornpanth, S., Wattanodorn, S., Theambooniers, A., Tantilertcharoen, R., Pattanarangsan, R., Arya, N., Ratanakorn, P., Osterhaus, D. M. and Poovorawan, Y. (2004). Avian influenza H5N1 in tigers and leopards. *Emerg Infect Dis* 10: 2189–2191.

Kenney, R. T., Frech, S. A., Muenz, L. R., Villar, C. P. and Glenn, G. M. (2004). Dose sparing with intradermal injection of influenza vaccine. *N Engl J Med* 351: 2295–2301.

Kida, H., Kawaoka, Y., Naeve, C. W. and Webster, R. G. (1987). Antigenic and genetic conservation of H3 influenza virus in wild ducks. *Virology* 159: 109–119.

Kida, H., Ito, T., Yasuda, J., Shimizu, Y., Itakura, C., Shortridge, K. F., Kawaoka, Y. and Webster, R. G. (1994). Potential for transmission of avian influenza viruses to pigs. *J Gen Virol* 75 (Pt 9): 2183–2188.

Klenk, H. D. and Garten, W. (1994). Host cell proteases controlling virus pathogenicity. *Trends Microbiol* 2: 39–43.

Kobasa, D., Takada, A., Shinya, K., Hatta, M., Halfmann, P., Theriault, S., Suzuki, H., Nishimura, H., Mitamura, K., Sugaya, N., Usui, T., Murata, T., Maeda, Y., Watanabe, S., Suresh, M., Suzuki, T., Suzuki, Y., Feldmann, H. and Kawaoka, Y. (2004). Enhanced virulence of influenza A viruses with the haemagglutinin of the 1918 pandemic virus. *Nature* 431: 703–707.

Kodihalli, S., Goto, H., Kobasa, D. L., Krauss, S., Kawaoka, Y. and Webster, R. G. (1999). DNA vaccine encoding hemagglutinin provides protective immunity against H5N1 influenza virus infection in mice. *J Virol* 73: 2094–2098.

Koopmans, M., Wilbrink, B., Conyn, M., Natrop, G., van der Nat, H., Vennema, H., Meijer, A., van Steenbergen, J., Fouchier, R., Osterhaus, A. and Bosman, A. (2004). Transmission of H7N7 avian influenza A virus to human beings during a large outbreak in commercial poultry farms in the Netherlands. *Lancet* 363: 587–593.

Krug, R. M., Yuan, W., Noah, D. L. and Latham, A. G. (2003). Intracellular warfare between human influenza viruses and human cells: the roles of the viral NS1 protein. *Virology* 309: 181–189.

Kuiken, T., Rimmelzwaan, G., van Riel, D., van Amerongen, G., Baars, M., Fouchier, R. and Osterhaus, A. (2004). Avian H5N1 influenza in cats. *Science* 306: 241.

Kurtz, J., Manvell, R. J. and Banks, J. (1996). Avian influenza virus isolated from a woman with conjunctivitis. *Lancet* 348: 901–902.

Le, Q. M., Kiso, M., Someya, K et al. (2005). Avian flu: isolation of drug-resistant H5N1 virus. *Nature* 437 (7062): 1108.

Lee, C. W., Suarez, D. L., Tumpey, T. M., Sung, H. W., Kwon, Y. K., Lee, Y. J., Choi, J. G., Joh, S. J., Kim, M. C., Lee, E. K., Park, J. M., Lu, X., Katz, J. M., Spackman, E., Swayne, D. E. and Kim, J. H. (2005). Characterization of highly pathogenic H5N1 avian influenza A viruses isolated from South Korea. *J Virol* 79: 3692–3702.

Leneva, I. A., Roberts, N., Govorkova, E. A., Goloubeva, O. G. and Webster, R. G. (2000). The neuraminidase inhibitor GS4104 (oseltamivir phosphate) is efficacious against A/Hong Kong/156/97 (H5N1) and A/Hong Kong/1074/99 (H9N2) influenza viruses. *Antiviral Res* 48: 101–115.

Leneva, I. A., Goloubeva, O., Fenton, R. J., Tisdale, M. and Webster, R. G. (2001). Efficacy of zanamivir against avian influenza A viruses that possess genes encoding H5N1 internal proteins and are pathogenic in mammals. *Antimicrob Agents Chemother* 45: 1216–1224.

Li, K. S., Guan, Y., Wang, J., Smith, G. J., Xu, K. M., Duan, L., Rahardjo, A. P., Puthavathana, P., Buranathai, C., Nguyen, T. D., Estoepangestie, A. T., Chaisingh, A., Auewarakul, P., Long, H. T., Hanh, N. T., Webby, R. J., Poon, L. L., Chen, H., Shortridge, K. F., Yuen, K. Y., Webster, R. G. and Peiris, J. S. (2004). Genesis of a highly pathogenic and potentially pandemic H5N1 influenza virus in eastern Asia. *Nature* 430: 209–213.

Li, S., Liu, C., Klimov, A., Subbarao, K., Perdue, M. L., Mo, D., Ji, Y., Woods, L., Hietala, S. and Bryant, M. (1999). Recombinant influenza A virus vaccines for the pathogenic human A/Hong Kong/97 (H5N1) viruses. *J Infect Dis* 179: 1132–1138.

Liem, N. T. and Lim, W. (2005). Lack of H5N1 avian influenza transmission to hospital employees, Hanoi, 2004. *Emerg Infect Dis* 11: 210–215.

Lin, Y. P., Shaw, M., Gregory, V., Cameron, K., Lim, W., Klimov, A., Subbarao, K., Guan, Y., Krauss, S., Shortridge, K., Webster, R., Cox, N. and Hay, A. (2000). Avian-to-human transmission of H9N2 subtype influenza A viruses: relationship between H9N2 and H5N1 human isolates. *Proc Natl Acad Sci U S A* 97: 9654–9658.

Lipatov, A. S., Krauss, S., Guan, Y., Peiris, M., Rehg, J. E., Perez, D. R. and Webster, R. G. (2003). Neurovirulence in mice of H5N1 influenza virus genotypes isolated from Hong Kong poultry in 2001. *J Virol* 77: 3816–3823.

Lipatov, A. S., Govorkova, E. A., Webby, R. J., Ozaki, H., Peiris, M., Guan, Y., Poon, L. and Webster, R. G. (2004). Influenza: emergence and control. *J Virol* 78: 8951–8959.

Lipatov, A. S., Andreansky, S., Webby, R. J., Hulse, D. J., Rehg, J. E., Krauss, S., Perez, D. R., Doherty, P. C., Webster, R. G. and Sangster, M. Y. (2005a). Pathogenesis of Hong Kong H5N1 influenza virus NS gene reassortants in mice: the role of cytokines and B- and T-cell responses. *J Gen Virol* 86: 1121–1130.

Lipatov, A. S., Webby, R. J., Govorkova, E. A., Krauss, S. and Webster, R. G. (2005b). Efficacy of h5 influenza vaccines produced by reverse genetics in a lethal mouse model. *J Infect Dis* 191: 1216–1220.

Liu, J. H., Okazaki, K., Mweene, A., Shi, W. M., Wu, Q. M., Su, J. L., Zhang, G. Z., Bai, G. R. and Kida, H. (2004). Genetic conservation of hemagglutinin gene of H9 influenza virus in chicken population in Mainland China. *Virus Genes* 29: 329–334.

Longini, I. M., Jr., Nizam, A., Xu, S., Ungchusak, K., Hanshaoworakul, W., Cummings, D. A. and Halloran, M. E. (2005). Containing pandemic influenza at the source. *Science* 309: 1083–1087.

Lu, B. L., Webster, R. G. and Hinshaw, V. S. (1982). Failure to detect hemagglutination-inhibiting antibodies with intact avian influenza virions. *Infect Immun* 38: 530–535.

Matrosovich, M. N., Gambaryan, A. S., Teneberg, S., Piskarev, V. E., Yamnikova, S. S., Lvov, D. K., Robertson, J. S. and Karlsson, K. A. (1997). Avian influenza A viruses differ from human viruses by recognition of sialyloligosaccharides and gangliosides and by a higher conservation of the HA receptor-binding site. *Virology* 233: 224–234.

Matrosovich, M., Zhou, N., Kawaoka, Y. and Webster, R. (1999). The surface glycoproteins of H5 influenza viruses isolated from humans, chickens, and wild aquatic birds have distinguishable properties. *J Virol* 73: 1146–1155.

Matrosovich, M. N., Krauss, S. and Webster, R. G. (2001). H9N2 influenza A viruses from poultry in Asia have human virus–like receptor specificity. *Virology* 281: 156–162.

Matrosovich, M. N., Matrosovich, T. Y., Gray, T., Roberts, N. A. and Klenk, H. D. (2004). Human and avian influenza viruses target different cell types in cultures of human airway epithelium. *Proc Natl Acad Sci U S A* 101: 4620–4624.

Mills, C. E., Robins, J. M. and Lipsitch, M. (2004). Transmissibility of 1918 pandemic influenza. *Nature* 432: 904–906.

Monto, A. S., Gravenstein, S., Elliott, M., Colopy, M. and Schweinle, J. (2000). Clinical signs and symptoms predicting influenza infection. *Arch Intern Med* 160: 3243–3247.

Morishima, T., Togashi, T., Yokota, S., Okuno, Y., Miyazaki, C., Tashiro, M. and Okabe, N. (2002). Encephalitis and encephalopathy associated with an influenza epidemic in Japan. *Clin Infect Dis* 35: 512–517.

Mounts, A. W., Kwong, H., Izurieta, H. S., Ho, Y., Au, T., Lee, M., Buxton Bridges, C., Williams, S. W., Mak, K. H., Katz, J. M., Thompson, W. W., Cox, N. J. and Fukuda, K. (1999). Case-control study of risk factors for avian influenza A (H5N1) disease, Hong Kong, 1997. *J Infect Dis* 180: 505–508.

Naeve, C. W., Hinshaw, V. S. and Webster, R. G. (1984). Mutations in the hemagglutinin receptor-binding site can change the biological properties of an influenza virus. *J Virol* 51: 567–569.

Nakajima, K., Desselberger, U. and Palese, P. (1978). Recent human influenza A (H1N1) viruses are closely related genetically to strains isolated in 1950. *Nature* 274: 334–339.

Nicholson, K. G., Wood, J. M. and Zambon, M. (2003). Influenza. *Lancet* 362: 1733–1745.

Ohuchi, R., Ohuchi, M., Garten, W. and Klenk, H. D. (1991). Human influenza virus hemagglutinin with high sensitivity to proteolytic activation. *J Virol* 65: 3530–3537.

Olofsson, S., Kumlin, U., Dimock, K. and Arnberg, N. (2005). Avian influenza and sialic acid receptors: more than meets the eye? *Lancet Infect Dis* 5: 184–188.

Orlich, M., Gottwald, H. and Rott, R. (1994). Nonhomologous recombination between the hemagglutinin gene and the nucleoprotein gene of an influenza virus. *Virology* 204: 462–465.

Oxford, J. S. (2000). Influenza A pandemics of the 20th century with special reference to 1918: virology, pathology and epidemiology. *Rev Med Virol* 10: 119–133.

Palladino, G., Mozdzanowska, K., Washko, G. and Gerhard, W. (1995). Virus–neutralizing antibodies of immunoglobulin G (IgG) but not of IgM or IgA isotypes can cure influenza virus pneumonia in SCID mice. *J Virol* 69: 2075–2081.

Paulsen, F., Thale, A., Kohla, G., Schauer, R., Rochels, R., Parwaresch, R. and Tillmann, B. (1998). Functional anatomy of human lacrimal duct epithelium. *Anat Embryol (Berl)* 198: 1–12.

Peiris, M., Yuen, K. Y., Leung, C. W., Chan, K. H., Ip, P. L., Lai, R. W., Orr, W. K. and Shortridge, K. F. (1999). Human infection with influenza H9N2. *Lancet* 354: 916–917.

Peiris, J. S., Guan, Y., Markwell, D., Ghose, P., Webster, R. G. and Shortridge, K. F. (2001). Cocirculation of avian H9N2 and contemporary "human" H3N2 influenza A viruses in pigs in southeastern China: potential for genetic reassortment? *J Virol* 75: 9679–9686.

Peiris, J. S., Yu, W. C., Leung, C. W., Cheung, C. Y., Ng, W. F., Nicholls, J. M., Ng, T. K., Chan, K. H., Lai, S. T., Lim, W. L., Yuen, K. Y. and Guan, Y. (2004). Re-emergence of fatal human influenza A subtype H5N1 disease. *Lancet* 363: 617–619.

Puthavathana, P., Auewarakul, P., Charoenying, P. C., Sangsiriwut, K., Pooruk, P., Boonnak, K., Khanyok, R., Thawachsupa, P., Kijphati, R. and Sawanpanyalert, P. (2005). Molecular characterization of the complete genome of human influenza H5N1 virus isolates from Thailand. *J Gen Virol* 86: 423–433.

Reid, A. H., Fanning, T. G., Hultin, J. V. and Taubenberger, J. K. (1999). Origin and evolution of the 1918 "Spanish" influenza virus hemagglutinin gene. *Proc Natl Acad Sci U S A* 96: 1651–1656.

Reid, A. H., Taubenberger, J. K. and Fanning, T. G. (2004). Evidence of an absence: the genetic origins of the 1918 pandemic influenza virus. *Nat Rev Microbiol* 2: 909–914.

Rimmelzwaan, G. F., Kuiken, T., van Amerongen, G., Bestebroer, T. M., Fouchier, R. A. and Osterhaus, A. D. (2001). Pathogenesis of influenza A (H5N1) virus infection in a primate model. *J Virol* 75: 6687–6691.

Rogers, G. N. and Paulson, J. C. (1983). Receptor determinants of human and animal influenza virus isolates: differences in receptor specificity of the H3 hemagglutinin based on species of origin. *Virology* 127: 361–373.

Rogers, G. N., Paulson, J. C., Daniels, R. S., Skehel, J. J., Wilson, I. A. and Wiley, D. C. (1983). Single amino acid substitutions in influenza haemagglutinin change receptor binding specificity. *Nature* 304: 76–78.

Rogers, G. N. and D'Souza, B. L. (1989). Receptor binding properties of human and animal H1 influenza virus isolates. *Virology* 173: 317–322.

Rowe, T., Abernathy, R. A., Hu-Primmer, J., Thompson, W. W., Lu, X., Lim, W., Fukuda, K., Cox, N. J. and Katz, J. M. (1999). Detection of antibody to avian influenza A (H5N1) virus in human serum by using a combination of serologic assays. *J Clin Microbiol* 37: 937–943.

Salomon, R., Franks, J., Govorkova, E. A., Ilyushina, N. A., Yen, H. L., Hulse-Post, D. J., Humberd, I., Trichet, M., Rehg, J. E., Webby, R. J., Webster, R. G. and Hoffmann, E. (2006). The polymerase complex genes contribute to the high virulence of the human H5NI influenza virus isolate A/Vietnam/1203/04. *J Exp Med* 203: 681–697.

Scholtissek, C., Koennecke, I. and Rott, R. (1978a). Host range recombinants of fowl plague (influenza A) virus. *Virology* 91: 79–85.

Scholtissek, C., von Hoyningen, V. and Rott, R. (1978b). Genetic relatedness between the new 1977 epidemic strains (H1N1) of influenza and human influenza strains isolated between 1947 and 1957 (H1N1). *Virology* 89: 613–617.

Scholtissek, C., Rohde, W., Von Hoyningen, V. and Rott, R. (1978c). On the origin of the human influenza virus subtypes H2N2 and H3N2. *Virology* 87: 13–20.

Schultsz, C., Dong, V. C., Chau, N. V. V., Le, N. T. H., Lim, W., Thanh, T. T., Dolecek, C., De Jong, M. D., Hien, T. T. and Farrar, J. (2005). Avian influenza H5N1 and health care workers. *Emerg Infect Dis* Online.

Schwartz, B. and Gellin, B. (2005). Vaccination strategies for an influenza pandemic. *J Infect Dis* 191: 1207–1209.

Senne, D. A., Panigrahy, B., Kawaoka, Y., Pearson, J. E., Suss, J., Lipkind, M., Kida, H. and Webster, R. G. (1996). Survey of the hemagglutinin (HA) cleavage site sequence of H5 and H7 avian influenza viruses: amino acid sequence at the HA cleavage site as a marker of pathogenicity potential. *Avian Dis* 40: 425–437.

Seo, S. H. and Webster, R. G. (2002). Tumor necrosis factor alpha exerts powerful anti-influenza virus effects in lung epithelial cells. *J Virol* 76: 1071–1076.

Seo, S. H., Hoffmann, E. and Webster, R. G. (2002). Lethal H5N1 influenza viruses escape host anti-viral cytokine responses. *Nat Med* 8: 950–954.

Seo, S. H., Hoffmann, E. and Webster, R. G. (2004). The NS1 gene of H5N1 influenza viruses circumvents the host anti–viral cytokine responses. *Virus Res* 103: 107–113.

Shinya, K., Ebina, M., Yamada, S., Ono, M., Kasai, N., Kawaoka, Y. (2006). Avian flu: influenza virus receptors in the human airway. *Nature* 440 (7083): 435–436.

Shinya, K., Hamm, S., Hatta, M., Ito, H., Ito, T. and Kawaoka, Y. (2004). PB2 amino acid at position 627 affects replicative efficiency, but not cell tropism, of Hong Kong H5N1 influenza A viruses in mice. *Virology* 320: 258–266.

Shortridge, K. F., Zhou, N. N., Guan, Y., Gao, P., Ito, T., Kawaoka, Y., Kodihalli, S., Krauss, S., Markwell, D., Murti, K. G., Norwood, M., Senne, D., Sims, L., Takada, A. and Webster, R. G. (1998). Characterization of avian H5N1 influenza viruses from poultry in Hong Kong. *Virology* 252: 331–342.

Snyder, M. H., Buckler-White, A. J., London, W. T., Tierney, E. L. and Murphy, B. R. (1987). The avian influenza virus nucleoprotein gene and a specific constellation of avian and human virus polymerase genes each specify attenuation of avian–human influenza A/Pintail/79 reassortant viruses for monkeys. *J Virol* 61: 2857–2863.

Songserm, T., Amonsin, A., Jam-On, R., Sae-Heng, N., Meemak, N., Pariyothorn, N., Payungporn, S., Theamboonlers, A. and Poororawan, Y. (2006). Avian influenza H5N1 in naturally infected domestic cat. *Emerging Infectious Diseases* 12: 681–683.

Steinhauer, D. A. (1999). Role of hemagglutinin cleavage for the pathogenicity of influenza virus. *Virology* 258: 1–20.

Stephenson, I., Nicholson, K. G., Wood, J. M., Zambon, M. C. and Katz, J. M. (2004). Confronting the avian influenza threat: vaccine development for a potential pandemic. *Lancet Infect Dis* 4: 499–509.

Stephenson, I., Bugarini, R., Nicholson, K. G., Podda, A., Wood, J. M., Zambon, M. C. and Katz, J. M. (2005). Cross-reactivity to highly pathogenic avian influenza H5N1 viruses after vaccination with nonadjuvanted and MF59-Adjuvanted Influenza A/Duck/Singapore/97 (H5N3) vaccine: a potential priming strategy. *J Infect Dis* 191: 1210–1215.

Stevens, J., Corper, A. L., Basler, C. F., Taubenberger, J. K., Palese, P. and Wilson, I. A. (2004). Structure of the uncleaved human H1 hemagglutinin from the extinct 1918 influenza virus. *Science* 303: 1866–1870.

Stohr, K. (2003). The global agenda on influenza surveillance and control. *Vaccine* 21: 1744–1748.

Stohr, K. and Esveld, M. (2004). Public health. Will vaccines be available for the next influenza pandemic? *Science* 306: 2195–2196.

Sturm-Ramirez, K. M., Ellis, T., Bousfield, B., Bissett, L., Dyrting, K., Rehg, J. E., Poon, L., Guan, Y., Peiris, M. and Webster, R. G. (2004). Reemerging H5N1 influenza viruses in Hong Kong in 2002 are highly pathogenic to ducks. *J Virol* 78: 4892–4901.

Suarez, D. L., Senne, D. A., Banks, J., Brown, I. H., Essen, S. C., Lee, C. W., Manvell, R. J., Mathieu-Benson, C., Moreno, V., Pedersen, J. C., Panigrahy, B., Rojas, H., Spackman, E. and Alexander, D. J. (2004). Recombination resulting in virulence shift in avian influenza outbreak, Chile. *Emerg Infect Dis* 10: 693–699.

Subbarao, E. K., London, W. and Murphy, B. R. (1993). A single amino acid in the PB2 gene of influenza A virus is a determinant of host range. *J Virol* 67: 1761–1764.

Subbarao, K., Klimov, A., Katz, J., Regnery, H., Lim, W., Hall, H., Perdue, M., Swayne, D., Bender, C., Huang, J., Hemphill, M., Rowe, T., Shaw, M., Xu, X., Fukuda, K. and Cox, N. (1998). Characterization of an avian influenza A (H5N1) virus isolated from a child with a fatal respiratory illness. *Science* 279: 393–396.

Sugaya, N. (2002). Influenza-associated encephalopathy in Japan. *Semin Pediatr Infect Dis* 13: 79–84.

Suzuki, Y., Kato, H., Naeve, C. W. and Webster, R. G. (1989). Single-amino-acid substitution in an antigenic site of influenza virus hemagglutinin can alter the specificity of binding to cell membrane-associated gangliosides. *J Virol* 63: 4298–4302.

Takada, A., Kuboki, N., Okazaki, K., Ninomiya, A., Tanaka, H., Ozaki, H., Itamura, S., Nishimura, H., Enami, M., Tashiro, M., Shortridge, K. F. and Kida, H. (1999). Avirulent Avian influenza virus as a vaccine strain against a potential human pandemic. *J Virol* 73: 8303–8307.

Tanaka, H., Park, C. H., Ninomiya, A., Ozaki, H., Takada, A., Umemura, T. and Kida, H. (2003). Neurotropism of the 1997 Hong Kong H5N1 influenza virus in mice. *Vet Microbiol* 95: 1–13.

Taubenberger, J. K., Reid, A. H., Krafft, A. E., Bijwaard, K. E. and Fanning, T. G. (1997). Initial genetic characterization of the 1918 "Spanish" influenza virus. *Science* 275: 1793–1796.

Taubenberger, J. K., Reid, A. H., Lourens, R. M., Wang, R., Jin, G., Fanning, T. G. (2005). Characterization of the 1918 influenza virus polymerase genes. *Nature* 437: 889–892.

Taylor, H. R. and Turner, A. J. (1977). A case report of fowl plague keratoconjunctivitis. *Br J Ophthalmol* 61: 86–88.

Terraciano, A. J., Wang, N., Schuman, J. S., Haffner, G., Panjwani, N., Zhao, Z. and Yang, Z. (1999). Sialyl Lewis X, Lewis X, and N-acetyllactosamine expression on normal and glaucomatous eyes. *Curr Eye Res* 18: 73–78.

To, K. F., Chan, P. K., Chan, K. F., Lee, W. K., Lam, W. Y., Wong, K. F., Tang, N. L., Tsang, D. N., Sung, R. Y., Buckley, T. A., Tam, J. S. and Cheng, A. F. (2001). Pathology of fatal human infection associated with avian influenza A H5N1 virus. *J Med Virol* 63: 242–246.

Treanor, J. J., Campbell, J. D., Zangwill, M., Rowe, T. and Wolff, M. (2006). Safety and immunogenicity of an inactivated subvirion influenza A (H5N1) vaccine. *N Eng J Med* 354: 1343–1351.

Treanor, J. J., Wilkinson, B. E., Masseoud, F., Hu–Primmer, J., Battaglia, R., O'Brien, D., Wolff, M., Rabinovich, G., Blackwelder, W. and Katz, J. M. (2001). Safety and immunogenicity of a recombinant hemagglutinin vaccine for H5 influenza in humans. *Vaccine* 19: 1732–1737.

Tweed, S. A., Skowroski, D. M., David, S. T., Larder, A., Petric, M., Lees, W., Li, Y., Katz, J., Krajden, M., Tellier, R., Halpert, C., Hirst, M., Astell, C., Lawrence, D. and Mak, A. (2004). Human illness from avian influenza H7N3, British Columbia. *Emerg Infect Dis* 10: 2196–2199.

Ungchusak, K., Auewarakul, P., Dowell, S. F., Kitphati, R., Auwanit, W., Puthavathana, P., Uiprasertkul, M., Boonnak, K., Pittayawonganon, C., Cox, N. J., Zaki, S. R., Thawatsupha, P., Chittaganpitch, M., Khontong, R., Simmerman, J. M. and Chunsutthiwat, S. (2005). Probable person-to-person transmission of avian influenza A (H5N1). *N Engl J Med* 352: 333–340.

van Riel, D., Munster, V. J., de Wit, E., et al. (2006). H5N1 Virus Attachment to Lower Respiratory Tract. *Science*, 312(5772): 399.

Walker, J. A. and Kawaoka, Y. (1993). Importance of conserved amino acids at the cleavage site of the haemagglutinin of a virulent avian influenza A virus. *J Gen Virol* 74 (Pt 2): 311–314.

Webby, R. J. and Webster, R. G. (2003). Are we ready for pandemic influenza? *Science* 302: 1519–1522.

Webby, R. J., Perez, D. R., Coleman, J. S., Guan, Y., Knight, J. H., Govorkova, E. A., McClain-Moss, L. R., Peiris, J. S., Rehg, J. E., Tuomanen, E. I. and Webster, R. G. (2004). Responsiveness to a pandemic alert: use of reverse genetics for rapid development of influenza vaccines. *Lancet* 363: 1099–1103.

Webster, R. G., Yakhno, M., Hinshaw, V. S., Bean, W. J. and Murti, K. G. (1978). Intestinal influenza: replication and characterization of influenza viruses in ducks. *Virology* 84: 268–278.

Webster, R. G., Geraci, J., Petursson, G. and Skirnisson, K. (1981). Conjunctivitis in human beings caused by influenza A virus of seals. *N Engl J Med* 304: 911.

Webster, R. G., Laver, W. G., Air, G. M. and Schild, G. C. (1982). Molecular mechanisms of variation in influenza viruses. *Nature* 296: 115–121.

Webster, R. G. and Rott, R. (1987). Influenza virus A pathogenicity: the pivotal role of hemagglutinin. *Cell* 50: 665–666.

Webster, R. G., Bean, W. J., Gorman, O. T., Chambers, T. M. and Kawaoka, Y. (1992). Evolution and ecology of influenza A viruses. *Microbiol Rev* 56: 152–179.

Webster, R. G. (2001). Virology. A molecular whodunit. *Science* 293: 1773–1775.

Webster, R. G., Guan, Y., Peiris, M., Walker, D., Krauss, S., Zhou, N. N., Govorkova, E. A., Ellis, T. M., Dyrting, K. C., Sit, T., Perez, D. R. and Shortridge, K. F. (2002). Characterization of H5N1 influenza viruses that continue to circulate in geese in southeastern China. *J Virol* 76: 118–126.

Weis, W., Brown, J. H., Cusack, S., Paulson, J. C., Skehel, J. J. and Wiley, D. C. (1988). Structure of the influenza virus haemagglutinin complexed with its receptor, sialic acid. *Nature* 333: 426–431.

WHO (2006). Cumulative number of confirmed human cases of avian influenza A/(H5N1) reported to WHO. Available at http://www.who.int/csr/disease/avian_influenza/country/cases_table_2005_06_08/en/index.html.

Wilson, I. A., Skehel, J. J. and Wiley, D. C. (1981). Structure of the haemagglutinin membrane glycoprotein of influenza virus at 3 A resolution. *Nature* 289: 366–373.

Wood, J. M. and Robertson, J. S. (2004). From lethal virus to life-saving vaccine: developing inactivated vaccines for pandemic influenza. *Nat Rev Microbiol* 2: 842–847.

Xu, X., Subbarao, Cox, N. J. and Guo, Y. (1999). Genetic characterization of the pathogenic influenza A/Goose/Guangdong/1/96 (H5N1) virus: similarity of its hemagglutinin gene to those of H5N1 viruses from the 1997 outbreaks in Hong Kong. *Virology* 261: 15–19.

Xu, X., Jin, M., Yu, Z., Li, H., Qiu, D., Tan, Y. and Chen, H. (2005). Latex agglutination test for monitoring antibodies to avian influenza virus subtype H5N1. *J Clin Microbiol* 43: 1953–1955.

Yen, H. L., Monto, A. S., Webster, R. G. and Govorkova, E. A. (2005). Virulence may determine the necessary duration and dosage of oseltamivir treatment for highly pathogenic A/Vietnam/1203/04 (H5N1) influenza virus in mice. *J Infect Dis* 192: 665–672.

Yuen, K. Y., Chan, P. K., Peiris, M., Tsang, D. N., Que, T. L., Shortridge, K. F., Cheung, P. T., To, W. K., Ho, E. T., Sung, R. and Cheng, A. F. (1998). Clinical features and rapid viral diagnosis of human disease associated with avian influenza A H5N1 virus. *Lancet* 351: 467–471.

Zitzow, L. A., Rowe, T., Morken, T., Shieh, W. J., Zaki, S. and Katz, J. M. (2002). Pathogenesis of avian influenza A (H5N1) viruses in ferrets. *J Virol* 76: 4420–4429.

Index

Page numbers followed by f and t indicate figures and tables, respectively.

A

African KS, 231, 234
AIDS-associated KS, 231–233
Antibody detection, for WNV disease; *see also* West Nile virus (WNV) infection
    IgG ELISA, 28
    IgM ELISA, 27–28
    neutralization test, 28
Antigen detection, for WNV disease; *see also* West Nile virus (WNV) infection
    antigen-capture ELISA, 29
    immunohistochemical staining, 29
Anti-apoptotic proteins, 216–217
Aseptic meningitis, 298
Athen's plague, 321
Atypical pneumonia, 159–160
Avian influenza viruses
    amantadine treatment, 344–345
    antigen detection, 343
    antiviral treatment, 344–346
    H5N1 viruses, 326, 329–330, 332, 336–341, 349–351, 360
    H7N3 viruses, 335
    H7N7 viruses, 326, 333–334
    H9N2 viruses, 335–336
    infecting humans, 330–341
    infection control and prophylaxis, 346–348
    infections in natural hosts, 326–327
    laboratory diagnosis of, 341–344
    neuraminidase treatment, 344–345, 347
    oseltamivir treatment, 344–346
    pandemic preparedness and future directives, 349–350
    pathogenesis, 326–330
    rimantadine treatment, 344–345
    RT-PCR diagnostic methods, 343
    serology diagnostic method, 343–344
    treatment and prevention, 344–348
    vaccination, 348
    viral determinants of pathogenicity of, 327–330
    virus isolation, 342
    zanamivir treatment, 344–346
Avipoxvirus, 128–129, 137, 152–153

B

Blood donations screening, for prevention of West Nile virus (WNV) infection, 36

C

Camelpox, 130, 132, 136, 138, 145
Capripoxviruses, 127–129, 150–151, 153
Cardiopulmonary failure, 299–300
Castleman disease, 235
Centers for Disease Control and Prevention, 78
Chordopoxviruses, 130, 133, 136, 138, 153
Chronic fatigue syndrome (CFS), 201
Cidofovir, 133
Clinical illness, 26–27
    in children, 26
    immunocompromised patients, 26–27
Clinical spectrum
    of hantavirus pulmonary syndrome (HPS), 71–75
    neuroinvasive disease, 19, 21–25
    ocular manifestations, 25–26
Community-acquired atypical pneumonia syndrome, 159
Convalescence and long-term sequelae, 300–301
Cowpox, 130, 136–137, 139, 143–144, 153
Coxsackievirus A16, 301

D

Dead bird surveillance, 36–37
Deerpoxvirus, 127–129, 153
    phylogenetic tree of, 129
Dengue viruses, 2, 3

E

Echoviruses, 290
Ectromelia virus, 144–145
Ehrlichiosis ewingii, *see* Human ehrlichioses

Electroencephalography, 32
El Niño Southern Oscillation (ENSO)
    phenomenon, 68
Encephalitis, 21–22
Endemic KS, 231–232, 234
Enterovirus 71 (EV71)
    antiviral agents, 304–308
    asymptomatic infection, 297
    capsid-binding agents for, 305
    cardiopulmonary failure, 299–300
    characteristics of, 290
    clinical spectrum, 296–301
    complicated illness with CNS involvement,
        298–299
    convalescence and long-term sequelae,
        300–301
    coxsackievirus A16 and, 301
    diagnosis, 302–303
    encephalomyelitis, 299
    epidemiology, worldwide, 294
    epidemiology in Taiwan, 294–296
    gene chips diagnosis, 302
    genotypes of, 291–292
    hand washing and isolation preventive
        measure, 308–309
    household transmission rate, 293
    IgM responses, 303
    image studies for CNS involvement, 299
    incubation period, 294
    inhibitors, uncoating for, 306
    inhibitors, virion attachment for, 305–306
    laboratory surveillance as preventive
        measure, 309
    management, 303–308
    neurovirulence of, 291–292
    neutralizing antibody, 302–303
    novel anti-EV71 agent, 306–308
    pathogenesis of, 300
    pleconaril anti-EV71 agent, 306–308
    poliomyelitis-like syndrome, 298–299
    prevention measures, 308–310
    pulmonary edema, 299–300
    replication cycle of, 291
    risk factors associated with complications,
        301
    route of transmission of, 292–293
    serology test, 302–303
    transmission of, 292–294
    uncomplicated illnesses, 297–298
    vaccination, 309–310
    virion structure of, 290–291
    virological classification of, 289
    virus isolation and identification, 302
Epidemic or AIDS-associated KS, 213–233

Epidemiology, of WNV infection, 7–18
    ecology, 7–10
    vectors, 7–10
    vertebrate hosts, 9–10
E-protein, of flavivirus genome, 1–4
    cell-membrane fusion (CMF)-competent, 2
    structure–function relationships, 3
    structure of, 3
EV71, *see* Enterovirus 71

F
Flaviviruses, 1
Flavivirus genome, 1
    E-protein, 1–4
    nonstructural proteins, 4–6
Fowlpox, 152–153

G
Genetics and virulence, 6–7
Genome, 1–6
    E-protein, 1–4
    nonstructural proteins, 4–6
Goatpox, 136, 150–151
Guillain–Barré syndrome, 22–23

H
Hantaan virus (HTN), 56
Hantavirus cardiopulmonary syndrome (HCPS)
    animal models, 67–68
    asymptomatic or mild infection, 71–72
    cardiopulmonary phase, 73–74
    classification and characteristics, 55–56
    clinical presentation of, 72–74
    clinical spectrum, 71–75
    convalescent phase, 74
    diagnosis of, 75
    discovery of, 55
    epidemiology, 68
    febrile phase, 72–73
    future directions, 79–80
    incubation period, 72
    management, 75–78
    pathophysiology, 59–67
    person-to-person transmission, 70
    prevention of, 78–79
    transmission, 68–70
    virology, 55–58
Hantaviruses (HV), 55–56
    associated with human infection, 57
    cellular targets, 61–62
    vaccines for, 78
Hantavirus pulmonary syndrome (HPS), 55
Hemorrhagic fever renal syndrome (HFRS), 55
    clinical presentation of, 74–75

Hendra virus infection
　clinical features, 274–275
　diagnosis, 275
　epidemiology, 274
　natural reservoir of, 274
　occurrence of, 273–274
　pathology, 275
Herpesvirus saimiri (HVS), 220
HHV, *see* Human herpesviruses
HHV-8
　anti-retroviral protease inhibitors, 238
　antivirals, 237
　assay development, 222–223
　biology, 204–222
　Castleman disease, 235
　cell tropism and viral entry, 204–205
　clinical spectrum, 230–237
　epidemiology, 222–230
　genotypes, 225–226
　geographical variation, 223–224
　host gene shutoff, 218
　immune response and immune evasion,
　　206–212
　infection by herpesvirus saimiri (HVS),
　　220–222
　infection by murine gammaherpesvirus 68,
　　218–220
　kaposin, 217–218
　kaposi sarcoma, 231–234
　latency and reactivation, 205–206
　latency-associated nuclear antigen (LANA),
　　213–214
　lymphoproliferative disorders, 236
　management, 237–238
　neoplastic disorders, 236
　nonsexual transmission, 228–230
　organ transplantation, 230
　parenteral transmission, 230
　pathogenesis, 212–218
　primary effusion lymphoma (PEL),
　　234–235
　primary infection, 230–231
　pulmonary hypertension associated with,
　　236
　rhadinovirus-encoded genes and,
　　208–209
　seroepidemiology, 222–225
　sexual transmission, 227–228
　subpopulations, 224–225
　transformation, 212–213
　transmission, 227–230
　vBcl2, vFLIP, K7 (Anti-apoptotic Proteins),
　　216–217
　vertical transmission, 228

HHV-6 and HHV-7
　animal model, 199
　antivirals, 204
　biology, 193–199
　cell tropism and viral entry, 193–194
　chronic fatigue syndrome (CFS), 201
　clinical spectrum, 201–203
　encephalitis, 202
　epidemiology, 199–201
　exanthem subitum (ES) (roseola), 201
　febrile convulsions, 202
　gene expression and replication,
　　194–195
　latency and reactivation, 195–197
　management and prevention, 204
　multiple sclerosis (MS), 201
　pathogenesis, 198–199
　pityriasis rosea (PR), 201
　post-transplantation disease, 202
　primary infections, 199–200
　proposed disease associations, 201
　solid organ transplantation, 203
　stem cell transplantation (SCT), 202–203
　transmission of, 201
　transplantation management, 204
H5N1 Avian influenza viruses, 326, 329–330,
　　332, 336–341, 360
Hong Kong influenza, pandemic of 1968,
　　331
Horsepox, 142
Human anaplasmosis
　antigenic characteristics, 106–108
　clinical spectrum, 113
　diagnosis, 113–114
　emergence, 112–113
　epidemiology, 112–113
　future directions, 115
　genetic characteristics, 106–108
　immunity, 108–111
　morphology, 105–106
　pathogenesis, 108–111
　phenotypic characteristics, 106–108
　prevention, 114–115
　taxonomy, 105
　transmission, 112–113
　treatment, 114–115
Human ehrlichioses
　antigenic characteristics, 94–96
　clinical spectrum, 102–103
　diagnosis, 103–104
　epidemiology, 100–102
　genetic characteristics, 94–96
　immunity, 96–100
　morphology, 91–94

Human ehrlichioses (*Cont'd*)
  pathogenesis, 96–100
  phenotypic characteristics, 94–96
  prevention, 104–105
  taxonomy, 91
  transmission, 100–102
  treatment, 104–105
Human granulocytotropic anaplasmosis
    (HGA), 105; *see also* Human
    anaplasmosis
Human granulocytotropic ehrlichiosis (HGE),
    105; *see also* Human anaplasmosis
Human herpesviruses (HHVs)
  antivirals, 204, 237
  biology, 191–199, 204–222
  cell tropism and viral entry, 193–194,
    204–205
  clinical spectrum, 201–203, 230–237
  epidemiology, 199–201, 222–230
  HHV-8, 204–238
  HHV-6 and HHV-7, 193–204
  latency and reactivation, 195–197, 205–206
  management and prevention, 204, 237–238
  pathogenic profiles of, 191–192, 198–199,
    212–218
  transmission, 201, 227–230
Human immunodeficiency virus (HIV)
    infection, 135
Human infection and disease, viruses
    associated with, 56–57
Human influenza viruses, *see* Influenza
    viruses
Human monocytotropic ehrlichiosis (HME),
    see Human ehrlichioses
Human neuroinvasive disease, 8
  incidence of, 10–11

I
Iatrogenic KS, 231, 234
Immunocompromised patients, 26–27
Infectious cDNA clone technology, 2
Influenza H5N1 viruses, 326, 329–330, 332,
    336–341, 349–351, 360; *see also*
    Aviation influenza viruses
  clinical spectrum of human H5N1
    infections, 337–340
  evolution of, 340–341
  outbreaks in poultry and humans, 336–337
Influenza viruses; *see also* Aviation influenza
    viruses; Influenza H5N1 viruses
  antigenic drift, 325
  antigenic shift, 325–326
  antigenic variation of, 325–326
  biological properties, 322

  classification, 323
  host-range, 323–325, 330
  natural hosts /reservoir of, 323
  pathogenesis of, 326–330
  transmission, 323
  virology, 322–326

J
Japanese encephalitis (JE), 276
  serocomplex, 1

K
K1, 214–215
K7, 216–217
K15, 214–215
Kaposi sarcoma–associated herpesvirus
    (KSHV), 191
Kaposi sarcoma (KS), 231–234
  classic, 231
  endemic or African, 231–232, 234
  epidemic or AIDS-associated, 231–233
  iatrogenic, 231, 234
KS, *see* Kaposi sarcoma
Kunjin (KUN) viruses, 1

L
Latency-associated nuclear antigen (LANA),
    213–214, 222
Leporipoxviruses, 128–129, 149–150, 153
Lymphoproliferative disorders, 236

M
Menangle viruses, 284
Meningitis, 21, 32
Molluscipoxvirus, 128–129, 133, 139,
    148–149, 154
Molluscum contagiosum virus (MCV)
    infection, 134–136, 139, 148–149
Monkeypox, 132, 138–139, 141–142
Mosquito control, for prevention of WNV
    infection, 35
Mousepox, 144–145
Multiple sclerosis (MS), 201
Murine gammaherpesvirus 68, 218–220
Murray valley encephalitis (MVE), 1

N
Neoplastic disorders, 236
Nephropathia epidemica (NE), 55
Neuroinvasive disease, 13–14
  clinical spectrum, 19, 21–25
  encephalitis, 21–22
  meningitis, 21
  weakness and paralysis in, 22–25

Neutralization mechanism, 4
Nipah virus infection
  cerebrospinal fluid (CSF) examination,
    279
  clinical features, 278–279
  electroencephalography (EEG) for, 280
  ELISA tests for, 279
  epidemiology, 276–278
  investigations, 279–280
  magnetic resonance imaging (MRI) brain
    scans for, 280
  pathogenesis, 283
  pathology, 281–283
  relapsed and late-onset encephalitis, 281
  reservoir for, 277
  spread of, 275–276
  treatment and outcome, 281
Non-mosquito transmission routes, 16–18
  aerosol transmission, 17
  blood transfusion, 16
  intrauterine transmission, 17
  lactating hamsters to suckling hamsters,
    17
  organ transplantation, 16–17
  through dialysis, 17
  West Nile virus (WNV), 16–18
Nucleic Acid Amplification Test (NAAT),
    29–31
Nucleic Acid Sequence-based Amplification
    (NASBA), 29
  in viral genomic sequences detection, 31

O

Ocular manifestations, in WNV infection,
    25–26
Orthopoxvirus, 128–129, 133, 138–146,
    153–154
  camelpox virus, 145
  cowpox virus, 139, 143–144
  disease in human, 138–146
  ectromelia virus, 144–145
  host processes targeted by, 135
  monkeypox virus, 139, 141–142
  phylogenetic tree of species in genus, 130
  vaccinia virus, 139, 142–143
  variola virus, 139–141

P

Pandemic influenza strains; *see also* Avian
    influenza viruses
  emergence of, 325–326
  preparedness and future directives for
    control of, 349–351
  of the 20th century, 330–332

Paralysis and weakness, 22–25
Parapoxvirus, 127–129, 133, 138–139,
    147–148, 153–154
Pathophysiology, 59–67
  animal models and, 67–68
  cell entry, 59–60
  cellular targets, 61–62
  immunity, 65–66
  pathology and pathogenesis, 62–63
  T-Cell response role, 63–66, 79
  virulence, 60
Picornavirus, 291
Pityriasis rosea (PR), 201
Plaque reduction neutralization test
    (PRNT), 56
Poxviruses
  avipoxvirus, 128–129, 137, 152–153
  capripoxvirus, 127–129, 150–151, 153
  co-evolution of, 133
  cross-species transmission, 131–132,
    136–138
  diseases in humans, 138–149
  family, 127–138·
  genera not causing diseases in humans,
    149–153
  leporipoxviruses, 128–129, 149–150, 153
  measures and countermeasures, 133–136
  molluscipoxvirus, 128–129, 133, 139,
    148–149, 154
  orthopoxvirus, 128–129, 133, 139–146,
    153–154
  parapoxvirus, 127–129, 133, 138–139,
    147–148, 153–54
  suipoxvirus, 128–129, 151–153
  survival strategy, 132–133, 136
  transmission patterns, 131–132, 136–138
  yatapoxvirus, 128–129, 138–139, 146–147,
    153
Primary effusion lymphoma (PEL), 234–235
Proteins for cellular activation signaling,
    214–215
Pulmonary edema, 299–300
Puumala virus, 60

R

Real-time 5′ exonuclease fluorogenic assays
    (TaqMan), 30
Reverse genetics technology, 60
Reverse transcriptase-polymerase chain
    reaction (RT-PCR), 30, 75, 161–162,
    169, 302, 342–343
Rhabdomyolysis, 26
Rhadinovirus-encoded genes, 208–209
Rhombencephalitis, 298

RT-PCR, *see* Reverse transcriptase-
polymerase chain reaction
Rubulavirus, 284

S

Saimiriine herpesvirus-2 (SaHV-2), 220
SARS, *see* Severe acute respiratory
syndrome
SARS-coronavirus (SARS-CoV), 161
classification of, 162–164
Koch's postulates for, 171–172
putative genes and annotation of, 167
virology, 162–167
Severe acute respiratory syndrome (SARS)
active and passive immunization for,
174–176
animal models for, 171–172
antivirals and immunomodulators,
173–174
clinical findings, 168–169
clinical management of, 172–178
community infection control, 178–179
epidemiologic characteristics, 160–162
hospital infection control, 178–179
Koch's postulates for, 171–172
laboratory diagnostics, 169–170
laboratory safety and infection control,
178–179
pathology and immunology, 170–171
sequence of emergence of, 159–160
virology, 162–167
virus epidemic in 2003, 349
Sheeppox, 150–151
Sin Nombre virus, 60
Smallpox, 130, 138, 140–141
Solid organ transplantation, 203
Spanish flu, 321, 331
St. Louis encephalitis (SLE), 1
Stem cell transplantation (SCT), 202–203
Suipoxvirus, 128–129, 151–153
Swinepox, 136, 151–152

T

Tanapoxvirus, 146
Taterapoxvirus, 145
Tick-borne ehrlichioses, of humans and
animals, 92t
Tickborne encephalitis (TBE) virus, 3
Tioman virus, 277, 284
Total leukocyte counts, 31
Tula virus, 60

U

Uasin Gishu virus, 145

V

Vaccinia virus, 139, 142–143
Variola, 138
virus, 139–141
vBcl2, 216–217
v-Cyclin, 214
vFLIP, 216–217
vGPCR, 214–215
Viral genomic sequences detection, 29–31
nucleic acid amplification test (NAAT),
29–31
nucleic acid sequence–based amplification
(NASBA), 31
real-time 5′ exonuclease fluorogenic assays
(TaqMan), 30
reverse transcriptase–polymerase chain
reaction (RT-PCR), 30
Viral modulation of innate immunity, 207–211
Viral modulation of the adaptive immune
response, 211–212
Virology
enterovirus 71, 289–292
hantavirus, 55–56, 57t, 58
influenza virus, 322–326
SARS, 162–163, 165
WNV, 1–7
Viruses, *see specific* viruses
Virus neutralizing monoclonal antibodies
(MAbs), 3
Virus transmission cycle, 7–8

W

West Nile fever (WN fever), 18–20
symptoms associated with, 19–20
West Nile poliomyelitis, 24
West Nile virus (WNV), neuroinvasive
disease of, 19, 20t, 21–25, 24t
West Nile virus (WNV) infection, 29
in children, 26
clinical manifestations, 25–26
clinical spectrum, 18–27
diagnosis, 27–32
diagnosis and treatment, 37
ecological surveillance for prevention of,
36–37
epidemiology, 7–18
genetics and virulence, 6–7
genome, 1–6
geographic spread, 10–13
human personal protection for prevention
of, 34–35
immunocompromised patients, 26–27
in Latin America, 11–13
management, 32–34

West Nile virus (WNV) infection (*Cont'd*)
  mosquito control for prevention of, 35
  neutralization mechanism, 4
  non-mosquito transmission routes, 16–18
  nucleotide sequences, 2
  ocular manifestations, 25–26
  organ transplant recipients risk of, 15
  prevention, 37–38
  rhabdomyolysis, 26
  risk factors for infection, severe disease,
      and death, 15–16
  screening of blood donations, 36
  in special population groups, 26–27

  total leukocyte counts, 31
  transmission of, 7–10
  in United States and Canada, 10–14
  vaccines for prevention of, 35–36
  vertebrate hosts, 9–10
  viral genomic sequences detection, 29–31
  virus structure of, 1
  virus transmission cycle, 7–8

Y
Yaba monkey tumor virus (YMTV), 146–147
Yatapoxvirus, 128–129, 138–139, 146–147,
      153